Evolutionary Psychiatry

'This is a fascinating read on a topic that, although has relevance, is not well known or understood in the mental health world. The book is stimulating, authoritative, and entertaining in tone and has the ability to motivate debate and provide some answers to issues we all struggle with. It is difficult to put down.'

Dr Adrian James, President, Royal College of Psychiatrists, UK

'Riadh Abed and Paul St John-Smith have provided a terrific service to the field of psychiatry to assemble a stimulating set of chapters exploring how psychiatric and neurodevelopmental conditions may be better understood through a Darwinian lens. Understanding poor mental health as an adaptive response to a toxic environment can lead to interventions focused on changing the environment rather than treating the patient. Understanding the genetic basis of neurodiversity encourages us to think about genotypes that may result in disabilities in certain environments and adaptive strengths in others. The challenge for researchers in the revolutionary field of evolutionary psychiatry is to come up with testable predictions to confirm or refute hypotheses. This volume will be welcomed by clinicians, research scientists, and students among others, who are interested in how psychiatry can be integrated within the broader framework of evolutionary biology.'

Professor Simon Baron-Cohen, University of Cambridge, UK

'Darwin's shocking discovery of the combined role of natural and sexual selection in shaping the evolution of homo sapiens revolutionized psychology every bit as much as biology. Freud was the first to apply Darwin's insights to the practice of clinical psychiatry, but many of his theories were limited by the science of his time. This book updates Darwin and Freud- providing a wonderful summary of how our evolutionary past inexorably influences our behavioural present. Great stuff for clinicians, patients, and anyone curious about human nature.'

Professor Allen Frances, Duke University, USA

'What is it to be psychologically normal, and when can we judge that something has gone wrong with an individual's mental functioning? Why do so many things seem to go wrong with our minds, anyway? The answers to these questions impact us not only socially, medically, and legally, but also very personally. Ultimately, the answers must be sought in an understanding of how our minds are biologically designed to function by evolutionary forces, and how and why those functions fail—for there is no further authority on who we are when functioning properly than our biological design by natural selection. This book presents a cornucopia of fresh and stimulating thought about these profound issues by an international group of researchers, both senior authorities and young-and-rising investigators who are among the most talented explorers of our evolutionary psychological heritage and its discontents. Consequently, the book is bursting with illuminating and often provocative insights into the possible sources and nature of mental disorders across the entire spectrum of disorder categories. The future of psychiatry belongs to an evolutionary understanding of the shaping of our minds, and this book takes the reader on the first step of the long journey to that future.'

Professor Jerome C. Wakefield, New York University, USA

'With a carefully thought-out sequence of chapters and an enviable roster of authors, this book is a superb invitation to evolutionary psychiatry for both researchers and practitioners in mental health. Readers will find a solid, concise introduction to the basic concepts; important but otherwise hard-to-find information (for example about mental illness in hunter-gatherers); and a range of thought-provoking hypotheses about the origins of specific conditions. As noted by the editors, this book exemplifies the power of evolutionary theory as a framework for "asking the right questions"; even better, it shows how an evolutionary approach can foster true interdisciplinary, and permit wide-ranging theoretical exploration while remaining firmly grounded in biological and psychological reality.'

Marco Del Giudice, Associate Professor of Psychology, University of New Mexico, USA

'In this remarkable book, the editors have brought together international leading thinkers and clinicians to illuminate how understanding the evolutionary history and functions of the mind provide crucial insights into our vulnerabilities to mental health difficulties and what we require to flourish. It is full of fascinating and detailed analyses of basic processes, from epigenetics, the role of hunter-gatherer societies in shaping our social motives, through to evolutionary conceptualisations of a range of different types of mental health problems and their treatment. With increasing recognition that progress in understanding, developing interventions for, and preventing mental health problems requires insight into how our brains, bodies, and minds came to be the way they are, this book makes an outstanding contribution and will be a major resource for clinicians and researchers for many years to come.'

Professor Paul Gilbert, PhD OBE, Author of human nature and suffering; Depression the evolution of powerlessness. Compassion focused therapy

Evolutionary Psychiatry

Current Perspectives on Evolution and Mental Health

Edited by

Riadh Abed
Retired Consultant Psychiatrist, Current Medical Member, Mental Health Tribunals,
Ministry of Justice

Paul St John-Smith
Retired Consultant Psychiatrist and Independent Scholar

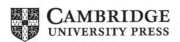
CAMBRIDGE
UNIVERSITY PRESS

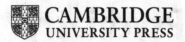

Shaftesbury Road, Cambridge CB2 8EA, United Kingdom

One Liberty Plaza, 20th Floor, New York, NY 10006, USA

477 Williamstown Road, Port Melbourne, VIC 3207, Australia

314–321, 3rd Floor, Plot 3, Splendor Forum, Jasola District Centre, New Delhi – 110025, India

103 Penang Road, #05–06/07, Visioncrest Commercial, Singapore 238467

Cambridge University Press is part of Cambridge University Press & Assessment, a department of the University of Cambridge.

We share the University's mission to contribute to society through the pursuit of education, learning and research at the highest international levels of excellence.

www.cambridge.org
Information on this title: www.cambridge.org/9781316516560

DOI: 10.1017/9781911623625

First published 2022

A catalogue record for this publication is available from the British Library

ISBN   978-1-316-51656-0   Hardback

Cambridge University Press & Assessment has no responsibility for the persistence or accuracy of URLs for external or third-party internet websites referred to in this publication and does not guarantee that any content on such websites is, or will remain, accurate or appropriate.

....

Every effort has been made in preparing this book to provide accurate and up-to-date information which is in accord with accepted standards and practice at the time of publication. Although case histories are drawn from actual cases, every effort has been made to disguise the identities of the individuals involved. Nevertheless, the authors, editors and publishers can make no warranties that the information contained herein is totally free from error, not least because clinical standards are constantly changing through research and regulation. The authors, editors and publishers therefore disclaim all liability for direct or consequential damages resulting from the use of material contained in this book. Readers are strongly advised to pay careful attention to information provided by the manufacturer of any drugs or equipment that they plan to use.

Contents

Contributors

Riadh Abed
Mental Health Tribunals, Ministry of Justice

Agnes Ayton
University of Oxford

Brian B. Boutwell
University of Mississippi Medical Center,
University of Mississippi

Martin Brüne
Department of Psychiatry, Psychotherapy and
Preventive Medicine,
Ruhr University Bochum

Nikhil Chaudhary
University of Cambridge

Robin I. M. Dunbar
Department of Experimental Psychology,
Radcliffe Observatory Quarter, University of
Oxford

Molly Fox
Departments of Psychiatry and Biobehavioral
Sciences, University of California, Los Angeles

Adam Hunt
Institute of Evolutionary Medicine, University of
Zurich

George Ikkos
Royal National Orthopaedic Hospital

Matthew M. Large
School of Psychiatry at the University of New
South Wales

John Launer
Tavistock and Portman NHS Foundation Trust

Severi Luoto
School of Psychology, University of Auckland

Graham Music
Tavistock and Portman NHS Foundation Trust

Randolph M. Nesse
Center for Evolution and Medicine, Arizona State
University

Pablo Malo Ocejo
Bizkaia Mental Health Network

Markus J. Rantala
Department of Biology, University of Turku

Michael J. Reiss
University College London Institute of
Education

Gul Deniz Salali
University College London

Todd K. Shackelford
Oakland University

Daniela F. Sieff
Independent Scholar

C. A. Soper
Psychotherapist and Independent Scholar

Paul St John-Smith
Retired Consultant Psychiatrist and Independent
Scholar

Megan Suprenant
University of Mississippi

Annie Swanepoel
North East London NHS Foundation Trust

Derek K. Tracy
West London NHS Trust

Alfonso Troisi
Department of Systems Medicine, University of
Rome Tor Vergata

Bernadette Wren
Tavistock and Portman NHS Foundation Trust

Foreword

As was common in the medical milieu of their times, both Emil Kraepelin (1856–1926) (Kraepelin, 1987) and Sigmund Freud (1856–1939) (Sulloway, 1980) had a strong interest in human evolution, the first pioneering the pursuit of psychiatric genetics in his university department and the second explicitly advocating the teaching of evolution in psychoanalytic training towards the end of his life. Unfortunately, the cruelties of eugenics and the malice of social Darwinism led to hideous practices, including the castration (Porter, 1999) and killing (Friedlander, 1995) of tens of thousands of disabled citizens with severe neuropsychiatric impairments. Regardless, the continuing confirmation of familial factors in the epidemiology of psychiatric syndromes and the scientific revolution in the understanding of DNA helped maintain active interest in psychiatric genetics. Probably and perhaps understandably, the hideous legacy and legitimate fear of 'just-so stories' (see Chapter 6) together with exciting advances in genetic techniques served to narrow the focus on genes and marginalise a broader evolutionary perspective in our speciality. This wide-ranging volume, which is guided by the needs of clinical practice, will serve to redress the balance. Crucially, all of the chapters are clearly written and pitched at a level that should engage psychiatric trainees (and interested others) and thus help future colleagues develop a deeper understanding of the diverse and multiply determined phenomena that we meet in the clinic or other settings.

In view of the history of the subject, it is important to note that the editors are firmly committed to hypothesis testing, not simply theory and interpretation. They also write of the potential of evolutionary theory to serve as a bridge between the biological and social understandings of mental health and illness – a necessary ambition. However, as Benedict Spinoza (Lloyd, 1996) argued more than 400 years ago and as these chapters make clear, matter and mind (biological and social) are two sides of a coin, and, like with a coin, we are so constituted as to be unable to look at both sides simultaneously. This cognitive and affective shortcoming of ours stands in the way of an even more ambitious aim: namely not simply a biopsychosocial but a truly pluralistic approach to psychiatry and mental health services. One of the volume's strengths – but not its only one – is its multidisciplinary authorship, including contributions from the perspectives of biology, psychology, anthropology and philosophy. What a hypothesis-testing evolutionary psychiatry promises with respect to pluralism is new questions as well as new understandings.

For the record, and as the only qualification for having been invited to contribute to this Foreword, I have been fortunate to know Dr Paul St John-Smith for decades as trainee, fellow specialist, co-author, intellectual sparring partner, evolutionary psychiatry mentor and friend. I am indebted to him and now to Dr Riadh Abed, too, for my continuing professional formation. It was Paul's suggestion that we invite Professor Randolph M. Nesse to speak on 'Evolutionary biology of attachment and depression' during the event on 'Emotion and Psychiatry: Neuroscience, History and Culture' that I co-organised with Professor Angelos Chaniotis and Dr Christos Sideras at the Royal Society of Medicine in London in May 2013. This in turn attracted Riadh, and he and Paul made each other's acquaintance. Their common enthusiasm led to the founding of the Evolutionary Psychiatry

Special Interest Group of the Royal College of Psychiatrists, which has developed into the foremost psychiatry organisation with such an interest worldwide. A key outcome of nearly a decade of common endeavour is this volume, whose merits include that it challenges oversimplifications, whether by psychiatrists or our critics.

George Ikkos
Royal National Orthopaedic Hospital

References

Friedlander, H. (1995) *The Origins of Nazi Genocide: From Euthanasia to the Final Solution*. Chapel Hill: University of North Carolina Press.

Kraepelin, E. (1987) *Memoirs*. Berlin: Springer Verlag.

Lloyd, G. (1996) *Spinoza and the Ethics*. Abingdon-on-Thames: Routledge.

Porter, D. (1999) The quality of population and family welfare: human reproduction, eugenics and social policy. In: *Health, Civilization and the State: A History of Public Health from Ancient to Modern Times*. Abingdon-on-Thames: Routledge, pp. 165–195.

Sulloway, F. J. (1980) Part two: Psychoanalysis: the birth of a genetic psychobiology. In *Freud, Biologist of the Mind: Beyond the Psychoanalytic Legend*. Cambridge, MA: Harvard University Press, pp. 135–416.

Preface

Riadh Abed and Paul St John-Smith

Thus, from the war of nature, from famine and death, the most exalted object which we are capable of conceiving, namely, the production of the higher animals, directly follows. There is grandeur in this view of life, with its several powers, having been originally breathed into a few forms or into one; and that, whilst this planet has gone cycling on according to the fixed law of gravity, from so simple a beginning endless forms most beautiful and most wonderful have been, and are being, evolved.

—*Charles Darwin,* On the Origin of Species
(1st ed., 1859)

Charles Darwin's momentous discovery that natural selection was the means through which complex traits are shaped, and species are differentiated by favouring traits that are advantageous to survival and reproduction over their alternatives, provided for the first time a fully naturalistic, non-miraculous explanation for the complexity and variety of life on Earth. Natural selection is nevertheless not the only mechanism involved in the process. Chance, in particular stochasticity, plays a central, even essential part in evolutionary processes, not least through the random process of mutation that is the only source of variation that selection must then work on – so much so that the French biochemist and Nobel Laureate Jacques Monod proclaimed that 'man was the product of an incalculable number of fortuitous events' (quoted in Carroll, 2020: 15). However, despite its random beginnings, further down the line there are also powerful non-random elements to selection (Dawkins, 1996).

In true Darwinian style, chance events have also played an important role in the production of this volume, as they have done in many of the other recent evolutionary endeavours of both the editors. Until recently, for many years we had both been practising clinicians within the NHS in different parts of the UK while also pursuing long-standing interests in evolution and mental health in relative isolation. However, things changed rather dramatically following a one-day conference in 2013 that we both attended at the Royal Society of Medicine organised by George Ikkos, where Randolph M. Nesse was speaking. Paul recognised Riadh from his name badge as the author of evolutionary papers on obsessive-compulsive disorder and schizophrenia that he had come across, and so he introduced himself. From that time onwards, we have kept in touch and have collaborated on a number of evolutionary projects, including meetings, articles and book chapters. Importantly, we also collaborated, together with colleagues, on the formation of the Evolutionary Psychiatry Special Interest Group (EPSIG) at the Royal College of Psychiatrists, which saw the light of day in 2016. And contrary to many gloomy predictions by colleagues (and sometimes even our own hunches) that psychiatrists would shun evolution, the membership of EPSIG has continued to grow and now exceeds 1,900. It is currently the largest evolutionary psychiatry group anywhere in the world. Since then we have organised, in collaboration with colleagues, four one-day international evolutionary psychiatry symposia where eminent evolutionists from around the world have presented their work, organised several half-day scientific meetings and webinars, set up a YouTube channel, established the Charles Darwin Essay Prize for psychiatric trainees and medical students and published more than 20 newsletters. This volume is the latest product of this collaboration. It was originally meant to mark the fifth anniversary of the formation of EPSIG, but it seems that by the time it is published it will coincide with the sixth.

Interestingly, the year of publication of this volume (2022) coincides, again purely by chance, with a propitious occasion for Darwinians, especially for those interested in human psychology, namely the 150th anniversary of the publication of Charles Darwin's only book on human psychology: *The Expression of Emotions in Man and Animals*. If Darwin were alive today, we think he would be pleased to see his world-changing theory being applied to the understanding of mental disorder. However, he might also be disappointed that psychiatry and medicine in general, unlike other life sciences, have been so slow to incorporate evolution into their mainstream.

We consider the current pre-Darwinian state of psychiatry to be an unfortunate anachronism and a hindrance to the future development of the field. It is therefore the aim of EPSIG, in collaboration with other evolutionarily minded psychiatrists around the world, to rectify this. However, we fully recognise that this will take time and effort. Most psychiatrists (and doctors generally), even if they accept evolution as a fact and the only scientific explanation for human origins, have given little thought to the profound consequences of evolution for the understanding of function, dysfunction, health and disease. As a result, evolutionary psychiatry remains a minority interest among clinicians, as only a few dozen psychiatrists scattered around the world are devoting significant time and energy to furthering the evolutionary understanding of mental disorders. This is only a tiny fraction of the psychiatrists who accept the reality of evolution.

We believe it is likely that many more psychiatrists will join the evolutionary psychiatry enterprise once they become better acquainted with its benefits and potential. The importance of population size (and critical mass) in advancing human knowledge and technology is well known. For example, the archaeological study of the island populations of Oceania at around the time of early European contact showed that the peoples of islands with small populations had less complicated marine foraging technology (Kline and Boyd, 2010). We also know that the population size of cities correlates positively with the production and exchange of knowledge and ideas (Bettencourt and West, 2010). Hence, the size of the evolutionary psychiatry community matters when it comes to the development and accumulation of knowledge. We therefore expect that greater dissemination of

evolutionary knowledge among psychiatrists internationally will lead to an exponential expansion of the range and sophistication of evolutionary theoretical models and to new, clinically relevant empirical data based on such models. We hope that this book will contribute to this vitally important process by showcasing the ideas and work of evolutionary psychiatrists from around the world, including many of the pioneers of the field, and by making these easily accessible in a single volume.

Our aim is to present readers with a cross section of a wide range of evolutionary thinking on mental health and human psychology that spans multiple disciplines, including psychiatry, psychology, anthropology and philosophy. While evolutionary science represents the foundational framework for all of the authors of this volume, there is ample room for disagreement on a whole range of issues, including on the nature of mental disorder itself. However, we consider this a sign of strength rather than a weakness, as evolutionary psychiatry is a science that will progress through proposing theories and hypotheses, testing their predictions and then accepting, rejecting or refining them in the light of empirical data. Thus, our evolutionary endeavour should, by its very nature, be correctable and dynamic as well as provisional and progressive. True science is neither a dogma nor a fixed body of information. Evolutionary psychiatry must be parsimonious, useful and pragmatic as well as consistent internally and externally and, importantly, ethical. We aspire to these goals. It is important, therefore, to underline that while the evolutionary approach is critical of the mainstream, it does not aim to replace current psychiatric knowledge and practice but to complement them. Evolutionists fully subscribe to the scientific method that forms the basis of modern medicine and, if anything, aim to strengthen and not to undermine it. However, evolutionists are critical of the exclusive focus of current psychiatry and medicine on proximate (mechanistic) explanations and models while neglecting ultimate or evolutionary causes (see Chapters 1 and 2). Hence, we suggest that evolution is to psychiatry what philosophy is to science: a framework that enables asking the right questions and not a means to obtain ready-made answers. Answers will only be obtained through analysing empirical evidence.

Therefore, this volume does not provide ready-made recipes regarding the nature and treatment of specific mental disorders but promotes and advocates a way of thinking and a framework for exploring and understanding human distress and suffering. The strength of evolution is that it places humans firmly within the complex web of life on Earth, not apart from it, and it provides understanding regarding our species' psychological traits and the vulnerabilities they give rise to in terms of the functions they served in the ancestral environment.

As to the future, we hope this book will be of interest not only to psychiatrists but also to psychologists, nurses, other mental health professionals and psychologically minded members of the health and caring professions. We also hope it will be of interest to academics in a range of fields, including philosophy, anthropology and biology, as well as the evolutionarily informed general public. We maintain that evolutionary thinking can help destigmatise mental dysfunction, and it has been our clinical experience that this is indeed the case. We especially hope that trainees in psychiatry and allied professions will take an interest in this topic and that evolutionary thinking will eventually become a part of the standard curricula and examinations.

Although the chapters of this volume may be read out of sequence as stand-alone evolutionary reviews of their respective subject matters, readers unfamiliar with the evolutionary literature will benefit from reading the introductory chapter first or, better still, the first five chapters. These should give the reader a good grounding in the basics of evolutionary medicine and human origins and provide explanations for some of the major benefits of applying evolutionary thinking to the understanding of mental disorder.

We are grateful for the support and encouragement we have received from a number of sources that helped us in this project. Randolph M. Nesse, the co-founder of the field of evolutionary medicine, has been generous with his time and advice. He volunteered to speak at our very first EPSIG symposium in 2016, altering his travel plans to stop in London and deliver his lecture at a time when we had no funds to cover any of his expenses. We have since kept in touch and met with him at other conference venues, and we continue to benefit from his sage advice. In addition, we are grateful to George Ikkos for his encouragement from the very inception of EPSIG and for chairing sessions at each of our four international symposia. We are especially grateful to Annie Swanepoel, the current EPSIG newsletter editor and our close collaborator on all matters relating to promoting evolution among colleagues and the general public. We are also grateful to our colleagues on the EPSIG executive committee and our evolutionary colleagues from the UK and around the world who have spoken at our symposia and/or contributed to this volume for sharing their evolutionary work and knowledge. We also wish to thank our colleagues at EPSIG who have kindly shared their time and clinical experience, not only encouraging us to organise this endeavour, but who also are assisting with the gradual clinical roll-out of these ideas. We also acknowledge that we are 'standing on the shoulders of giants'[1] and recognise the huge contributions made by authors of books on evolution and psychiatry, in particular Randolph M. Nesse, John Price, Alfonso Troisi, Martin Brüne and Marco Del Giudice, without whose books the field would be greatly diminished.

In addition, special thanks are given to Cambridge University Press and the Royal College of Psychiatrists Publishing Board for agreeing to publish this title and to the anonymous reviewers for their positive feedback and encouragement. Furthermore, our thanks go to the past and present administrative staff at the Royal College of Psychiatrists, Catherine Langley and Kelsey Henschel, respectively, who have offered us day-to-day support at EPSIG regarding keeping in touch with our membership and have helped to organise our evolutionary events. Our thanks also go to Lindsey Edwards, who kindly proofread our chapters, to Harley St John-Smith,

---

[1] 'If we see more and farther than our predecessors, it is not because we have keener vision or greater height, but is because we are lifted up and borne aloft on their gigantic stature' (Bernard of Chartres, twelfth century, quoted by Isaac Newton, 1675).

who designed and drafted the cover illustration and EPSIG logo, and to David Geaney, who reviewed Chapter 12 on substance abuse. Finally, we wish to thank Olivia Boult, Jessica

Papworth and Saskia Pronk at Cambridge University Press for their help and support in the production of this volume.

References

Bettencourt, L. and West, G. A. (2010). A unified theory of urban living. *Nature*, 467, 912–913.

Carroll, S. B. (2020). *A Series of Fortunate Events*. Princeton, NJ: Princeton University Press.

Dawkins, R. (1996). *Climbing Mount Improbable*. London: Norton.

Kline, M. A. and Boyd, R. (2010). Population size predicts technological complexity in Oceania. *Proceedings of the Royal Society B: Biological Sciences*, 277, 2559–2564.

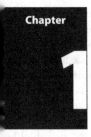
Introduction to Evolutionary Psychiatry

Riadh Abed and Paul St John-Smith*

Abstract

This introductory chapter serves multiple purposes. Its primary aim is to introduce psychiatrists and other mental health professionals who are new to Darwinian thinking to some of the basic concepts and terminology of evolutionary science in order to ease their progress through the remaining chapters of this volume. Another aim is to provide a distillation and update of some significant theoretical and other developments in a variety of evolutionary disciplines relevant to psychiatry and psychology that would be of benefit to all readers, including existing evolutionists. Given the constraints of space, there will inevitably be significant omissions. We have elected to cover the basics of standard evolutionary theory, as well as some of the basic principles of evolutionary psychology and medicine. We also briefly survey some of the recent developments in the evolutionary literature on cultural evolution and related fields. We recognise that a balance needs to be struck between covering as wide an area as possible without the chapter becoming a glossary of terms. Readers unfamiliar with specialised evolutionary terms are advised to consult the glossary on the Evolutionary Psychiatry Special Interest Group at the Royal College of Psychiatrists' website: www.epsig.org (click on 'About us' then 'Resources').

Keywords

EEA, evolutionary medicine, evolutionary psychiatry, evolutionary psychology, Tinbergen

Key Points

- Darwinian theory is the organising framework for all life sciences.
- Evolutionary thinking can transform our understanding of causality in medicine and psychiatry through the application of Tinbergen's four questions.
- Without evolution, our understanding of the causes of disease is necessarily incomplete.
- The evolutionary perspective can help us understand human vulnerability to disease and disorder.
- Evolutionary psychiatry complements and augments mainstream psychiatry and does not seek to replace it.
- Evolution can also help us understand human uniqueness and especially the role of cumulative culture and gene–culture co-evolution in shaping the human body and mind.

* We are grateful to Lindsey Edwards, Adam Hunt and Annie Swanepoel for providing valuable comments on previous drafts of this chapter.

1.1 Introduction to Evolutionary Theory

1.1.1 Background

Charles Darwin made two distinct and revolutionary proposals in 1859. The first was that all living organisms shared a common ancestor and the second was that natural selection was the mechanism through which all the diversity of life on Earth arose (Nesse and Stein, 2019).

These insights set in motion one of the greatest scientific revolutions in history. Whereas other major scientific paradigm shifts occurred in the physical sciences (e.g. those of Copernicus, Newton, Einstein and Heisenberg), they had few conspicuous implications outside their specialist fields. Darwinism, however, challenged deeply entrenched assumptions in multiple fields of enquiry and belief, ranging from biology to geology, as well as having profound meta-scientific consequences in its challenge to creationism, essentialism and anthropocentrism

(Mayr, 1971). Yet despite being part of the life sciences, psychiatry (as well as much of medicine) has remained largely pre-Darwinian in its approach. In this book, evolutionary scholars of various disciplines, including psychiatrists, philosophers, anthropologists and psychologists, aim to rectify this, not by rejecting or replacing current mainstream psychiatry, but through the addition of the evolutionary perspective, which should provide the discipline with a more contemporary, sound scientific foundation.

Psychiatry is the branch of medicine that deals with mental disorders that manifest themselves through disturbances in cognition, emotions and behaviour. However, the failure of psychiatry to make significant progress in understanding the aetiology of mental disorders has been described as a 'crisis' by leading evolutionists (Brüne et al., 2012) – a fact that has also been acknowledged in an article in *Science* that stated that there have been no major breakthroughs either in the treatment of schizophrenia for 50 years or in the treatment of depression for 20 years (Akil et al., 2010). Evolutionists would contend that this is partly because mainstream psychiatry focuses exclusively on proximate causation and favours mechanistic explanations of disease and disorder. However, unlike medicine, where human physiology provides clear reference points for normal functioning, psychiatry has attempted to identify disorder and dysfunction without a coherent theory of normal human psychology (Nesse, 2016). Also, even on the rare occasions when the vital questions of function and the role of evolution are considered by mainstream psychiatrists, they stop well short of exploring the full implications of such a radical shift in thinking and approach (e.g. Kendler, 2008). Evolutionary psychiatrists argue that Darwinian theory can serve as the essential, missing basic science for psychiatry (Nesse, 2019).

Psychiatry's pre-Darwinian state may be changing very gradually with the development of evolutionary models for a number of psychiatric disorders and the publication of a number of influential evolutionary psychiatric texts over the past couple of decades (Baron-Cohen, 1997; Brüne, 2015; Del Giudice, 2018; Gilbert and Bailey, 2000; McGuire and Troisi, 1998; Nesse, 2019; Stevens and Price, 2000).

In its development, evolutionary psychiatry has benefited from work in two closely related fields. The first field is evolutionary medicine, which has seen a massive expansion since the publication of Nesse and Williams' (1994) foundational work (preceded by an article by Williams and Nesse (1991) and an American Association for the Advancement of Science symposium on evolutionary medicine in 1993) followed by many others (e.g. Gluckman et al., 2009; Trevathan et al., 2008). The other field is the now highly accomplished and rapidly expanding domain of evolutionary psychology. This was heralded as an academic discipline by the publication of the highly influential *Adapted Mind* (Barkow et al., 1992) followed by the publication of many influential texts and specialised academic journals, as well as the voluminous scientific output of numerous university departments across the Western world. Furthermore, evolutionary anthropologists have had a significant impact on these academic strands, especially on the development of evolutionary medicine (Trevathan et al., 2008).

In this book, we provide reasons as to why evolution is ideally placed to guide psychiatrists in determining what the phenotypic end products of neurobiological systems are (these are the genetically based, behavioural and psychological traits that have been shaped by selection). Importantly, the evolutionary emphasis on function can provide the scientific basis for a non-reductionist expansion of the concept of the biological to encompass the psychological, social and cultural domains (Abed and St John-Smith, 2021). Hence, in contrast with mainstream biological psychiatry's narrow 'decontextualized' view of mental disorder as brain disorder (or brain circuit disorder) (Insel and Cuthbert, 2015), evolutionists consider the environmental context to be of paramount importance in determining the existence and nature of mental disorder (Nesse, 2019).

Thus, evolutionists consider Darwinian theory to be the fundamental organising framework or meta-theory underpinning the whole of the life sciences and not simply one perspective to be considered alongside many others. Evolutionary psychiatry is the application of modern evolutionary theory to the scientific understanding of mental health and disease. The goal of evolutionary psychiatry then is to understand why people get sick as well as how they get sick.

The remainder of this introductory chapter will provide a survey of some of the fundamentals of evolutionary science relevant to the understanding of health and disease in humans.[1]

1.1.2 Evolution, Natural Selection and Adaptation

What is evolution? Evolution may be defined as any net directional change or any cumulative change in the characteristics of organisms or populations over many generations – in other words, descent with modification. When individuals in a population vary in ways that influence their genetic contribution to future populations, the average characteristics of the population will change.

It is essential to understand that biologists recognise many ways in which evolution can occur, evolution by natural selection being just one of them, although it is often held to be the most important. Other basic evolutionary processes include genetic drift, mutation, migration and sexual and social selection.

Natural selection can lead to speciation, where one species gives rise to a new and distinctly different species. This is one of the processes that drives evolution and helps to explain the diversity of life on Earth. Natural selection is the process through which populations of living organisms adapt and change. Natural selection, however, involves no foresight, planning or goal. Hence, any heritable (genetically based) phenotypic trait that confers a reproductive advantage in competition with alternatives within a population will spread, and given enough time the trait may become fixed as a species-wide characteristic. The measure of reproductive success is referred to as 'fitness'. Repeated cycles of natural selection lead to the preservation of successful variants and the elimination of less successful ones, leading to the appearance of design and the shaping of traits that increase the organism's fitness. These are referred to in the evolutionary literature as 'adaptations'. Although Darwin was unaware of the existence of genes or how variation came about, we now know that variation arises as a result of mutations, which are copying errors in the DNA sequence that occur during cell division (NIH, 2020). When mutations occur in germ-line cells as opposed to somatic cells they can be transmitted to offspring.

The basic Darwinian ideas (variation, inheritance and natural selection) were enhanced in the twentieth century by what was called the 'modern synthesis'. This involved the incorporation of the modern science of genetics, which included the concepts of genes, mutation and Mendelian inheritance, into evolutionary theory.

The modern synthesis led to the insight that while the primary mechanism that generates variation is random (mutations), the success or failure of the different variants depends on the fitness they confer and is not at all random. Thus, natural selection shapes adaptive and functional systems that aid survival and reproduction through favouring certain phenotypic traits over others and leads to the spread of the underlying genes within the population. Nevertheless, the same evolutionary processes that shape functional adaptations, paradoxically and inevitably, produce maladaptations (Brady et al., 2019) as well as vulnerabilities to disease and disorder (Nesse, 2019) (see Box 1.1). However, before tackling the evolutionary causes of the persistence of disease and disorder, we will first explore how evolutionary thinking can transform our understanding of causality followed by a brief discussion of a range of other important evolutionary concepts.

> **Box 1.1 Evolutionary pathways for the persistence of disease and disorder (adapted from Crespi (2016) and Gluckman et al. (2009))**
>
> - Mismatch
> - Life history factors
> - Overactive defence mechanisms
> - Co-evolutionary considerations: consequences of the arms race against pathogens
> - Constraints imposed by evolutionary history
> - Trade-offs
> - Sexual selection and its consequences
> - Balancing selection and heterozygote advantage
> - Demographic history and its consequences
> - Selection favours reproductive success at the expense of health
> - Deleterious alleles
> - Extremes of adaptations

---

[1] Readers interested in a more detailed introduction to evolutionary science relevant to medicine may wish to consult *Principles of Evolutionary Medicine* (Gluckman et al., 2009) or later editions.

1.1.3 Tinbergen's Causal Framework

One of the most significant implications of evolutionary theory is in the understanding of causality in the biological sciences. In his seminal paper on the subject, Nikolaas Tinbergen, Nobel Laureate and co-founder of the science of ethology, proposed a causal system that is now known as 'Tinbergen's four questions' (Tinbergen, 1963). Building on the distinction between proximate (mechanistic) and ultimate (evolutionary) causation made by Mayr (1961), Tinbergen proposed that a complete understanding of any biological system, trait or organ requires an understanding of all four categories of its causation (Table 1.1). These are the mechanisms that make it work (physiology, structure), the developmental processes that form the system during the lifetime of the organism, the phylogenetic history of the system and the function that the system served the organism in its natural environment. In Table 1.1, boxes (1) and (2) correspond to the proximate causes and boxes (3) and (4) correspond to the ultimate causes according to Mayr's classification. It is important to note that all four causes apply simultaneously to all biological phenomena and are not alternatives to each other, and that neglecting any of these four causal elements necessarily results in an incomplete understanding of the given system or trait.

As diseases and disorders are phenomena affecting biological systems, they should plainly benefit from the application of Tinbergen's system by asking 'why' questions that supplement the more traditional 'how' questions (see Chapter 2 for a detailed discussion of some clinical applications).

Focusing exclusively on the proximate (as is currently the case in mainstream psychiatry) is akin to a technician's view of a machine, whereas considering ultimate causation as well is more like an engineer's view (Nesse, 2019). Evolutionists consider that a clinician skilled in the recognition of distressing emotional states who also understands why we have such emotions and how emotional systems interact with people's current lives is likely to have a deeper understanding of the patient's distress and is able to take greater account of the circumstances that may be contributing to the patient's current state (Abed and St John-Smith, 2021). In addition, importantly, evolutionary considerations have the potential for influencing research agendas through testing hypotheses regarding what is the normal function of the system that is giving rise to psychopathology; questions that are seldom asked by mainstream psychiatry (Brüne, 2015).

1.1.4 Darwinian Fitness and Inclusive Fitness

Fitness is a central concept in evolutionary theory. Darwinian fitness is a measure of reproductive success and can be defined either with respect to a genotype or to a phenotype in a given environment. This is measured by the average contribution to the gene pool of the next generation that is made by an individual of the specified genotype or phenotype. Where fitness is affected by differences between various alleles of a given gene, the relative frequency of those alleles will change across generations through selection, and alleles with greater positive effects on individual fitness will become more common over time.

As alluded to earlier, the integration of modern genetics with Darwinian theory led to the 'modern synthesis' and the formulation of the concept of 'inclusive fitness' (Hamilton, 1964). According to Hamilton's formulation, fitness should be measured not only through the number of direct descendants who carry copies of one's genes, but also through the number of non-descendant kin who also carry copies of the

Table 1.1 Tinbergen's four questions (adapted from Nesse, 2013)

	Developmental/historical	Characteristics of the trait/system
Proximate causation	(2) Ontogeny: how does the trait develop during the lifetime of the organism?	(1) Mechanism: how does it work?
Evolutionary or ultimate causation	(3) Phylogeny: what is the phylogenetic history of the trait? (*Why* is the trait/system the way it is?)	(4) Adaptive function: how has the trait or system contributed to the organism's inclusive fitness in its natural environment? (*Why* does the trait/system exist?)

same genes. It follows that behaving altruistically towards kin can improve one's overall fitness or inclusive fitness (the sum total of descendant and non-descendant kin who carry copies of one's genes) provided that the fitness cost to the altruist is lower than the fitness gain to kin multiplied by the coefficient of relatedness (this is also known as Hamilton's rule). This provides a basis for the understanding of the evolution of altruism and of the conditions that would give rise to competition and cooperation (Del Giudice, 2018). 'Kin selection' is the term that is used for the evolutionary strategy that increases inclusive fitness through the application of Hamilton's rule.

1.1.5 Evolution and the Concept of Psychological Mechanisms

Natural and sexual selection are the only known causal processes capable of producing complex functional mechanisms (also known as adaptations). An adaptation may be defined as an inherited characteristic that came into existence as a feature of a species through natural selection because it facilitated survival and reproduction during the period of its evolution (Tooby and Cosmides, 1992). Solving a recurrent adaptive problem is the function of any given adaptation. There must be genes for any adaptation because they are axiomatically required for the passage of the adaptation from parents to offspring. Therefore, evolutionary psychologists/psychiatrists start from the position that all brain neurobiological mechanisms/systems have been shaped through a long process of selection within a particular set of environmental conditions (see Section 1.1.8) (Buss, 2009).

Psychological mechanisms are viewed as specialised neurobiological systems shaped by selection to solve recurrent problems of survival and reproduction faced by ancestral humans over evolutionary history (Tooby and Cosmides, 1992). An understanding of the function and phylogeny of evolved mechanisms thereby provides unique insights into both their adaptive output as well as how and why these mechanisms can misfire, leading to maladaptive responses (e.g. in novel environmental conditions; see Section 1.2.1). Examples of evolved psychological mechanisms include: fear, attachment, security, status, mating and caregiving (Del Giudice, 2018).

An illustrative example of the derailing of an evolved mechanism is the way in which the cuckoo chick exploits the innate parental feeding mechanism of certain bird species. The hatching cuckoo chick provides a supernormal stimulus that triggers a (parental) feeding response through its huge gaping beak despite being in the nest of a different species (such as a great reed warbler), which induces the warbler to feed the cuckoo chick to the detriment of its own offspring (e.g. Tanaka et al., 2011). Similarly, evolved psychological mechanisms in humans can be derailed and produce maladaptive responses when exposed to novel environmental conditions, leading to mental disorder in some individuals (see Section 1.2.1).

1.1.6 Parental Investment Theory and Parent–Offspring Conflict

Parental investment is the investment that parents make in an offspring that increases that offspring's chances of surviving. By definition, such investment imposes a cost on the parents as measured by their ability to invest in other offspring, current and future. Components of fitness include the well-being of existing offspring, parents' future reproduction and inclusive fitness through aid to kin (Hamilton, 1964; Trivers, 1972). Parental investment may be performed by both males and females (biparental care), females alone (exclusive maternal care) or males alone (exclusive paternal care). Care can be provided at any stage of the offspring's life, from prenatal (e.g. egg guarding and incubation in birds and placental nourishment in mammals) to postnatal (e.g. food provisioning and protection of offspring).

Parental investment theory predicts that, on average, the sex that invests more in its offspring, including the size of gametes, gestation, lactation and child rearing, will be more selective when choosing a mate, and the less-investing sex will engage in more intra-sexual competition for access to mates. This theory has been influential in explaining sex differences in sexual selection and mate preferences throughout the animal kingdom, including humans. Trivers (1974) extended parental investment theory to explain parent–offspring conflict: the conflict between optimal investment from the parent's versus the offspring's perspective.

A further complication in nurturing occurs with parent–offspring conflict. This is a biological process that can start from the moment of conception. This conflict, which occurs exclusively in sexually reproducing species, is based on the fact that while the mother (or father) is related to their offspring by 50%, the foetus is 100% related to itself. This is used to signify the evolutionary conflict arising from differences in optimal parental investment to an offspring from the standpoint of both the parent and the offspring (Trivers, 1974).

Similarly, each sibling is only 50% related to any of their full siblings, and so they have a propensity to attempt to acquire more than their fair share of parental investment and more than the parents are willing to provide. However, parent–offspring conflict is functionally and statistically counterbalanced by the processes related to inclusive fitness and thus limited by the close genetic relationship between parent and offspring as additional parental investment obtained by one offspring at the expense of its siblings can decrease the number of its surviving siblings and reduce inclusive fitness. This leads to the prediction that, all other things being equal, parent–offspring conflict will be stronger among half-siblings than among full siblings. These observations and models may have significant effects relevant to child psychiatry (see Chapters 14 and 15).

1.1.7 Phenotypic Plasticity, Canalisation and Differential Susceptibility

Plasticity is an evolutionary adaptation to environmental variation that is reasonably predictable and occurs within the lifespan of an individual organism as it allows individuals to 'fit' their phenotype to different environments. Phenotypic plasticity describes the possibility of modifying developmental trajectories in response to specific environmental cues and also the ability of an individual organism to change its phenotypic state or activity (e.g. its metabolism) in response to variations in environmental conditions (Garland and Kelly, 2006).

Phenotypic plasticity can evolve if Darwinian fitness is increased by changing the phenotype. However, the fitness benefits of plasticity may be limited by the trade-off of the costs of plastic responses (e.g. synthesising new proteins, adjusting expression ratios of isozyme variants,

maintaining sensory machinery to detect changes) as well as the predictability and reliability of environmental cues. Canalisation is the converse of plasticity and refers to developmental stability that resists both genetic and environmental disruption or perturbation. Canalisation mechanisms are vitally important and ensure that an organism's traits demonstrate robustness and develop reliably. However, their drawback is that they limit plasticity (Haltigan et al., 2021; Waddington, 1942).

Another interpretation of psychological findings that are traditionally discussed according to the diathesis–stress model is differential susceptibility (Belsky, 1997). Both models suggest that development can be differentially susceptible to experiences or qualities of the environment. Whereas the diathesis–stress model suggests a distinct and mostly negativity-sensitive response, Belsky describes a group that is sensitive to adverse experiences but also to positive experiences. These models may be complementary if some individuals are dually or uniquely positivity-sensitive while others are uniquely negativity-sensitive.

Bakermans-Kranenburg and van IJzendoorn (2006) were the first to test the differential susceptibility hypothesis as a function of genetic factors, examining the moderating effect of the dopamine receptor D4 seven-repeat polymorphism (DRD4-7R) on the association between maternal sensitivity and externalising behaviour problems in 47 families. Children with the DRD4-7R allele and 'insensitive mothers' displayed significantly more externalising behaviours than children with the same allele but with 'sensitive' mothers. Children with the DRD4-7R allele and sensitive mothers had the fewest externalising behaviours of all, whereas maternal sensitivity had no effect on children without the DRD4-7R allele.

Research has also demonstrated that possessing at least one s-allele of the serotonin transporter gene HTTLPR confers an increased risk of developing depression when facing adverse events. However, the same variation is linked to superior cognitive performance in several domains and increases social conformity (Homberg and Lesch, 2011).

These examples serve as evidence against simple genetic determinism and also provide indications that naïvely aspiring to alter genes alone in order to treat disorders may not be in an individual's best interest as differing circumstances alter the harmfulness or benefits of such a gene.

1.1.8 The Ancestral Environment or Environment of Evolutionary Adaptedness

The concept of the environment of evolutionary adaptedness (EEA) was first proposed by John Bowlby (1969) of attachment theory fame. Broadly speaking, the EEA refers to the overall ancestral human environment during which the distinctive traits of modern humans were shaped. It is sometimes referred to incorrectly as if it were a single, uniform time and place. However, it is more appropriately conceptualised as 'a statistical composite of the adaptation-relevant properties of the ancestral environments encountered by members of ancestral populations, weighted by their frequency and fitness consequences' (Tooby and Cosmides, 1990: 386–387). The EEA is therefore a compound idea representing the sum of a population's exposure, over a given time frame, to external conditions and stimuli, threats and opportunities, including nutrients, social pressures, threats from parasites, predators and competitors as well as climate and general habitat (Gluckman et al., 2009). Thus, it may be considered as a 'composite of environmental properties of the most recent segment of a species' evolution that encompasses the period during which its modern collection of adaptations assumed their present form' (Tooby and Cosmides, 1990: 388). It is important to note that 'different adaptations will have different EEAs. Some, like language, are firmly anchored in approximately the last two million years; others, such as infant attachment, reflect a much lengthier evolutionary history' (Durrant and Ellis, 2003: 10).

Critics of the concept of the EEA have argued that we do not know much about how our remote ancestors lived, and they claim that this makes the concept of the EEA a highly speculative and unscientific premise (Hagen, 2016). Critics such as Gould (1997), Buller (2005) and Laland and Brown (2011) also objected to the use of the concept of the EEA because they assumed that we are unable to specify the living conditions of our ancestors with sufficient precision. There is no doubt that some of these concerns are legitimate and should be seriously considered. However, if their assertions are true, such that we can never know anything about how our ancestors lived and will never be able to do so, then an evolutionary approach could not ascertain the exact function of any somatic or brain system. As all functions are adaptations shaped by selection in response to past environments, discovering facts about past environments remains an important part of the evolutionary endeavour and a prerequisite to understanding current function and dysfunction.

The assertion that we cannot know much about the past is nowadays no longer tenable and contradicts a wide range of academic disciplines whose focuses are entirely on investigating the past. These fields include archaeology, palaeontology, palaeoanthropology, history and cosmology, which now include not only research into fossils and artefacts, but also sequencing the DNA of ancient and extinct species (Hagen, 2020). This has allowed enormous progress and clearly and decisively demonstrates that scientific research aimed at discovering facts about the past is capable of producing rigorous, testable and falsifiable models of past environments (e.g. Dunbar, 2014). Without knowledge of the past, evolutionary science simply cannot progress, and hence a concept of the EEA or ancestral human environment is essential. This does not mean that statements about human evolutionary history should be accepted blindly or uncritically. All such claims should be stated as hypotheses that can be supported or falsified by the evidence, and a similar level of scientific rigour should also apply to hypotheses about human psychological adaptations and their functions.

1.2 The Evolutionary Pathways for the Persistence of Disease and Disorder

As we have seen, natural selection produces bodies and brains with assortments of adaptations shaped over thousands of generations to enhance reproductive success (fitness) but not necessarily well-being or happiness. The explanation for the conundrum of why evolution has left humans so vulnerable to disease and disorder has itself been evolving ever since it was first posed by the

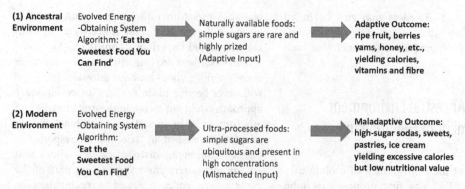

Figure 1.1 Illustration of nutritional mismatch in the modern environment (adapted from Li et al., 2018)

founders of modern evolutionary medicine (Nesse and Williams, 1994). Accordingly, a range of pathways have been proposed by which evolutionary processes can lead to the existence and persistence of disease or disorder, as presented in Box 1.1.

Some of these pathways are more relevant than others to psychiatry, and they are not mutually exclusive. Several may be implicated concurrently or sequentially in the origin of mental disorders. They represent a list of ultimate/evolutionary causes of our vulnerability to disease and disorder, including mental disorder.

1.2.1 Mismatch

Mismatch is arguably one of the most important insights of evolutionary medicine and is indispensable to the understanding of a range of diseases and disorders prevalent in the modern environment, such as the increased prevalence of coronary artery disease, hypertension, obesity, type 2 diabetes, depression, alcoholism and eating disorders, to name a few (Nesse and Williams, 1994; Pollard, 2008). The idea of mismatch is based on the fact that adaptations are shaped by selection within a given environment. If the environment changes rapidly and radically, some biological systems run the risk of becoming mismatched to the new environment. This is also referred to as 'genome lag' (Li et al., 2018). Given that the modern human environment has undergone a radical change from that of our ancestors in a number of ways, this has led to some systems becoming mismatched to this novel environment, giving rise to dysfunctional outcomes, including a range of mental disorders (see Chapter 2 for

further discussion). Examples of mental disorders arising/increasing in the modern environment include eating disorders (Rantala, 2019; Russell, 2000) and drug and alcohol addictions (Nesse, 2005) (see Figure 1.1 for an illustration of nutritional mismatch). However, while humans may be mismatched to certain aspects of the modern environment (e.g. the constant abundance of nutrients and especially of ultra-processed foods), we are well matched to the majority of modern conditions, as humans are clearly thriving and not becoming extinct (Hagen, 2020).

1.2.2 Life History Theory

Life history theory (LHT) deals with species' typical solutions to problems associated with survival and reproduction that change over an individual's lifespan (Brüne, 2015). Hence, LHT provides a framework for understanding how organisms allocate time and energy in achieving core biosocial goals across their lifespan. Life history strategies involve a series of trade-offs that shape important biological developments, including the timing of sexual maturity and the number and quality of offspring, as well as the length of lifespan (Stearns, 1992). The application of LHT demonstrates that these trade-offs yield a spectrum of life history strategies, and the trade-offs include somatic versus reproductive effort, present versus the future and quality versus quantity of offspring. The 'fast' end of the spectrum is characterised by a shorter lifespan, faster growth, earlier maturation and reproduction and a larger number of offspring, while those at the 'slow' end of the life history spectrum show the opposite characteristics (Del Giudice, 2018). The idea of a fast–slow spectrum of life history has been proposed as a framework for understanding individual differences, including vulnerability to mental disorders (Del Giudice, 2018). Differences in life history strategies are partly under genetic control, but it appears that the nature and quality of an individual's early environment may also be important (Belsky et al., 1991; Ellis et al., 2011). The application of LHT to trait variations between individuals as opposed to between species has recently come under critical scrutiny (e.g. Zietsch and Sidari, 2020). As a result, this area of research is undergoing considerable revision regarding both its methodology and its theoretical assumptions (Del Giudice, 2020; Young et al., 2020).

1.2.3 Overactive Defences

Defences such as the mood- and anxiety-regulating systems can become overactive or dysregulated, resulting in harmful outcomes and leading to defence activation disorders (Del Giudice, 2018; Nesse, 2019). Examples of defences in general medicine include pain, diarrhoea, vomiting and pyrexia, for which similar principles apply. Importantly, all defences – whether in biologically evolved or human-made systems – have a common design feature such that they are designed to allow false alarms (also known as false positives), as these are far less costly than failure to activate (false negatives) when the risk is present (usually with catastrophic results; imagine, for example, ingesting a toxin and failing to vomit). This is referred to as the 'smoke detector principle' and explains why all bodily defences (including aversive emotions) can activate excessively (Nesse, 2019). The excessive tendency for false alarms that characterises all defence systems is akin to a strategy of 'better safe than sorry' (Blumstein, 2020) and explains why it is usually safe to block a defence once it is established that the response is not necessary or even counterproductive.

1.2.4 Co-evolutionary Considerations (Arms Races between Pathogens and Hosts)

Humans as hosts have been and continue to be engaged in an unending arms race with rapidly evolving pathogens such as bacteria and viruses (Ewald, 1994). This means that increasingly innovative host defences (e.g. increasingly sophisticated immune responses) are matched by even more novel ways of evading such defences. Also, increasing numbers of pathogens have become resistant to antimicrobial therapy, which poses an increasingly serious hazard to human health. In this arms race, pathogens, as rapid replicators, have the advantage because of their much faster capacity to evolve (Nesse, 2005). The recent Covid-19 pandemic is a vivid example of a newly evolved virus jumping species and spreading globally through the human population, taking a massive toll in terms of human life and livelihoods, and there seems no doubt that there will be other such pandemics in the future. This is undoubtedly a massive problem for medicine in general, but examples in mental health appear more limited. For example, obsessive-compulsive disorder (OCD) can arise as a result of streptococcal-induced autoimmune disease (Swedo et al., 1994), and there have been ongoing suggestions of a link between *Toxoplasma gondii* and schizophrenia (Fuglewicz et al., 2017) (see Chapter 10).

1.2.5 Constraints Arising from Evolutionary History

Unlike a human designer, evolution cannot go back to the drawing board and start afresh. This is called 'path dependency' and explains poor 'designs' such as why human eyes have blood vessels that occlude portions of the retina (Nesse, 2005), why the light receptors in the human retina face the wrong way (Lents, 2020), the tortuous path of the recurrent laryngeal nerve and why our bipedal skeleton – a modified version of a quadrupedal design plan – creates myriad vulnerabilities from ubiquitous back problems to birth canals too narrow to admit a foetal head (Pavličev et al., 2020; Taylor, 2015). It is also why phylogenetic history and the EEA matter so much. Evolution must work with what has gone before; complex systems are not created out of nothing. Evolution has been described as a tinkerer, shaping adaptations (from available biological systems) that work just well enough for survival and reproduction (Jacobs, 1977). Hence, evolution is a process that shapes adaptations through historical constraints, multiple trade-offs and (genetic) errors (Nesse, 2005). Evolutionary thinking, therefore, explains the flaws, quirks and tortuous complexity that is ubiquitous in biological systems, all of which can create vulnerabilities to dysfunction and disorder.

1.2.6 Trade-Offs

It is necessary to appreciate that all biologically evolved adaptations, traits and systems represent trade-offs, as increasing one trait is often at the expense of worsening the performance of another. For example, increasing resistance to infections increases the risk of autoimmune diseases. Also, this explains why improving energy conservation and famine resistance increases the risk of obesity when food becomes plentiful and why the reciprocal trade-off between body size/muscle bulk and speed of movement has an optimum balance such that increasing one can lead to a decrease in the other.

1.2.7 Sexual Selection and Its Consequences

Sexual selection was described by Darwin (1871) to explain the evolution of traits that do not aid survival and may even be detrimental to it. The canonical example of a sexually selected trait is the peacock's tail, which serves no survival purpose but is an attractor of peahens. Sexually selected traits are those that improve reproductive success through increased attractiveness to the opposite sex. Sexual selection occurs in all sexually reproducing organisms, including humans, and usually involves the display of costly and extravagant traits that are difficult to fake and can therefore act as honest markers of good health and high-quality genes. Sexual selection tends to shape traits that are gender divergent and to specifically target the preferences of the opposite sex. The evolution of sexually selected traits can create particular kinds of vulnerabilities to mental disorders, which are often skewed in their sex ratios. Examples of mental disorders where sexual selection may play an important role include eating disorders (Abed, 1998) (see Chapter 11), sexual dysfunction and schizophrenia (Del Giudice, 2017).

1.2.8 Balancing Selection and Heterozygote Advantage

In diploid species such as humans, the two alleles can be identical (homozygote) or different

(heterozygote). The classical example in medicine of a heterozygote advantage is sickle cell anaemia, where the heterozygote state confers immunity to malaria (which is a major advantage in parts of the world where malaria is endemic), whereas the homozygote state causes sickle cell anaemia, a serious and debilitating disease (Gluckman et al., 2009). In this example, the benefits of the heterozygote state are counterbalanced by the deleterious effect of the homozygote state. Other examples of heterozygote advantage in medicine are more speculative (e.g. cystic fibrosis). There are currently no examples of this process relevant to mental health.

1.2.9 Demographic History and Its Consequences

Human migrations out of Africa took place around 70,000 years ago onwards. They took place in successive waves and in doing so human populations frequently passed through impediments or bottlenecks (due to famine, disease, etc.) that caused significantly reduced genetic diversity (Henn et al., 2012). Such scenarios also include small populations that become isolated through chance events and continue living in small, isolated communities where otherwise-rare mutations can become unusually prevalent as a result of a 'founder effect' (Gluckman et al., 2009). Such chance events are also referred to as genetic drift. Examples of rare harmful genes becoming prevalent as a result of the founder effect include Tay–Sachs disease, which exclusively affects Ashkenazi Jews, and Gaucher's disease, which is found disproportionately in French Canadians. Interestingly, recent findings suggest that globally, human populations, in their migration out of Africa, have been subject to serial bottlenecks (and founder effects) that increased the further away they travelled from the African continent, as a result of which genetic diversity successively declined (Henn et al., 2012). This phenomenon may also explain the high prevalence rates of Huntington's disease in Venezuela, Colombia, Peru and Brazil (Kay et al., 2017).

1.2.10 Selection Favours Reproductive Success over Health

The basic tenet of Darwinian theory is that selection works through reproductive success and not necessarily through good health and well-being. Therefore, a gene that reduces health and well-being but increases reproductive success will nonetheless spread within the population (Nesse, 2005). Hence, high levels of competitiveness, reduced cooperativeness, increased jealousy, greed and envy and unquenchable sexual desire will spread despite their potential adverse effects on the health and well-being of self and others because of their positive effects on reproductive success (Buss, 2000).

1.2.11 Deleterious Alleles

Deleterious genes that allow survival beyond reproductive age and do not manifest themselves until later life may remain within the population, such as those responsible for Huntington's disease. Such alleles/mutations can remain at low levels in the population as selection is limited in its ability to eliminate them. Also, non-fatal *de novo* mutations (mutations that arise in the germ line during the lifetime of a parent and where the parent is unaffected by the mutation) will be passed on to offspring. Such mutations are invisible to selection in the first generation and will only be subject to selection in subsequent generations if they are compatible with survival to reproductive age.

1.2.12 The Extreme Ends of Functional Adaptations

Functionally adaptive traits such as anxiety, fear or fastidiousness can become dysfunctional and maladaptive at the extreme end of the spectrum, where they present as generalised anxiety disorder, phobia or OCD (Abed and De Pauw, 1998; Crespi, 2016). Similarly, the extreme ends of adaptive personality traits can lead to dysfunctional and maladaptive states (Trull and Widiger, 2013). Maladaptive extremes can be dysfunctional at both ends (i.e. where the trait is too low as well as too high). This can apply to any biologically based trait, such as mentalising (theory of mind), where both overactivity and underactivity have been implicated in mental disorders (schizophrenia and autistic spectrum disorder, respectively) (Crespi, 2016).

Hence, taking an evolutionary perspective provides a key insight that mental distress can arise from functional systems (e.g. overactive

defences or mismatch) (Abed et al., 2019). It therefore follows that undesirable conditions, which should still warrant intervention by healthcare professionals, may result from a variety of situations that may but do not necessarily involve true biological dysfunction. In addition, an evolutionary analysis provides a theoretical framework that enables us to distinguish states of mental distress and mental disorder that arise from functional or dysfunctional systems and also provides a more effective way of understanding the role of environmental context (see Chapter 2 for a discussion of harmful dysfunction).

1.3 Evolution, Human Uniqueness and the Role of Culture

1.3.1 The Social and Cultural Brain

The human brain accounts for 2% of body weight but consumes 15–20% of the total energy required by the body (Brüne, 2015). This striking fact requires an evolutionary explanation as such an energetically expensive organ could only evolve if its benefits outweighed its costs (Aiello and Wheeler, 1995). The most compelling and empirically supported explanation for this is that the demands of the social environment were the main drivers of the increase in brain size over the course of human evolutionary history (Dunbar, 2003a; Humphrey, 1976).

The social brain refers to a network of neurobiological systems that specialise in the processing of information relating to the social domain (Brothers, 1997; Dunbar, 2003b). There appears to be a quantitative relationship between a species' brain size and the average size of its social groups that holds true across species (Dunbar, 2014). However, the relationship between brain size and group size (strictly speaking the volume of the neocortex) applies only to species that have bonded social relationships and form highly structured groups. These social bonds manifest in the form of friendships – intense, emotionally close relationships that are similar to pair-bonds but do not involve sex and reproduction. Such complex social arrangements contrast sharply with the fleeting and ephemeral interactions of herd animals that do not form lasting bonds (Dunbar, 2014).

The social organisation of hunter-gatherers appears to have been characterised by a nested hierarchy of groups starting with bands of 30–50 people, bonded communities of 150 people, endogamous communities of 500 people and ethnolinguistic units (tribes) of 1,500 people (Dunbar, 2014). Interestingly, these various levels of organisation are still evident in modern-day humans in the concentric 'circles of acquaintance-ship' (Dunbar, 2014).

Such an increase in social complexity would not have been possible without language, which is one of the most distinctive human traits (Del Giudice, 2018; Pinker, 1994). This has enabled unprecedented levels of information and knowledge transfer that laid the groundwork for cumulative culture (see Section 1.3.2). The scaling up of human social organisation into mega-groups comprising millions (even hundreds of millions in modern nation states) would not have been possible without the human facility for culture acquisition and transmission on a massive scale (Henrich, 2016). Understanding the functions and dysfunctions of the social brain may be relevant to a number of mental disorders involving impairments to sociality, including schizophrenia (Burns, 2007) and autistic spectrum disorders (Baron-Cohen, 1994).

1.3.2 Cultural Evolution and Gene–Culture Co-evolution

Humans, unlike other organisms, have two parallel and interacting inheritance systems, namely genes and culture. Although culture of sorts is present in a wide range of species and is not unique to humans, cumulative cultural evolution, which involves cumulative improvement over many generations that could not be achieved by any one individual alone (sometimes referred to as the cultural ratchet effect; Tomasello, 1990), is widely considered to be unique to our species (Dean et al., 2014). Cumulative cultural evolution creates changes in the environment that produce selection pressures on genes. In addition, culturally evolved social environments favour the possession of an inherited psychology that is suited to such environments (Richerson and Boyd, 2005). The consequences of gene–culture co-evolution for modern humans is related to the phenomenon of 'self-domestication' described by some authors (e.g. Brüne, 2007). The existence of these two evolving and interacting systems running in parallel (genes and culture) has been referred to as the 'dual inheritance system'.

The role of culture in shaping humans both behaviourally and morphologically cannot be overestimated. For example, while we do not know what the last common ancestor (LCA) of chimpanzees and humans (who lived about 7 million years ago) looked like, one influential view suggests that the LCA was a chimpanzee-like ape (Pilbeam and Lieberman, 2017). If this is so, then humans would have undergone a truly radical behavioural and morphological transformation since the LCA, whereas chimpanzees appear to have changed very little during the same period. Similarly, without cumulative culture or gene–culture co-evolution, gorillas (who resemble overgrown chimpanzees morphologically) have not altered significantly over even longer evolutionary timescales (humans shared a common ancestor with gorillas around 10 million years ago). One plausible explanation for this is that humans have been subject to sustained and prolonged gene–culture co-evolution while there is no evidence of any such effects in the chimpanzee (including bonobo) lineage or the lineages of other great apes (Henrich and Tennie, 2017). Hence, it may not be an exaggeration to suggest that gene–culture co-evolution has shaped the human mind, the human body and human social structures. It is ultimately worth considering how culture can and has influenced gene frequencies, as culture is in itself an environment and thus becomes part of selection processes.

In addition to culture's influence on gene selection over evolutionary timescales, it appears that cultural practices can lead to the rewiring of our brains during an individual's lifespan (Henrich, 2020). The example that has been studied extensively is literacy, where it has been shown that the literate have brains that differ significantly from the illiterate, with a thicker corpus callosum, the shifting of the processing of faces to the right hemisphere, an impairment in face recognition and an improvement in verbal memory (Dehaene et al., 2015).

A salient example of the influence of gene–culture co-evolution on modern humans is the shaping of our digestive system. Our digestive system is unusual for an organism of our size with a small mouth, small teeth, small stomach and a short colon, all of which have evolved as a result of the cultural practices of food preparation and the use of fire in cooking in the human lineage (Wrangham, 2009). Also, the culturally influenced, unique human ability to accurately use projectiles in hunting and fighting over human evolutionary timescales has been proposed as an explanation for the reduction in the physical robustness of modern humans who no longer needed to hunt or fight at close quarters (Richersen and Boyd, 2005). Other more evolutionarily recent consequences of gene–culture co-evolution include the evolution of lactase persistence (lactose tolerance), which occurs in populations descended from ancestors with a dairying culture (mainly in northern Europe and parts of the Middle East and Africa). These populations carry a mutation that arose 6,000–7,000 years ago that enables individuals to digest lactose in adulthood (Cavali-Sforza et al., 1994). Culture has also shaped human psychology, making us 'cultural addicts' through weeding out norm violators and rewarding sociable, docile conformists. Humans have also evolved the capacity for accurate learning from members of our in-group so that we developed what might be called 'collective brains' (Henrich, 2016).

A recent study, taking a metabolic approach in an attempt to tease out ecological, social and cultural factors over human evolutionary history, suggests that ecological rather than social challenges played the crucial role and that the extraordinary brain growth in the human lineage was strongly promoted by culture (Gonzalez-Forero and Gardner, 2018). This finding is consistent with the cultural hypotheses of human brain evolution (Henrich, 2016; Laland, 2017).

Interestingly, a novel theory was recently proposed regarding human evolution that may have a direct bearing on the unique human phenomenon of cumulative cultural evolution. This is the proposal that sometime between 70,000 and 100,000 years ago modern humans evolved a 'systemising mechanism' that uniquely enables humans to detect patterns in the world that are hidden from other species (Baron-Cohen, 2020). The claim is made that this mechanism uniquely endowed humans with the talent for 'generative inventiveness', which has resulted in the extraordinary diversification in cultural/artistic/utilitarian artefacts in the archaeological record from around 50,000 years ago onwards and contrasts sharply with the long periods of cultural stasis before then (Baron-Cohen, 2020). It is claimed that the extreme variant of the systemising mechanism is evident in individuals with autistic spectrum disorders. The theory has clear implications for the

phenomenon of cumulative cultural evolution as the systemising mechanism provides the engine for the continuous production of new inventions (cultural variants) that is present in humans and absent in other species.

However, with the exception of Baron-Cohen's recently proposed link between autistic spectrum disorders and the systemising mechanism, the implications for mental health of the recent cultural evolution models and gene–culture co-evolution, as well as recent research findings on the developmental influences of cultural practices, remain largely unexplored and deserve further attention from evolutionary psychologists and psychiatrists.

1.3.3 Mental Disorder and the Relaxation of Natural Selection Pressures Model

One recently published evolutionary theory attempts to explain the emergence of mental disorders in humans as being the result of the relaxation of natural selection pressures (RNSP) (Fuchs, 2019). This is an interesting and novel idea that proposes that, over thousands of generations of evolutionary history, humans have constructed around them an environment that shielded them from a wide range of hazards (e.g. predation), and this has resulted in what the author has termed 'diversification of human instinctual drives'. The author bases his assumption on a range of sound evolutionary and ethological ideas and concepts, including the differentiation/diffusion of instinctual drives, open and closed genetic instinctual programmes (Mayr, 1974), active versus reactive behaviours and the consequences of frustration of instinctual drives that include vacuous behaviour, displacement, aggression and dysphoria. His ideas on the human construction of a shielding environment are closely related to both the concepts of 'niche construction' and gene–culture co-evolution. Interestingly, in their discussion of niche construction, Laland et al. (2017) placed this phenomenon somewhere between natural and artificial selection, and they considered that niche construction would lead to reduced genetic diversity but not to the extent that artificial selection does. This view seems to contradict Fuchs' RNSP model.

Nevertheless, the relaxation of particular natural selection pressures is an observable phenomenon that has clear consequences on the traits that are freed from specific selection pressures. This is demonstrated in cavefish (Calderoni et al., 2016), who not only lose their eyesight, as imperfect structures are no longer eliminated (as it is not disadvantageous to have no eyesight in complete darkness and maintaining eyesight is costly), but the absence of daylight leads also to the degradation of their biological clocks. The effects of RNSP are also evident in humans (and many other primates), where the loss of function of the *GULO* gene, due to the wide availability of vitamin C from plant sources, has resulted in the loss of the ability to synthesise vitamin C (unlike the majority of mammals) and thus has given rise to humans' susceptibility to the risk of scurvy (Lents, 2020).

Fuchs argues that RNSP was exploited during human evolution to shape useful human adaptations, but that the extremes of these diversified adaptations led to dysfunctional forms of behaviour and to various forms of mental disorder. The merits and implications of Fuchs' novel theory for the understanding of mental disorder remain largely unexplored and deserve further attention from evolutionists.

When applying Fuchs' RNSP model to present-day culture, and to medicine in particular, we should note that while selection pressures are relaxed in some areas, such as the risk from predators and many infectious diseases, new selection pressures arise in other areas. Humans, of course, remain vulnerable to old threats such as microorganisms (old and new), while new pressures such as the stresses of modern life and technology are having currently unknown effects on fitness and hence on the composition of the human genome of future generations. Therefore, selection pressures are different, not absent.

1.4 Implications and Conclusions

1.4.1 Opportunities

We have argued in this chapter that evolutionary science presents a range of advantages for psychiatry. The advantages can be summarised as follows (Nesse, 2005):

(1) Asking new questions about why evolution has left us all vulnerable to mental disorders;

(2) Providing a way to think clearly about development and the ways in which early experiences influence later characteristics;

(3) Providing a foundation for understanding emotions and their regulation;

(4) Providing a foundation for a scientific diagnostic system;

(5) Providing a framework for incorporating multiple causal factors that explain why some people get mental disorders while others do not.

However, it is important to emphasise that evolutionary psychiatry does not seek to replace mainstream psychiatry. It supplements, informs and augments mainstream psychiatric thinking. Evolutionists fully accept the current ethical principles that govern the practice of psychiatry in which the interests of individual patients, their welfare and the reduction of harm to patients and others remain the central concerns. Furthermore, evolutionary psychiatrists fully subscribe to the principles of evidence-based medicine and do not suggest or prescribe untested treatments to patients based on purely theoretical formulations. Evolutionary thinking can and does generate theories regarding causation that can lead to proposals for novel treatments. However, any such treatments should be subjected to the same rigorous assessments using the standard scientific methodology currently in use in mainstream medicine and psychiatry. Evolutionary psychiatry has no connection to the ideological and unscientific doctrines of social Darwinism and eugenics (see Wilson, 2019). Hence, evolutionary psychiatry aims to utilise our understanding of human vulnerabilities arising from evolutionary processes to help alleviate distress and aid the recovery of individual patients in every ethical and evidenced-based way possible (Troisi, 2015).

1.4.2 Clinical Utility

There are currently only a few examples of psychological/psychiatric interventions based on evolutionary theory. These include compassion-focused therapy (Gilbert, 2020) as well as a new type of cognitive behavioural therapy (Abrams, 2020). Nevertheless, we would argue that evolutionary knowledge can be useful to both the patient and the clinician in clinical practice even when not administering specific therapies (e.g. through enhancing empathy, greater attention to context and deeper understanding of the evolved function(s) of emotions). However, evolution's main utility is in helping us to understand health and disease in populations rather than individuals. Evolutionary science is therefore more analogous to epidemiology than therapeutics. It is important to appreciate that, like all models of health and disease, evolutionary theory does not instantly solve all outstanding problems. Issues in psychiatry are particularly complex, and therefore expansive claims of the efficacy of any particular approach are simply not credible. However, evolutionary theory has already been of immense value in multiple areas of biology. As a greater understanding of the human genome will take medicine towards individualised treatments, taking an evolutionary approach can offer invaluable insights. For example, evolution reminds us that there is no such thing as a normal genome. There are only genes that construct phenotypes that result in higher or lower reproductive success in a given environment (Nesse and Dawkins, 2010).

1.4.3 Research Implications

An evolutionary approach suggests a new class of questions about the aetiology of disease. Research to answer these questions should eventually allow the psychiatric literature to provide evolutionary considerations for each disease (Nesse and Dawkins, 2010). The strategies for formulating such questions and hypotheses remain unsettled, and the methods for testing evolutionary hypotheses are unfamiliar to many in medicine. Nesse (2011) has suggested a structure for appropriate evolutionary research that uses recent examples to illustrate successful strategies as well as some common challenges. He identifies appropriate questions to consider in testing evolutionary hypotheses. Addressing them systematically can help minimise confusion and errors.

1.4.4 Conclusion

We recognise that providing an introduction to a volume on evolutionary psychiatry that hopes to cater for both the newcomer to evolution as well as evolutionary scholars was going to be a challenge. We aimed to cover the basics of evolutionary theory while presenting current, up-to-date thinking on the subjects included. We particularly hope that those new to evolution feel better prepared to tackle the rest of this volume as a result of reading this introduction and also perhaps interested in consulting some of the references to this chapter and/or reading more widely around the rich and fascinating literature on evolutionary psychology and psychiatry.

References

Abed, R. (1998). The sexual competition hypothesis for eating disorders. *British Journal of Medical Psychology*, 71, 525–547.

Abed, R. and De Pauw, K. W. (1998). An evolutionary hypothesis for obsessive-compulsive disorder: a psychological immune system? *Behavioural Neurology*, 11, 245–250.

Abed, R. and St John-Smith, P. (2021). Evolutionary psychology and psychiatry. In T. K. Shackleford (ed.), *The Sage Handbook of Evolutionary Psychology: Applications of Evolutionary Psychology* (pp. 24–50). London: Sage.

Abed, R., Ayton, A., St John-Smith, P., Swanepoel, A. and Tracy, D. (2019). Evolutionary biology: an essential basic science for the training of the next generation of psychiatrists. *British Journal of Psychiatry*, 215, 699–701.

Abrams, M. (2020). *The New CBT: Clinical Evolutionary Psychology*. San Diego, CA: Cognella Academic Publishing.

Aiello, L. C. and Wheeler, P. (1995). The expensive tissue hypothesis – the brain and the digestive-system in human and primate evolution. *Current Anthropology*, 36, 199–221.

Akil, H., Brenner, S., Kandel, E., Kendler, K. S., King, M.-C., Scolnick, E., Watson, J. D. and Zoghby, H. Y. (2010). The future of psychiatric research: genomes and neural circuits. *Science*, 327, 1580–1581.

Bakermans-Kranenburg, M. J. and van IJzendoorn, M. H. (2006). Gene–environment interaction of the dopamine D4 receptor (DRD4) and observed maternal insensitivity predicting externalizing behavior in preschoolers. *Developmental Psychobiology*, 48, 406–409.

Barkow, J. H., Cosmides, L. and Tooby, J. (1992). *The Adapted Mind: Evolutionary Psychology and the Generation of Culture*. New York: Oxford University Press.

Baron-Cohen, S. (1994). How to build a baby that reads minds: cognitive mechanisms in mindreading. *Current Psychology of Cognition*, 13, 513–552.

Baron-Cohen, S. (1997). *The Maladapted Mind: Classic Readings in Evolutionary Psychopathology*. Hove: Psychology Press.

Baron-Cohen, S. (2020). *The Pattern Seekers: How Autism Drives*

Human Invention. New York: Basic Books.

Belsky, J. (1997). Variation in susceptibility to rearing influences: an evolutionary argument. *Psychological Inquiry*, 8, 182–186.

Belsky, J., Steinberg, L. and Draper, P. (1991). Childhood experience, interpersonal development and reproductive strategy: an evolutionary theory of socialization. *Child Development*, 62, 647–670.

Blumstein, D. (2020). *The Nature of Fear: Survival Lessons from the Wild*. Cambridge, MA: Harvard University Press.

Bowlby, J. (1969). *Attachment and Loss, Vol. 1: Attachment*. New York: Basic Books.

Brady, S. P., Bolnick, D. I., Angert, A. L., Gonzalez, A., Barrett, R. D. H., Crispo, E., Derry, A. M., Eckert, C. G., Fraser, D. J., Fussmann, G. F., Guichard, F., Lamy, T., McAdam, A. G., Newman, A. E. M., Paccard, A., Rolshausen, G., Simons, A. M. and Hendry, A. P. (2019). Causes of maladaptation. *Evolutionary Applications*, 12, 1229–1242.

Brothers, L. (1997). *Friday's Footprint: How Society Shapes the Human Mind*. Oxford: Oxford University Press.

Brüne, M. (2007). On human self-domestication, psychiatry and eugenics. *Philosophy, Ethics and Humanities in Medicine*, 2, 21.

Brüne, M. (2015). *Textbook of Evolutionary Psychiatry & Psychosomatic Medicine: The Origins of Psychopathology*. Oxford: Oxford University Press.

Brüne, M., Belsky, J., Fabrega, H., Feierman, H. R., Gilbert, P., Glantz, K., Polimeni, J., Price, J. S., Sanjuan, J., Sullivan, R., Troisi, A. and Wilson, D. R. (2012). The crisis of psychiatry – insights and prospects from evolutionary theory. *World Psychiatry*, 11, 55–57.

Buller, D. J. (2005). *Adapting Minds: Evolutionary Psychology and the Persistent Quest for Human Nature*. Cambridge, MA: MIT Press.

Burns, J. (2007). *The Descent of Madness: Evolutionary Roots of Psychosis and the Social Brain*. London: Routledge.

Buss, D. M. (2000). The evolution of happiness. *American Psychologist*, 55, 15–23.

Buss, D. M. (2009). The great struggles of life: Darwin and the emergence of evolutionary psychology. *American Psychologist*, 64, 140–148.

Calderoni, L., Rota-Stabelli, O., Frigato, E., Panziera, A., Kirchner, S., Foulkes, N. S., Kruckenhauser, L., Bertolucci, C. and Fuselli, S. (2016). Relaxed selective constraints drove functional modifications in peripheral photoreception of the cavefish *P. andruzzii* and provide insight into the time of cave colonization. *Heredity*, 117, 383–392.

Cavali-Sforza, L., Menozzi, P. and Piazza, A. (1994). *The History and Geography of Human Genes*. Princeton, NJ: Princeton University Press.

Crespi, B. J. (2016). The evolutionary aetiologies of autism spectrum and psychotic affective spectrum disorders. In A. Alvergne, C. Jenkinson and C. Faurie (eds.), *Evolutionary Thinking in Medicine: From Research to Policy and Practice* (pp. 299–327). Cham: Springer.

Darwin, C. (1859). *On the Origin of Species by Means of Natural Selection*. London: Murray.

Darwin, C. (1871). *On the Descent of Man, and Selection in Relation to Sex*. London: Murray.

Dean, L. G., Vale, G. L., Laland, K. N., Flynn, E. and Kendal, R. L. (2014). Human cumulative culture: a comparative perspective. *Biological Reviews*, 89, 284–301.

Dehaene, S., Cohen, L., Morris, J. and Kolinsky, R. (2015). Illiterate to literate: behavioural to cerebral changes induced by reading acquisition. *Nature Reviews: Neuroscience*, 16, 234–244.

Del Giudice, M. (2017). Mating, sexual selection, and the evolution of schizophrenia. *World Psychiatry*, 16, 141–142.

Del Giudice, M. (2018). *Evolutionary Psychopathology: A Unified Approach*. New York: Oxford University Press.

Del Giudice, M. (2020). Rethinking the fast–slow continuum of individual differences. *Evolution and Human Behavior*, 41, 536–549.

Dunbar, R. (2003a). Evolution of the social brain. *Science*, 302, 1160–1161.

Dunbar, R. (2003b). The social brain: mind language and society in evolutionary perspective. *Annual Review of Anthropology*, 32, 163–181.

Dunbar, R. (2014). *Human Evolution: A Pelican Introduction*. London: Pelican.

Durrant, R. and Ellis, B. (2003). Evolutionary psychology: core assumptions and methodology. In M. Gallagher and R. Nelson (eds.), *Comprehensive Handbook of Psychology. Vol. 3: Biological Psychology* (pp. 1–35). New York: John Wiley and Sons.

Ellis, B. J., Shirtcliff, E. A., Boyce, W. T., Deardorff, J. and Essex, M. J. (2011). Quality of early family relationships and the timing and tempo of puberty: effects depend on biological sensitivity to context. *Developmental Psychopathology*, 23, 85–99.

Ewald, P. W. (1994). *Evolution of Infectious Disease*. Oxford: Oxford University Press.

Fuchs, I. (2019). *The Evolutionary Mechanism of Human Dysfunctional Behavior*. New York: Radius Book Group.

Fuglewicz, A. J., Piotrowski, P. and Stodolak, A. (2017). Relationship between toxoplasmosis and schizophrenia: a review. *Advances in Clinical and Experimental Medicine*, 26, 1031–1036.

Garland, T., Jr and Kelly S. A. (2006). Phenotypic plasticity and experimental evolution. *Journal of Experimental Biology*, 209, 2344–2361.

Gilbert, P. (2020). Compassion: from its evolution to a psychotherapy. *Frontiers in Psychology*, 11, 1–31.

Gilbert, P. and Bailey, K. (2000). *Genes on the Couch: Explorations in Evolutionary Psychotherapy*. Hove: Brunner-Routledge.

Gluckman, P. D., Beedle, A. S. and Hanson, M. A. (2009). *Principles of Evolutionary Medicine*. Oxford: Oxford University Press.

Gonzalez-Forero, M. and Gardner, A. (2018). Inference of ecological and social drivers of brain size evolution. *Nature*, 557, 554–557.

Gould, S. J. (1997). Evolution: the pleasures of pluralism. *New York Review of Books*, 44, 47–52.

Hagen, E. H. (2016). Evolutionary psychology and its critics. In D. Buss (ed.), *Handbook of Evolutionary Psychology*, Vol. 1, 2nd Ed. (pp. 136–160). Hoboken, NJ: Wiley.

Hagen, E. H. (2020). Is evolutionary psychology impossible? https://thisviewoflife.com/is-evolutionary-psychology-impossible/ (accessed 30 November 2020).

Haltigan, J., Del Giudice, M. and Khorsand, S. (2021). Growing points in attachment disorganization: looking back to advance forward. *Attachment and Human Development*, 23, 438–454.

Hamilton, W. D. (1964). The genetical evolution of social behaviour. I. *Journal of Theoretical Biology*, 7, 1–16.

Henn, B. M., Cavalli-Sforza, L. L. and Feldman, M. W. (2012). The great human expansion. *Proceedings of the National Academy of Sciences of the United States of America*, 109, 17758–17764.

Henrich, J. (2016). *The Secret of Our Success: How Culture Is Driving Human Evolution, Domesticating Our Species, and Making Us Smarter*. Princeton, NJ: Princeton University Press.

Henrich, J. (2020). *The Weirdest People in the World: How the West Became Psychologically Peculiar and Peculiarly Prosperous*. London: Allen Lane.

Henrich, J. and Tennie, C. (2017). Cultural evolution in chimpanzees and humans. In M. Muller, R. Wrangham and D. Pilbeam (eds.), *Chimpanzees and Human Evolution* (pp. 645–702). Cambridge, MA: Belknap Press of Harvard University Press.

Homberg, J. R. and Lesch, K. P. (2011). Looking on the bright side of serotonin transporter gene variation. *Biological Psychiatry*, 69, 513–519.

Humphrey, N. K. (1976). The social function of intellect. In P. P. G. Bateson and R. A. Hinde (eds.), *Growing Points in Ethology* (pp. 303–317). Cambridge: Cambridge University Press.

Insel, T. R. and Cuthbert, B. N. (2015). Brain disorders? Precisely. *Science*, 348, 499–500.

Jacobs, F. (1977). Evolution as tinkering. *Science*, 169, 1161–1166.

Kay, C., Tirado-Hurtado, I., Cornejo-Olivas, M., Collins, J. A., Wright, G., Inca-Martinez, M., Veliz-Otani, D., Ketelaar, M. E., Slama, R. A., Ross, C. J., Mazzetti, P. and Hayden, M. R. (2017). The targetable A1 Huntington disease haplotype has distinct Amerindian and European origins in Latin America. *European Journal of Human Genetics*, 25, 332–340.

Kendler, K. S. (2008). Explanatory models for psychiatric illness. *American Journal of Psychiatry*, 165, 695–702.

Laland, K. (2017). *Darwin's Unfinished Symphony: How Culture Made the Human Mind*. Princeton, NJ: Princeton University Press

Laland, K. and Brown, G. (2011). *Sense and Nonsense: Evolutionary Perspectives on Human Behaviour* (2nd Ed.). Oxford: Oxford University Press.

Laland, K., Odling-Smee, J. and Endler, J. (2017). Niche construction, sources of selection and trait coevolution. *Interface Focus*, 7, 20160147.

Lents, N. H. (2020). *Human Errors: A Panorama of Our Glitches from Pointless Bones to Broken Genes*. London: Weidenfeld and Nicholson.

Li, N. P., van Vugt, M. and Colarelli, S. M. (2018). The evolutionary mismatch hypothesis: implications for psychological science. *Current Directions in Psychological Science*, 27, 38–44.

Mayr, E. (1961). Cause and effect in biology. *Science*, 134, 1501–1506.

Mayr, E. (1971). The nature of the Darwinian revolution. *Science*, 176, 981–989.

Mayr, E. (1974). Behavior programs and evolutionary strategies. *American Scientist*, 62, 650–659.

McGuire, M. T. and Troisi, A. (1998). *Darwinian Psychiatry*. New York: Oxford University Press.

Nesse, R. M. (2005). Maladaptation and natural selection. *Quarterly Review of Biology*, 80, 62–70.

Nesse, R. M. (2011). Ten questions for evolutionary studies of disease vulnerability. *Evolutionary Applications*, 4, 264–277.

Nesse, R. M. (2013) Tinbergen's four questions organized: a response to Bateson and Laland. *Trends in Ecology & Evolution*, 28, 681–682.

Nesse, R. M. (2016). Evolutionary psychology and mental health. In D. Buss (ed.), *Handbook of Evolutionary Psychology*, Vol. 2, 2nd Ed. (pp. 1007–1026). Hoboken, NJ: Wiley.

Nesse, R. M. (2019). *Good Reasons for Bad Feelings: Insights from the Frontiers of Evolutionary Psychiatry*. London: Allen Lane.

Nesse, R. M. and Dawkins, R. (2010). Evolution: medicine's most basic science. In D. A. Warrell, T. M. Cox, J. D. Firth and E. J. J. Benz (eds.), *Oxford Textbook of Medicine*, 5th Ed. (pp. 12–15). Oxford: Oxford University Press.

Nesse, R. M. and Stein, D. (2019). How evolutionary psychiatry can advance psychopharmacology. *Dialogues in Clinical Neuroscience*, 21, 167–175.

Nesse, R. M. and Williams, G. (1994). *Why We Get Sick: The New Science of Darwinian Medicine*. New York: Times Books.

NIH (2020) National Human Genome Research Institute. www.genome.gov/genetics-glossary/Mutation (accessed 30 November 2020).

Pavličev, M., Romero, R. and Mitteroecker, P. (2020). Evolution of the human pelvis and obstructed labor: new explanations of an old obstetrical dilemma. *American Journal of Obstetrics and Gynecology*, 222, 3–16.

Pilbeam, D. R. and Lieberman, D. E. (2017). Reconstructing the last common ancestor of chimpanzees and humans. In M. Muller, R. Wrangham and D. Pilbeam (eds.), *Chimpanzees and Human Evolution* (pp. 22–141). Cambridge, MA: Belknap Press of Harvard University Press.

Pinker, S. (1994). *The Language Instinct: How the Mind Creates Language*. New York: Harper Collins.

Pollard, T. (2008). *Western Diseases: An Evolutionary Perspective*. Cambridge: Cambridge University Press.

Rantala, M. J., Luoto, S., Krama, T. and Krams, I. (2019). Eating disorders: an evolutionary psychoneuroimmunological approach. *Frontiers in Psychology*, 10, 2200.

Richerson, P. and Boyd, R. (2005). *Not by Genes Alone: How Culture Transformed Human Evolution*. Chicago, IL: University of Chicago Press.

Russell, G. (2000). Disorders of eating. In M. G. Gelder, J. J. Lopez-Ibor Jr and N. C. Andreasen (eds.), *New Oxford Textbook of Psychiatry*, Vol. 1 (pp. 835–855). Oxford: Oxford University Press.

Stearns, S. C. (1992). *The Evolution of Life Histories*. Oxford: Oxford University Press.

Stevens, A. and Price, J. (2000). *Evolutionary Psychiatry: A New Beginning*, 2nd Ed. London: Routledge.

Swedo, S., Leonard, H. and Kiessling, L. S. (1994). Speculations on anti-neuronal antibody-mediated neuropsychiatric disorders of childhood. *Pediatrics*, 93, 323–326.

Tanaka, K. D., Morimoto, G., Stevens, M. and Ueda, K. (2011). Rethinking visual supernormal stimuli in cuckoos: visual modeling of host and parasite signals. *Behavioral Ecology*, 22, 1012–1019.

Taylor, J. (2015). *Body by Darwin: How Evolution Shapes our Health and Transforms Medicine*. Chicago, IL: University of Chicago Press.

Tinbergen, N. (1963). On aims and methods of ethology. *Zeitschrift Für Tierpsychologie*, 20, 410–433.

Tomasello, M. (1990). Cultural transmission in tool use and communicatory signaling of chimpanzees? In S. Parker and K. Gibson (eds.), *'Language' and Intelligence in Monkeys and Apes: Comparative Developmental Perspectives* (pp. 274–311). Cambridge: Cambridge University Press.

Tooby, J. and Cosmides, L. (1990). The past explains the present: emotional adaptions and the structure of ancestral environments. *Ethology and Sociobiology*, 11, 375–424.

Tooby, J. and Cosmides, L. (1992). The psychological foundations of culture. In J. H. Barkow, L. Cosmides and J. Tooby (eds.), *The Adapted Mind: Evolutionary Psychology and the Generation of Culture* (pp. 19–136). New York: Oxford University Press.

Trevathan, W. R., Smith, E. O. and McKenna, J. J. (2008). *Evolutionary Medicine and Health: New Perspectives*. New York: Oxford University Press.

Trivers, R. L. (1972). Parental investment and sexual selection. In B. Campbell (ed.), *Sexual Selection and the Descent of Man, 1871–1971* (pp. 136–179). Chicago, IL: Aldine.

Trivers, R. L. (1974). Parent–offspring conflict. *American Zoologist*, 14, 249–264.

Troisi, A. (2015). The evolutionary diagnosis of mental disorder. *WIREs Cognitive Science*, 6, 323–331.

Trull, T. J. and Widiger, T. A. (2013). Dimensional models of personality: the five-factor model and the DSM-5. *Dialogues in Clinical Neuroscience*, 15, 135–146.

Waddington, C. H. (1942). Canalization of development and the inheritance of acquired characters. *Nature*, 150, 563–565.

Williams, G. C. and Nesse, R. M. (1991). The dawn of Darwinian medicine. *Quarterly Review of Biology*, 66, 1–22.

Wilson, D. S. (2019). *This View of Life: Completing the Darwinian Revolution*. New York: Pantheon Books.

Wrangham, R. (2009). *Catching Fire: How Cooking Made Us Human*. London: Profile Books.

Young, E. S., Frankenhuis, W. E. and Ellis, B. J. (2020). Theory and measurement of environmental unpredictability. *Evolution and Human Behavior*, 41, 550–556.

Zietsch, B. P. and Sidari, M. J. (2020). A critique of life history approaches to human trait covariation. *Evolution and Human Behavior*, 41, 527–535.

Chapter

The Biopsychosocial Model Advanced by Evolutionary Theory

Adam Hunt, Paul St John-Smith and Riadh Abed

Abstract

The currently dominant model of health and disease in psychiatry and medicine is Engel's biopsychosocial (BPS) model, proposed in the 1970s to advance reductionistic biomedicine by integrating psychological and social factors. Although the BPS model represented progress, its scientific and philosophical foundations remain questionable and it cannot be considered complete or sufficient. In this chapter, we provide a historical and conceptual analysis of the BPS model before showing that the integration of evolutionary theory can provide a suitable next step from the BPS model, much as the BPS model was a step forward from the biomedical approach. Evolutionary theory justifies and enhances the BPS model's recognition of multiple levels of causation and expands it by recognising both ultimate and proximate causation. It allows a clearer distinction of biological function from dysfunction and encourages a phylogenetic perspective on biology, which can guide research in new directions. In connecting the model of health with the most fundamental theory of biology, this approach provides the philosophical and scientific coherence that the BPS model sorely lacked.

Keywords

biopsychosocial model, evolutionary causation, evolutionary theory, harmful dysfunction

Key Points

- The biopsychosocial model was an advance on the dominant, reductionist, biomedical model.
- The evolutionary perspective exposes the limitations of the reductionist biomedical approach.
- Evolutionary theory extends the biopsychosocial model by integrating analysis of function and phylogeny.
- Evolutionary theory provides a superior scientific basis for understanding biological function and dysfunction.

2.1 The Modern Medical Model

2.1.1 Introduction of the Biomedical

In Britain, the term 'biomedicine' first appeared in Dorland's 1923 medical dictionary (Quirke and Gaudillière, 2008), meaning 'clinical medicine based on the principles of physiology and biochemistry'. Twentieth-century medicine became progressively associated with laboratory science, leading health research towards more stringent experimental methods (Bynum et al., 2006) and 'evidence-based medicine'. Contemporary regulatory authorities require scientific justification of therapies referring to biochemical or other pathophysiological pathways and pharmacological mechanisms for approval (Van Norman, 2016). Medicine in general has thereby become a practice associated with biological alteration and intervention, after centuries of being associated with conjurations including humours and spiritual maladies, which spawned treatments with considerable potential for harm (Wootton, 2006).

This repositioning towards defining disease in terms of dysfunctional biological (henceforth 'somatic') processes came later to mainstream psychiatry than medicine. Having been dominated by psychoanalysis for the first half of the twentieth century (Shorter, 1997), psychiatry moved towards a biomedical approach with the publication of *The Diagnostic and Statistical*

Manual of Mental Disorders, Third Edition (DSM-III) in 1980. This shift took place under the direction of Robert Spitzer, who aimed at emulating the model that had proven so successful in the rest of medicine (Surís et al., 2016). Advocates of this biomedical approach are sometimes known as 'biological psychiatrists'.

The reductionist biomedical approaches entering psychiatry in the 1970s elicited powerful opposition from 'antipsychiatry' (Pilgrim, 2002), most famously articulated by Thomas Szasz. Szasz argued that 'mental illness' was purely a metaphor for human problems in living – whilst people behave and think in socially disturbing ways, what we call mental illnesses are not 'illnesses' in the sense of physical illnesses, except for a few identifiable brain diseases (e.g. Alzheimer's disease, Huntington's disease). Szasz noted that there are 'neither biological or chemical tests nor biopsy or necropsy findings for establishing a diagnosis' (Szasz, 2008: 2–5).

One method of deflecting such criticism has been the proclamation that research into neuroscience and genetics would soon adequately explain psychiatric disorders by reliably demonstrating the disease process. This has remained a common position for almost 50 years (Linden, 2012), but confidence in the notion that such simplistic reductionist biomedical explanations await discovery is dwindling, particularly when we consider complex interacting networks of factors that defy reductionist analysis (Borsboom et al., 2019). Within healthcare, the most widely acknowledged and adopted advance from the reductionist biomedical model remains George Engel's 'biopsychosocial' (BPS) model (Engel, 1977, 1980), described as 'the status quo of contemporary psychiatry' (Ghaemi, 2009).

2.1.2 Origins and Basis of Engel's BPS Model

Engel based the BPS model on the theoretical model of systems theory (von Bertalanffy, 1968; Weiss, 1969), identifying a hierarchy of physical systems at different levels of interacting organisation: subatomic particles; atoms; molecules; organelles; cells; tissues; organs/organ systems; the nervous system; the person; two persons; the family; the community; culture–subculture; society–nation; biosphere. Each level in the hierarchy was taken to represent an organised dynamic whole. The biomedical model,

in its extreme, makes a physician merely a seeker of biomarkers and fixer of broken physiological states (e.g. Andreasen, 1984). Engel argued that this could only be true of levels below that of the 'person', being ignorant of the relationships, families, communities and cultures that human beings are situated within, which have downward effects on the hierarchies below them and so are key concerns in healthcare. To take depression as an example (which will be returned to throughout this chapter), Engel's gripe would be with perspectives that treat depression as solely a brain disorder involving, for example, some unusual fluctuation in serotonin uptake – he would claim that this ignores the many instances of depression caused by factors easily observed at the psychosocial level (see Chapter 8).

Engel's original two papers, arguably inspired by the political purposes of uniting psychoanalysts with the new breed of biomedical researchers (Shorter, 2005), emphasised the importance of observing and potentially intervening at the psychosocial level as well as the somatic level. Unlike recent updates to the BPS model (e.g. Bolton and Gillett, 2019), this original formulation was unconcerned with precisely defining and delineating the 'bio' from the 'psycho' and the 'social'. Engel avoided philosophical arguments beyond a stance against reductionism and biomedical dogmatism – his simple point was that proper care and a fuller understanding of ill health requires recognising a patient's psychological state and social situation. Even perfect understanding of the neurological changes associated with depression could miss basic information about the causes of those changes, such as whether the person had recently lost their job or been divorced. Engel also emphasised that even if biomedical approaches could succeed in altering certain conditions, a patient should be considered an agent with their own mental states and social situations that bear relevance to their health. This is uncontroversial, even amongst critics of the BPS model (Borell-Carrió et al., 2004), and is today reflected (even if unsystematically) in much of current treatment and research. Psychological processes and placebo responses are accepted as common relevant factors in medical interventions, and furthermore the health consequences of social circumstances are widely recognised (Braveman and Gottlieb, 2014).

In fact, the present-day exploration of the relationship between social circumstances and health has notably broadened, with extensive separate investigations from public health scholars (Smith, 2000), epidemiologists (Syme, 1987), anthropologists (Hoke and McDade, 2014), social scientists (Conrad and Kern, 1981) and others. This research is spread across various sub-disciplines, commonly introducing alternative terminology such as 'social determinants of health' (Braveman and Gottlieb, 2014), 'political economy of health' (Doyal, 1979), 'social epidemiology' (Krieger, 2001), 'ecosocial' (Krieger, 1994), 'biosocial' (Hoke and McDade, 2014) and 'biocultural' (McElroy, 1990), often with no mention of the term 'biopsychosocial' in title or text, despite its direct relevance. This research, like Engel's, is cited in international and national public health agendas (Kelly et al., 2009; Marmot, 2005), noting the multiple social factors that affect physical and mental health, such as stress, early-life adversity, social exclusion, work, unemployment, social support, addictions, nutrition and diet, transport (Marmot and Wilkinson, 1999), social status (Marmot, 2006), racism (Harrell et al., 2011), debt (Sweet et al., 2013), and neighbourhood (Ludwig et al., 2011, 2012). Even though this body of research notably exceeds the number of published articles using the expression 'biopsychosocial' (Álvarez et al., 2012), 'biopsychosocial' remains the term of choice used to describe the general concept of multidimensional healthcare by various large institutions (Alonso, 2004), in medical schools and in psychiatry (Adler, 2009; Mai, 1995; Pilgrim, 2002).

2.1.3 Criticisms of and Updates to the BPS Model

Most authors, including critics (Sadler and Hulgus, 1990; Suls and Rothman, 2004), concur with Engel that solely biomedical healthcare tends towards excessive reductionism. However, two main categories of criticism have been raised against the BPS model (Bolton and Gillett, 2019). The first is that it lacks philosophical clarity or scientific validity. The second is that it is too vague and therefore clinically unworkable.

Firstly, the philosophical and scientific merits of the BPS model have been interrogated by various authors (e.g. Benning, 2015). It has been criticised for not meeting the criteria of a scientific theory or model (McLaren, 1998) and called an attempt to preserve psychoanalysis 'through the back door' (Shorter, 2005). Furthermore, the

'social' dimension seemingly leaves out important environmental elements of public health concerns (Kelly et al., 2009), such as pollution, radiation, noxious substances, infection, noise and diet. This has led recent proponents to make environmental factors an addendum (Bolton and Gillett, 2019) in an attempt to make the model more complete. Arguably, and importantly, philosophical validity was not Engel's primary concern (Álvarez et al., 2012). His concern was that biomedicine undervalued certain factors, and he proposed the BPS model as a timely criticism of medical practise, not a theoretical model of health issues in its own right.

The second area of criticism, regarding the BPS model's vagueness and clinical impracticality, derives from observations that the BPS model is neither prescriptive nor precise (Sadler and Hulgus, 1992). Beyond recognising that interacting levels cause sickness, Engel provides no clear guidance for the clinician as to diagnostic and treatment approaches for a given patient (although recent authors have attempted to formalise and exemplify this process; e.g. Evers et al., 2014; Smith et al., 2013). Ghaemi (2009, 2010), a prominent critic of the BPS model, notes that it can devolve into essentially arbitrary treatment methods, with individual clinicians justified in concentrating on the 'bio', 'psycho' or 'social' however they see fit. This vagueness also contributes to difficulty in developing research agendas (Pilgrim, 2002). Although the term 'biopsychosocial' is now widely given lip service, biomedical research agendas remain dominant; little has changed since Engel's publications (Alonso, 2004; Suls and Rothman, 2004), causing researchers within and outside of psychiatry to voice their concerns and to label psychiatry as a discipline in crisis (Bracken et al., 2012; Deacon, 2013).

Bolton and Gillett (2019) recently attempted to update the BPS model and to address these criticisms, giving philosophical arguments seeking to justify the distinctions between and definitions of the 'bio', 'psycho' and 'social'. We agree with Frazier (2020) that this is a 'somewhat narrow philosophical evaluation' that fails to truly advance the BPS model and is subject to many new criticisms. For example, Bolton and Gillett (2019) introduce a singular concept of 'agency' in defining the psychological domain of the BPS model, but this seems disconnected from the full scope of important psychological processes, including inner conflict, subconscious processes and so forth. In our eyes, Bolton and Gillett's attempt presents *post hoc* arguments attempting to patch up the gaps in a model intended as a practical action plan rather than a stringent scientific theory. They complicate the BPS model but fail to justify it as a rigorous and comprehensive model of health. We venture here that to move towards a model of health and disease that is not only clinically useful but also theoretically coherent and scientifically informative, such philosophical arguments are fatally lacking in a key scientific insight that has transformed all biological sciences – namely Darwin's theory of evolution by natural selection (Darwin, 1859).

2.2 Going Beyond the BPS Model

2.2.1 From Biomedical to BPS to Evolutionary

As explored in Chapter 1, Charles Darwin's *On the Origin of Species* introduced the theory of evolution by natural selection, causing a paradigm shift in the biological sciences. In biology, evolutionary theory is essentially an inescapable law of nature, applying to all forms of life regardless of time and place. Causation in biology then involves multiple levels (Mayr, 1961), with complex systems including interacting amino acids, proteins, RNA, DNA, cells, microstructures, organelles, organs and organisms (see Chapter 1). Engel's BPS model incorporated these interacting levels within system theory and on that basis justified the BPS model's superiority over the purely biomedical approach, while acknowledging that this complex causation excludes the possibility that biomedical reductionism is fully informative. Recent network models (Barabási and Oltvai, 2004; Borsboom et al, 2019) are more contemporary versions of this view of causation within the context of interacting multilevel complexity.

Engel's purpose in proposing the BPS model was to draw attention to levels of causation and intervention beyond the biomedical, but his dimension of concern was of microscopic to macroscopic effects, cellular to society wide, a recognition of multiple levels of spatial analysis. However, causation in biology is also necessarily understood temporally, as the product of a historical process: from mechanism to individual development, to the history of evolutionary function, in multiple species diverging over millions of years. These have been recognised by evolutionary scientists in Tinbergen's four questions (Tinbergen, 1963; see Chapter 1 of this volume for more details), which were further iterations of Mayr's distinction between proximate and ultimate causation (Mayr, 1961).

In Table 2.1 we provide a tabulation inspired by Medicus (2005), creating cells from Tinbergen's four questions and Engel's three levels for an evolutionary–biopsychosocial picture of depression. It depicts how the BPS advanced the biomedical (extending proximate questions of mechanism and development to the psychological and social levels) and how the evolutionary advances the BPS (extending ultimate questions of function and phylogeny for all levels of analysis).

In the biomedical framework, the top-left 'somatic–proximate' causes are the primary concern. Engel's BPS model advanced the paradigm by extending this proximate column down to include the 'psychological–proximate' and 'social–proximate'. These include the areas of psychological and social analysis and their consequent applications, which is where the BPS model encouraged a more holistic role for practitioners, opening the door to public health research and interventions on the social level.

Evolutionary medicine and psychiatry extend all three levels to include the 'ultimate' analysis of function and phylogeny, with relevance to research and treatment at each level. Note that the ultimate analysis of the somatic level is already of practical utility in medical research – researchers recognise that key molecules are present throughout the body and that our biology is comparable to other species. This opens the door to understanding the side effects of interventions and to experimentation using animal models. However, this practise has developed without appreciating that evolution by natural selection explains *why* side effects are the norm rather than the exception (evolution co-opts existing molecules and systems for new functions) and that animal models are useful (biological systems are shared across phylogenies, so experimentation on non-human animals allows us to predict outcomes in humans). More explicit recognition of this explanatory theory may lead to better prediction and mitigation of side effects and superior use of animal models.

Table 2.1. Mapping depression with Engel's BPS levels and Mayr and Tinbergen's evolutionary questions

| | Evolutionary questions | | | |
| | Proximate | | Ultimate | |
BPS levels	Mechanism	Development	Function	Phylogeny
Somatic				
Area of research	Relevant brain circuits; receptors and genes; neurotransmitter system properties (e.g. serotoninergic system)	Neurotransmitter system development and genetic developmental plasticity (e.g. DNA methylation modifications)	Function of key molecules or hormones throughout the body (e.g. serotonin in the gut, heart and reproductive system)	Shared neurotransmitter pathways and molecular mechanisms with other species (e.g. serotoninergic system in mammals)
Application	Identify targets for drugs; possible discovery of biomarkers	Identify individuals at risk for developing condition; intervene in pathways before health problems present	Predict side effects of drugs and possible extraneous harms of treatment	Identify homologous systems in animal models for drug testing
Psychological				
Area of research	Psychological processes experienced as debilitating (e.g. anhedonia, rumination, pessimism)	Development and history of the individual's problem (e.g. learned helplessness, attachment problems)	Dysfunctioning adaptive process or harmful functions (e.g. low mood system over-activated; functional disengaging)	Psychological and behavioural correlates in other species (e.g. low mood and subdual in primates)
Application	Identify harmful thoughts, moods and behaviours as therapeutic targets	Pre-empt onset and intervene in harmful circumstances or psychological processes	Normalise and destigmatise; inform therapy (e.g. encourage improving social standing)	Inform therapy by observing natural triggers and alleviators of related mood states in other species
Social				
Area of research	Social triggers of the phenomenon; social perception and reaction to the phenomenon (e.g. bereavement, divorce, job loss)	Debilitating social environments and relationships (e.g. chronic stress, low social support)	Ancestral social environments shaped functional psychological traits (e.g. hierarchy recognition and reaction, conflict reduction)	Social situations that trigger analogous states in other species (e.g. hierarchy status in primates)
Application	Identify scenarios suitable for short-term social intervention, find depressed individuals	Identify areas for social reform, pre-empt at-risk individuals and groups	Inform public health measures and social reform interventions with better understanding of natural human social environment	Identify optimal and suboptimal social conditions in related species, directing effective social prevention and intervention

Research at the psychological and social levels of relevance to health has been largely bereft of the potential benefits of an evolutionary analysis. This is perhaps partly a result of the philosophical, psychological and sociological perspectives that dominate theorising at these levels being largely disconnected from evolutionary theory and comparative cross-species research. Evolutionary psychology, evolutionary anthropology and primatology have in turn been largely non-medical and have concentrated on apparent function rather than dysfunction. Therefore, this remains a largely untapped field of research.

2.2.2 Ultimate Understanding of the Psychosocial

Chapter 1 provided an overview of the cultural evolution of humanity and the social brain, a topic of relevance in considering how an evolutionary approach enhances the psychological and social analysis of depression.

The study of hunter-gatherers suggests that our ancestors lived in fairly egalitarian small-scale societies. Despite the egalitarian nature of most hunter-gatherers, social hierarchies and a degree of inequality existed (Boehm, 2012; Chagnon, 2013), and these affected reproductive success (Alami et al., 2020; von Rueden and Jaeggi, 2016). These selection pressures plausibly encouraged psychological adaptations related to in-group social hierarchies, such as causing low mood after status decline to reduce the risk of futile and/or dangerous contests (Price et al., 1994; also see Chapter 8 of this volume). Mismatch could cause this natural propensity for low mood to develop into clinical depression in modern societies – modern social mobility is constrained, and a loss of status may be due to unalterable modern variables, such as the loss of certain professions during a severe economic recession or technological shift. In hunter-gatherer societies such systemic problems did not exist – the individual could react to low mood to improve their situation such as by moving to another band, performing some admirable feat or forming a new alliance. As such, the low mood could be productive and self-limiting rather than persistently deepening and even paralysing, as is seen in clinical depression. In the ancestral environment, the availability of multiple sources of social support could

ameliorate the duration and intensity of low mood and hence reduce the possibility of progressing into pathological states of depression (Rantala, 2018).

Of course, evolutionary approaches to understanding health problems encourage not just consideration of natural human habitats and humanity's evolutionary history, but also phylogenetic comparison with other species. The tendency for depressed mood in the wake of social defeat may have been functional in ancestral contexts of close bands of co-living primates in conflict over mates and resources, serving a protective purpose by encouraging disengagement from further conflict (Gilbert and Allan, 1998; Sloman et al., 2003). Work on primates has shown that levels of circulating glucocorticoids (markers of stress) increase progressively with decline in social rank. However, this occurs only if the subordinate individual is subjected to aggression from dominants and has no supportive social connections or relatives present nearby (Abbott et al., 2003). Stress and depressive behaviours can be observed in non-human primates, with implications for understanding their causes and possible mitigating factors (Shively and Willard, 2012). Such phylogenetic work could point towards potentially toxic and beneficial social arrangements for humans.

Although the BPS model improved upon the biomedical model by leading researchers to recognise, for example, that strong social networks can mitigate certain health problems, its shallowness of explanation can lead to uninformed and fruitless responses. For example, if depression often follows the loss of a job, a reasonable assumption from a modern perspective might be that the depression is caused by the financial loss – the implication being that improving the individual's financial situation (e.g. with unemployment benefits) should help their depression. It may also be assumed that the depressed and unemployed will respond to normal interventions for depression, such as cognitive behavioural therapy. But if the depression is related primarily to the loss of status and social network (which an evolutionary perspective recognises as more psychologically relevant than finances), then we would expect financial improvement or therapy alone to have little effect on the depression – it needs to be accompanied by a lifestyle change recouping the lost status and social connections, probably by finding another job. This indeed seems to be the case (Moore et al., 2017).

Beyond specific examples, evolutionary theory can be used to understand general mechanisms relating psychosocial factors to health outcomes. For example, developmental plasticity (see Chapter 1) has been shaped by selection and could help to account for disparate factors affecting health that are still not well understood in terms of pathogenesis, including social status, self-esteem, identity, divorce, bereavement, job loss, arrest or retirement (Cohen et al., 2019). Ultimate evolutionary questions must be applied to understand the fundamental mechanisms that lead to these negative health consequences (Troisi, 2020). If humans are developmentally plastic (Lea et al., 2017) or have differential levels of susceptibility (Albott et al., 2018), this adaptive process could malfunction. For plasticity to evolve, it needed to provide reproductive success on average ancestrally, but it need not have been infallible. Disorders might arise as occasional, unfortunate by-products, such as when a stressor passes a threshold of longevity or severity. Plasticity (especially neurological plasticity) might inevitably be error-prone – and this error-proneness could be magnified in modern mismatched environments. Note that this analysis complements research on the proximate neurobiological systems behind plasticity and disorder. The evolutionary perspective then explains *why* those systems and their vulnerabilities exist and speaks to the extensive behavioural genetics research linking quantitative genetics to environmental exposure (Assary et al., 2018). Where the BPS model expanded public health considerations to include proximate psychosocial factors, evolutionary medicine and psychiatry deepen our understanding of these systems.

2.2.3 The Placebo Effect and Defences

The study of the placebo effect is the study of the psychosocial context specific to a particular trial situation that includes the expectation of clinical improvement and conditioning and that results in positive health outcomes (Colloca and Benedetti, 2005; Finniss and Benedetti, 2005). The placebo effect is stark proof of the porousness of the boundaries between somatic, environmental, psychological and social: environmental and psychosocial events induce biochemical changes in a patient's brain and body that in turn affect disease course and therapeutic outcome (Benedetti, 2008). In the placebo effect, interpersonal relationships and the social environment become essential components in explaining how healing and caring work (McQueen et al., 2013).

Placebo responses permit mammals to modify internal processes and behaviours, and multiple adaptive advantages could accrue from these abilities to modify our internal environment in the light of accurate positive evaluations of our external environments, social interactions and appraisals of future environments (McQueen et al., 2013). Nesse (2019) stresses that placebo responses primarily entail modification of the body's defences rather than altering disease processes (see Box 2.1). Evolution has selected for biological mechanisms that defend against injury, infection or poisoning, and the regulation of these defences is influenced by appraisals of the environment. However, many defences appear to be over-expressed, which is understandable within the framework of 'signal detection analysis'. When an organism can react in a protective way for little cost but potentially huge benefit (e.g. avoiding death), the optimal system expresses many false alarms. Vomiting may cost only a few hundred calories and a few minutes, whereas not vomiting risks death from poisoning. This has been dubbed the 'smoke detector principle' (Nesse, 2001; see Chapter 7 of this volume). The regulation of defences also allows otherwise 'protective' defences to be turned off in situations of extreme danger to facilitate escape and in situations propitious for recovery where they are no longer necessary. Understanding this complex and ubiquitous element of human healthcare from an evolutionary perspective provides a useful insight missing from modern medical discourse.

> **Box 2.1 Examples of the body's defences**
> - *Somatosensory:* pain, lethargy, nausea, anxiety, depression, fever, itching
> - *Skeletal/motor responses:* flight, freezing
> - *Visceral:* sneezing, coughing, vomiting, diarrhoea
> - *Humoral responses:* immune modulation, regulation of the hypothalamic–pituitary–adrenal axis

2.3 Justifying Non-reductionism

A concern of modern psychiatrists is that Engel's proposed BPS model has not had enough of an effect on psychiatric research or practise (Deacon, 2013). To some extent, this has been an inevitable consequence of its philosophical and scientific flaws – its influence has been limited by its theoretical shortcomings. Here we consider how evolutionary medicine can both justify and extend a core tenet of the BPS model – the interacting levels of the somatic, psychological and social – in a way that is more theoretically satisfying.

2.3.1 Bidirectional Causation

Evolutionary theory recognises bidirectional causation between the somatic, psychological and social levels: the psychological and social alter the somatic over generations via selection pressures whilst being constantly mediated by somatic processes (neurobiological, genetic and so forth). For example, the serotonergic system is created by genes that affect mood and psychological and social interactions, and whether those psychological and social effects are fitness enhancing affects the evolution of the serotonergic system. The somatic system thus exists for good evolutionary reasons related to its psychological and social effects (Andrews et al., 2015). Taking an evolutionary perspective in medicine is tantamount to turning genetics on its head: while a non-evolutionary biomedical view of depression may consider specific DNA sequences as the primary biological causes of the condition, an evolutionary approach also seeks to understand the selection pressures over evolutionary history that led to the persistence of these genes throughout the generations (e.g. Raison and Miller, 2013).

2.3.2 Multiple Realisability

One of the major strengths of the evolutionary approach is that it enables the identification of the end products of selection through identifying traits that contributed to an organism's inclusive fitness (in its natural environment). The insight that the selected phenotype may be multiply realised at lower levels of organisation further justifies non-reductive analysis (Borsboom et al., 2019; Krakauer et al., 2017). Examples of multiple realisability abound. One such group of examples are phenotypes that have evolved to prevent or mitigate malaria infection, which are achieved through multiple molecular arrangements of haemoglobin with distinct genetic inheritance (Weatherall and Clegg, 2001). Pure reductionism would mistake these as different phenomena – an evolutionary analysis of the individual-level traits in malaria-rich environments is required to recognise their shared ultimate cause. Critical functions can go unrecognised unless the phenomenon is explored through an evolutionary lens and within its full social/environmental context. Hence, the recognition that agriculture encourages mosquitos and thus malaria (Janko et al., 2018) is also required to fully understand malaria's global mortality rates, not just a reductionist analysis of *Plasmodium* parasites.

Other salient examples exist of multiple somatic realisations for the same adaptive functions. Lactase persistence, allowing the lactase enzyme to persist into adulthood, evolved repeatedly and independently in several populations and via different mechanisms within those populations (Campbell and Ranciaro, 2021). Pale skin evolved independently in the low-UV-ray regions of north-east Asian and north-west European populations with distinct genetic causations (Hider et al., 2013; Norton et al., 2007). The adaptation to live in low-oxygen conditions at high altitudes evolved through different pathways in Andean (Bolivia and Chile), Tibetan and Ethiopian highlanders (Beall, 2007; Bigham et al., 2010; Scheinfeldt et al., 2012; Xu et al., 2011). Note that although all of these examples are functional adaptations, they can also lead to health problems: haemoglobin-related diseases such as sickle cell disease; lactose intolerance; folate and vitamin D deficiency; and polycythaemia. These examples demonstrate the limitations of reductionist explanations, justifying the necessity of viewing health problems at a simultaneously somatic, psychological and social level and highlighting that such health problems are also better understood when viewed through the lens of evolutionary theory.

2.3.3 Multilevel Mismatch

As discussed in Chapter 1, our genes, bodies and brains primarily evolved within hunter-gatherer life, but today they are born into the novel conditions of modern societies, and this 'mismatch' can

Table 2.2. Examples of mismatch and consequences across BPS domains

Area of concern	Conditions humans are adapted to	Conditions humans are not adapted to	Consequences of mismatch
Somatic – immune system	High infectious burden with active immune system (Rubio-Ruiz et al., 2015)	Low-grade chronic inflammation, ubiquitous in modern environments (Rubio-Ruiz et al., 2015)	Increased risk of metabolic syndrome, type 2 diabetes, autoimmune diseases and depression (Bullmore, 2019)
Psychological – stress and depression	Low levels of chronic stress and chronic depression (Rantala et al., 2018)	High levels of chronic stress and chronic depression (Brenner et al., 2015)	Increased risk of hypertension 5–16 years later (Brown et al., 2004), increased risk of diabetes and cancer (McGee et al., 1994; Pollard, 2008)
Social – community	High levels of social integration and support from kin and in-group (Hamilton et al., 2007)	Involuntary social isolation and loneliness prevalent in modern settings (Heinrich and Gullone, 2006)	Increased risk of coronary heart disease, stroke and increased mortality (Elovainio et al., 2017; Valtorta et al., 2016)

have negative health consequences. Table 2.2 lists examples where novel living conditions (either absent or rare during human evolutionary history) have cross-domain effects: social or psychological factors can cause somatic disorders and vice versa. Recognising this mismatch allows a depth of explanation beyond the scope of either biomedicine or the BPS model for a variety of adverse health outcomes whilst justifying the necessity of non-reductive analysis.

2.4 Problems with Current Disorder Categories

Oversimplification is a problem throughout the current psychiatric paradigm. The Diagnostic and Statistical Manual of Mental Disorders (DSM) is a descriptivist system of creating, validating, studying and employing a diagnostic system in clinical psychiatric practice. Although attempting to be atheoretical, it carries a crucial presupposition on the nature of mental disorder: it dictates that the psychiatric disorders it distinguishes and labels are distinct syndromes. In formulating these syndromes as clusters of regularly co-occurring symptoms, it was hoped that homogeneous groups of patients with unifying pathological processes would be studied; specific psychotherapies and pharmacotherapies could then be developed. However, psychiatric illness does not follow simple categorical – or syndromal – constructs (Zachar and Kendler, 2017). Symptoms are shared between multiple disorders,

appear in subclinical forms in the healthy population and vary in character and severity, both within individuals over time and between individuals given the same diagnosis. The brain does not function or dysfunction within the distinct categories of the DSM system (Schwartz, 2013), yet the DSM encourages psychiatrists to treat based upon a patient's categorical diagnosis, as in general medicine. This approach makes sense in homogeneous populations, as would be the case if each schizophrenic or each depressive was identical in symptoms, psychology, social connectedness and underlying biological brain functioning. Psychiatric conditions are not homogeneous in this way.

Engel's BPS model encouraged more individualised treatment than the biomedical approach because at psychosocial levels individual differences are obvious. Somatic differences between individuals within the same disorder categories undoubtedly exist but are not identifiable within a normal psychiatric assessment. The evolutionary advance on the BPS model has practical implications here by justifying the recognition of the inherent complexity, interaction and context dependency of evolved systems across all of the BPS levels. Mental disorders are not simple diseases, as would suit a DSM-type descriptivist categorisation. In the future, an evolutionarily informed psychiatrist should be able to utilise genotypic, endophenotypic and psychosocial findings to tailor initial psychopharmacological regimens and management to more directly target appropriate neuropathways, normalise endophenotypes, suggest lifestyle changes and facilitate symptom resolution. A 'circuits driving symptoms' theoretical approach may actually mimic brain function more than the DSM-validated syndromal diagnostic approach.

2.5 Function, Dysfunction and the Concept of Harmful Dysfunction

Finally, we note a unique theoretical strength of evolutionary medicine and psychiatry that justifies their suitability as the guiding paradigms of healthcare. The concepts of disease and disorder are inextricably linked with assumed biological dysfunction. The BPS model of health is, in this sense, a model through which to identify and treat biological dysfunction either by restoring function or by alleviating symptoms of dysfunction. An evolutionary perspective can advance the BPS model by grounding concepts of function and dysfunction in evolutionary theory.

In common parlance, the terms 'functional' and 'dysfunctional' are loosely defined. 'Functional' broadly refers to normal, working or good states, whilst 'dysfunctional' refers to abnormal, disrupted or bad states. These are defined by norms rather than truly objective standards. This looseness of definition is also present in medicine and psychiatry (Boyd, 2000). The terms 'illness', 'disease', 'ill health', 'condition', 'disorder', 'dysfunction', 'pathology' and 'sickness' are used essentially interchangeably for biological states we deem as bad and of medical relevance without clear definitions or distinctions between them (although undoubtedly carrying different connotations; see Box 2.2). However, biological function can be defined evolutionarily, lending greater clarity to medical terminology.

Unlike the objects and processes of physics and chemistry, which cannot strictly be said to be either functioning or dysfunctioning (Bolton and Gillett, 2019), biological systems are the products of evolution by natural selection, and so their 'function' and 'dysfunction' can be related to that evolutionary process. The concept of evolutionary function is tied to the reproductive success brought about by the phenotypes that caused genes to be propagated. Eyes evolved to see – the function of the eyes is to see – so dysfunctional eyes are those that cannot see. This sense of function is defined by the evolutionary history of

> **Box 2.2 Connotations of current terminology in medicine and psychiatry**
>
> *Disease:* an objective biological abnormality, dysfunction or condition of the organism, in medicine understood somatically and pathophysiologically.
> *Disorder:* a normative dysfunction, in psychiatry understood to be characterised by combinations of psychosocial problems with abnormal thoughts, emotions, behaviour and relationships with others.
> *Illness:* a subjective experience, particularly distress, which includes symptomatic manifestations of disease and disorder to be understood phenomenologically.
> *Condition:* a particular state of being; when used as a noun in medicine, this is understood as a negative situation or predicament that can include diseases, diagnoses, disabilities, illnesses and so on.
> *Disability:* an enduring physical or mental condition that restricts a person in their ability to function.
> *Health:* an organism's overall state of well-being, understood as suitable functioning in their current environment without normative dysfunction, unhelpful subjective distress or somatic indisposition, permitting optimal performance.

eyesight providing reproductive success, not current cultural opinions of normality and abnormality on which common conceptions of health and disorder often depend (Fabrega and Brüne, 2017). The important fact is the evolutionary history, not the modern assessment. This makes evolutionary theory uniquely ideal for objectively defining dysfunction and, by extension, medical terminology.

Jerome Wakefield's influential 'harmful dysfunction' model of disease and disorder (Wakefield, 1992, 1997, 2015) utilises this evolutionary framing, defining genuine disorder as a hybrid concept with two components. The first component is the existence of dysfunction, based on the biological criterion of failure of a system to perform its evolved function. The second, non-biological criterion is that the dysfunction causes harm to the individual as judged by prevailing sociocultural standards. Hence forms of depression that served no adaptive purpose to our ancestors and reduced reproductive success are true disorders, but depressive states (more akin to normal low mood), which served an adaptive purpose (say, of preventing dangerous antagonistic behaviour after social defeat; Gilbert and Allan, 1998), would be considered harmful in the modern environment but are not dysfunctional, thus not classifying as a true disorder.

Despite the theoretical coherence of the harmful dysfunction model and its reliance on explicitly biological rather than cultural antecedents, it suffers from its own practical difficulties. The most important scientific difficulty is that the function of the majority of neurobiological systems involved in mental disorder remain poorly understood, and the fact that our evolutionary history is obscured by the past makes scientific assessment of cognitive function difficult. The second is a more practical difficulty related to the appropriate application of medical treatment. Distress, debilitation and psychic pain can arise both as features of functional systems or from functional systems producing maladaptive outcomes in unfamiliar mismatched environments (Del Giudice, 2018; Nesse, 2019). Medical and psychiatric intervention is justifiably offered in a range of situations involving distress without genuine biological dysfunction. Such situations have been labelled 'conditions of psychiatric interest' (Fabrega and Brüne, 2017) instead of disorders. Before the terminology used by psychiatry and medicine can be sufficiently clarified with evolutionary theory, these two issues require significant theoretical work.

This concern is not merely terminological. Correctly identifying the functional status of the system could have an important bearing on the type of intervention required and the condition's prognosis. If certain forms of depression are normal responses to recent life events with recognisable adaptive evolutionary histories (e.g. following status loss; Sloman et al., 2003), then different psychosocial interventions might be advisable. It may be useful in clinical and research settings to apply terminology upon evolutionary lines (e.g. calling truly dysfunctional depression a 'disease' and functional yet harmful depression a 'disorder'). Evolutionary perspectives accounting for ultimate causes allow more meaningful subtyping of broad heterogeneous labels such as 'depression' (Rantala et al., 2018; see also Chapter 8 of this volume). Introducing this objective standard of 'dysfunction' would also distance psychiatry from the patently unscientific practices of recent history, such as labelling homosexuality as a mental disorder until cultural attitudes changed and then removing it from the DSM by vote (Drescher, 2015).

2.6 Conclusion

Commenting on the state of mental health research, Thomas Insel, the American neuroscientist and biological psychiatrist who led the National Institute of Mental Health between 2002 and 2015, said, 'Whatever we've been doing for five decades, it ain't working ... When I look at the numbers – the number of suicides, the number of disabilities, the mortality data – it's abysmal, and it's not getting any better. Maybe we just need to rethink this whole approach ... With no validated biomarkers and too little in the way of novel medical treatments since 1980 ... it is time to rethink mental disorders' (Greenberg, 2013). We believe rethinking mental disorders, and indeed setting medicine in general upon a more productive path (even paradigm), will require integrating the fundamental theory of all biology: evolutionary theory.

Whilst the BPS model was an important step encouraging medicine and psychiatry to go beyond the reductionist biomedical model, it did not go far enough. Evolutionary psychiatry provides the scientific basis for expanding the concept of the biological to encompass the psychological, social and cultural domains (Abed and St John-Smith, 2016), in contrast with mainstream biological psychiatry's narrow 'decontextualised' view of mental disorder simply as brain disorder (Andreasen, 1984). Evolutionarily informed researchers can recognise the multiple levels of relevance to any given condition and start to predict, understand and propose changes to ameliorate the effects of such factors. Grounding healthcare in evolutionary theory gives the pivotal considerations of the BPS model a solid scientific and philosophically coherent base. The evolutionary advance on the BPS model then allows for a definition of dysfunction that is not merely normative; opens up medical research to recognising novel mismatched environments in understanding the causes of disease; and directs treatment and prevention efforts in several ways, partly by encouraging the understanding and mitigation of certain aspects of the modern environment to which humans are poorly adapted.

Many more examples of potential benefits, both theoretical and practical, shall be found in the various chapters of this volume.

Engel proposed the BPS model as an action plan for practitioners; theoretical coherence was not his aim. Although his work is laudable, this blind spot is likely the reason why biomedical approaches retain disproportionate dominance. The spurious claims made from psychosocial perspectives made the BPS model less scientifically appealing, and philosophical reassessments have not helped. We contend that an evolutionary re-conceptualisation is highly scientifically appealing, embedding medicine and psychiatry in biological theory. Where the biomedical practitioner may give primacy to brain processes and little weight to a patient's unique psychological or social state, the BPS practitioner recognises psychosocial aspects, but without deep explanatory knowledge. Evolutionary theory provides that deeper understanding. One immediate consequence may be in enhancing the therapeutic relationship and in playing a part in cognitive behavioural therapy; a recent publication has provided initial guidelines for this application under the label of 'ICT' (informed cognitive therapy) (Abrams, 2020).

As Darwin wrote in the conclusion of the first edition of *On the Origin of Species*, 'In the distant future I see open fields for far more important researches' (Darwin, 1859). The evolutionary sciences hold great importance for understanding complex health problems and inspiring novel solutions, especially in relation to the ongoing research in the areas of genetics, epigenetics and developmental plasticity, as well as in the fundamental theoretical work from evolutionary medicine and evolutionary psychiatry as found in this volume. This represents a serious scientific advance to the field of medicine, which for most of its history has been concerned with practise over theory. As Frazier (2020) states, the BPS model was not exactly a Kuhnian paradigm shift so much as a move towards a more holistic view of medicine. The move towards evolutionary medicine and psychiatry, however, could much more reasonably be called a paradigm shift, explaining health problems within a superior theoretical framework and connecting the practise of medicine with the science of biology.

References

Abbott, D. H. et al. (2003) 'Are subordinates always stressed? A comparative analysis of rank differences in cortisol levels among primates', *Hormones and Behavior*, 43, pp. 67–82.

Abed, R. and St John-Smith, P. (2016) 'Evolutionary psychiatry: a new College special interest group', *BJPsych Bulletin*, 40, pp. 233–236.

Abrams, M. (2020) *The New CBT: Evolutionary Clinical Psychology*. San Diego, CA: Cognella Press.

Adler, R. H. (2009) 'Engel's biopsychosocial model is still relevant today', *Journal of Psychosomatic Research*, 67, pp. 607–611.

Alami, S. et al. (2020) 'Mother's social status is associated with child health in a horticulturalist population', *Proceedings of the Royal Society B: Biological Sciences*, 287, p. 20192783.

Albott, C. S., Forbes, M. K. and Anker, J. J. (2018) 'Association of childhood adversity with differential susceptibility of transdiagnostic psychopathology to environmental stress in adulthood', *JAMA Network Open*, 1, p. e185354.

Alonso, Y. (2004) 'The biopsychosocial model in medical research: the evolution of the health concept over the last two decades', *Patient Education and Counseling*, 53, pp. 239–244.

Álvarez, A. S., Pagani, M. and Meucci, P. (2012) 'The clinical application of the biopsychosocial model in mental health: a research critique', *American Journal of Physical Medicine and Rehabilitation*, 91, pp. S173–S180.

Andreasen, N. C. (1984) *The Broken Brain: The Biological Revolution in Psychiatry*. New York: Harper & Row. Available at: https://cmc .marmot.org/Record/.b11138543 (accessed 10 May 2019).

Andrews, P. W. et al. (2015) 'Is serotonin an upper or a downer? The evolution of the serotonergic system and its role in depression and the antidepressant response', *Neuroscience and Biobehavioral Reviews*, 51, pp. 164–188.

Assary, E. et al. (2018) 'Gene–environment interaction and psychiatric disorders: review and future directions', *Seminars in Cell and Developmental Biology*, 77, pp. 133–143.

Barabási, A. L. and Oltvai, Z. N. (2004) 'Network biology: understanding the cell's functional organization', *Nature Reviews Genetics*, 5, pp. 101–113.

Beall, C. M. (2007) 'Two routes to functional adaptation: Tibetan and Andean high-altitude natives', *Proceedings of the National Academy of Sciences of the United States of America*, 104, pp. 8655–8660.

Benedetti, F. (2008) 'Mechanisms of placebo and placebo-related effects across diseases and treatments', *Annual Review of Pharmacology and Toxicology*, 48, pp. 33–60.

Benning, T. (2015) 'Limitations of the biopsychosocial model in psychiatry', *Advances in Medical Education and Practice*, 6, p. 347.

Bigham, A. et al. (2010) 'Identifying signatures of natural selection in Tibetan and Andean populations using dense genome scan data', *PLoS Genetics*, 6, p. e1001116.

Boehm, C. (2012) 'Costs and benefits in hunter-gatherer punishment', *Behavioral and Brain Sciences*, 35, pp. 19–20.

Bolton, D. and Gillett, G. (2019) *The Biopsychosocial Model of Health and Disease: New Philosophical and Scientific Developments*. London: Palgrave Macmillian.

Borell-Carrió, F., Suchman, A. L. and Epstein, R. M. (2004) 'The biopsychosocial model 25 years later: principles, practice, and scientific inquiry', *Annals of Family Medicine*, 2, pp. 576–582.

Borsboom, D., Cramer, A. O. J. and Kalis, A. (2019) 'Brain disorders? Not really: why network structures block reductionism in psychopathology research', *Behavioral and Brain Sciences*, 42, pp. 1–54.

Boyd, K. M. (2000) 'Disease, illness, sickness, health, healing and wholeness: exploring some elusive concepts', *Medical Humanities*, 26, pp. 9–17.

Bracken, P. et al. (2012) 'Psychiatry beyond the current paradigm', *British Journal of Psychiatry*, 201, pp. 430–434.

Braveman, P. and Gottlieb, L. (2014) 'The social determinants of health: it's time to consider the causes of the causes', *Public Health Reports*, 129, pp. 19–31.

Brenner, S. L. et al. (2015) 'Evolutionary mismatch and chronic psychological stress', *Journal of Evolutionary Medicine*, 3, p. 11.

Brown, E. S., Varghese, F. P. and McEwen, B. S. (2004)

'Association of depression with medical illness: does cortisol play a role?', *Biological Psychiatry*, 55, pp. 1–9.

Bullmore, E. T. (2019) *The Inflamed Mind: A Radical New Approach to Depression*. London: Short Books Ltd.

Bynum, W. F. et al. (2006) *The Western Medical Tradition: 1800 to 2000*. Cambridge: Cambridge University Press.

Campbell, M. C. and Ranciaro, A. (2021) 'Human adaptation, demography and cattle domestication: an overview of the complexity of lactase persistence in Africa', *Human Molecular Genetics*, 30, pp. 98–109.

Chagnon, N. A. (2013) *Noble Savages: My Life among Two Dangerous Tribes – The Yanamamö and the Anthropologists*. New York: Simon & Schuster.

Cohen, S., Murphy, M. L. M. and Prather, A. A. (2019) 'Ten surprising facts about stressful life events and disease risk', *Annual Review of Psychology*, 70, pp. 577–597.

Colloca, L. and Benedetti, F. (2005) 'Placebos and painkillers: is mind as real as matter?', *Nature Reviews Neuroscience*, 6, pp. 545–552.

Conrad, P. and Kern, R. (1981) *The Sociology of Health and Illness: Critical Perspectives*. New York: St. Martin's Press.

Darwin, C. (1859) *On the Origin of Species by Means of Natural Selection, or the Preservation of Favoured Races in the Struggle for Life*. Available at: http://darwin-online.org.uk/Variorum/1866/1866-576-c-1859.html (accessed 10 August 2019).

Deacon, B. J. (2013) 'The biomedical model of mental disorder: a critical analysis of its validity, utility, and effects on psychotherapy research', *Clinical Psychology Review*, 33, pp. 846–861.

Del Giudice, M. (2018) *Evolutionary Psychopathology: A Unified Approach*. New York: Oxford University Press.

Doyal, L. (1979) *The Political Economy of Health*. London: Pluto Press.

Drescher, J. (2015) 'Out of DSM: depathologizing homosexuality', *Behavioral Sciences*, 5, pp. 565–575.

Elovainio, M. et al. (2017) 'Contribution of risk factors to excess mortality in isolated and lonely individuals: an analysis of data from the UK Biobank cohort study', *Lancet Public Health*, 2, pp. e260–e266.

Engel, G. L. (1977) 'The need for a new medical model: a challenge for biomedicine', *Science*, 196, pp. 129–136.

Engel, G. L. (1980) 'The clinical application of the biopsychosocial model', *American Journal of Psychiatry*, 137, pp. 535–544.

Evers, A. W. M. et al. (2014) 'Incorporating biopsychosocial characteristics into personalized healthcare: a clinical approach', *Psychotherapy and Psychosomatics*, 83, pp. 148–157.

Fabrega, H. and Brüne, M. (2017) 'Evolutionary foundations of psychiatric compared to nonpsychiatric disorders', in T. K. Shackelford and V. Zeigler-Hill (eds.), *The Evolution of Psychopathology*. Cham: Springer, pp. 1–35.

Finniss, D. G. and Benedetti, F. (2005) 'Mechanisms of the placebo response and their impact on clinical trials and clinical practice', *Pain*, 114, pp. 3–6.

Frazier, L. D. (2020) 'The past, present, and future of the biopsychosocial model: a review of *The Biopsychosocial Model of Health and Disease: New Philosophical and Scientific Developments* by Derek Bolton and Grant Gillett', *New Ideas in Psychology*, 57, p. 100755.

Ghaemi, S. N. (2009) 'The rise and fall of the biopsychosocial model', *British Journal of Psychiatry*, 195, pp. 3–4.

Ghaemi, S. N. (2010) *The Rise and Fall of the Biopsychosocial Model: Reconciling Art and Science in Psychiatry*. Baltimore, MD: Johns Hopkins University Press.

Gilbert, P. and Allan, S. (1998) 'The role of defeat and entrapment (arrested flight) in depression: an exploration of an evolutionary view', *Psychological Medicine*, 28, pp. 585–598.

Greenberg, G. (2013) 'The Rats of N.I.M.H.', *The New Yorker*. Available at: www.newyorker.com/tech/annals-of-technology/the-rats-of-n-i-m-h (accessed 15 June 2020).

Hamilton, M. J. et al. (2007) 'The complex structure of hunter-gatherer social networks', *Proceedings of the Royal Society B: Biological Sciences*, 27, pp. 2195–2203.

Harrell, C. J. P. et al. (2011) 'Multiple pathways linking racism to health outcomes', *Du Bois Review*, 8, pp. 143–157.

Heinrich, L. M. and Gullone, E. (2006) 'The clinical significance of loneliness: A literature review', *Clinical Psychology Review*, 26, pp. 695–718.

Hider, J. L. et al. (2013) 'Exploring signatures of positive selection in pigmentation candidate genes in populations of East Asian ancestry', *BMC Evolutionary Biology*, 13, p. 150.

Hoke, M. K. and McDade, T. (2014) 'Biosocial inheritance: a framework for the study of the intergenerational transmission of health disparities', *Annals of Anthropological Practice*, 38, pp. 187–213.

Janko, M. M. et al. (2018) 'The links between agriculture, *Anopheles* mosquitoes, and malaria risk in children younger than 5 years in the Democratic Republic of the Congo: a population-based, cross-sectional, spatial study', *Lancet Planetary Health*, 2, pp. e74–e82.

Kelly, M. P. et al. (2009) 'A conceptual framework for public health: NICE's emerging approach', *Public Health*, 123, pp. e14–e20.

Krakauer, J. W. et al. (2017) 'Neuroscience needs behavior: correcting a reductionist bias', *Neuron*, 93, pp. 480–490.

Krieger, N. (1994) 'Epidemiology and the web of causation: has anyone seen the spider?', *Social Science and Medicine*, 39, pp. 887–903.

Krieger, N. (2001) 'A glossary for social epidemiology', *Journal of Epidemiology and Community Health*, 55, pp. 693–700.

Lea, A. J. et al. (2017) 'Developmental plasticity: bridging research in evolution and human health', *Evolution, Medicine, and Public Health*, 2017, pp. 162–175.

Linden, D. E. J. (2012) 'The challenges and promise of neuroimaging in psychiatry', *Neuron*, 73, pp. 8–22.

Ludwig, J. et al. (2011) 'Neighborhoods, obesity, and diabetes – a randomized social experiment', *New England Journal of Medicine*, 365, pp. 1509–1519.

Ludwig, J. et al. (2012) 'Neighborhood effects on the long-term well-being of low-income adults', *Science*, 337, pp. 1505–1510.

Mai, F. M. (1995) 'Clinical and basic science aspects of the biopsychosocial model', *Journal of Psychiatry & Neuroscience*, 20, pp. 335–336.

Marmot, M. (2005) 'Social determinants of health inequalities', *Lancet*, 365, pp. 1099–1104.

Marmot, M. (2006) 'Status syndrome: a challenge to medicine', *Journal of the American Medical Association*, 295, pp. 1304–1307.

Marmot, M. and Wilkinson, R. (eds.) (1999) *Social Determinants of Health*. Oxford: Oxford University Press.

Mayr, E. (1961) 'Cause and effect in biology', *Science*, 134, pp. 1501–1506.

McElroy, A. (1990) 'Biocultural models in studies of human health and adaptation', *Medical Anthropology Quarterly*, 4, pp. 243–265.

McGee, R., Williams, S. and Elwood, M. (1994) 'Depression and the development of cancer: a meta-analysis', *Social Science and Medicine*, 38, pp. 187–192.

McLaren, N. (1998) 'A critical review of the biopsychosocial model', *Australian & New Zealand Journal of Psychiatry*, 32, pp. 86–92.

McQueen, D. et al. (2013) 'Rethinking placebo in psychiatry: how and why placebo effects occur', *Advances in Psychiatric Treatment*, 19, pp. 171–180.

Medicus, G. (2005) 'Mapping transdisciplinarity in human sciences', in J. W. Lee (ed.), *Focus on Gender Identity*. New York: Nova Science Publishers, pp. 95–114.

Moore, T. H. M. et al. (2017) 'Interventions to reduce the impact of unemployment and economic hardship on mental health in the general population: a systematic review', *Psychological Medicine*, 47, pp. 1062–1084.

Nesse, R. M. (2001) 'The smoke detector principle. Natural selection and the regulation of defensive responses', *Annals of the New York Academy of Sciences*, 935, pp. 75–85.

Nesse, R. M. (2019) *Good Reasons for Bad Feelings: Insights from the Frontier of Evolutionary Psychiatry*. London: Allen Lane.

Norton, H. L. et al. (2007) 'Genetic evidence for the convergent evolution of light skin in Europeans and East Asians',

Molecular Biology and Evolution, 24, pp. 710–722.

Pilgrim, D. (2002) 'The biopsychosocial model in Anglo-American psychiatry: past, present and future?', *Journal of Mental Health*, 11, pp. 585–594.

Pollard, T. M. (2008) *Western Diseases: An Evolutionary Perspective*. Cambridge: Cambridge University Press.

Price, J. et al. (1994) 'The social competition hypothesis of depression', *British Journal of Psychiatry*, 164, pp. 309–315.

Quirke, V. and Gaudillière, J. P. (2008) 'The era of biomedicine: science, medicine, and public health in Britain and France after the Second World War', *Medical History*, 52, pp. 441–452.

Raison, C. L. and Miller, A. H. (2013) 'The evolutionary significance of depression in Pathogen Host Defense (PATHOS-D)', *Molecular Psychiatry*, 18, pp. 15–37.

Rantala, M. J. et al. (2018) 'Depression subtyping based on evolutionary psychiatry: proximate mechanisms and ultimate functions', *Brain, Behavior, and Immunity*, 69, pp. 603–617.

Rubio-Ruiz, M. E. et al. (2015) 'An evolutionary perspective of nutrition and inflammation as mechanisms of cardiovascular disease', *International Journal of Evolutionary Biology*, 2015, p. 179791.

Sadler, J. Z. and Hulgus, Y. F. (1990) 'Knowing, valuing, acting: clues to revising the biopsychosocial model', *Comprehensive Psychiatry*, 31, pp. 185–195.

Sadler, J. Z. and Hulgus, Y. F. (1992) 'Clinical problem solving and the biopsychosocial model', *American Journal of Psychiatry*, 149, pp. 1315–1323.

Scheinfeldt, L. B. et al. (2012) 'Genetic adaptation to high altitude in the Ethiopian highlands', *Genome Biology*, 13, p. R1.

Schwartz, T. (2013) 'Psychopharmacological practice: the DSM versus the brain', *Mens Sana Monographs*, 11, pp. 25–41.

Shively, C. A. and Willard, S. L. (2012) 'Behavioral and neurobiological characteristics of social stress versus depression in nonhuman primates', *Experimental Neurology*, 233, pp. 87–94.

Shorter, E. (1997) *A History of Psychiatry: From the Era of the Asylum to the Age of Prozac*. Hoboken, NJ: John Wiley & Sons.

Shorter, E. (2005) 'The history of the biopsychosocial approach in medicine: before and after Engel', in P. White (ed.), *Biopsychosocial Medicine: An Integrated Approach to Understanding Illness*. New York: Oxford University Press, pp. 1–19.

Sloman, L., Gilbert, P. and Hasey, G. (2003) 'Evolved mechanisms in depression: the role and interaction of attachment and social rank in depression', *Journal of Affective Disorders*, 74, pp. 107–121.

Smith, G. D. (2000) 'Learning to live with complexity: ethnicity, socioeconomic position, and health in Britain and the United States', *American Journal of Public Health*, 90, pp. 1694–1698.

Smith, R. C. et al. (2013) 'An evidence-based patient-centered method makes the biopsychosocial model scientific', *Patient Education and Counseling*, 91, pp. 265–270.

Suls, J. and Rothman, A. (2004) 'Evolution of the biopsychosocial model: prospects and challenges for health psychology', *Health Psychology*, 23, pp. 119–125.

Surís, A., Holliday, R. and North, C. S. (2016) 'The evolution of the classification of psychiatric disorders', *Behavioral Sciences*, 6, p. 5.

Sweet, E. et al. (2013) 'The high price of debt: household financial debt and its impact on mental and physical health', *Social Science and Medicine*, 91, pp. 94–100.

Syme, S. (1987) 'Social determinants of disease', *Annals of Clinical Research*, 19, pp. 44–52.

Szasz, T. (2008) *Psychiatry: The Science of Lies*. Syracuse, NY: Syracuse University Press.

Tinbergen, N. (1963) 'On aims and methods of ethology', *Zeitschrift für Tierpsychologie*, 20, pp. 410–433.

Troisi, A. (2020) 'Social stress and psychiatric disorders: evolutionary reflections on debated questions', *Neuroscience and Biobehavioral Reviews*, 116, pp. 461–469.

Valtorta, N. K. et al. (2016) 'Loneliness and social isolation as risk factors for coronary heart disease and stroke: systematic review and meta-analysis of longitudinal observational studies', *Heart*, 102, pp. 1009–1016.

Van Norman, G. A. (2016) 'Drugs, devices, and the FDA: part 1: an overview of approval processes for drugs', *JACC: Basic to Translational Science*, 1, pp. 170–179.

von Bertalanffy, L. (1968) *General System Theory*. New York: Braziller.

von Rueden, C. R. and Jaeggi, A. V. (2016) 'Men's status and reproductive success in 33 nonindustrial societies: effects of subsistence, marriage system, and reproductive strategy', *Proceedings of the National Academy of Sciences of the United States of America*, 113, pp. 10824–10829.

Wakefield, J. C. (1992) 'The concept of mental disorder: on the boundary between biological facts and social values', *American Psychologist*, 47, pp. 373–388.

Wakefield, J. C. (1997) 'When is development disordered?

Developmental psychopathology and the harmful dysfunction analysis of mental disorder', *Development and Psychopathology*, 9, pp. 269–290.

Wakefield, J. C. (2015) 'Biological function and dysfunction: conceptual foundations of evolutionary psychopathology', in D. M. Buss (ed.), *The Handbook of Evolutionary Psychology*. Hoboken, NJ: John Wiley & Sons, pp. 1–19.

Weatherall, D. J. and Clegg, J. B. (2001) 'Inherited haemoglobin disorders: an increasing global health problem', *Bulletin of the World Health Organization*, 79, pp. 704–712.

Weiss, P. A. (1969) 'The living system: determinism stratified', in A. Koestler and J. R. Smythies (eds.), *Beyond Reductionism: New Perspectives in the Life Sciences*. London: Hutchinson, pp. 3–55.

Wootton, D. (2006) *Bad Medicine: Doctors Doing Harm since Hippocrates*. Oxford: Oxford University Press.

Xu, S. et al. (2011) 'A genome-wide search for signals of high-altitude adaptation in Tibetans', *Molecular Biology and Evolution*, 28, pp. 1003–1011.

Zachar, P. and Kendler, K. S. (2017) 'The philosophy of nosology', *Annual Review of Clinical Psychology*, 13, pp. 49–71.

Chapter 3

Hominin Evolution I

The Origins of Homo sapiens

Derek K. Tracy

Abstract

Just over 50,000 years ago – a blink in evolutionary time – there were at least six, possibly seven, human species alive: *sapiens, neanderthal, denisova, floresiensis, luzonensis,* remnants of *erectus* and, perhaps, the last of *Homo naledi*. This is similar to contemporary primates, with chimpanzees, gorillas, baboons and so forth all living side by side. It underlines the important fact that *sapiens* is one hominin species among many and that it is firmly part of nature and does not stand apart from it. However, we are used to occupying a unique solo position as the only humans, though such a situation accounts for less than 1% of the time since we separated from our last common ancestor with chimpanzees. This has led to the conceit and falsehood that evolution is a linear trail, marked through ever greater brain growth, leading to us. It also adds to the challenge when looking at the fossil record to determine whether some ancient species were indeed our ancestors or just side chains in a rich hominin tree. A further difficulty is that taxonomic descriptions imply clean leaps from species to species, such as between *Homo habilis* and *Homo erectus*. However, each child is a close genetic variant of its parents, and there are no hard borders as changes accrue across millennia. Late *Australopithecus* looks closer to the genus *Homo* than to early Australopithecines. Determining 'when is a species a species' is difficult (Barraclough, 2019). Adding to the uncertainty, interbreeding between different human species appears to be the rule rather than the exception, with there being complex flows of genetic material. It is a jigsaw for which we do not know how many pieces there are, nor how they might interlink. Further, the pieces are often found in fragments of single bones, and they can be so rare that many finds remain known by their 'site name'. The last 10 years have seen enormous leaps in palaeoanthropology, from the discovery of previously unknown (and entirely unexpected) human species, to advances in molecular biology that have allowed us to sequence the Neanderthal genome and better estimate temporal links between fossils. Genetic data tell us that there are several other hominin species as yet undiscovered, whose ghostly footprints are currently seen only through a unique genetic imprint across some human populations.

Keywords

Australopithecus, bipedalism, Denisova, *Homo sapiens*, human origins, Neanderthal

I believe a blade of grass no less than the journeywork of the stars.
—*Walt Whitman,* Song of Myself

Key Points

- Human evolution has not been a 'linear' process to *Homo sapiens*; for most of our existence multiple human species have been alive at the same time.

- Bipedalism was a critical evolutionary response to environmental shifts, and one that would enable greater resource mastery.
- Greater opposable thumb grip, tool use and eventually cooking of food developed alongside bipedalism, further facilitating brain growth.
- Three major hominin species coexisted for most of the past 200,000 years – *sapiens*,

neanderthal and *denisova* – with interbreeding occurring when they met.

- The survival of *sapiens* and the demise of other hominin species is incompletely understood but may involve environmental and demographic issues as much as any physiological or cognitive differences.

3.1 Genus *Homo*: The Birth of Humans

3.1.1 The First Steps to Genus *Homo*

The genus *Australopithecus* survived for about 2 million years, encompassing five or six species before giving rise to the genus *Homo*. Although still quite ape-like, Australopithecines were the first definite obligatory bipeds, walking entirely on two legs. Their foramen magnum had fully rotated to the base of their skulls and they had the beginnings of a spinal curve. Their jaws were wide and teeth thick, suited to heavy chewing of vegetative matter. At their origins their brains were little bigger than a chimpanzee's; by their transition to *Homo* they exceeded that of all apes, approaching 500 cc, with heights and weights of perhaps 150 cm and 40 kg in males and 110 cm and 30 kg in females.

It is unclear which Australopiths gave rise to other members of the genus. The earliest ancestral example appears to be *A. anamensis*, dated to 4.2–3.9 Ma (Ma = millions of years ago). It appears that *A. anamensis* evolved into *A. afarensis* (Kimbel et al., 2006), the best-known Australopithecine following the seminal find of the largely complete skeleton 'Lucy' by Johanson et al. (1982). From *afarensis*, possibly two distinct subsequent east African lineages appear: one to *A. aethiopicus* and then *A. boisei*, which appears to be non-ancestral; and another to *Homo habilis*.

In southern Africa, *A. africanus* seems similar to *afarensis* and has proposed separate lineages to *A. robustus* and *A. sediba*. *A. sediba* was only discovered in 2008 (Berger et al., 2010) and was proposed as an alternative link to what would become the genus *Homo*. However, recent work has shown that *sediba* lived alongside early *Homo erectus*, and at this time the evidence is most supportive of it being the east African *A. afarensis* that led to the genus *Homo*.

3.1.1.1 Homo habilis

Linnaeus (1735) formalised the binomial nomenclature we still use today in naming organisms. When it came to describing our genus *Homo* and its then sole species *sapiens*, he said simply '*nosce te ipsum*' – know thyself. Almost 230 years later, a landmark paper by Louis Leakey et al. in *Nature* (1964) described a new find from the Olduvai Gorge that the authors proposed could not fit into the genus *Australopithecus*. They named it *Homo habilis*, or 'handy man', referencing their use of primitive tools. Until quite recently, there had been a significant time gap between the last *A. afarensis* and the first *H. habilis*. However, in 2015, a remarkable *habilis* find from Ethiopia was dated to 2.75–2.80 Ma (Villmoore et al., 2015), 400,000 years older than the previously oldest known *Homo* but, crucially, still after the youngest known *A. afarensis*.

This transitional period is notable for climate variability, which may have been a key evolutionary driver. The landscape cooled and changed dramatically from a mixture of woods and grasslands to a drier, more open savannah favouring grazers such as gazelles, with considerable local instability, including monsoons and volcanism. Versatility and adaptability, including growing sociality, were selected for in our ancestors.

It remains unclear whether *habilis* is a single species or two subspecies: *H. rudolfensis* is the name sometimes used for a seemingly later version of *habilis*, though this remains debated. The holotype of *habilis* ('holotype' is the first specimen found of a species, upon which its description becomes based) shows very primitive long and narrow dentition closer to *A. afarensis* than later derived forms, but virtual skull reconstruction estimated a cranial volume of 729–824 cc (Spoor et al., 2015), about 30% greater than Australopithecines. When compared with *Australopithecus*, *H. habilis* has a flatter face and smaller teeth, a higher skull and the emergence of a forehead; its longer legs were better for walking, but its arms were still relatively long and archaic. The 'handy man' is considered the first hominin to consistently use tools.

3.1.1.2 Homo erectus

If longevity is a marker of a species, then *Homo erectus* is the greatest hominin, surviving for 2 million years. With *erectus* we see a 'grade shift' towards modern humans (Foley et al., 2016). 'Java man' was the original holotype name. 'Java man' was discovered in 1891 by Eugène Dubois, who was searching in the Far East for the 'missing link' between humans and apes. Later it was renamed *erectus* as it was thought to be the first fully upright hominin.

The post-cranial skeleton is similar to that of modern humans, including essentially modern hands and shortened arms, though their thoraces were stockier and the pelvises still somewhat Australopithecine (Bastir et al., 2020). Their feet were fundamentally modern, their legs long and they had our familiar spinal curvature. Their loco-motion was probably very similar to ours, and in *erectus* we see an endurance runner. This human appears more predator than scavenger: one who could track and kill, with footprint evidence showing them hunting in groups (Bennett et al., 2009). Inferentially, the need to lose heat suggests that this is when our ancestors became 'hairless'. However, all of these morphological changes represent gradual shifts across 2 million years of this great human ancestor.

The skull of *erectus* is robust and low, with a thick brow ridge, though with the flat face and projecting nose common to all subsequent humans. The cranial volume eventually reached 800–1,000 cc (Anton et al., 2014). The cranial limit that can be passed through the pelvis in childbirth is about 500 cm; therefore, from *erectus* onwards, significant brain development would have to occur after birth. Teeth growth suggests an extended childhood compared with other apes, though conversely, when compared with *sapiens*, they were adults by the age of about 11. Furthermore, beyond cranial capacities of about 700 cc, it seems hominins cannot reproduce sufficiently quickly to replace population numbers without group support – *alloparenting* (Isler and van Schaik, 2012) – implying growth in sociality.

Erectus was the first hominin to leave Africa, being found across much of Europe and Asia by about 1.3 Ma and surviving in Java until about 100,000 years ago (Rizal et al., 2020). Their walking and running abilities increased their range, and their wide range of abilities seemed to propel them to travel and thrive across a wide swathe of the planet. With *erectus* we truly see a great generalist that foreshadows us. Rather than having evolved a niche kit of very specific adaptations, its success was due to its flexibility across many different physical environments.

3.1.1.3 The Muddle in the Middle Pleistocene

From *erectus* to us is surprisingly unclear in terms of lineage; several candidate ancestors emerge, but it remains uncertain which species directly preceded us. Between about 800,000 and 300,000 years ago has been described as the 'muddle in the Middle Pleistocene'. *Sapiens*, *Neanderthal* and *Denisovans* share a common ancestor after *erectus* until about 750,000 years ago, when *Neanderthal* and *Denisova* split from our lineage, but no currently known species fully matches its expected morphology (Gomez-Robles et al., 2013).

Homo heidelbergensis is one candidate. In the 1980s, this name was used in an attempt to classify some fossil specimens from Europe, Asia and Africa that had common features that appeared to be derived from *erectus*. *Heidelbergensis* had heavy brows and low foreheads, but their brain volumes were in the range of 1,125–1,390 cc (Arsuaga et al., 1993). Their bodies were similar to ours in height, but more robust and stockier and with shorter limbs. The initial timing of these fossils, typically between about 200,000 and 600,000 years ago, fitted a gap in the fossil record, although some of these fossils, particularly from the important site at Atapuerca in Spain, have been argued to be more related to *Neanderthal*.

Homo rhodesiensis is sometimes considered the 'African form' of *heidelbergensis* and thus the one that putatively evolved into *sapiens* (with the 'European/Asian' *heidelbergensis* becoming Neanderthal and Denisovan). However, there are a couple of key issues that undermine the claim that *heidelbergensis* is ancestral to us. The *rhodesiensis* Kabwe 1 skull from Zambia was long assumed to be approximately half a million years old, but reanalysis has shown it to be far younger than expected at just under 300,000 years old (Grun et al., 2020), at which point early *Homo sapiens* were already emerging. Furthermore, data now also suggest that *heidelbergensis* might not have evolved until about 700,000 years ago, which follows the separation of what would become *sapiens* from the ancestors of *Neanderthal–Denisovan*.

Homo antecessor emerged about 1.2 million to 800,000 years ago and seems the best current candidate for the last common ancestor of *sapiens, neanderthal* and *denisova*. As well as fitting the appropriate time frames, it shares morphological features with *sapiens*, notably in its dentition and facial structure. Proteomic analysis from *antecessor* dental enamel shows it to be closely related to a last common ancestor of *sapiens, neanderthal* and *denisova* (Welker et al., 2020). However, another possibility is that *antecessor* was actually another sister species, with all four sharing an as-yet unidentified common parent.

The predecessor of Neanderthal and Denisovans instigated the *second* great human migration out of Africa, starting from 1.2 Ma. The western-spreading populations would evolve with time into *Neanderthal* and the eastern-spreading populations into *Denisovans*.

3.2 Bipedalism, Tools and Fire

3.2.1 The Tale of a Toe, the Angle of an Arch

The uniqueness of our upright posture is perhaps lost on us through familiarity, yet there is no other animal that moves like humans. Consider the *least* stable way to arrange an animal's body: it would be to stand it upright. To see the biomechanics of a human skeleton walk and run – to stand on one foot and not fall, as most humans can easily do – is to witness a marvel of motion and balance, as robot engineers are learning to their cost.

Bipedalism was the *enabler* of subsequent brain growth. Climate change, forest shrinkage and a growing of savannah were the evolutionary pressures; walking upright, then running, gave our ancestors an advantage over other primates. We were standing taller, with longer-ranged visual fields, and we were less exposed to the sun, allowing more time for walking/foraging over greater distances on our long legs without overheating. Once mastered, bipedalism is exceptionally energetically efficient: chimpanzees typically cover 3–4 km per day, compared with the 9–15 km of a hunter-gatherer, and it takes chimpanzees twice as much energy (per unit mass) to cover a given distance.

The key components are two foot arches – the longitudinal and transverse – and a great toe that, with connecting ligaments, absorb shock, store energy and act as a rigid propulsive lever when moving forward. By *A. afarensis*, the foot had developed a straight-pointing toe, demonstrated in one of the most important and beautiful finds in palaeoanthropology: the footprints at Laetoli, Tanzania. However, the shorter Australopithecine legs that made these footprints meant that the stride gait was initially shorter, and they appear to have had less developed Achilles tendons, so Australopithecines likely could not run efficiently (Latimer and Lovejoy, 1989). Other skeletal parts evolved bipedal adaptations, with knees almost identical to our own, with larger articular surfaces providing greater support between the tibia and femur; femurs angling inwards to places the legs under the body; and a lower and wider pelvis dropping the centre of gravity. The spine began to move towards the modern S shape. Human spinal curvature might at first seem 'odd' – why would it not just be straight? But back arches beautifully distribute forces, like a spring, during walking and running (Been et al., 2017).

By genus *Homo*, other changes particularly selected for endurance running emerge: enlarged gluteus maximum muscles, better inner-ear balance systems and elongated Achilles tendons. This has led to the endurance running hypothesis positing that we became persistence hunters (Bramble and Lieberman, 2004). Quadrupeds, once they break from a trot into a gallop, lack adequate mechanisms for cooling down over longer periods – if they can be kept at a gallop pace, they eventually become hyperthermic and die. Humans avoid this through significant sweating abilities (far more than most other animals) and by being hairless. Despite sweating, we still use 30–50% less water per day than extant apes through much more efficient water conservation abilities (aided by the shape of our noses) (Pontzer et al., 2021).

However, there are evolutionary pressures *against* bipedalism: a loss of agility and speed in forest environments and a proneness to tripping injuries (non-trivial problems in predator landscapes), as well as lower back pain, with the spinal 'S' curvature making us prone to spondylolysis and spondylolisthesis. The greatest challenge, though, is childbirth – and the 'obstetric dilemma' (Wells et al., 2012). If *sapiens* followed typical mammalian patterns, we might be expected to have an *in utero* gestation of perhaps 21 months (consider that chimpanzee pregnancies last a year) (Portmann, 1990). The biomechanical demands of bipedalism put significant restraints on the need for pelvic stability, limiting the size of the pelvic outlet and thus the foetus. Even at a 9-month gestation, humans have exceptional labour difficulties and maternal mortality rates. There can be few evolutionary pressures against a new mutation greater than increasing maternal or infant death. However, this hypothesis has faced push back (Pavlicev et al., 2020); a counterargument, the 'metabolic crossover hypothesis', argues that it becomes ever more energetically demanding on a mother to provide nutrition to an enlarging baby, thus 'forcing' a 9-month delivery time (Dunsworth, 2018). The 'obstetric dilemma' remains unresolved.

3.2.2 Technology: Tools and Weapons

Humans have moved from 'object-assisted' to an 'object-dependent' species (Plummer, 2004), and this has bidirectionally influenced brain development, notably visuospatial integration in the parietal lobes. The archaeological challenges are that non-stone tools, such as wood, were likely more common, but they are perishable, and stone tools can be difficult to date and ascribe with certainty to a given population. Human hands evolved with the development of tools, selecting for ever stronger and more precise grip. Virtual modelling of the opponens pollicis muscle with ancient bone anatomy suggests that the torque required for biomechanically efficient thumb opposition arose about 2 million years ago (Karakostis et al., 2021); therefore, this was *not* fully present, but was developing, in Australopithecines. Nevertheless, whilst traditionally a defining feature of *Homo*, we now recognise simple tool use in Australopithecines.

Stone knapping, using a hard 'hammerstone' to strike the edge of a more brittle core rock (such as quartz or flint) to induce sharp conchoidal fractures, requires considerable cognitive and sensorimotor abilities. These include choosing the right source stones, appreciating their fracture mechanics and striking with appropriate force in the correct location (Lewis and Harmand, 2016). Stone tools have been reliably dated to 3.3 million years old, when *A. afarensis* was beginning to butcher bones (McPherron et al., 2010). However, it increases with early *Homo*, initially reflecting *occasional* stone tool use (Cerling et al., 2011). Early examples – 'Oldowan technology' – are sometimes called 'pebble tools', as the 'blanks' from which they were made already look somewhat like the final product.

'Acheulean tools' are a refinement, utilising larger flakes and producing a large core from which tools would be shaped, necessitating the creation of a mental template over such blank cores. Their manufacture is a skilled operation, and it has been demonstrated that individuals cannot reproduce them without instruction (Shea, 2015). This implies a considerable cultural component in terms of teaching instruction and copying technique (Morgan et al., 2015). Stone tool production requires the complex integration of visual, auditory and sensorimotor information across the temporal cortices, as well as memory and action planning. This 'technocomplex' phase, begun by *H. erectus*, was the longest-lasting technological phase in human history, dating from about 1.7 Ma until a few hundred thousand years ago. In this period, tool use moves to *habitual*, generating further selective pressures towards an efficient bipedal gait (Carvalho et al., 2012).

Hunting weapons appear around 400,000–500,000 years ago – the era of *heidelbergensis*. The earliest were spears that were thrust and not thrown, which is a riskier form of hunting. The killing of large animals with such weaponry suggests cooperative hunts and forward planning – tool use thus became *obligatory* (Shea, 2017). From around 300,000 years ago, there was a considerable increase in diversity of tools, including composite tools that had more than one component, such as a wooden handle and a stone head. 'Digging sticks' were made from hard, heavy boxwood that was charred with fire to peel their bark and toughen them. The Pinnacle Point caves in South Africa show heat treating to attain finer flakes in blade technology (Brown et al., 2009). Such pyro-technology requires burial in a hearth at a high temperature for several hours, necessitating planning and experiment, and is not something that occurs accidentally. Humans were learning to experiment with materials.

3.2.3 Food and Fire

Ancestral diets can be assayed through: the shapes, structure and chemistry of teeth and bones; plants stuck on tooth plaque, particularly hardened microscopic 'phytoliths'; tools and fire; and butchery marks on animal bones.

Australopithecus was likely an omnivore but primarily frugivorous (fruit eating), similar to chimpanzees. It had very strong chewing muscles, implying that much of its day was spent eating energy-poor sources of food (chimpanzees can spend 11 hours a day eating). Meat accounts for about 3% of a chimp's diet, though this includes scarce micronutrients – many vital to brain functioning – including vitamins A, B6, B12 and K, iron, zinc, sodium, potassium and calcium. It seems reasonable to imagine that *Australopithecus* would also consume this energy-rich source opportunistically.

Our brain accounts for 20% of our energy requirements (the equivalent of all skeletal muscle at rest). The other energetically expensive tissue is the gastrointestinal tract (GIT). Both contain enormous numbers of neurons that need to be kept in a primed, ready-to-fire state. The 'expensive tissue hypothesis' relates these two (Aiello and Wheeler, 1995): meat's concentrated protein and fat does not need a long digestive tract for absorption, allowing GIT shrinkage ('freeing' more energy) and supporting any mutations facilitating brain growth.

Early meat acquisition was through scavenging. Experimental data suggest that there is actually quite a lot of meat left after group carnivore feeds. A typical zebra kill by lions leaves 95% of bones abandoned with at least some flesh on them, and 50% have significant meat remnants. An average zebra carcass leaves behind 15 kg of meat: this equates to 60,000 calories, or enough to meet the requirements of 27 adult male *H. erectus* for a day (Pobiner, 2020). *Persistent carnivory* appears to be the domain of the genus *Homo*. From about 2 Ma we see evidence of a decrease in rib and pelvis size in *H. erectus*, implying a smaller, more efficient digestive tract, and by then they were proficient *hunters* of antelope and zebra (Bunn and Kroll, 1986). By 1.5 Ma, butchery marks show that *erectus* was going for the 'choicest cuts' on the animal (Pobiner et al., 2008). Evidence of aquatic animals being part of our diet comes from around this time (Braun et al., 2010), and their long-chain polyunsaturated fatty acids might have particularly supported brain growth.

However, cranial size tracked body size until about 1 Ma, at which point brain growth really took off. This is most likely accounted for by the acquiring of mastery over fire and cooking of food. Cooking sterilises food, breaks down toxins and makes plant material digestible (consider potatoes), it makes material easier to chew and it liberates up to 40% more energy. Wrangham's 'cooking hypothesis' (2009) argues that it was *H. erectus* that first adapted to a cooked diet and therefore controlling fire, pushing the emergence of this skill to about 1.9 Ma.

The use of fire – 'anthropogenic fire' – is a much-debated area. Initially hominins were attracted to natural fire sites with exposed, injured or killed (and cooked) bounty – *opportunistic* use. Learning to track smoke signals might have been a universal skill. The next achievement was *conserving* fire using slow-burning materials such as plant tapers, then to a final step of the *kindling* of fire (Gowlett, 2016). The first unambiguous evidence that human *controlled* fires is from 1 Ma at the Wonderwerk Cave in South Africa (Berna et al., 2012), but it is really only in the last half a million years or so that we see convincing evidence of true mastery and regular use of fire. Large hearths, which can sustain warmth and cooking for a community group, require significant daily quantities of wood, the maintenance of which seems unlikely without at least some proto-language.

3.3 The Last of the Other Humans

Two hundred thousand years ago, three cognitively advanced hominin species walked the earth: *sapiens*, *Neanderthal* and *Denisovans*. But we have learned in the last decade of three other coexisting human species: *floresiensis*, *luzonensis* and *naledi*. Genetic data also tell of 'ghost' populations, for whom we lack physical evidence but whose unique patterns are still seen within our own DNA. Within about 160,000 years, all but *sapiens* would be extinct.

3.3.1 An Unexpected Party: New Hominin Cousins

3.3.1.1 Homo floresiensis

Floresiensis is a remarkable twenty-first-century fossil find. It was the first of several new species that recalibrated our sense of what it meant to be human, shaking a linear narrative marching 'to' *sapiens*. In a cave on the island of Flores, Indonesia (Brown et al., 2004; Morwood et al., 2004), a skeleton only three feet six inches tall and with disproportionally large feet was found, perhaps inevitably being dubbed 'the hobbit'. The complete holotype skull, 'LB1', was undoubtedly from an adult despite its small size – dentition and cranial epiphyseal plate closure confirm this – but there was much debate as to whether this 30-year-old female, nicknamed the 'little lady of Flores' or 'Flo', was an isolated, perhaps pathological or genetic abnormality. But more research, and the subsequent discovery of a second, older site, confirmed this as a new species. *Floresiensis* appeared to be an example of the phenomenon of 'insular dwarfism', where there are selective evolutionary island pressures for ever smaller sizes.

Floresiensis had a cranial capacity of about 420 cc – half that of *erectus*. However, the sites showed evidence of carcass butchery with tools and the use of fire, bringing *floresiensis* into the genus *Homo* whilst challenging us on what the cognitive capacity of this diminutive human might have been. *Floresiensis* was bipedal, though with long curved toes, a short big toe and a weak flattened arch suggesting a slower gait, and one unsuited to distance running (Jungers et al., 2009). Its face shows the transition to *Homo*, but some features appear more closely related to *habilis* than *erectus* (Argue et al., 2017).

Controversially, initial dating put the first specimens at just 12,000 years old. There had been long-standing local folklore of short human-like creatures named 'Ebu Gogo' ('gluttonous granny') whose description fitted somewhat with *floresiensis*. These were spoken of as hairy with wide faces and big mouths, and while having some language of their own, they would try to mimic the sounds of locals. Debate raged as to whether the Ebu Gogo were actually folk memories of *floresiensis*. However, more recent analysis has now dated those first fossils at closer to 60,000–100,000 years old (Sutikna et al., 2016), taking the Ebu Gogo out of the mainstream.

These data align the disappearance of *floresiensis* with the estimated arrival of *sapiens*, though notably there is evidence for regional environmental changes at this time, and the extinction of *floresiensis* may be multifactorial (Sutikna et al., 2018). It would appear that the two species did overlap, at least for a time. Genomic analysis (Teixeira et al., 2021) shows no evidence for any interbreeding between *floresiensis* (or *luzonensis*; see Section 3.3.1.2) and *sapiens*. This is an interesting break in the seemingly inevitable mating that occurs when any human groups meet, though it remains possible that this did occur but did not produce viable offspring or led to a lineage that died out.

The second *floresiensis* site dates back 700,000 years, demonstrating its longevity as a species and

an earlier-than-expected acquisition of its dwarf aspects (van den Bergh et al., 2016). Each of the two current competing evolutionary theories for *floresiensis* has a very significant problem. If it derived from *erectus*, a subpopulation needed to shrink to about half its body (and brain) mass in just a few hundred thousand years. This also does not address the question of the occurrence of some of the more archaic features of *floresiensis* not seen in *erectus*. However, if it evolved directly from a more ancient ancestor, it must have left Africa and travelled to Flores, but there is no physical evidence for this at this time.

3.3.1.2 Homo luzonensis

Another recent unexpected discovery occurred in the neighbouring Philippines. *Homo luzonensis* is currently known only through some finger and toe bones, a thigh bone and teeth that have been dated to 50,000–67,000 years ago (Detroit et al., 2019). We lack cranial remains, but the indications are of a human with a mix of modern and archaic features. The foot bones appear closer to *Australopithecus* than *Homo*, suggesting it was also of a small size, with a height of about three feet. This has drawn obvious comparisons with *floresiensis*, though even the limited current skeletal remains show sufficient morphological variations to differentiate them as species.

Hominin activity has been dated in the Philippines to over 700,000 years ago, with evidence of butchery of a now-extinct species of rhinoceros, alongside multiple stone tools made using a simple knapping technique (Ingicco et al., 2018). It remains unclear if *luzonensis* will remain in genus *Homo* if it shows neither tool use nor significant cranial capacity (and indeed it was not definitively bipedal).

3.3.1.3 Homo naledi

Homo naledi was discovered in the Rising Star caves in South Africa (Berger et al., 2015). Over 1,500 bone fragments have been recovered from six adults and nine juveniles. The physiology of *naledi* quite uniquely combines a range of primitive and advanced characteristics. It has a small head and brain (about 450–600 cc), yet interestingly the brain shows a modern asymmetry and frontal lobe structure. Their teeth and jaws suggest a diet that did not require significant chewing, but the teeth are pitted, chipped and worn in a manner indicating considerable grit in their food, potentially from underground sources such as tubers (Davies et al., 2020). Their shoulders were narrow, with long arms and curved finger bones, indicating adaptations to an arboreal or climbing life (Kivell et al., 2015). However, their legs, ankles and feet were not dissimilar to later hominins, signifying clear bipedality, and they stood about five feet tall and weighed 40–45 kg. We do not see this combination of 'old' and 'new' in any other members of the genus *Homo*.

Surprisingly, analyses give an age range for *H. naledi* of 236,000–335,000 years old (Dirks et al., 2017), though its morphology had suggested a far more archaic human. The precise place of *naledi* on our hominin tree remains unanswered: how long did it exist, and from which predecessor did it evolve? Two possibilities emerge: the first is that it is an archaic species with a unique evolutionary path perhaps back to late Australopiths or very early *Homo* (its tooth morphology supports this, with *habilis* as a likely ancestor; Davies et al., 2020); the second is that it has a more recent hominin ancestor such as *erectus*, but if so its evolutionary path led to reductions in brain volume akin to *floresiensis*. Another interesting aspect to *naledi* is that it lived for some considerable time alongside other hominins. This suggests that it had found a unique evolutionary niche; perhaps an arboreal or climbing lifestyle and diet that kept it sufficiently out of the way of larger-brained hominins.

It is also not clear how these bodies ended up in chambers that are exceptionally hard to reach and lack natural light. Suggestions included an intentional depository for the dead, supported by the subsequent discovery of a second chamber in the system with a similar array of bodies. However, this necessitates considerable cognition in a small-brained human. A recent paper has proposed that the shoulder girdle of *naledi* was particularly adapted to rock climbing, which the authors note was a more common landscape in southern Africa at that time (Voisin et al., 2020). If inherently a rock climber, perhaps cave exploration was a more normalised behaviour for this human, even if it seems alien to us.

3.3.2 Neanderthal: War, Pestilence or Famine?

No other hominin has captured the public imagination or been more misunderstood than *Homo neanderthalensis*. Discovered in 1856, it was originally regarded as a pathological human skeleton, but it was subsequently recognised and named as the first other member of our genus.

Sequencing of its genome generated the famous statistic[1] that individuals of European heritage typically have about 2% Neanderthal DNA. Interbreeding appears to have occurred rapidly with the earliest *sapiens* populations in Europe (ancestral to contemporary Europeans) some 42,000–45,000 years ago (Hajdinjak et al., 2021). How consensual and enduring any such relationships might have been are unknown, though clearly at least some of these offspring were cared for, raised in their communities and reproduced in their own turn. Nevertheless, there is more Neanderthal DNA in *non-coding* regions of *sapiens* today, showing negative selection and implying that hybrids were genetically less fit (Jegou et al., 2017).

Physically, Neanderthals were simultaneously similar to yet different from us. Short and stocky, barrel-chested and with reduced limb length, Neanderthals showed adaptations to the series of ice ages Europe had been going through. Their skulls had projecting midfaces, big noses and big brow ridges and were elongated from front to rear. Their brain volumes fell within that of the recent *sapiens* range (VanSickle et al., 2020). Their eye sockets and occipital cortices were big, suggesting enhanced eyesight and visual processing, or at least compensatory mechanisms to overcome any deficits endured by evolving in northern latitudes. Neanderthal teeth equating to developmental ages 4, 11 and 16 in *sapiens* were in fact chronologically 3, 8 and 12 years old (Smith et al., 2010). A faster maturation to adulthood came at a cost of a foreshortened childhood and likely cognitive and behavioural development, possibly representing a trade-off for growing more rapidly in a tougher environment.

Neanderthals were found from the Iberian Peninsula to Uzbekistan and as far north as Siberia. Why did they go extinct? There is no

---

[1] It is perhaps difficult to appreciate what an unexpected and paradigm-shifting finding this was. As with *floresiensis*, it shook the bedrock of the 'march of progress' to *sapiens*, showing that our history was far more complex. The finding was one that many thought technically impossible (sequencing such ancient DNA) and culturally impossible (that we bred with Neanderthals).

evidence for direct warfare between *sapiens* and Neanderthals. Perhaps they did not recognise each other as 'different' and 'distinct'; however, some conflict seems inevitable, but perhaps within more indirect arenas such as attaining resources. The total Neanderthal population may have been as small as 10,000 individuals across the entire continent, and their genome shows evidence of 'bottlenecking' that is hypothesised to have occurred from considerable shrinkage in numbers during climate extremes and a gradual population decline over time (Rogers et al., 2020). Thus, they might have been on the brink of collapse when our arrival coincided with another very cold period. Current estimates suggest that they had disappeared from northwest Europe between 40,000 and 44,000 years ago (Deviese et al., 2021), with the very last of the Neanderthals surviving in small numbers in the Iberian Peninsula until perhaps about 28,000 years ago. *Sapiens* appeared to survive the harshest weather better, possibly through technological advancements. Animals associated with fur production were found with both species but in greater numbers with *sapiens*. Neanderthals appear to have more often employed cape-like clothing without the sewing or weaving employed by *sapiens*. Bone needles from about 40,000 years ago have not been found with Neanderthals, and they might have lacked the technological development of stitching and thus more fitted winter gear. Their lung capacities were about 20% greater than those of *sapiens*, indicating greater oxygen needs resulting from a higher metabolic drive, probably due to their proportionally greater muscle bulk (Garcia-Martinez et al., 2018). Neanderthals' muscle mass necessitated 100–350 kcal more per person per day than *sapiens*, hindering their competitive advantages (Froehle and Churchill, 2009).

Neanderthals generally lacked 'blade tools' – those twice as long as they are wide. This mattered insofar as blade tools can be usefully modified into awls to make holes in leather and clothing and into microliths to embed into bone and make composite tools for the development of harpoons and so forth. *Sapiens* was producing these, particularly during harsher weather conditions, yet Neanderthals have been described as demonstrating 'technological inertia' across 200,000 years (Bocquet-Appel and Tuffreau, 2009). A fascinating recent study analysed differences between the hands and loading pressures of Neanderthals and *sapiens* (Bardo et al., 2020): the remains of *sapiens* are more consistent with forceful 'pad-to-pad' thumb–finger precision grips, while Neanderthal remains are more consistent with a habitually more adducted transverse power squeeze grip, as occurs when one grasps hafted tools such as an axe.

Achilles tendon characteristics suggest Neanderthals were less efficient runners than *sapiens* (Raichlen et al., 2011). Their straighter spine alignment made their gait less 'springy' when running, but had advantages for carrying heavier loads and walking on rugged terrain (Been et al., 2017). Neanderthals appear less competent at adopting the persistence hunting common to early *sapiens*, and so *sapiens* might have better exploited the same environments. Relative isotope distributions in bones and teeth make clear that Neanderthals were big game hunters, relying on mammoth, bison and deer for much of their meat intake. Interestingly, many remains around hearths show animals that were eaten raw, and Neanderthals showed less diversification outside of these high-calorie but higher-risk food sources, including less exploitation of seafood, freshwater fish and waterfowl (Guillaud et al., 2021). However, glaciation would have destroyed much coastal site evidence, and a Neanderthal site on the Portuguese Atlantic (Zilhao et al., 2020) shows shells of crabs, molluscs and tortoises and bones of fish and marine birds.

Cave art in Spain has been dated to about 65,000 years old (Hoffmann et al., 2018), predating the arrival of *sapiens*, and thus being of presumed Neanderthal origin. These red and black paintings of animals, geometric shapes and handprints provide evidence of some symbolic behaviour. Nevertheless, Neanderthal art, as well as being far less common, lacks much of the richness and perspective of the work of *sapiens* and is generally more simplistic in manner.

There is evidence that Neanderthals buried their dead (Balzeau et al., 2020), though typically sites show more ambiguous evidence of the placement of bodies rather than the more ritualistic processes and 'grave goods' of early modern *sapiens*. However, Neanderthals clearly cared for their sick: the Shanidar 1 skeleton is a good example of this, demonstrating an individual who survived serious head and body injuries for many years, necessitating a considerable social matrix (Trinkaus and Villotte, 2017).

Ultimately, we do not know why Neanderthals perished. An emerging consensus amongst palaeoanthropologists is that their demise was primarily a demographic issue (Vaesen et al., 2021), but our coming seems to have pushed them over the edge. They appeared able to do most of the things we did, though their proficiency perhaps did not quite match ours. We seem to have shown greater innovation and cognitive flexibility when they were most required. However, over the past decade, emerging evidence has closed the gap between us considerably, and there is a counterpoint that there might have been very little to separate them from us.

3.3.3 Homo denisova

The Denisova cave in the Siberian Altai Mountains produced a most unexpected find: a third modern hominin living alongside and interbreeding with *sapiens* and Neanderthals and whose genetic footprints would subsequently be found through a huge swathe of modern humans. The cave had been an archaeological site since the 1980s, when two unexceptional human-looking teeth and a finger bone, originally described in 1988 as Neanderthal, were reanalysed. The mitochondrial DNA showed them to be neither Neanderthal nor *sapiens*. They were assigned the name *Homo denisova* (Reich et al., 2010). Since then, about 14 fragmentary fossils have been extracted, including some skull parietal bones sufficiently large to allow an estimate of the overall skull shape (Viola et al., 2019). It appears more angular and lower than Neanderthal and about 10% larger than early *sapiens*. It is a risk to extrapolate too much from single specimens, but these data support Denisovans being larger and more robust than us.

This is supported by genomic analysis showing Denisovans to be closest relatives to Neanderthals, diverging from them 381,000–473,000 years ago. Nuclear DNA sequence diversity found in the cave specimens is low, inferring that the population in that region was a small one (Slon et al., 2017). However, more recent finds outside the Altai Mountains have confirmed that Denisovans had wide genetic variation (far more than Neanderthals), with perhaps three distinct population lineages covering almost all of Asia (Jacobs et al., 2019). In 2018, a 2.5-cm bone fragment

caused a sensation when it was shown to be from a first-generation child of a Neanderthal mother and a Denisovan father who died 90,000–100,000 years ago (Slon et al., 2018).

The first non-Siberian Denisovan fossil is a Neanderthal-like jawbone initially found in Tibet in the 1980s that was ignored for some years. DNA could not be extracted, but bone collagen proteins confirmed it as Denisovan (Chen et al., 2019). Genetic data also confirmed Denisovan adaptations to low-oxygen environments, which has passed, through interbreeding, to modern Tibetans, who carry the Denisovan *EPAS1* gene that improves erythrocytes' oxygen-carrying efficiency (Huerta-Sanchez et al., 2014). Denisovan DNA is found in almost all Asian populations; the largest proportions occur in Australian aboriginal people and Melanesians, accounting for up to 5% of their genomes (Vernot et al., 2016). Somewhat controversially, work has suggested that the last admixture might have been as recent as 15,000 years ago, which, if correct, would make Denisovans the latest-surviving humans besides us (Jacobs et al., 2019). There has been very rapid growth in our knowledge of Denisovans, yet much remains unknown, including the causes of their demise, owing to a bewildering lack of fossils for a human species so widespread and recent.

3.3.4 The Ghost Introgressors

There is evidence for several distinct hominin populations identifiable only through their genetic fingerprints within us. The genomes of people living in the Middle East 3,400–14,000 years ago showed that about half of their ancestry came from a 'basal Eurasian' lineage that showed no signs of interbreeding with Neanderthals. It had been isolated for an adequately long period of time to develop unique genetic markers, but there are no archaeological or fossil traces of this human population.

Three quite different and geographically very dispersed African hunter-gatherer populations (the Baka from Cameroon, the Khoisan-speaking Hadza and the Sandawe from Tanzania) contain an unknown hominin genetic signature (Lachance et al., 2012). As this is not found in any Eurasian populations, it implies introgression *after* those populations left Africa – meaning within the past 30,000 years (Hsieh et al., 2016). Fascinatingly, this introgressor appears genetically as different from *sapiens* as Denisovans or Neanderthals. It has been shown that 2–19% of the DNA of four West African populations comes from an archaic hominin, possibly *rhodesiensis/heidelbergensis* (Durvasula and Sankararaman, 2020).

In the modern Asian population, there are genetic remnants from several other archaic populations, with at least one introgression proposed to have occurred across all Asian populations (Mondal et al., 2019).

References

Aiello, L. C. and Wheeler, P. 1995. The expensive-tissue hypothesis: the brain and the digestive system in human and primate evolution. *Curr Anthropol*, 36, 199–221.

Anton, S. C., Potts, R. and Aiello, L. C. 2014. Human evolution. Evolution of early *Homo*: an integrated biological perspective. *Science*, 345, 1236828.

Argue, D., Groves, C. P., Lee, M. S. Y. and Jungers, W. L. 2017. The affinities of *Homo floresiensis* based on phylogenetic analyses of cranial, dental, and postcranial characters. *J Hum Evol*, 107, 107–133.

Arsuaga, J. L., Martinez, I., Gracia, A., Carretero, J. M. and Carbonell, E. 1993. Three new human skulls from the Sima de los Huesos Middle Pleistocene site in Sierra de Atapuerca, Spain. *Nature*, 362, 534–537.

Balzeau, A., Turq, A., Talamo, S., Daujeard, C., Guerin, G., Welker, F., Crevecoeur, I., Fewlass, H., Hublin, J. J., Lahaye, C., Maureille, B., Meyer, M., Schwab, C. and Gomez-Olivencia, A. 2020. Pluridisciplinary evidence for burial for the La Ferrassie 8 Neandertal child. *Sci Rep*, 10, 21230.

Bardo, A., Moncel, M. H., Dunmore, C. J., Kivell, T. L., Pouydebat, E. and Cornette, R. 2020. The implications of thumb movements for Neanderthal and modern human manipulation. *Sci Rep*, 10, 19323.

Barraclough, T. G. 2019. *The Evolutionary Biology of Species*. Oxford: Oxford University Press.

Bastir, M., Garcia-Martinez, D., Torres-Tamayo, N., Palancar, C. A., Beyer, B., Barash, A., Villa, C., Sanchis-Gimeno, J. A., Riesco-Lopez, A., Nalla, S., Torres-Sanchez, I., Garcia-Rio, F., Been, E., Gomez-Olivencia, A., Haeusler, M., Williams, S. A. and Spoor, F. 2020. Rib cage anatomy in *Homo erectus* suggests a recent evolutionary origin of modern human body shape. *Nat Ecol Evol*, 4, 1178–1187.

Been, E., Gomez-Olivencia, A., Shefi, S., Soudack, M., Bastir, M. and Barash, A. 2017. Evolution of spinopelvic alignment in hominins. *Anat Rec (Hoboken)*, 300, 900–911.

Bennett, M. R., Harris, J. W., Richmond, B. G., Braun, D. R., Mbua, E., Kiura, P., Olago, D., Kibunjia, M., Omuombo, C., Behrensmeyer, A. K., Huddart, D. and Gonzalez, S. 2009. Early hominin foot morphology based on 1.5-million-year-old footprints from Ileret, Kenya. *Science*, 323, 1197–1201.

Berger, L. R., De Ruiter, D. J., Churchill, S. E., Schmid, P., Carlson, K. J., Dirks, P. H. and Kibii, J. M. 2010. *Australopithecus sediba*: a new species of *Homo*-like australopith from South Africa. *Science*, 328, 195–204.

Berger, L. R., Hawks, J., De Ruiter, D. J., Churchill, S. E., Schmid, P., Delezene, L. K., Kivell, T. L., Garvin, H. M., Williams, S. A., Desilva, J. M., Skinner, M. M., Musiba, C. M., Cameron, N., Holliday, T. W., Harcourt-Smith, W., Ackermann, R. R., Bastir, M., Bogin, B., Bolter, D., Brophy, J., Cofran, Z. D., Congdon, K. A., Deane, A. S., Dembo, M., Drapeau, M., Elliott, M. C., Feuerriegel, E. M., Garcia-Martinez, D., Green, D. J., Gurtov, A., Irish, J. D., Kruger, A., Laird, M. F., Marchi, D., Meyer, M. R., Nalla, S., Negash, E. W., Orr, C. M., Radovcic, D., Schroeder, L., Scott, J. E., Throckmorton, Z., Tocheri, M. W., Vansickle, C., Walker, C. S., Wei, P. and Zipfel, B. 2015. *Homo naledi*, a new species of the genus *Homo* from the Dinaledi Chamber, South Africa. *Elife*, 4, e09560.

Berna, F., Goldberg, P., Horwitz, L. K., Brink, J., Holt, S., Bamford, M. and Chazan, M. 2012. Microstratigraphic evidence of *in situ* fire in the Acheulean strata of Wonderwerk Cave, Northern Cape province, South Africa. *PNAS*, 109, E1215–E1220.

Bocquet-Appel, J. P. and Tuffreau, A. 2009. Technological responses of Neanderthals to macroclimatic variations (240,000–40,000 BP). *Hum Biol*, 81, 287–307.

Bramble, D. M. and Lieberman, D. E. 2004. Endurance running and the evolution of Homo. *Nature*, 432, 345–352.

Braun, D. R., Harris, J. W., Levin, N. E., Mccoy, J. T., Herries, A. I., Bamford, M. K., Bishop, L. C., Richmond, B. G. and Kibunjia, M. 2010. Early hominin diet included diverse terrestrial and aquatic animals 1.95 Ma in East Turkana, Kenya. *PNAS*, 107, 10002–10007.

Brown, K. S., Marean, C. W., Herries, A. I., Jacobs, Z., Tribolo, C., Braun, D., Roberts, D. L., Meyer, M. C. and Bernatchez, J. 2009. Fire as an engineering tool of early modern humans. *Science*, 325, 859–862.

Brown, P., Sutikna, T., Morwood, M. J., Soejono, R. P., Jatmiko, Saptomo, E. W. and Due, R. A. 2004. A new small-bodied hominin from the Late Pleistocene of Flores, Indonesia. *Nature*, 431, 1055–1061.

Bunn, H. T. and Kroll, E. M. 1986. Systematic butchery by Plio-Pleistocene hominids at Olduvai Gorge, Tanzania. *Curr Anthropol*, 27, 431–452.

Carvalho, S., Biro, D., Cunha, E., Hockings, K., Mcgrew, W. C., Richmond, B. G. and Matsuzawa, T. 2012. Chimpanzee carrying behaviour and the origins of human bipedality. *Curr Biol*, 22, R180–R181.

Cerling, T. E., Wynn, J. G., Andanje, S. A., Bird, M. I., Korir, D. K., Levin, N. E., Mace, W., Macharia, A. N., Quade, J. and Remien, C. H. 2011. Woody cover and hominin environments in the past 6 million years. *Nature*, 476, 51–56.

Chen, F., Welker, F., Shen, C. C., Bailey, S. E., Bergmann, I., Davis, S., Xia, H., Wang, H., Fischer, R., Freidline, S. E., Yu, T. L., Skinner, M. M., Stelzer, S., Dong, G., Fu, Q., Dong, G., Wang, J., Zhang, D. and Hublin, J. J. 2019. A late Middle Pleistocene Denisovan mandible from the Tibetan Plateau. *Nature*, 569, 409–412.

Davies, T. W., Delezene, L. K., Gunz, P., Hublin, J. J., Berger, L. R., Gidna, A. and Skinner, M. M. 2020. Distinct mandibular premolar crown morphology in *Homo naledi* and its implications for the evolution of *Homo* species in southern Africa. *Sci Rep*, 10, 13196.

Detroit, F., Mijares, A. S., Corny, J., Daver, G., Zanolli, C., Dizon, E., Robles, E., Grun, R. and Piper, P. J. 2019. A new species of *Homo* from the Late Pleistocene of the Philippines. *Nature*, 568, 181–186.

Deviese, T., Abrams, G., Hajdinjak, M., Pirson, S., De Groote, I., Di Modica, K., Toussaint, M., Fischer, V., Comeskey, D., Spindler, L., Meyer, M., Semal, P. and Higham, T. 2021.

Reevaluating the timing of Neanderthal disappearance in northwest Europe. *PNAS*, 118, e2022466118.

Dirks, P. H., Roberts, E. M., Hilbert-Wolf, H., Kramers, J. D., Hawks, J., Dosseto, A., Duval, M., Elliott, M., Evans, M., Grun, R., Hellstrom, J., Herries, A. I., Joannes-Boyau, R., Makhubela, T. V., Placzek, C. J., Robbins, J., Spandler, C., Wiersma, J., Woodhead, J. and Berger, L. R. 2017. The age of *Homo naledi* and associated sediments in the Rising Star Cave, South Africa. *Elife*, 6, e24231.

Dunsworth, H. M. 2018. There Is no "obstetrical dilemma": towards a braver medicine with fewer childbirth interventions. *Perspect Biol Med*, 61, 249–263.

Durvasula, A. and Sankararaman, S. 2020. Recovering signals of ghost archaic introgression in African populations. *Sci Adv*, 6, eaax5097.

Foley, R. A., Martin, L., Mirazon Lahr, M. and Stringer, C. 2016. Major transitions in human evolution. *Philos Trans R Soc Lond B Biol Sci*, 371, 20150229.

Froehle, A. W. and Churchill, S. E. 2009. Energetic competition between Neandertals and anatomically modern humans. *Palaeoanthropology*, 2009, 96–116.

Garcia-Martinez, D., Torres-Tamayo, N., Torres-Sanchez, I., Garcia-Rio, F., Rosas, A. and Bastir, M. 2018. Ribcage measurements indicate greater lung capacity in Neanderthals and Lower Pleistocene hominins compared to modern humans. *Commun Biol*, 1, 117.

Gomez-Robles, A., Bermudez De Castro, J. M., Arsuaga, J. L., Carbonell, E. and Polly, P. D. 2013. No known hominin species matches the expected dental morphology of the last common ancestor of Neanderthals and modern humans. *PNAS*, 110, 18196–18201.

Gowlett, J. A. 2016. The discovery of fire by humans: a long and convoluted process. *Philos Trans R Soc Lond B Biol Sci*, 371, 27216521.

Grun, R., Pike, A., Mcdermott, F., Eggins, S., Mortimer, G., Aubert, M., Kinsley, L., Joannes-Boyau, R., Rumsey, M., Denys, C., Brink, J., Clark, T. and Stringer, C. 2020. Dating the skull from Broken Hill, Zambia, and its position in human evolution. *Nature*, 580, 372–375.

Guillaud, E., Bearez, P., Daujeard, C., Defleur, A. R., Desclaux, E., Rosello-Izquierdo, E., Morales-Muniz, A. and Moncel, M. H. 2021. Neanderthal foraging in freshwater ecosystems: a reappraisal of the Middle Paleolithic archaeological fish record from continental Western Europe. *Quat Sci Rev*, 252, 106731.

Hajdinjak, M., Mafessoni, F., Skov, L., Vernot, B., Hubner, S., Fu, Q., Essel, E. S. N., Meyer, M., Skoglund, P., Kelso, J. and Paabo, S. 2021. Initial Upper Palaeolithic humans in Europe had recent Neanderthal ancestry. *Nature*, 592, 253–257.

Hoffmann, D. L., Standish, C. D., Garcia-Diez, M., Pettitt, P. B., Milton, J. A., Zilhao, J., Alcolea-Gonzalez, J. J., Cantalejo-Duarte, P., Collado, H., De Balbin, R., Lorblanchet, M., Ramos-Munoz, J., Weniger, G. C. and Pike, A. W. G. 2018. U–Th dating of carbonate crusts reveals Neandertal origin of Iberian cave art. *Science*, 359, 912–915.

Hsieh, P., Woerner, A. E., Wall, J. D., Lachance, J., Tishkoff, S. A., Gutenkunst, R. N. and Hammer, M. F. 2016. Model-based analyses of whole-genome data reveal a complex evolutionary history involving archaic introgression in Central African Pygmies. *Genome Res*, 26, 291–300.

Huerta-Sanchez, E., Jin, X., Asan, Bianba, Z., Peter, B. M., Vinckenbosch, N., Liang, Y., Yi, X., He, M., Somel, M., Ni, P.,

Wang, B., Ou, X., Huasang, Luosang, J., Cuo, Z. X., Li, K., Gao, G., Yin, Y., Wang, W., Zhang, X., Xu, X., Yang, H., Li, Y., Wang, J., Wang, J. and Nielsen, R. 2014. Altitude adaptation in Tibetans caused by introgression of Denisovan-like DNA. *Nature*, 512, 194–197.

Ingicco, T., Van Den Bergh, G. D., Jago-On, C., Bahain, J. J., Chacon, M. G., Amano, N., Forestier, H., King, C., Manalo, K., Nomade, S., Pereira, A., Reyes, M. C., Semah, A. M., Shao, Q., Voinchet, P., Falgueres, C., Albers, P. C. H., Lising, M., Lyras, G., Yurnaldi, D., Rochette, P., Bautista, A. and De Vos, J. 2018. Earliest known hominin activity in the Philippines by 709 thousand years ago. *Nature*, 557, 233–237.

Isler, K. and Van Schaik, C. P. 2012. How our ancestors broke through the gray ceiling: comparative evidence for cooperative breeding in early Homo. *Curr Anthropol*, 53, S453–S465.

Jacobs, G. S., Hudjashov, G., Saag, L., Kusuma, P., Darusallam, C. C., Lawson, D. J., Mondal, M., Pagani, L., Ricaut, F. X., Stoneking, M., Metspalu, M., Sudoyo, H., Lansing, J. S. and Cox, M. P. 2019. Multiple deeply divergent Denisovan ancestries in Papuans. *Cell*, 177, 1010–1021. e32.

Jegou, B., Sankararaman, S., Rolland, A. D., Reich, D. and Chalmel, F. 2017. Meiotic genes are enriched in regions of reduced archaic ancestry. *Mol Biol Evol*, 34, 1974–1980.

Johanson, D. C., Taieb, M. and Coppens, Y. 1982. Pliocene hominids from the Hadar Formation, Ethiopia (1 973–1 977): stratigraphic, chronologic, and paleoenvironmental contexts, with notes on hominid morphology and systematics. *Am J Phys Anthropol*, 57, 373–402.

Jungers, W. L., Harcourt-Smith, W. E., Wunderlich, R. E., Tocheri, M. W., Larson, S. G., Sutikna, T., Due, R. A. and Morwood, M. J. 2009. The foot of *Homo floresiensis*. *Nature*, 459, 81–84.

Karakostis, F. A., Haeufle, D., Anastopoulou, I., Moraitis, K., Hotz, G., Tourloukis, V. and Harvati, K. 2021. Biomechanics of the human thumb and the evolution of dexterity. *Curr Biol*, 31, 1317–1325.e8.

Kimbel, W. H., Lockwood, C. A., Ward, C. V., Leakey, M. G., Rak, Y. and Johanson, D. C. 2006. Was *Australopithecus anamensis* ancestral to *A. afarensis*? A case of anagenesis in the hominin fossil record. *J Hum Evol*, 51, 134–152.

Kivell, T. L., Deane, A. S., Tocheri, M. W., Orr, C. M., Schmid, P., Hawks, J., Berger, L. R. and Churchill, S. E. 2015. The hand of *Homo naledi*. *Nat Commun*, 6, 8431.

Lachance, J., Vernot, B., Elbers, C. C., Ferwerda, B., Froment, A., Bodo, J. M., Lema, G., Fu, W., Nyambo, T. B., Rebbeck, T. R., Zhang, K., Akey, J. M. and Tishkoff, S. A. 2012. Evolutionary history and adaptation from high-coverage whole-genome sequences of diverse African hunter-gatherers. *Cell*, 150, 457–469.

Latimer, B. and Lovejoy, C. O. 1989. The calcaneus of *Australopithecus afarensis* and its implications for the evolution of bipedality. *Am J Phys Anthropol*, 78, 369–386.

Leakey, L. S., Tobias, P. V. and Napier, J. R. 1964. A new species of the genus *Homo* from Olduvai Gorge. *Nature*, 202, 7–9.

Lewis, J. E. and Harmand, S. 2016. An earlier origin for stone tool making: implications for cognitive evolution and the transition to *Homo*. *Philos Trans R Soc Lond B Biol Sci*, 371, 20150233.

Linnaeus, C. 1735. *Systema naturae per regna tria naturae, secundum classes, ordines, genera, species cum characteribus, differentiis, synonymis, locis*. Stockholm: Laurentii Salvii.

Mcpherron, S. P., Alemseged, Z., Marean, C. W., Wynn, J. G., Reed, D., Geraads, D., Bobe, R. and Bearat, H. A. 2010. Evidence for stone-tool-assisted consumption of animal tissues before 3.39 million years ago at Dikika, Ethiopia. *Nature*, 466, 857–860.

Mondal, M., Bertranpetit, J. and Lao, O. 2019. Approximate Bayesian computation with deep learning supports a third archaic introgression in Asia and Oceania. *Nat Commun*, 10, 246.

Morgan, T. J., Uomini, N. T., Rendell, L. E., Chouinard-Thuly, L., Street, S. E., Lewis, H. M., Cross, C. P., Evans, C., Kearney, R., De La Torre, I., Whiten, A. and Laland, K. N. 2015. Experimental evidence for the co-evolution of hominin tool-making teaching and language. *Nat Commun*, 6, 6029.

Morwood, M. J., Soejono, R. P., Roberts, R. G., Sutikna, T., Turney, C. S., Westaway, K. E., Rink, W. J., Zhao, J. X., Van Den Bergh, G. D., Due, R. A., Hobbs, D. R., Moore, M. W., Bird, M. I. and Fifield, L. K. 2004. Archaeology and age of a new hominin from Flores in eastern Indonesia. *Nature*, 431, 1087–1091.

Pavlicev, M., Romero, R. and Mitteroecker, P. 2020. Evolution of the human pelvis and obstructed labor: new explanations of an old obstetrical dilemma. *Am J Obstet Gynecol*, 222, 3–16.

Plummer, T. 2004. Flaked stones and old bones: biological and cultural evolution at the dawn of technology. *Am J Phys Anthropol*, 125, 118–164.

Pobiner, B. L. 2020. The zooarchaeology and paleoecology of early hominin scavenging. *Evol Anthropol*, 29, 68–82.

Pobiner, B. L., Rogers, M. J., Monahan, C. M. and Harris, J.

W. 2008. New evidence for hominin carcass processing strategies at 1.5 Ma, Koobi Fora, Kenya. *J Hum Evol*, 55, 103–130.

Pontzer, H., Brown, M. H., Wood, B. M., Raichlen, D. A., Mabulla, A. Z. P., Harris, J. A., Dunsworth, H., Hare, B., Walker, K., Luke, A., Dugas, L. R., Schoeller, D., Plange-Rhule, J., Bovet, P., Forrester, T. E., Thompson, M. E., Shumaker, R. W., Rothman, J. M., Vogel, E., Sulistyo, F., Alavi, S., Prasetyo, D., Urlacher, S. S. and Ross, S. R. 2021. Evolution of water conservation in humans. *Curr Biol*, 31, 1804–1810.e5.

Portmann, A. 1990. *A Zoologist Looks at Humankind*. New York: Columbia University Press.

Raichlen, D. A., Armstrong, H. and Lieberman, D. E. 2011. Calcaneus length determines running economy: implications for endurance running performance in modern humans and Neandertals. *J Hum Evol*, 60, 299–308.

Reich, D., Green, R. E., Kircher, M., Krause, J., Patterson, N., Durand, E. Y., Viola, B., Briggs, A. W., Stenzel, U., Johnson, P. L., Maricic, T., Good, J. M., Marques-Bonet, T., Alkan, C., Fu, Q., Mallick, S., Li, H., Meyer, M., Eichler, E. E., Stoneking, M., Richards, M., Talamo, S., Shunkov, M. V., Derevianko, A. P., Hublin, J. J., Kelso, J., Slatkin, M. and Paabo, S. 2010. Genetic history of an archaic hominin group from Denisova Cave in Siberia. *Nature*, 468, 1053–1060.

Rizal, Y., Westaway, K. E., Zaim, Y., Van Den Bergh, G. D., Bettis, E. A., 3Rd, Morwood, M. J., Huffman, O. F., Grun, R., Joannes-Boyau, R., Bailey, R. M., Sidarto, Westaway, M. C., Kurniawan, I., Moore, M. W., Storey, M., Aziz, F., Suminto, Zhao, J. X., Aswan, Sipola, M. E., Larick, R., Zonneveld, J. P., Scott, R., Putt, S. and Ciochon, R. L. 2020. Last appearance of *Homo erectus* at Ngandong, Java,

117,000–108,000 years ago. *Nature*, 577, 381–385.

Rogers, A. R., Harris, N. S. and Achenbach, A. A. 2020. Neanderthal–Denisovan ancestors interbred with a distantly related hominin. *Sci Adv*, 6, eaay5483.

Shea, J. J. 2015. Making and using stone tools: advice for learners and teachers and insights for archaeologists. *Lithic Technol*, 40, 231–248.

Shea, J. J. 2017. Occasional, obligatory, and habitual stone tool use in hominin evolution. *Evol Anthropol*, 26, 200–217.

Slon, V., Mafessoni, F., Vernot, B., De Filippo, C., Grote, S., Viola, B., Hajdinjak, M., Peyregne, S., Nagel, S., Brown, S., Douka, K., Higham, T., Kozlikin, M. B., Shunkov, M. V., Derevianko, A. P., Kelso, J., Meyer, M., Prufer, K. and Paabo, S. 2018. The genome of the offspring of a Neanderthal mother and a Denisovan father. *Nature*, 561, 113–116.

Slon, V., Viola, B., Renaud, G., Gansauge, M. T., Benazzi, S., Sawyer, S., Hublin, J. J., Shunkov, M. V., Derevianko, A. P., Kelso, J., Prufer, K., Meyer, M. and Paabo, S. 2017. A fourth Denisovan individual. *Sci Adv*, 3, e1700186.

Smith, T. M., Tafforeau, P., Reid, D. J., Pouech, J., Lazzari, V., Zermeno, J. P., Guatelli-Steinberg, D., Olejniczak, A. J., Hoffman, A., Radovcic, J., Makaremi, M., Toussaint, M., Stringer, C. and Hublin, J. J. 2010. Dental evidence for ontogenetic differences between modern humans and Neanderthals. *PNAS*, 107, 20923–20928.

Spoor, F., Gunz, P., Neubauer, S., Stelzer, S., Scott, N., Kwekason, A. and Dean, M. C. 2015. Reconstructed *Homo habilis* type OH 7 suggests deep-rooted species diversity in early Homo. *Nature*, 519, 83–86.

Sutikna, T., Tocheri, M. W., Faith, J. T., Jatmiko, Due Awe, R., Meijer, H. J. M., Wahyu Saptomo, E. and Roberts, R. G. 2018. The spatio-temporal distribution of archaeological and faunal finds at Liang Bua (Flores, Indonesia) in light of the revised chronology for *Homo floresiensis*. *J Hum Evol*, 124, 52–74.

Sutikna, T., Tocheri, M. W., Morwood, M. J., Saptomo, E. W., Jatmiko, Awe, R. D., Wasisto, S., Westaway, K. E., Aubert, M., Li, B., Zhao, J. X., Storey, M., Alloway, B. V., Morley, M. W., Meijer, H. J., Van Den Bergh, G. D., Grun, R., Dosseto, A., Brumm, A., Jungers, W. L. and Roberts, R. G. 2016. Revised stratigraphy and chronology for *Homo floresiensis* at Liang Bua in Indonesia. *Nature*, 532, 366–369.

Teixeira, J. C., Jacobs, G. S., Stringer, C., Tuke, J., Hudjashov, G., Purnomo, G. A., Sudoyo, H., Cox, M. P., Tobler, R., Turney, C. S. M., Cooper, A. and Helgen, K. M. 2021. Widespread Denisovan ancestry in Island Southeast Asia but no evidence of substantial super-archaic hominin admixture. *Nat Ecol Evol*, 5, 616–624.

Trinkaus, E. and Villotte, S. 2017. External auditory exostoses and hearing loss in the Shanidar 1 Neandertal. *PLoS ONE*, 12, e0186684.

Vaesen, K., Dusseldorp, G. L. and Brandt, M. J. 2021. An emerging consensus in palaeoanthropology: demography was the main factor responsible for the disappearance of Neanderthals. *Sci Rep*, 11, 4925.

Van Den Bergh, G. D., Kaifu, Y., Kurniawan, I., Kono, R. T., Brumm, A., Setiyabudi, E., Aziz, F. and Morwood, M. J. 2016. *Homo floresiensis*-like fossils from the early Middle Pleistocene of Flores. *Nature*, 534, 245–248.

Vansickle, C., Cofran, Z. D. and Hunt, D. 2020. Did Neandertals have large brains? Factors affecting endocranial volume comparisons. *Am J Phys Anthropol*, 173, 768–775.

Vernot, B., Tucci, S., Kelso, J., Schraiber, J. G., Wolf, A. B., Gittelman, R. M., Dannemann, M., Grote, S., Mccoy, R. C., Norton, H., Scheinfeldt, L. B., Merriwether, D. A., Koki, G., Friedlaender, J. S., Wakefield, J., Paabo, S. and Akey, J. M. 2016. Excavating Neandertal and Denisovan DNA from the genomes of Melanesian individuals. *Science*, 352, 235–239.

Villmoare, B., Kimbel, W. H., Seyoum, C., Campisano, C. J., Dimaggio, E. N., Rowan, J., Braun, D. R., Arrowsmith, J. R. and Reed, K. E. 2015. Paleoanthropology. Early *Homo* at 2.8 Ma from Ledi-Geraru, Afar, Ethiopia. *Science*, 347, 1352–1355.

Viola, B., Gunz, P., Neubauer, S., Slon, V., Kozlikin, M. B.,

Shunkov, M. V., Mayer, M., Paabo, S. and Derevianko, A. P. 2019. A parietal fragment from Denisova cave. *Am J Phys Anthropol*, 168, 258.

Voisin, J.-L., Feuerriegel, E. M., Churchill, S. E. and Berger, L. R. 2020. The *Homo naledi* shoulder girdle: an adaptation to boulder climbing. *L'Anthropologie*, 124, 102783.

Welker, F., Ramos-Madrigal, J., Gutenbrunner, P., Mackie, M., Tiwary, S., Rakownikow Jersie-Christensen, R., Chiva, C., Dickinson, M. R., Kuhlwilm, M., De Manuel, M., Gelabert, P., Martinon-Torres, M., Margvelashvili, A., Arsuaga, J. I., Carbonell, E., Marques-Bonet, T., Penkman, K., Sabido, E., Cox, J., Olsen, J. V., Lordkipanidze, D., Racimo, F., Lalueza-Fox, C., Bermudez De Castro, J. M., Willerslev, E. and Cappellini, E. 2020. The dental proteome of

Homo antecessor. *Nature*, 580, 235–238.

Wells, J. C., Desilva, J. M. and Stock, J. T. 2012. The obstetric dilemma: an ancient game of Russian roulette, or a variable dilemma sensitive to ecology? *Am J Phys Anthropol*, 149, 40–71.

Wrangham, R. 2009. *Catching Fire. How Cooking Made Us Human.* London: Profile Books.

Zilhao, J., Angelucci, D. E., Igreja, M. A., Arnold, L. J., Badal, E., Callapez, P., Cardoso, J. L., D'Errico, F., Daura, J., Demuro, M., Deschamps, M., Dupont, C., Gabriel, S., Hoffmann, D. L., Legoinha, P., Matlas, H., Monge Soares, A. M., Nabais, M., Portela, P., Queffelec, A., Rodrigues, F. and Souto, P. 2020. Last Interglacial Iberian Neandertals as fisher-hunter-gatherers. *Science*, 367, eaaz7943.

Hominin Evolution II

Sapiens, *Masters of the Known Universe*

Derek K. Tracy

Abstract

Our immediate ancestry remains uncertain at this time, but what is clear is that we are all African. This chapter will start with the current debates on the emergence of *Homo sapiens* and the changes we see in the subsequent 200,000 years in terms of our behavioural and cultural development. We have already shown that the 'march of progress' image – so culturally famous from t-shirts to posters – of a line of ever more upright and 'civilised' walking ape-to-man creatures is wrong. There has never been a single line, and we are not the apotheosis of evolution. A second myth is that 'we evolved' 200,000–300,000 years ago and since then have been static, with only technology progressing. However, humans have continued to change with time. The third conceit is the focus on 'our' move 'out of Africa' 50,000–60,000 years ago. This idea is problematic: it culturally assumes a non-African terminus as our destiny and is a very Eurocentric view of the world. It is true that a subpopulation of hunter-gather *sapiens*, most likely Yoruba peoples from around what is now Tanzania, left that continent at around that time, and from that group the rest of the world's populations emerge. But this is to downplay the fact that for 80% of our species' existence we have all been entirely African, and a genetically small subgroup left for the last 20% of that time. History is written by the 'victors', and much anthropology has been written by Western academia. In 2020, it was estimated that fewer than 2% of whole sequenced genomes have as yet come from Africa (Maxmen, 2020), and we lack ancient DNA from Africa greater than 15,000 years old (partially due to climactic reasons). However, the tide has begun to turn, and the next 10 years look very exciting in this regard.

Keywords

brain evolution, grandmother hypothesis, language origins, recent African origin, social brain hypothesis

Ex Africa semper aliquid novi [Out of Africa there is always something new]
—*Pliny the Elder*

Key Points

- Genetic data indicate *Homo sapiens* emerged between 250,000 and 350,000 years ago in Africa, but there is likely no single 'birthplace of humanity'.
- Contemporary data do not support rapid biological changes driving an apparent 'behavioural modernity' in the past 50,000 years.
- The social brain hypothesis, grandmother hypothesis and hunting hypothesis are

complementary models describing the emerging complexity in *Homo sapiens*.

4.1 Our African Origins

4.1.1 The Emergence of *Sapiens*

Homo sapiens had, for some time, an estimated upper age of about 200,000 years, but the astonishing find at Jebel Irhoud in the 1960s, when re-dated in 2017, pushed this back to 315,000 years (Hublin et al., 2017). There is no definitive model on the emergence of *sapiens*, though several hypotheses exist. Henn et al. (2018) summarised the major possible hypotheses, none of which has universal support. The first is 'African multiregionalism', with different populations arising in parallel across different sites and with interbreeding between them. The others posit a single group emerging and dominating and replacing other subpopulations, with differing levels of gene flow between them. At this time, the evidence suggests that there was not a single 'birthplace of humanity', but rather the emergence of a mosaic 'meta-population' across the entire continent from diverse, interbreeding populations (Scerri et al., 2019).

Using mitochondrial DNA (mtDNA), which has a solely maternal inheritance, the landmark paper by Cann et al. in *Nature* (1987) established the first human genetic tree and the famous 'mitochondrial Eve', or so-called mother of all *sapiens*, dating back to about 200,000 years ago in Africa. There was clearly not a 'single mother' of us all: most ancestors do not leave a genetic trace, and 'Eve' is a useful marker but not the 'first' actual human. The most ancient mtDNA haplotype, 'L', is found in most African populations: the oldest sub-branch, L_0, occurs in the Khoisan people of southern Africa, L_1 in central and West Africans and L_2 – the most common type – in west and south-eastern Africa. L_3, widespread across sub-Saharan Africa, led to the most recent 'M' and 'N' haplotypes found in non-Africans.

mtDNA work is inherently limited, and subsequent exploration included the more complex Y chromosome and autosomal DNA lineages. Y chromosome work tracks male populations, adding in the complicating though sociologically interesting variance in mating patterns between men and women.[1] However, the richest data come from whole-genome autosomal DNA, though it has only been in the last decade that technological advances have made this approach both rapid and cheap, allowing estimation of common ancestry back several million years. This approach estimates the first modern human emergence at 260,000–350,000 years ago. The San/Khoisan

people of southern Africa show the most ancient ancestry, diverging from other branches starting perhaps 150,000–200,000 years ago (Gronau et al., 2011). Indeed, for most of our existence, they have been the largest human population on Earth (Kim et al., 2014), and they show the greatest genetic diversity of any people: for almost as long as there have been *Homo sapiens*, there have been the San – may that always be so.

4.1.2 'Out of Africa'

The third great human migration from Africa (following *Homo erectus* and later the Neanderthal/Denisovan ancestor) was the spread of *sapiens* around the world, facilitated via ecologically very different grasslands: 'green Sahara' (Blanchet et al., 2021) and 'green Arabia' (Roberts et al., 2018). The famous Skhul and Qafzeh fossils show evidence of *sapiens* in what is now Israel by 100,000 years ago, but current thinking is that excursions prior to about 65,000 years ago were smaller and non-ancestral. The main exodus, which might have involved just a few thousand people, occurred at about 60,000–65,000 years ago from a group of Yoruba people that would become the ancestors of all non-Africans. These lineages show a very considerable population bottlenecking, and non-Africans are essentially a small genetic subset of those whose ancestors remained on the continent (Skoglund et al., 2017).

Some *sapiens* migrated east, meeting and mating with Denisovans on the way. There was a northern route avoiding the Himalayas to northern China and Mongolia (Zwyns et al., 2019). Some fossils in China have been dated to 80,000–120,000 years old (Liu et al., 2015), but more recent analysis indicates a more modest figure closer to 45,000–50,000 years of age might be more accurate (Sun et al., 2021). *Sapiens* may have made it to Australia by 65,000 years ago (Clarkson et al., 2017), though this figure, which is based on the stratigraphy of stone tool assemblages, is not without challenge, with genetic data from Aboriginal Australasians suggesting a founding population closer to 32,000 years ago. These timings are not irreconcilable if the earlier dispersal is due to a non-ancestral group that died out.

Fascinatingly, given its far greater proximity, the move into Europe is relatively more recent, occurring about 45,000 years ago (Hublin et al.,

---

[1] The 'Genghis Khan lineage' is interesting in this regard: it has been shown that perhaps 8% of men in Asia (0.5% worldwide) have a lineage tracking back to around 1,000 years ago in Mongolia. This is considered to be an outcome of Khan's conquering and pillaging of huge swathes of that part of the world, fathering enormous numbers of children on the way (as did his immediate male descendants) (Zerjal et al., 2003).

2020). It is not clear whether the Neanderthal presence in Europe had a chilling impact on the initial migrations of *sapiens* there. Interestingly, it is perhaps only in the last 8,000 years, or about 3% of human existence, that a Eurasian subpopulation first evolved depigmented ('white') skin (Mathieson et al., 2015; see also Chapter 2 of this volume).

4.2 Cognitive Changes

As we move beyond 'bones and stones', it becomes a challenge to try to inferentially interpret cognitive, behavioural and social interactions from archaeological finds. There are risks in assigning meaning that may be biased by our current societal practices or thoughts, or by assuming that modern hunter-gatherers necessarily behave exactly as our ancestors did.

Much evidence points towards an apparent change in *sapiens* about 50,000 years ago, with a blossoming of cultural artefacts, often referenced as 'behavioural modernity': an emergence of planned funerals and burial goods; huts for different activities such as tool making, food preparation and sleeping; long-distance transport of valuable materials such as amber and beads; more complex food gathering such as fishing nets; and higher population densities. The question arises as to why this change occurred. A potential answer, notably advanced by Klein (1995), is a rapid change in brain structure, perhaps through a fortuitous genetic mutation, quickly transmitted through sexual selection. One such candidate, *FOXP2*, has been linked with the emergence of language and subsequently far greater symbolic expression.

However, there are strong counterarguments. As noted by Powell et al. (2009), Henrich's transmission model has demonstrated that a critical population mass or density optimises the attainment of new knowledge (see also Chapter 1 of this volume on cumulative cultural evolution). Earlier developments might have been lost in small population groups with solely oral transmission of knowledge, which are vulnerable to population crashes. Fitting with this, many of the technologies postulated to have suddenly emerged were actually present in African societies tens of thousands of years earlier, from long-distance trade through blade technology to systematic use of art and decoration (McBrearty and Brooks,

2000). Intentional collection of non-utilitarian objects (crystals and ostrich shells) have been dated to 105,000 years ago (Wilkins et al., 2021); a 100,000-year-old ochre-processing workshop has been described in South Africa (Henshilwood et al., 2011); and the rich Panga ya Saidi cave site in Kenya has abundant collections of cultural and technological innovations dating back 78,000 years (d'Errico et al., 2020). The protected cave location of the latter is perhaps telling: Africa's climates are less helpful for archaeological and fossil preservation than, say, the Siberian plateaus. Much evidence is likely lost, and as mentioned elsewhere, historically, there has often been less focus on even searching for such evidence across the vast African continent.

Genetic data are perhaps the strongest rebuttal to the suggestions of a recent rapid biological 'switch'. *Sapiens* populations began to separate from each other at least 160,000 years ago, yet any crucial behavioural changes appear universal in all *sapiens* populations. The current evidence shows perhaps more convincingly that 50,000 years ago marks a demographic moment and a critical mass for the rapid spreading of technology, demonstrating the pivotal role of cultural evolution in the history of *sapiens* (see Chapter 1).

4.2.1 Anatomical Brain Changes

Studying brain changes over evolutionary time is challenging: soft tissue does not usually fossilise; cranial fossil numbers are small and fragmentary; we can only judge superficial brain shapes that might be secondary to cranial constraints; and size is not the sole marker of complexity. However, one can make inferential approaches along several lines: allometric (disproportionate growth of particular regions) sulcal pattern changes; associated cultural evidence from archaeological digs; and cross-comparisons of ontological development *in utero* with other species (sometimes called 'evo-devo').

The vertebrate brain has a widely conserved morphogenetic plan, particularly across subcortical structures such as the brainstem, cerebellum, hypothalamus, olfactory bulb and mesencephalon/midbrain, including the basal ganglia, thalamus and so forth (Karten, 2015). Primate volumetric analysis shows that the human limbic system is considerably larger than predicted even when adjusted for brain volume (Barger et al.,

2014), speaking to the fact that emotional and memory processing became ever more important to us as we evolved.

The mammalian six-layered neocortex represents a critical break from other animal classes (Hughlings Jackson, 1884), emerging in the Triassic–Jurassic. Much is common across mammals, with grey matter being about 70–80% excitatory glutamatergic and most of the rest being inhibitory GABAergic neurons modulating efficient cortical processing. Interestingly, our cortex is only about twice as thick as that of a mouse – growth in surface area, not depth, underlies hominin brain expansion. Gyrencephaly – folding of the cortex into gyri and sulci – is a phylogenetically ancient feature from an early mammalian ancestor (Sun and Hevner, 2014). Our pyramidal projection neurons are larger, with more complex dendritic arborisation and density of spines (Sousa et al., 2017) and more short-range cortico-cortical connections from layers II and III than in other primates (van den Heuvel et al., 2016).

Developmentally, the radial unit hypothesis proposes a mechanism for translating neuron proliferation into forming parcellated ontogenetic columns (Rakic, 1988), with species-specific functionally distinct regions regulated by patterning centres that secrete signalling molecules (Rakic, 2009). The evolutionary growth in the convoluted cortical surface area has required ever greater connectivity and patterns of connections between regions (Krubitzer and Kaas, 2005). However, there are also dangers that, without effective organisation, growth in neuron numbers and connections could reduce brain efficiency (Hofman, 2001).

The neocortex arises from the pallium, and ancient mutations in secreted morphogens have produced a wide range of adaptive changes in its size and organisation, to the point that we have over three times as many neurons as extant great apes. Increased neocortical volumes and surface areas are particularly related to the growth in progenitor cells during development, especially in the outer subventricular zone (OSVZ), which directs migrating neuron trajectory and increases neuron numbers (Lui et al., 2011). The OSVZ in primates is different from all other animals in that it has a much greater diversity of precursors, with unique cell-cycle regulatory loops, including crucial intermediate progenitor cells that contribute

enormously to radial expansion and gyrification (Vasistha et al., 2015). Ultimately, these considerably influence the positions, lamination and connectivity of neurons (Garcia-Moreno and Molnar, 2020). Early primates showed significant growth of visual and somatosensory association cortices, with an allometric growth in size and cellular density of the frontal and parietal areas (Collins et al., 2010), in particular deep layer III pyramidal neurons that form complex connections with other brain areas and are essential to cognitive functioning (Molnar et al., 2019).

The genetics of the prefrontal cortex (PFC) have shone a focus particularly upon epigenetics and promotor regions that expand the neocortex and increase neuronal spinal density. Segmental duplications (SDs) have occurred in a non-random manner in our evolutionary lineage, and SDs show greater differences in content and structure between us and extant great apes than other regions (Dennis and Eichler, 2016). Recent examples include: the *ARHGAP11B* gene, which has been shown to increase the number of basal radial glia progenitors and upper-layer neurons and to induce PFC folding (Heide et al., 2020); and the determination that some transcription factor binding sites, which regulate neuronal gene expression, have been highly conserved from an evolutionary perspective (Liu and Robinson-Rechavi, 2020). Work on brain organoids has shown that the ZEB2 epithelial–mesenchymal transition regulator promotes neuroepithelial transition and the acquisition of a human-like architecture compared with extant apes (Benito-Kwiecinski et al., 2021).

It is difficult to recognise specialist developments in early hominin brains. Recent work has shown that *Australopithecus afarensis* endocasts sulcal imprints were very ape-like, though comparison across ages shows more protracted brain growth, implying longer childhoods (Gunz et al., 2020). Early *Homo* species similarly retained a more primitive, ape-like organisation within their frontal lobes, but later *erectus*, from about 1.5 Ma, demonstrates changes, particularly in Broca's cap and the posterior parietal and occipital cortices (Ponce de Leon et al., 2021). Broca's cap is a fronto-orbital bulge with different underlying areas in *sapiens* and extant great apes: for us, it is a neurofunctional substrate for social cognition, tool making and language production and comprehension. Thus, the reorganisation of the frontal lobe appears to be a relatively late development, challenging the view that our current brain structure emerged with the first *Homo* species. There appear to be few obvious differences between *erectus* and *heidelbergensis* beyond an isometric growth in size (Bruner et al., 2015).

Neanderthals' brains have wider frontal and parietal lobes (though *not* greater in volume) and larger occipital cortices (Bruner, 2021); *sapiens*, meanwhile, have comparatively longer and larger temporal lobes, larger cerebella and expanded orbitofrontal cortices (Eisova et al., 2019). Both have (differential) enlargement of their parietal lobes over earlier hominins, an area that has crucial sensorimotor integrative functions. The medial and superior parietal lobes of *sapiens* are relatively large (Bruner et al., 2003) and with more connections with the frontal and temporal lobes (Preuss, 2017) than Neanderthals, though there is no current evidence of distinguishing lobe reorganisation between the two species (Bruner, 2018). The parietal lobes are notably connected with language and (particularly the precuneus) visuospatial and integrative processing. Whilst we cannot know how these changes differentially impacted Neanderthals' cognitive functioning, it has been argued (see Section 4.3.1) that the relative reduction in the orbitofrontal cortex in particular might have limited some of their social functioning in comparison with *sapiens*.

4.2.2 Language

We do not know when language emerged; it 'fossilises' only through writing. There are different streams of enquiry into this, from linguistic approaches that can track language families' divergence in a manner akin to genetic approaches through to anthropological approaches that look for proxy markers. There are about 7,000 extant languages, down from possibly 20,000 at the start of the Neolithic (Pagel, 2000). We are familiar with clustered language 'families' (e.g. Romance, Germanic) and how words can be similar in different tongues. Some 'primal' words, such as 'mother', appear to have great commonality, with Swadesh (1952) first proposing a (now heavily critiqued) 'fundamental vocabulary' of perhaps 200 very slowly changing words. As well as phonemes and word meaning (vocabulary), languages can be compared via grammar and semantic structure, such as variance in the sentence ordering of subject–verb–object. However appealing, tracing backwards via linguistics has been argued to have an information ceiling of about 6,000–10,000 years (Greenhill et al., 2010). Baker et al. (2017) compared the genomic data of almost 6,000 individuals from 282 global samples with language families; their data support 21 historical ancestries independent of self-identified ethnolinguistic labels. These largely map onto known genetic migration patterns, and again southern African languages, and specifically the Khoisan languages, appear to be most ancient.

One can speculate on the iterative steps in language origins from the various calls we see in primates through more complex protolanguages of increasing complexity and how various co-evolving processes such as group hunting and tool making would favour selection for greater social communicative skills. Such skills require physical control of the larynx, mouth, tongue and diaphragm through to cognitive aspects of reception, understanding and replicating sounds, semantics and syntax, which could have evolved in a gradual manner (Jarvis, 2019). It is hard to imagine that Australopithecines had anything less than the communication repertoire seen in contemporary great apes, and some have argued that protolanguages may have emerged by *erectus*, but we cannot be sure. Although Neanderthals' inner ears were different from ours, modelling has shown that their 'occupied bandwidth', which is directly related to vocal communication efficiency, was very similar to *sapiens*, implying that they at least had the auditory physiology to support speech equivalent to ours (Conde-Valverde et al., 2021). Certainly, language must have been present for all of the 'behavioural modernism' of the last 50,000 years, as many such behaviours involve the types of symbolism that require explanation and storytelling.[2]

---

[2] Readers may be familiar with the debated concept of 'universal grammar' first proposed by Noam Chomsky in the 1960s. It argues that syntactic knowledge is innate from birth, with children just needing to learn their language-specific rules and vocabulary thereafter. Controversially for evolutionists, Chomsky saw no real role for evolutionary processes in sculpting this. Much cross-disciplinary academic ink has been spilt on the topic.

Several candidate elements of a protolanguage have been proposed. Laughter is seen in primates at play; it is a teeth-baring activity, and humour and laughter might have been a mechanism of sublimating aggression. It is also a contagious, endorphin-releasing group activity that reinforces social bonding (see Chapter 13). 'Motherese', the universal song-like cooing mothers and infants share, might be another, arising from strategies to help reassure, silence and control the behaviours of infants unable to cling to their mothers' bodies (Falk, 2004). Dunbar (2016) advanced this with *gossip* being a sophisticated way to replace peer grooming and to enhance social ties. A neat experiment by Redhead and Dunbar (2013) tested different functions of language to see which were more easily recalled and hence might be deeper and stronger underpinnings of its evolutionary selection. Participants were told short stories that differentially involved social relationships ('gossip'), social contracts (declarative information) and complexity (the 'Scheherazade' sexual selection hypothesis of language projecting intelligence to potential mates); gossip was best recalled, implying – the authors propose – its deeper root in language evolution and selection.

The *FOXP2* gene has attracted much debate since 2001 when a rare mutation in a large, three-generation British family resulted in normal-range intelligence but considerable deficits of receptive–expressive language and grammar (Lai et al., 2001). The gene is ancient and shared by many species; however, mouse data show that *FOXP2* deletions in the key speech regions of the cortex, striatum and cerebellum are not enough to explain the vocalisation deficits found, implying that the gene's effects might be mediated by other anatomical regions necessary for vocalising (Urbanus et al., 2020).

4.3 Behavioural Changes

4.3.1 The Social Brain Hypothesis (and Grandmothers)

Grooming is the primary hominid behaviour for group cohesion, releasing reinforcing endorphins, including oxytocin; as group sizes increase, so does the amount of time spent grooming and ensuring group stability. Our faces show evolutionary changes linked to prosociality: decreases in canine sizes; the sclerae of our eyes becoming white to highlight where we are looking (other primates have brown sclerae); and emotion-displaying eyebrows.

The cultural or social brain hypothesis states that growing social requirements were a strong evolutionary driver for our enlarging brains – more than a 'general intelligence' need – and that these emerge early in human ontogeny. Herrmann et al. (2007) showed that children as young as 2.5 years old have more sophisticated cognitive skills than adult primates in dealing with the social world. Originally proposed by Byrne and Whiten (1988), but considerably expanded upon and popularised by Dunbar (1998), the social brain hypothesis robustly links brain volumes with social functioning, including the size of social groups. Dunbar's work notes how much time hominids have to allocate to different daily tasks, including feeding, travel, sleeping and social bonding; with the growth in calorie-rich meat eating, especially once the meat is cooked, more time was released for this last aspect. This links with the interplaying increase in brain volumes to manage these ever more complex social behaviours and groups. *Dunbar's number* is the maximum size of a group that an individual can successfully interact with whilst maintaining stable social functioning and relationships. For contemporary *sapiens*, this is about 150 (West et al., 2020), nesting within bigger and more distant social circles of several communities that might identify as a wider clan that occasionally comes together in groups of, say, 500 or so (e.g. at feasts) and broader self-identifying tribal groups of perhaps 1,500 or so individuals whose faces we can put names to (Hamilton et al., 2007). The nesting can be reversed to layers of 'intimate friends' (n = 5), 'best friends' (n = 15) and 'good friends' (n = 50), and the amount of social capital expended is related to the intimacy of the grouping (Dunbar, 2016). Larger networks clearly offer societal protection and support but practically require work and cognitive load to manage. Interestingly, the calculated 'Dunbar number' is lower for Neanderthals and *heidelbergensis*, implying that their social groups were about a third smaller and less complex than ours.

The growth in hominin socialisation can be linked with the development of greater abilities of mentalising – the recursive understanding of another's intent. This can be measured more formally by orders or degrees of intentionality (Dennett, 1983).[3] We see a growth in the degrees of intentionality that can be held in terms of ontogenesis across the lifespan (attaining 'theory of mind' being indeed a childhood test), as well as – putatively – through phylogenesis across our ancestry. This is processed by the orbito- and dorsomedial prefrontal cortices (Jamali et al., 2021), though a wide network is involved, including the temporal and parietal cortices (Barrett et al., 2003; Koster-Hale and Saxe, 2013), and higher-order intentionality tasks have been shown to be cognitively more demanding than 'factual' ones (Lewis et al., 2017).

If we take extant hominids, there is a linear relationship between frontal cortex volume and degree of intentionality that can be held in mind (and group size that can be maintained). In particular, the orbitofrontal cortex appears key, with volume across different species mediating social cognitive skills and network sizes (Powell et al., 2012) (though at the individual level there have been fewer supporting data that this holds for variance between people; Lin et al., 2020). Dunbar (2016) proposed that extrapolating this to hominin cranial endocasts would have Australopithecines attaining at most second-order intentionality (similar to the great apes today), with erectus at third-order intentionality and subsequent hominins, including Neanderthals and heidelbergensis, likely maximally at fourth-order intentionality: sapiens alone appears to reach fifth-order intentionality and beyond. If correct – and Dunbar acknowledged the limitations of applying this to extinct species – this alters some

of the debate on language from 'when did it first arise?' and 'which species could talk?' to considering the nature and complexity of any language. Fifth-order mentalisation and metacognition would provide an animal – sapiens – with far more nuanced abilities to consider deeper and more profound aspects of its environment and interactions with others.

Sapiens spent the first 95% of our existence as hunter-gatherers until the Neolithic ushered in the Agricultural Revolution at the beginning of the Holocene. Work on contemporary !Kung hunter-gatherers in southern Africa has shown how important night-time fireside conversations are: they shift from economic matters and gossip more commonly seen during the day to singing, dancing and storytelling about known people (Wiessner, 2014). Wiessner argued that such night talk invokes higher orders of mentalising through imaginative evocations of virtual 'big picture' communities, and that this assists in important regional-level processes such as cooperation and trust between tribes.

Hunter-gatherer societies show unique cultural transmission and cooperation with non-kin groups not seen in any other species, including cooperative group acquisition and sharing of food, significant alloparental care and maintenance of living spaces. This facilitates longer juvenile development, later sexual maturity and fecundity and larger numbers surviving to adulthood and post-reproductive ages. Interestingly, work by Hill et al. (2011) evaluating contemporary hunter-gatherer societies suggests that close groups are typically made up of individuals either distantly related or not related at all, not the patrilocal bands of close kin often assumed. They argue that the unique group selection undergone by sapiens may have spread innovations, cooperative institutions and prosocial, social learning mechanisms, and that modelling suggests that these are required to support large interaction networks.

Several other behavioural aspects of sapiens are comparatively 'abnormal': our early weaning age, late first reproduction, short inter-birth intervals (a female chimpanzee can only rear a new child about every six years) and long lifespan beyond reproductive years (Smith et al., 2010; Williams, 1957). These issues are combined in the 'grandmother hypothesis' (Hawkes, 2020). Data on contemporary hunter-gatherer societies

---

[3] For example, consider if you and I were conversing together: 'I hope you found my book chapters interesting' might be my second-order intentionality musing (as I try to 'read your mind' while we discuss evolutionary psychiatry). 'It seems to me he is wondering if I found his boring discursive footnotes interesting' could be your third-order intentionality thought (note how you are now anticipating my thoughts of you). 'I think that patently disinterested person has figured out that Derek is trying to establish if he was intrigued by the anecdote of the Ebu Gogo in the last chapter' might be fourth-order intentionality contemplated by Drs Abed and St John-Smith, the editors of this volume, as they watched what was happening. Indeed, you are now utilising fifth-degree intentionality in holding all of these people and permutations in your head!

show that older women have enormous productivity, facilitating alloparenting and allowing daughters to focus on having more children. From an evolutionary perspective, the grandmother is supporting her own genes and also selecting for female longevity, which may explain their typically longer lives over less essential grandfathers. This is presented as an alternative to the 'hunting hypothesis' predicated on primarily male provisioning of food. Such hunting is a rich but erratic and unreliable food source, with high rates of failure – perhaps less than 4% of hunts result in large carcass acquisitions (Hawkes et al., 2001). This is a rich bounty when it occurs, often being shared between a community, but female gathering is a far more reliable 'income' for families; further, the tubers commonly found in this way are typically easily turned into starchy pastes that can support weaning infants. In reality, however, the two hypotheses are not mutually exclusive. Human behavioural ecological research has emphasised how flexibility and adaptability are the keys to hunter-gatherer societies. It is seductively easy to take contemporary southern African populations and ethnographically project a continuous model back over 200,000 years. However, there are hunter-gatherer societies that have attained most of their caloric intakes from red meat, from fish and from non-meat-based foods. From the Arctic to the Equator, *sapiens'* greatness has been in its ability to master all domains. Ethnographic data do, however, align with the Dunbar number: populations of 25–30, with 4–7 active hunters, appear optimal for maintaining adequate hunting returns whilst having a surrounding environment adequate for localised foraging. Once groups exceed this, pressures on gathering foods within a reasonable radius from home are unsustainable.

Once hominids begin to form groups, they tend to form either alpha-male harem societies or monogamous ones.[4] Data from 230 primate species have suggested that the most compelling argument for the emergence of social monogamy

is male infanticide (Opie et al., 2013). Infanticide is common amongst primates, as it will return a female to a fertile state. The long period of care required by our infants has made them especially vulnerable to infanticide, but bi-parental care significantly reduces this, increasing the likelihood of an individual infant's survival and of the rearing of a greater number of them (and thus perpetuating genes associating with male care behaviour and monogamy). Monogamous pair-bonded animals have larger brains than those that are not, likely due to the cognitive and social demands on the brain, and Dunbar has argued that 'there is no route out of monogamy' once a species has adopted it due to the evolutionary pressures that got it there in the first instance. An interesting addendum to human mating has been the question as to why, atypically for primates, female ovulation is concealed. The long-dominant 'male investment hypothesis' argued that this was to ensure continued investment and support from males in phases when women were not fertile. More recent analysis better supports a 'female rivalry' hypothesis (Krems et al., 2021), arguing that concealed ovulation minimises aggression from other women and enhances intra-sexual social relationships.

Baron-Cohen (2020) has recently argued that a less appreciated aspect of our cognitive development has been our ability to see patterns and draw inferences from these. He proposes that these 'if-and-then' algorithms allowed us to problem solve with systemising that ultimately led to the invention of (as an exceptional example) agriculture and that underpins philosophical and scientific thinking (see Chapter 1). Data from the UK Brain Types Study have shown a normal distribution for the so-called Systemizing Quotient (SQ) and a separate phenomenon for the Empathy Quotient (EQ) (Greenberg et al., 2018), together demonstrating different emergent personality patterns.

4.3.2 Art and Culture

The oldest human art yet identified comes from Blombos Cave in South Africa, where an ochre crayon etched a hatched symbol onto rock 73,000 years ago (Henshilwood et al., 2011). Much cave art has been found across all continents, and no doubt much remains to be discovered: accurate dating is a challenge, not least as the materials used to make the art (e.g. charcoal) might be far

---

[4] Gorillas provide an interesting counterpoint to humans. They have both male protection/monogamy and harem groups. It would seem that the sexual dimorphism of this species, with males being so much larger than females, may perpetuate this. This is not typically seen in primates with less dimorphism.

older than the image created. However, transmission of cultural knowledge appears to be a uniquely human attribute (Csibra, 2007).

In 1940, a dog, Robot, stumbled into a cave at Lascaux in the Dordogne, France. As his owners followed him in, they found hundreds of ancient images in what would become the most famous site of cave art. Against a white calcite background were horses, bulls (aurochs) and deer on a huge scale (one bull is over five metres long). This art was commenced about 17,000 years ago, and it involves a succession of paintings over many generations. Older discovered European art includes that from Chauvet in France and El Castillo in Spain, dated at over 30,000 years old, and both are notable for their many animal outlines. More recently, pieces of cave art at least 40,000 years old from Borneo and 44,000–45,000 years old from Sulawesi in Indonesia have been identified as the oldest currently known *narrative* art, with scenes including a 4.5-metre-long pig and buffalo hunt and drawings of warty pigs (Aubert et al., 2019; Brumm et al., 2021). As well as their antiquity, their importance is due to them upending the idea that figurative art necessarily began in Europe.

Both the Lascaux and Sulawesi sites have human figures with animal traits, such as a human with a bird's head in the former and humans with tails and snouts in the latter. It is clearly impossible to know what the artists were thinking, but they are conceiving of things that do not exist, implying mythologies, belief in the supernatural and storytelling. This is amplified by the consideration of the cave sites and attempting to imagine what these sites meant to our ancient ancestors. Without natural light, they were illuminated by fire hearths on the floor or lamps, the flickers creating shadows and movement, the caves echoing sounds. Of the cave in Lascaux, Picasso said 'they've invented everything'.

The sites are commonly very deep in caves, beyond where one would expect humans to live; they appear almost intentionally difficult to access (though it is possible that only art in such inaccessible places survives). Certainly, they were found and created through intentional exploration and deposition, and it required planning and effort to source and bring in the necessary equipment such as pigments, which sometimes came from many kilometres away. These must have had importance and meaning to the people

of the time, and many of the caves' paintings have been shown to have been painted across millennia, demonstrating these caves' long-term significance as cultural hubs. One possible explanation for this is that, like other Palaeolithic monuments, they served as aggregation sites and events, bringing together disparate populations separated for periods of the year due to hunting expeditions on propitious occasions to mix and to share knowledge and stories, and providing opportunities for mating across groups (Clottes, 2016).

The Aurignacian period of about 35,000–43,000 years ago shows some of the oldest flourishing of *sapiens'* culture, with figurative art, musical instruments and personal ornaments often intricately carved from bone and ivory and often coloured with iron oxide red ochre (Velliky et al., 2021). Female 'Venus' figurines occurred from about 30,000 years ago all across Europe, from southern Spain to Siberia.

4.4 Conclusion: *Ecce Homo* – Behold the Man

What a piece of work is a man! How noble in reason, how infinite in faculty! In form and moving how express and admirable! In action how like an angel, in apprehension how like a god! The beauty of the world. The paragon of animals. And yet, to me, what is this quintessence of dust?
—Hamlet, *II, ii, William Shakespeare*

And so we have this magnificent, ultimate generalist. Neither the fastest nor the strongest, yet able to live and thrive in every environment on the planet, utilising any and all resources and foods it can find. Our incredible bodies, born to run, to hunt and to gather. Beautifully evolved to prioritise the calorie-richest foods, to store excess energy as fat on the occasions we managed to obtain it, to rid ourselves of expensive muscle when we were not using it and to rest when we could. Our incredible minds, seeing patterns and connections everywhere, seeking and embracing the company of others, the telling of tales and the metacognitive imagining of things that had not been, stamped by language, art and culture. A ranging, enquiring animal that could foresee its own death and consider life beyond it.

I sometimes imagine *sapiens* just before the Neolithic Agricultural Revolution, so like us in every way – enjoying the draw of a fire, with food, at night, and storytelling, dance and feasting. We are drawn to these still. The great questioner, the social animal, in a limitless world of mystery, intrigue and dangers. Why did the sun rise and fall and influence the growth of plants and food? What were the stars that moved silently through the sky and the planets that wandered[5] between them? What had happened to our relatives who had died, or what would happen to our children in the future? What excitement and wonder when they met an outside group, tried to communicate and exchanged and bartered goods, hearing tales of other lands and frightening beasts. As metaphorical orphans on a planet unknowable in scale and scope, how could we not answer the mysteries of life and our world through storytelling and imagination, captured in our early art and cultural artefacts. How could we not link coincidences, climactic and environmental occurrences as causal in life events and meanings?

I have questioned how close I could ever really come to appreciating their world when watching a London sunrise from my sheltered existence where water boils at the click of a switch to infuse coffee beans flown halfway around a planet in an apartment of instant light and heat. Yet they were simply us: they loved and laughed and fought and forgave and worried and cared. They shared every emotion you have ever felt, from guilt and despair to joy and ecstasy. I am reminded of James Joyce's line in *Ulysses* where Stephen Dedalus says, 'Famine, plague, and slaughters. Their blood is in me, their lusts my waves' (Joyce, 1922).

Richard Dawkins noted that every living organism can trace its origin, in a clear sequence, straight back to that last universal common ancestor, LUCA. Clear differences between species only occur over considerable periods of time, but these have, perhaps misleadingly, been our focus. Instead, the emerging picture is of fuzzy, gradual changes over time – sometimes so distinct that a new name is applied – with a consistent picture of the interbreeding of similar groups.

I predict that across the next 10–20 years a revolution in genomics will rewrite much of this history. It will change our understanding of the 'muddle in the Middle Pleistocene', clarifying *sapiens*' emergence and helping us better understand that 80% of our common history when we all lived in Africa. There are limits to DNA survival to perhaps 1 Ma, and thus we are unlikely to ever have, for example, direct Australopithecine genetic material. However, this might be replaced by the growth in importance of proteomics and ancient protein analysis: proteins, those transcribed outputs of DNA, are often quite rugged and enduring, and their changes over time can also be measured (Hendy, 2021).

Our erstwhile preponderance of fossil findings in caves and sites such as the Great Rift Valley is not accidental. These preserve via climate or sediment, and much has been lost – and, just perhaps, hidden – elsewhere. I am reminded of the joke about a drunk man found looking for his keys under a street light by a passing policeman; the policeman asks him where he lost them, and the man replies, 'In the park, but the lighting is better here'. Our myth of 'cavemen' comes from findings in caves: a future species might just as well consider that contemporary humans all appeared to live in graveyards. But palaeoanthropology is shifting focus. Eastwards, there is much current interest in Denisovans, where much is yet to be discovered. Equally, focus is shifting towards our African home, where to date only approximately 10% of sites with stone tools have any fossils. South East Asia has shown itself to be a hotbed of hominin diversity, and new island finds seem inevitable.

It is not currently clear whether, with time, we will more generally consider Neanderthals and Denisovans to be 'fully human' in the sense of being a diverse part of a broader *sapiens* grouping rather than a different species. The answer is as likely to be a cultural and philosophical one as much as a genetic or palaeoanthropological one. The technical aspects of this are likely to matter little to most of us. However, whilst the famous ladder-like 'march of progress' image may not die easily, what is more important is that there will be wider understanding and appreciation of the 'hominin bush'.

---

[5] It is perhaps harder to imagine in our contemporary world that has less exposure to vast open skies unaffected by light pollution, but ancient peoples were very familiar with the 'fixed' nature of the stars that slowly wheeled across the night sky. Amongst them, ever changing, were 'wandering stars', which is exactly what the Greek word 'planet' (πλάνητες ἀστέρες) means. Like the other great celestial bodies, societies would imbue these with cultural and spiritual meanings.

We are the sole hominin survivors, but not the inevitable masters. Luck, as much as biology, might have been key to *sapiens'* place in the world. Our existence as a species is due to a series of devastating, largely random catastrophes, each of which overhauled the planet and its ecosystems, providing new opportunities: from the meteorite impact that killed the dinosaurs but unleashed mammals through to climate change in Africa some 2 million years ago and the emergence of the great savannahs. Extinction is common – indeed, it is the norm for most species that have ever lived – and rapid climactic change has often driven it. We have just entered the geological epoch of the Anthropocene, marked by the commencement of significant, non-random, human-created impacts on our own ecology and climate. Evolutionary changes are unlikely to save our species this time, but that mercurial, quick, meta-cognitive neocortex just might, if we listen to it and try override our deep-seated propensity to preferentially take immediate gratification.

References

Aubert, M., Lebe, R., Oktaviana, A. A., Tang, M., Burhan, B., Hamrullah, Jusdi, A., Abdullah, Hakim, B., Zhao, J. X., Geria, I. M., Sulistyarto, P. H., Sardi, R. and Brumm, A. 2019. Earliest hunting scene in prehistoric art. *Nature*, 576, 442–445.

Baker, J. L., Rotimi, C. N. and Shriner, D. 2017. Human ancestry correlates with language and reveals that race is not an objective genomic classifier. *Sci Rep*, 7, 1572.

Barger, N., Hanson, K. L., Teffer, K., Schenker-Ahmed, N. M. and Semendeferi, K. 2014. Evidence for evolutionary specialization in human limbic structures. *Front Hum Neurosci*, 8, 277.

Baron-Cohen, S. 2020. *The Pattern Seekers. A New Theory of Human Invention*. London: Allen Lane.

Barrett, L., Henzi, P. and Dunbar, R. 2003. Primate cognition: from 'what now?' to 'what if?'. *Trends Cogn Sci*, 7, 494–497.

Benito-Kwiecinski, S., Giandomenico, S. L., Sutcliffe, M., Riis, E. S., Freire-Pritchett, P., Kelava, I., Wunderlich, S., Martin, U., Wray, G. A., Mcdole, K. and Lancaster, M. A. 2021. An early cell shape transition drives evolutionary expansion of the human forebrain. *Cell*, 184, 2084–2102.e19.

Blanchet, C. L., Osborne, A. H., Tjallingii, R., Ehrmann, W., Friedrich, T., Timmermann, A., Bruckmann, W. and Frank, M. 2021. Drivers of river reactivation in North Africa during the last glacial cycle. *Nat Geosci*, 14, 97–103.

Brumm, A., Oktaviana, A. A., Burhan, B., Hakim, B., Lebe, R., Zhao, J. X., Hadi Sulistyarto, P., Ririmasse, M., Adhityatama, S., Sumantri, I. and Aubert, M. 2021. Oldest cave art found in Sulawesi. *Science*, 7, eabd4648.

Bruner, E. 2018. Human paleoneurology: shaping cortical evolution in fossil hominids. *J Comp Neurol*, 527, 1753–1765.

Bruner, E. 2021. Evolving Human Brains: Paleoneurology and the Fate of Middle Pleistocene. *J Archaeol Method Theory*, 28, 76–94.

Bruner, E., Grimaud-Herve, D., Wu, X., De La Cuetara, J. M. and Holloway, R. L. 2015. A paleoneurological survey of *Homo erectus* endocranial metrics. *Quat Int*, 368, 80–87.

Bruner, E., Manzi, G. and Arsuaga, J. L. 2003. Encephalization and allometric trajectories in the genus *Homo*: evidence from the Neandertal and modern lineages. *PNAS*, 100, 15335–15340.

Byrne, R. E. and Whitten, A. 1988. *Machiavellian Intelligence: Social Expertise and the Evolution of Intellect in Monkeys, Apes, and Humans*. Oxford: Clarendon Press/Oxford University Press.

Cann, R. L., Stoneking, M. and Wilson, A. C. 1987. Mitochondrial DNA and human evolution. *Nature*, 325, 31–36.

Clarkson, C., Jacobs, Z., Marwick, B., Fullagar, R., Wallis, L., Smith, M., Roberts, R. G., Hayes, E., Lowe, K., Carah, X., Florin, S. A., Mcneil, J., Cox, D., Arnold, L. J., Hua, Q., Huntley, J., Brand, H. E. A., Manne, T., Fairbairn, A., Shulmeister, J., Lyle, L., Salinas, M., Page, M., Connell, K., Park, G., Norman, K., Murphy, T. and Pardoe, C. 2017. Human occupation of northern Australia by 65,000 years ago. *Nature*, 547, 306–310.

Clottes, J. 2016. *What Is Palaeolithic Art? Cave Paintings and the Dawn of Human Creativity*. Chicago, IL: University of Chicago Press.

Collins, C. D., Airey, D. C., Young, N. A., Leitch, D. B. and Kaas, J. H. 2010. Neuron densities vary across and within cortical areas in primates. *PNAS*, 107, 15927–15932.

Conde-Valverde, M., Martinez, I., Quam, R. M., Rosa, M., Velez, A. D., Lorenzo, C., Jarabo, P., Bermudez De Castro, J. M., Carbonell, E. and Arsuaga, J. L. 2021. Neanderthals and *Homo sapiens* had similar auditory and speech capacities. *Nat Ecol Evol*, 5, 609–615.

Csibra, G. 2007. Teachers in the wild. *Trends Cogn Sci*, 11, 95–96.

D'Errico, F., Pitarch Marti, A., Shipton, C., Le Vraux, E., Ndiema, E., Goldstein, S., Petraglia, M. D. and Boivin, N.

2020. Trajectories of cultural innovation from the Middle to Later Stone Age in Eastern Africa: personal ornaments, bone artifacts, and ocher from Panga ya Saidi, Kenya. *J Hum Evol*, 141, 102737.

Dennett, D. 1983. Intentional systems in cognitive ethology: the 'Panglossian paradigm' defended. *Behav Brain Sci*, 6, 343–390.

Dennis, M. Y. and Eichler, E. E. 2016. Human adaptation and evolution by segmental duplication. *Curr Opin Genet Dev*, 41, 44–52.

Dunbar, R. I. M. 1998. The social brain hypothesis. *Evol Anthropol*, 6, 178–190.

Dunbar, R. I. M. 2016. *Human Evolution. Our Brains and Behaviour*. Oxford: Oxford University Press.

Eisova, S., Veleminsky, P. and Bruner, E. 2019. The Neanderthal endocast from Ganovce (Poprad, Slovak Republic). *J Anthropol Sci*, 96, 139–149.

Falk, D. 2004. Prelinguistic evolution in early hominins: whence Motherese? *Behav Brain Sci*, 27, 491–503; discussion 503–583.

Garcia-Moreno, F. and Molnar, Z. 2020. Variations of telencephalic development that paved the way for neocortical evolution. *Prog Neurobiol*, 194, 101865.

Greenberg, D. M., Warrier, V., Allison, C. and Baron-Cohen, S. 2018. Testing the empathizing–systemizing theory of sex differences and the extreme male brain theory of autism in half a million people. *PNAS*, 115, 12152–12157.

Greenhill, S. J., Atkinson, Q. D., Meade, A. and Gray, R. D. 2010. The shape and tempo of language evolution. *Proc Biol Sci*, 277, 2443–2450.

Gronau, I., Hubisz, M. J., Gulko, B., Danko, C. G. and Siepel, A. 2011. Bayesian inference of ancient human demography from individual genome sequences. *Nat Genet*, 43, 1031–1034.

Gunz, P., Neubauer, S., Falk, D., Tafforeau, P., Le Cabec, A., Smith, T. M., Kimbel, W. H., Spoor, F. and Alemseged, Z. 2020. *Australopithecus afarensis* endocasts suggest ape-like brain organization and prolonged brain growth. *Sci Adv*, 6, eaaz4729.

Hamilton, M. J., Milne, B. T., Walker, R. S., Burger, O. and Brown, J. H. 2007. The complex structure of hunter-gatherer social networks. *Proc Biol Sci*, 274, 2195–2202.

Hawkes, K. 2020. Cognitive consequences of our grandmothering life history: cultural learning begins in infancy. *Philos Trans R Soc Lond B Biol Sci*, 375, 20190501.

Hawkes, K., O'Connell, J. F. and Blurton Jones, N. G. 2001. Hunting and nuclear families: some lessons from the Hadza about men's work. *Curr Anthropol*, 42, 681–709.

Heide, M., Haffner, C., Murayama, A., Kurotaki, Y., Shinohara, H., Okano, H., Sasaki, E. and Huttner, W. B. 2020. Human-specific ARHGAP11B increases size and folding of primate neocortex in the fetal marmoset. *Science*, 369, 546–550.

Hendy, J. 2021. Ancient protein analysis in archaeology. *Sci Adv*, 7, eabb9314.

Henn, B. M., Steele, T. E. and Weaver, T. D. 2018. Clarifying distinct models of modern human origins in Africa. *Curr Opin Genet Dev*, 53, 148–156.

Henshilwood, C. S., D'Errico, F., Van Niekerk, K. L., Coquinot, Y., Jacobs, Z., Lauritzen, S. E., Menu, M. and Garcia-Moreno, R. 2011. A 100,000-year-old ochre-processing workshop at Blombos Cave, South Africa. *Science*, 334, 219–222.

Herrmann, E., Call, J., Hernandez-Lloreda, M. V., Hare, B. and Tomasello, M. 2007. Humans have evolved specialized skills of social cognition: the cultural intelligence hypothesis. *Science*, 317, 1360–1366.

Hill, K. R., Walker, R. S., Bozicevic, M., Eder, J., Headland, T., Hewlett, B., Hurtado, A. M., Marlowe, F., Wiessner, P. and Wood, B. 2011. Co-residence patterns in hunter-gatherer societies show unique human social structure. *Science*, 331, 1286–1289.

Hofman, M. 2001. Brain evolution in hominids: are we at the end of the road? In: K. R. Gibson and D. Falk (eds.), *Evolutionary Anatomy of the Primate Cerebral Cortex*. Cambridge: Cambridge University Press, pp. 113–130.

Hublin, J. J., Ben-Ncer, A., Bailey, S. E., Freidline, S. E., Neubauer, S., Skinner, M. M., Bergmann, I., Le Cabec, A., Benazzi, S., Harvati, K. and Gunz, P. 2017. New fossils from Jebel Irhoud, Morocco and the pan-African origin of *Homo sapiens*. *Nature*, 546, 289–292.

Hublin, J. J., Sirakov, N., Aldeias, V., Bailey, S., Bard, E., Delvigne, V., Endarova, E., Fagault, Y., Fewlass, H., Hajdinjak, M., Kromer, B., Krumov, I., Marreiros, J., Martisius, N. L., Paskulin, L., Sinet-Mathiot, V., Meyer, M., Paabo, S., Popov, V., Rezek, Z., Sirakova, S., Skinner, M. M., Smith, G. M., Spasov, R., Talamo, S., Tuna, T., Wacker, L., Welker, F., Wilcke, A., Zahariev, N., Mcpherron, S. P. and Tsanova, T. 2020. Initial Upper Palaeolithic *Homo sapiens* from Bacho Kiro Cave, Bulgaria. *Nature*, 581, 299–302.

Hughlings Jackson, J. 1884. Evolution and dissolution of the nervous system, Croonian Lectures at the Royal College of Physicians. *Lancet*, 123, 649–652.

Jamali, M., Grannan, B. L., Fedorenko, E., Saxe, R., Baez-Mendoza, R. and Williams, Z. M.

2021. Single-neuronal predictions of others' beliefs in humans. *Nature*, 591, 610–614.

Jarvis, E. D. 2019. Evolution of vocal learning and spoken language. *Science*, 366, 50–54.

Joyce, J. 1922. *Ulysses*. Paris: Shakespeare and Company.

Karten, H. J. 2015. Vertebrate brains and evolutionary connectomics: on the origins of the mammalian 'neocortex'. *Philos Trans R Soc Lond B Biol Sci*, 370, 20150060.

Kim, H. L., Ratan, A., Perry, G. H., Montenegro, A., Miller, W. and Schuster, S. C. 2014. Khoisan hunter-gatherers have been the largest population throughout most of modern-human demographic history. *Nat Commun*, 5, 5692.

Klein, R. G. 1995. Anatomy, behavior, and modern human origins. *J World Prehistory*, 9, 167–198.

Koster-Hale, J. and Saxe, R. 2013. Theory of mind: a neural prediction problem. *Neuron*, 79, 836–848.

Krems, J. A., Claessens, S., Fales, M. R., Campenni, M., Haselton, M. G. and Aktipis, A. 2021. An agent-based model of the female rivalry hypothesis for concealed ovulation in humans. *Nat Hum Behav*, 5, 726–735.

Krubitzer, L. and Kaas, J. 2005. The evolution of the neocortex in mammals: how is phenotypic diversity generated? *Curr Opin Neurobiol*, 15, 444–453.

Lai, C. S., Fisher, S. E., Hurst, J. A., Vargha-Khadem, F. and Monaco, A. P. 2001. A forkhead-domain gene is mutated in a severe speech and language disorder. *Nature*, 413, 519–523.

Lewis, P. A., Birch, A., Hall, A. and Dunbar, R. I. M. 2017. Higher order intentionality tasks are cognitively more demanding. *Soc Cogn Affect Neurosci*, 12, 1063–1071.

Lin, C., Keles, U., Tyszka, J. M., Gallo, M., Paul, L. and Adolphs, R. 2020. No strong evidence that social network index is associated with gray matter volume from a data-driven investigation. *Cortex*, 125, 307–317.

Liu, J. and Robinson-Rechavi, M. 2020. Robust inference of positive selection on regulatory sequences in the human brain. *Sci Adv*, 6, eabc9863.

Liu, W., Martinon-Torres, M., Cai, Y. J., Xing, S., Tong, H. W., Pei, S. W., Sier, M. J., Wu, X. H., Edwards, R. L., Cheng, H., Li, Y. Y., Yang, X. X., De Castro, J. M. and Wu, X. J. 2015. The earliest unequivocally modern humans in southern China. *Nature*, 526, 696–699.

Lui, J. H., Hansen, D. V. and Kriegstein, A. R. 2011. Development and evolution of the human neocortex. *Cell*, 146, 18–36.

Mathieson, I., Lazaridis, I., Rohland, N., Mallick, S., Patterson, N., Roodenberg, S. A., Harney, E., Stewardson, K., Fernandes, D., Novak, M., Sirak, K., Gamba, C., Jones, E. R., Llamas, B., Dryomov, S., Pickrell, J., Arsuaga, J. L., De Castro, J. M., Carbonell, E., Gerritsen, F., Khokhlov, A., Kuznetsov, P., Lozano, M., Meller, H., Mochalov, O., Moiseyev, V., Guerra, M. A., Roodenberg, J., Verges, J. M., Krause, J., Cooper, A., Alt, K. W., Brown, D., Anthony, D., Lalueza-Fox, C., Haak, W., Pinhasi, R. and Reich, D. 2015. Genome-wide patterns of selection in 230 ancient Eurasians. *Nature*, 528, 499–503.

Maxmen, A. 2020. The next chapter for African genomics. *Nature*, 578, 350–354.

Mcbrearty, S. and Brooks, A. S. 2000. The revolution that wasn't: a new interpretation of the origin of modern human behavior. *J Hum Evol*, 39, 453–563.

Molnar, Z., Clowry, G. J., Sestan, N., Alzu'Bi, A., Bakken, T., Hevner, R. F., Huppi, P. S., Kostovic, I., Rakic, P., Anton, E. S., Edwards, D., Garcez, P., Hoerder-Suabedissen, A. and Kriegstein, A. 2019. New insights into the development of the human cerebral cortex. *J Anat*, 235, 432–451.

Opie, C., Atkinson, Q. D., Dunbar, R. I. and Shultz, S. 2013. Male infanticide leads to social monogamy in primates. *PNAS*, 110, 13328–13332.

Pagel, M. 2000. The history, rate and pattern of world linguistic evolution. In: C. Knight, M. Studdert-Kennedy and J. Hurford (eds.), *The Evolutionary Emergence of Language*. Cambridge: Cambridge University Press, pp. 391–416.

Ponce De Leon, M. S., Bienvenu, T., Marom, A., Engel, S., Tafforeau, P., Warren, J. L. A., Lordkipanidze, D., Kurniawan, I., Murti, D. B., Suriyanto, R. A., Koesbardiati, T. and Zollikofer, C. P. E. 2021. The primitive brain of early Homo. *Science*, 372, 165–171.

Powell, A., Shennan, S. and Thomas, M. G. 2009. Late Pleistocene demography and the appearance of modern human behavior. *Science*, 324, 1298–1301.

Powell, J., Lewis, P. A., Roberts, N., Garcia-Finana, M. and Dunbar, R. I. 2012. Orbital prefrontal cortex volume predicts social network size: an imaging study of individual differences in humans. *Proc Biol Sci*, 279, 2157–2162.

Preuss, T. M. 2017. The human brain: evolution and distinctive features. In: M. Tibayrenc and F. J. Ayala (eds.), *On Human Nature: Biology, Psychology, Ethics, Politics, and Religion*. Cambridge, MA: Academic Press, pp. 125–149.

Rakic, P. 1988. Specification of cerebral cortical areas. *Science*, 241, 170–176.

Rakic, P. 2009. Evolution of the neocortex: a perspective from developmental biology. *Nat Rev Neurosci*, 10, 724–735.

Redhead, G. and Dunbar, R. I. 2013. The functions of language: an experimental study. *Evol Psychol*, 11, 845–854.

Roberts, P., Stewart, M., Alagaili, A. N., Breeze, P., Candy, I., Drake, N., Groucutt, H. S., Scerri, E. M. L., Lee-Thorp, J., Louys, J., Zalmout, I. S., Al-Mufarreh, Y. S. A., Zech, J., Alsharekh, A. M., Al Omari, A., Boivin, N. and Petraglia, M. 2018. Fossil herbivore stable isotopes reveal middle Pleistocene hominin palaeoenvironment in 'Green Arabia'. *Nat Ecol Evol*, 2, 1871–1878.

Scerri, E. M. L., Chikhi, L. and Thomas, M. G. 2019. Beyond multiregional and simple out-of-Africa models of human evolution. *Nat Ecol Evol*, 3, 1370–1372.

Skoglund, P., Thompson, J. C., Prendergast, M. E., Mittnik, A., Sirak, K., Hajdinjak, M., Salie, T., Rohland, N., Mallick, S., Peltzer, A., Heinze, A., Olalde, I., Ferry, M., Harney, E., Michel, M., Stewardson, K., Cerezo-Roman, J. I., Chiumia, C., Crowther, A., Gomani-Chindebvu, E., Gidna, A. O., Grillo, K. M., Taneli Helenius, I., Hellenthal, G., Helm, R., Horton, M., Lopez, S., Mabulla, A. Z. P., Parkington, J., Shipton, C., Thomas, M. G., Tibesasa, R., Welling, M., Patterson, N., Morris, A. G., Boivin, N., Pinhasi, R., Krause, J. and Reich, D. 2017. Reconstructing prehistoric African population structure. *Cell*, 171, 59–71.

Smith, T. M., Tafforeau, P., Reid, D. J., Pouech, J., Lazzari, V., Zermeno, J. P., Guatelli-Steinberg, D., Olejniczak, A. J., Hoffman, A., Radovcic, J., Makaremi, M., Toussaint, M., Stringer, C. and Hublin, J. J. 2010. Dental evidence for ontogenetic differences between modern humans and Neanderthals. *PNAS*, 107, 20923–20928.

Sousa, A. M. M., Meyer, K. A., Santpere, G., Gulden, F. O. and Sestan, N. 2017. Evolution of the human nervous system function, structure, and development. *Cell*, 170, 226–247.

Sun, T. and Hevner, R. F. 2014. Growth and folding of the mammalian cerebral cortex: from molecules to malformations. *Nat Rev Neurosci*, 15, 217–232.

Sun, X. F., Wen, S. Q., Lu, C. Q., Zhou, B. Y., Curnoe, D., Lu, H. Y., Li, H. C., Wang, W., Cheng, H., Yi, S. W., Jia, X., Du, P. X., Xu, X. H., Lu, Y. M., Lu, Y., Zheng, H. X., Zhang, H., Sun, C., Wei, L. H., Han, F., Huang, J., Edwards, R. L., Jin, L. and Li, H. 2021. Ancient DNA and multimethod dating confirm the late arrival of anatomically modern humans in southern China. *PNAS*, 118, e2019158118.

Swadesh, M. 1952. Lexico-statistic dating of prehistoric ethnic contacts. *Proc Am Phil Soc*, 96, 453–463.

Urbanus, B. H. A., Peter, S., Fisher, S. E. and De Zeeuw, C. I. 2020. Region-specific Foxp2 deletions in cortex, striatum or cerebellum cannot explain vocalization deficits observed in spontaneous global knockouts. *Sci Rep*, 10, 21631.

Van Den Heuvel, M. P., Bullmore, E. T. and Sporns, O. 2016. Comparative connectomics. *Trends Cogn Sci*, 20, 345–361.

Vasistha, N. A., Garcia-Moreno, F., Arora, S., Cheung, A. F., Arnold, S. J., Robertson, E. J. and Molnar, Z. 2015. Cortical and clonal contribution of Tbr2 expressing progenitors in the developing mouse brain. *Cereb Cortex*, 25, 3290–3302.

Velliky, E. C., Schmidt, P., Bellot-Gurlet, L., Wolf, S. and Conard, N. J. 2021. Early anthropogenic use of hematite on Aurignacian ivory personal ornaments from Hohle Fels and Vogelherd caves,

Germany. *J Hum Evol*, 150, 102900.

West, B. J., Massari, G. F., Culbreth, G., Failla, R., Bologna, M., Dunbar, R. I. M. and Grigolini, P. 2020. Relating size and functionality in human social networks through complexity. *PNAS*, 117, 18355–18358.

Wiessner, P. W. 2014. Embers of society: firelight talk among the Ju/'hoansi Bushmen. *PNAS*, 111, 14027–14035.

Wilkins, J., Schoville, B. J., Pickering, R., Gliganic, L., Collins, B., Brown, K. S., Von Der Meden, J., Khumalo, W., Meyer, M. C., Maape, S., Blackwood, A. F. and Hatton, A. 2021. Innovative *Homo sapiens* behaviours 105,000 years ago in a wetter Kalahari. *Nature*, 592, 248–252.

Williams, G. C. 1957. Pleiotropy, natural selection, and the evolution of senescence. *Evolution*, 11, 398–411.

Zerjal, T., Xue, Y., Bertorelle, G., Wells, R. S., Bao, W., Zhu, S., Qamar, R., Ayub, Q., Mohyuddin, A., Fu, S., Li, P., Yuldasheva, N., Ruzibakiev, R., Xu, J., Shu, Q., Du, R., Yang, H., Hurles, M. E., Robinson, E., Gerelsaikhan, T., Dashnyam, B., Mehdi, S. Q. and Tyler-Smith, C. 2003. The genetic legacy of the Mongols. *Am J Hum Genet*, 72, 717–721.

Zwyns, N., Paine, C. H., Tsedendorj, B., Talamo, S., Fitzsimmons, K. E., Gantumur, A., Guunii, L., Davakhuu, O., Flas, D., Dogandzic, T., Doerschner, N., Welker, F., Gillam, J. C., Noyer, J. B., Bakhtiary, R. S., Allshouse, A. F., Smith, K. N., Khatsenovich, A. M., Rybin, E. P., Byambaa, G. and Hublin, J. J. 2019. The Northern Route for human dispersal in central and northeast Asia: new evidence from the site of Tolbor-16, Mongolia. *Sci Rep*, 9, 11759.

Hunter-Gatherers, Mismatch and Mental Disorder

Nikhil Chaudhary and Gul Deniz Salali

Abstract

For most of human evolutionary history our species lived as hunter-gatherers; hence, much of our cognition and behaviour is adapted to this way of life. Given the magnitude of the sociocultural, economic and lifestyle changes experienced by *Homo sapiens* over the last 10,000 years, in particular the last several hundred years, aspects of human psychology may be maladapted to modern ways of life. This process of maladaptation following changes in the physical or social environment is referred to as 'evolutionary mismatch' and has been hypothesised to contribute to the high prevalence of mental disorders in industrialised societies. However, very few studies have examined the prevalence of these pathologies among contemporary hunter-gatherer populations; thus, empirical support for such *diseases of modernity* hypotheses is lacking. In this chapter, we review the limited existing research and theorise about the key differences between hunter-gatherer and industrialised societies that are likely to have profound implications for mental health. Specifically, we contrast the strong social support networks, egalitarianism, explorative modes of learning, sensitive child-rearing practices and present orientation of hunter-gatherers with corresponding features of industrialised populations. We argue that mismatches in these domains are partially responsible for of a vast array of mental illnesses, ranging from common mood disorders to behavioural pathologies and psychotic spectrum disorders. We hope that this chapter stimulates the generation and testing of mismatch hypotheses and, eventually, trials of interventions based on mismatch reduction. We end by offering suggestions for methodological approaches to this future research.

Keywords

child development, diseases of civilization, egalitarianism, evolutionary mismatch, human life history, hunter-gatherers, mental health

Key Points

- Differences between the physical and social environment in contemporary industrialised societies and those experienced by our hunter-gatherer ancestors can result in maladaptive cognition or behaviour. This process is referred to as 'evolutionary mismatch'.
- Modern environments may produce novel pathological phenotypes that did not occur among hunter-gatherers (phenotypic mismatch). Additionally, some phenotypes that were adaptive in a hunter-gatherer context have not changed but are maladaptive or pathological in modern environments (environmental mismatch).

- Research with contemporary hunter-gatherers is scarce but indicates that their prevalence rates of various mental disorders may be lower – and level of psychological well-being higher – than in industrialised populations.
- Compared to hunter-gatherers, industrialised societies are characterised by smaller social support networks, increased social and economic inequality, less sensitive child-rearing, high-pressured didactic education and the requirement for long-term planning. All of these differences likely increase our vulnerability to an array of mental disorders.

5.1 Introduction

5.1.1 Mismatch and Its Relevance to Disease

Evolutionary mismatch refers to a scenario where there is a discrepancy between the physical or social environmental conditions an organism currently faces and past conditions in which some trait of that organism originally evolved – its *environment of evolutionary adaptedness* (EEA) – resulting in physical, cognitive or behavioural maladaptation (Barkow et al., 1992; Bowlby, 1969; also see Chapters 1 and 2 of this volume). Mismatch occurs because natural selection is a blind process relying on random mutations, of which an infinitesimally small proportion provide any adaptive benefit, and those that do are then selected for over extended time frames before reaching fixation. Therefore, there is often an *adaptive lag* after environmental changes.

Whilst the 'goals' of natural selection certainly do not always align with optimisation of health or well-being (Nesse, 2019), they often do. Given the magnitude of the sociocultural, economic and lifestyle changes experienced by our species over the last 10,000 years, and especially the last several hundred years, there has been growing interest in the potential of mismatch to explain a range of pathologies. A classic example is the ubiquitous preference for foods high in sugar and fat (see Figure 1.1). These preferences evolved to motivate the acquisition of such foods in ancestral environments where they were scarce and provided invaluable nutritional benefits; conversely, in present-day industrialised societies they are abundant and readily available. High consumption driven by the mismatched taste preferences and low physical activity levels characteristic of modern lifestyles has significantly contributed to epidemics of obesity, diabetes and cardiovascular disease in WEIRD (Western Educated Industrialised Rich Democratic) populations (O'Keefe and Cordain, 2004). Taking a mismatch perspective may offer unique preventative solutions and remedies by encouraging the replication of relevant aspects of ancestral lifestyles, thereby attenuating the mismatch.

5.1.2 Hunter-Gatherers and Mismatch

Given the explanatory potential of mismatch thinking, there has been growing interest among public health researchers in the use of extant hunter-gatherer populations as models of ancestral lifestyles (Pontzer et al., 2018). The premise of this approach is that a hunter-gatherer lifestyle is likely to resemble the EEA for many traits relevant to health; for more than 95% of human evolutionary history, prior to the Neolithic Revolution, we occupied this mode of subsistence (Kelly, 2013). Broadly speaking, hunter-gatherer societies are defined by a primary reliance on the foraging of wild foods via hunting, gathering or fishing and a lack of domestication of plants or animals except dogs (Kelly, 2013).

Typologies usually divide such populations into *immediate-* versus *delayed-return* hunter-gatherers or *simple* versus *complex* hunter-gatherers. In each typology, the former lack food storage mechanisms, live in small, highly mobile groups and are politically egalitarian, whereas the latter store food, live in larger, more sedentary groups and have recognised social and economic inequalities (Woodburn, 1982). Compared to simple hunter-gatherers, evidence for the presence of complex hunter-gatherers appears much more recently in the archaeological record and tends to be confined to coastal regions (Arnold et al., 2016; Marlowe, 2005). Therefore, many anthropologists agree that the former are more representative of our species' evolutionary history (Marlowe, 2005; Shultznier et al., 2010). Correspondingly, herein, our discussion of foraging societies and their relevance to mismatch refers to simple hunter-gatherers unless otherwise stated.

Epidemiological work has demonstrated an extremely low prevalence or a complete absence of various non-communicable diseases among contemporary hunter-gatherers (Pontzer et al., 2018), and less than 10% of deaths are caused by chronic disease (Gurven and Kaplan, 2007). Numerous promising mismatch hypotheses of mental disorder have also been put forward, pertaining to depression (Chapter 8 of this volume), schizophrenia (Abed and Abbas, 2014; Chapter 10 of this volume), attention deficit hyperactivity disorder (ADHD; Chapter 15 of this volume), eating disorders (Chapter 11 of this volume) and post-partum depression (PPD; Hahn-Holbrook and Haselton, 2014). However, epidemiological studies among hunter-gatherers, which test empirically whether these disorders are in fact *diseases of modernity*, are extremely scarce. In

Section 5.3, we briefly review the limited existing hunter-gatherer research relevant to mental illness and psychological well-being.

Given the current dearth of epidemiological work, in Section 5.4 we discuss various aspects of hunter-gatherer existence – principally related to social organisation and child-rearing – that are notably different from WEIRD populations and likely have profound implications for mental health; we do not attend to lifestyle factors such as physical activity levels or diet since these have been discussed extensively elsewhere (e.g. Gurven and Lieberman, 2020). Importantly, there are two distinct routes by which such mismatches may contribute to psychiatric illness. Firstly, via the generation of novel pathological cognitive or behavioural patterns that would not manifest in a hunter-gatherer context, we suggest such cases are referred to as *phenotypic mismatch* (an environmental change has produced a novel maladaptive/pathological phenotype). Alternatively, it may be that the same 'symptoms' do occur among hunter-gatherers but in such contexts are considered neither pathological, because they do not impede an individual's ability to function in society, nor maladaptive, because they are not associated with reduced reproductive success. We propose the term *environmental mismatch* to describe this second form of mismatch (the phenotype has not changed but is maladaptive/pathological in the new environment). For instance, some scholars have suggested that psychosis would have been less likely to occur in hunter-gatherer societies for reasons relating to social organisation (Abed and Abbas, 2014); using our classification scheme this would be a phenotypic mismatch hypothesis. Conversely, others have suggested that what we now call psychosis did occur in foraging societies, but rather than negatively impacting functionality, it was spiritually valued and a precursor to gaining prestigious shamanic status (Polimeni and Reiss, 2002); we consider this an environmental mismatch hypothesis. As said by one Inuit, 'when the shaman is healing he is out of his mind, *but he is not crazy*' (Murphy, 1976, p. 1022, emphasis in original).

We hope this chapter encourages anthropological research that can meaningfully contribute to the developing field of evolutionary psychiatry via the generation and testing of mismatch hypotheses. Additionally, we aim to equip

clinicians with a basic understanding of the lifestyle that much of our cognition and behaviour is adapted to, which may reframe how one thinks about the aetiology of mental disorder. In fact, it has been suggested that providing patients with evolutionary explanations for mental disturbances can have a therapeutic effect in and of itself (Nesse, 2019).

5.2 The Validity of Our Approach

Here, we briefly respond to potential objections to our approach, which have two key themes: the validity of using contemporary hunter-gatherers as a model for prehistoric societies and the relevance of mismatch within the domains of cognition and behaviour.

5.2.1 Are Hunter-Gatherers Useful Models of Prehistoric Human Societies?

Arguments that extant hunter-gatherers are not representative of ancestral societies are often focused around the impact of modern outside influences. This perspective was stressed in the *Kalahari Debate* by the *revisionists* who argued that the !Kung San Bushmen of southern Africa are no longer operating in an independent foraging economy but represent an underclass in an increasingly integrated market economy (Wilmsen et al., 1990). Indeed, most studied forager populations have a non-trivial level of interaction with the outside world. That said, an imperfect model is not a useless one, and many features of contemporary hunter-gatherer life discussed below likely approximate those of our ancestors (Gray, 2013; Shultziner et al., 2010).

Others have argued that contemporary hunter-gatherers are marginal remnants of ancestral societies that have been displaced and forced into low-productivity regions (Lee and DeVore, 1968). However, what constitutes productive land for foragers and non-foragers is not the same, and regardless, the lands inhabited by warm-climate foragers have higher net primary productivity than those occupied by non-foragers (Porter and Marlowe, 2007).

Some scholars have criticised the concept of a 'hunter-gatherer way of life' altogether, highlighting the substantial inter-population variation that exists (Bailey and Milner, 2002). There is certainly variability across numerous domains, especially when comparing simple and complex hunter-gatherers. Nevertheless, there are many shared features among simple hunter-gatherers that distinguish them from societies practising other forms of subsistence. A lack of food storage, egalitarianism and high mobility are uniform features of simple hunter-gatherers (Woodburn, 1982). Given that the distribution of food, social hierarchy and foraging mobility are considered by many ethologists as the most important selective pressures acting on primate behaviour (Wrangham, 1980), the shared features listed above are certainly sufficient to qualify the (simple) hunter-gatherer way of life as a meaningful construct.

5.2.2 Is Human Psychology Subject to Evolutionary Mismatch?

There is also disagreement between scholars of the evolutionary social sciences regarding the occurrence and extent of mismatch in the domains of cognition and behaviour. Evolutionary psychologists argue in favour, asserting that inflexible genetic mechanisms underpin psychological processes; these mechanisms are thus subject to the aforementioned adaptive lags, resulting in a mismatch between modernity and our *Stone Age minds* (Barkow et al., 1992). Conversely, human behavioural ecologists take an adaptationist stance and make the *behavioural and phenotypic gambits* (Nettle et al., 2013). That is to say, they emphasise the plasticity of behaviour, assuming it can respond flexibly to environmental changes unconstrained by any underlying neurological mechanisms or genetic architecture. Finally, cultural evolutionists emphasise the importance of social learning as the foundation of behaviour (Henrich and McElreath, 2003). This perspective assumes that behavioural mismatch, as defined here, is less important since learned behaviour can change multiple times even within one lifetime, permitting far more rapid adaptation than genetic selection. In reality, these are not truly mutually exclusive approaches, but rather differences in emphasis. Distinct cognitive and behavioural processes unequivocally differ in the extent to which they are genetically, epigenetically or culturally determined. Therefore, to rule out the utility of any one approach or to assume that mismatch is a categorically redundant concept would certainly

diminish the explanatory power of the evolutionary perspective.

Evolutionary psychologists have also been criticised for generating *just-so stories* (i.e. reverse engineering explanations for a given psychological feature based on unsubstantiated assumptions about its EEA and, in turn, the nature of mismatch) (Richardson, 2007). It is true that some of the literature presents a picture of hunter-gatherer life that seems to be a caricature of 'tribal' peoples and has no anthropological or archaeological evidence base. However, by premising our discussion on our own experience of fieldwork with hunter-gatherers as well as the wider ethnographic literature, this chapter does not suffer from this flaw. In fact, we hope it serves to correct any inaccurate perceptions of foraging societies that readers may have acquired elsewhere.

5.3 Existing Research

Psychiatric epidemiological research with hunter-gatherer populations is limited to a handful of studies. There are equally few non-medical studies examining subjective well-being and happiness (see Section 5.3.2). In this section, we provide a detailed review of these studies, interpret them within a mismatch framework and summarise the methods employed that may be of use to researchers planning to conduct similar work in the future.

5.3.1 Mental Illness in Contemporary Hunter-Gatherers

A study of PPD among the Hadza of Tanzania represents the most direct application of a clinical screening tool from Western psychiatry to a hunter-gatherer population (Herlosky et al., 2020). Herlosky and colleagues administered the Edinburgh Postnatal Depression Scale (EPDS) – which has been validated cross-culturally and used in rural settings (January and Chimbari, 2018; Small et al., 2007) – to 23 Hadza women with infants less than a year old. A total of 52% of the Hadza women scored above 12, which is commonly used as the threshold for probable depression. These rates are very high in comparison with industrialised populations: PPD prevalence rates average approximately 19% in low- and middle-income countries (Woody et al., 2017). Complementary data indicated among the Hadza that the EPDS score was not associated with any measures of social support, including presence of a husband, which have been identified as major risk factors in WEIRD populations (Boyce, 2003). This may reflect the fact that in hunter-gatherer societies everyone has adequate access to social support derived from community living (see Section 5.4.1).

Several responses alluded to anxieties relating to offspring health, which is understandable given the Hadza experience an infant mortality rate of approximately 21% (Blurton-Jones et al., 1992) and that rates among hunter-gatherers tend to range between 20% and 35% (Hewlett, 1991). These findings highlight that even when mismatches do not increase the prevalence of a given mental disorder, they may affect the relevant risk factors. In the case of PPD, among WEIRD populations a lack of social support may have become a novel risk factor, whereas the high infant mortality rates experienced by ancestral populations are no longer primary drivers of maternal anxiety. Alternatively, PPD, whilst distressing, may have evolved as an adaptation to focus maternal behaviour on mitigating the high infant mortality risk faced by our ancestors. Despite the low risk in contemporary industrialised settings, the condition persists due to adaptive lag (i.e. it is an environmental mismatch).

Another study examined the distribution of dopamine receptor gene D4 (*DRD4*) variants among South Amerindian populations with a recent history of either agricultural or foraging subsistence (Tovo-Rodrigues et al., 2010). The *7R* variant has been associated with novelty-seeking, impulsivity and hyperactivity (Tovo-Rodrigues et al., 2010). Accordingly, in a meta-analytic review of candidate genes associated with childhood ADHD, this polymorphism had the largest association of all genes examined (Gizer et al., 2009). Interestingly, in the study of South Amerindian populations, the frequency of the *7R* allele at this locus averaged 0.58 across the populations with a recent history of hunting and gathering compared to 0.48 across recent farmers (Tovo-Rodrigues et al., 2010). Moreover, genetic analyses indicate that the *7R* allele has undergone strong positive selection since its origin approximately 40,000 years ago, which also coincides with a period of major human expansion (Ding et al., 2002).

One interpretation of these findings is that personality and behavioural traits such as novelty-seeking and hyperactivity, which are now considered symptoms of ADHD, provided fitness-related benefits in a hunter-gatherer context. They may have encouraged nomadic foragers to explore new environments and, in turn, facilitated more effective resource exploitation. However, following the Neolithic Revolution, as sedentism and resource intensification became the norm, such traits were no longer adaptive. Hyperactivity and a reduced ability to pay attention to the same thing for extended periods are particularly mismatched to modern classroom environments. Therefore, ADHD fits neatly into the category of environmental mismatch; we continue this discussion in Section 5.4.2.1.

The final two epidemiological studies examined the prevalence and correlates of major depressive disorder (MDD) among the Tsimane of lowland Bolivia. The Tsimane are usually categorised as forager-horticulturalists rather than hunter-gatherers, since approximately two-thirds of their diet is derived from non-intensive farming and only a third is from foraging (Stieglitz et al., 2015b). Nevertheless, given their high physical activity levels, small community residences and relatively egalitarian political organisation, these studies still offer insight into mismatch.

Stieglitz and colleagues tested the host-defence hypothesis of depression, which proposes that depression is a 'sickness behaviour' and part of a coordinated response to infection (Stieglitz et al., 2015b). Depressive symptoms such as hypersomnia, social withdrawal, fatigue and anhedonia facilitate recovery from infection or tissue injury by promoting the reallocation of energy to immune function (Raison and Miller, 2012). Stieglitz and colleagues (2015b) examined associations between depressive symptoms and immune biomarkers and responses among the Tsimane (n = 249). A structured interview examining the emotional, cognitive and somatic symptoms of depression was constructed by adapting items from Beck's Depression Inventory, Hamilton's Depression Rating Scale and the Center for Epidemiologic Studies Depression Scale. A total of 10% of the sample were classified as depressed, of which 90%, 86% and 84% experienced emotional, somatic and cognitive symptoms, respectively.

A 10% point-prevalence of depression is relatively low in comparison to most South American countries (mean = 20.6%) (Lim et al., 2018). Nevertheless, this non-trivial prevalence highlights that the high physical activity levels, community living and egalitarianism characteristic of foraging life are not sufficient to eliminate depression. This is to be expected if one driver of depression is in fact infection, as proposed by the host-defence hypothesis and supported by this study's subsequent analysis. Baseline concentrations of tumour necrosis factor alpha (TNF-α), interlukin-1 beta (IL-1β), interleukin-6 (IL-6) and C-reactive protein (CRP) were the immune biomarkers measured. Additionally, the proinflammatory cytokine responses of the first three of these to *ex vivo* antigen stimulation were examined. Across each domain of depressive symptoms – emotional, somatic and cognitive – associations with immune activation at baseline were found; and consistent with the hypothesis, the somatic symptoms showed the strongest relationship with antigen stimulation.

Another study examined other predictors of Tsimane depression scores using the same scale (Stieglitz et al., 2015a). Stieglitz and colleagues' productive value hypothesis posits that depression may occur when an individual's ability to produce fitness-enhancing resources for self and kin is reduced. This may explain why feeling burdensome in old age and unemployment in general are major predictors of depression in WEIRD societies (Liang et al., 2001; McGee, 2015). Similarly, among the Tsimane, lower functional ability – measured using modified exercises from the MacArthur Studies of Successful Aging – and reduced involvement in subsistence were associated with high depression scores. However, there was no association between higher scores and older age.

This may reflect a generalised difference between foraging and WEIRD societies, which is driven by others' perceptions and self-perceptions of elder members of the community and their value. In WEIRD contexts, the pace of technological change is now so fast that in many industries an individual's skill base becomes redundant quickly, and older members of society do not participate in the workforce at all. Conversely, in foraging societies, the contribution of the elderly is irreplaceable due to the extensive ecological knowledge accumulated over the life course. For instance, Hadza women's foraging productivity increases continuously and into old age because

identifying where to find carbohydrate-rich tubers is an experience-dependent skill (Kaplan et al., 2000). This vital contribution of elderly women has been proposed as a leading driver of human longevity and our extended post-reproductive lifespan, since it allowed elderly hunter-gatherer women to substantially enhance the survival prospects of younger generations (Hawkes, 2003). Similarly, in many hunting and gathering societies elders contribute traditional medical knowledge. We conducted a study with the BaYaka hunter-gatherers residing in the rainforests of northern Congo and found participants in the oldest age category (45+) had the greatest knowledge of medicinal plants (Salali et al., 2016). Therefore, old-age depression may be a form of phenotypic mismatch caused by the productive redundancy among the elderly in WEIRD societies.

The findings of these studies make clear that mental disorders, as we conceptualise and define them clinically, do occur among hunter-gatherers, highlighting that the romantic notions of ancestral utopias pervading popular culture should be discarded. This does not negate the explanatory value of mismatch, and the exiting studies discussed have already offered some intriguing insights. The prevalence of MDD, especially among the elderly, may have been lower in foraging societies and principally driven by infection rather than the common risk factors in industrialised contexts such as social isolation, low physical activity levels and unemployment. In contrast, the prevalence of PPD may have actually been higher among hunter-gatherers due to considerable infant mortality but is now redundant in WEIRD societies and only persists due to adaptive lag. Similarly, genes contributing to ADHD may have encouraged adaptive exploration and novelty-seeking among ancestral foragers, but such behaviours are dysfunctional in the context of modern education systems. Based on this work, public health scholars may test novel interventions for improving psychiatric outcomes in industrialised societies; we consider potential avenues in Section 5.5.

5.3.2 Happiness and Subjective Well-Being among Hunter-Gatherers

Two recent studies have examined happiness in hunter-gatherers, both of which suggest foragers have relatively high subjective psychological well-being. The first examined scores on items from the Subjective Happiness Scale that address generalised happiness on a seven-point Likert scale (Frackowiak et al., 2020). The Hadza (n = 145) scored 1.28 points higher than the Polish respondents (n = 156). Moreover, the Hadza score of 5.83 is significantly higher than scores from *all* 12 industrialised societies where the same scale has been previously applied. There was also a significant decline in happiness among older Polish participants, whereas age had no effect among the Hadza, offering further support to the relationship between mood and old age discussed in Section 5.3.1.

Another study examined subjective reports of general well-being (Reyes-Garcia et al., 2021). The following single question was asked: 'Taking everything into consideration would you say your life is . . .' Responses were on a Likert scale from 1 (very bad) to 5 (very good). Participants were from three populations: the Baka, Penan and Tsimane. The Baka and Penan are hunter-gatherers residing in the forests of Cameroon and Brunei, respectively. Good (3) was the modal response in all three populations. The authors also note that participants tended to provide justifications, usually related to health, for low scores, but were less likely to provide reasons for high scores. They interpret this as moderate happiness being the baseline state in these societies such that respondents only felt compelled to justify sadness, not happiness.

The studies reviewed in this section suggest that moderately positive life satisfaction may be the baseline state among foragers, and their self-reported happiness is higher than those living in industrialised societies. Moreover, the prevalence of maladaptive mental pathologies appears to be lower among hunter-gatherers. In the next section, we outline key differences between foraging and WEIRD lifestyles that may be responsible for these trends and provide preliminary hypotheses to direct future research.

5.4 Differences between Hunter-Gatherer Life and Modernity with Implications for Mental Health

5.4.1 Social Organisation

5.4.1.1 Social Structure and Community Living

Simple hunter-gatherers live in multi-household camps, with an average camp size of 37.5 individuals (Marlowe, 2005) (see Figure 5.1). The composition of each household tends to resemble a nuclear family, though it is not uncommon for some extended family members such as a grandparent to co-reside in the same household; most households have five to six residents (Dyble et al., 2016). A common misconception is that camps are composed only of closely related individuals. In fact, the genetic relatedness between adult camp mates is low; from the perspective of the average adult resident, only 7% of co-resident adults are close kin (siblings or parents) and only 25% are distant kin (r ≥ 0.03125, equivalent to third cousins) (Hill et al., 2011).

To understand the tight relationships between mental health and sociality, it is necessary to consider the *ultimate* drivers of the social organisation outlined above. In comparison with other primates, our species has traditionally occupied a high-risk foraging niche. Chimpanzee diets are composed of approximately 95% predictable and easy-to-collect foods such as leaves and fruits; in contrast, hunter-gatherers rely on unpredictable resources, which require both high skill and good luck to obtain (Kaplan et al., 2000). For instance, in some foraging societies, successful acquisition of meat occurs on fewer than 20% of hunting trips (Biesele and Barclay, 2001). However, when it does occur, it produces large nutrient-dense food packages, which provide more meat than the hunter's household can consume before it rots. This diet drives hunter-gatherer group living because on days when one hunter is successful they can share meat with those lacking food at a low cost; this donation will then be reciprocated and provide a large benefit when the same hunter is unsuccessful (Dyble et al., 2016). For instance, without food sharing, isolated Ache households would have less than 1,000 kcal/person on approximately 30% of days, but with food sharing, this figure drops to 3% of days (Kaplan et al., 1990); and within BaYaka camps, individuals with larger social networks have a higher body mass index and greater fertility (Chaudhary et al., 2016).

Thus, for our ancestors, social networks were a matter of life and death, group living was the norm and social isolation was rare, carrying fatal risks. In turn, psychological mechanisms promoting the maintenance of social relationships have been heavily favoured by natural selection. Social

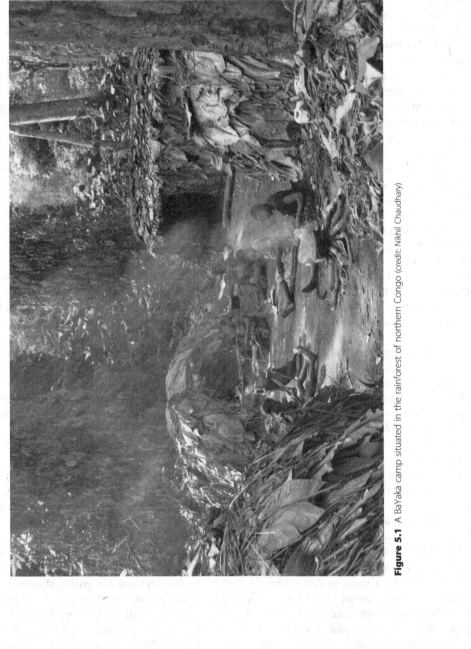

Figure 5.1 A BaYaka camp situated in the rainforest of northern Congo (credit: Nikhil Chaudhary)

exclusion shares the neural underpinnings of physical pain, altering activity in the dorsal anterior cingulate cortex and the anterior insula (Eisenberger, 2012). In combination with changes in affect, such as loneliness, these proximate mechanisms have evolved as a kind of behavioural homeostasis, producing an aversive and corrective response to isolation. Such is the magnitude of our evolved psychological dependence on social interaction that, even when surrounded by individuals who have committed the most heinous crimes, solitary confinement for more than 15 days is considered psychological torture by the United Nations (2015).

In contrast to foragers, social isolation is common among members of WEIRD societies. They rarely live in close proximity to any natal kin and often have no relationships with extended kin and their friendships are not characterised by the same commitment or frequency of interaction as in foragers. We suspect that the driver of this decline in high-quality social support networks relates to changes in subsistence interdependence. Hunter-gatherers have obligate group living due to their risky foraging niche and requirement for daily food sharing and cooperation. At the other end of the spectrum, those participating in market economies usually have reliable and predictable access to income and nutrition and engage in specialised individual-based labour tasks, shrinking their residential and high-quality networks to the nuclear family.

This enormous increase in social isolation has likely resulted in overexpression of the aforementioned aversive psychological responses. Loneliness is associated with increased stress, anxiety and hypervigilance, partially mediated via heightened cortisol levels (Hawkley and Cacioppo, 2010; Steptoe et al., 2004). Due to the rarity and substantial danger associated with isolation for our ancestors, such considerable responses were acute, appropriate and served an important function. However, given the high frequency and low danger of isolation in industrialised societies, they can now be considered pathological and a form of environmental mismatch. Moreover, chronic loneliness – affecting 15–30% of those living in economically developed populations (Hawkley and Cacioppo, 2010) – results in overstimulation of these psychological responses to isolation, representing a form of phenotypic mismatch. Correspondingly, social isolation is associated with a vast number of psychiatric problems, including increased risk of personality disorders, psychosis, MDD, PPD, Alzheimer's disease and suicide (Hawkley and Cacioppo, 2010; Leigh-Hunt et al., 2017).

Beyond the size and quality of social networks, their structure among hunter-gatherers is more conducive to mental well-being relative to WEIRD societies. Being part of a community – a social network, often with some shared goal or interest, in which one's social partners are themselves social partners with one another – provides a sense of belonging, purpose and mental well-being (Tajfel and Turner, 2019). Spiritual communities in particular create a strong sense of group identity via ritual practices that bond participants. It is no coincidence that across the world, from football fans to devout members of the Abrahamic religions, group-based rituals share the same highly conserved ingredients: synchronous chanting and movement. These synchronous activities have been shown to lower cortisol and increase oxytocin levels, to stimulate the release of beta-endorphins and to increase trust, entitativity and cooperation among group members (Beck et al., 2000; Fischer et al., 2013; Pearce et al., 2015; also see Chapter 13 of this volume). Such rituals were likely selected via cultural evolution since they enhanced the functioning and resilience of ancestral groups, which were so heavily dependent on cooperation and group cohesion.

Our experience of living with the BaYaka highlighted the fundamental importance of ritual in building community. The BaYaka practice *massana*. These are rituals comprised polyphonic singing, dancing and synchronous swaying and clapping (see Figure 5.2), which *all* camp members – from infants to the elderly – are present for. They have a spiritual focus, and each *massana* is associated with a particular *mokondi* – spirit of the forest – and aims to achieve some mutual goal such as bringing fortune in an upcoming hunt or ensuring the successful passing of a recently deceased individual. *Massana* can go on for days and sometimes stimulate trance-like states among participants. In contrast, ritual engagement in WEIRD populations has declined rapidly. For instance, in the UK, less than 1% of the population attends church on a weekly basis, of which a third are over the age of 70 (Church of England Research and Statistics 2019).

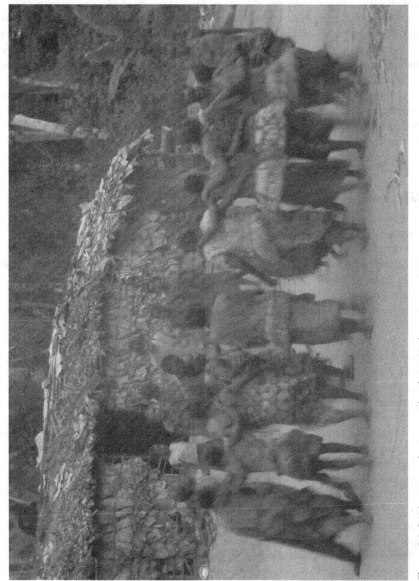

Figure 5.2 BaYaka women dancing together during *Ngoku massana* (credit: Nikhil Chaudhary)

The void of spiritual-based communities appears to have drastic consequences for mental well-being. A study of completed suicides in New York found that the odds of dying by suicide were six times higher for individuals not engaged in any form of religious congregation (Duberstein et al., 2004). Such insights offer unintuitive remedies to the phenotypic mismatch resulting from an absence of ritual practice. Further work is required, but one study examined the outcomes of a charity programme in which individuals with chronic mental illness or issues with substance abuse participated in weekly choir groups (i.e. synchronous singing) (Dingle et al., 2004). Participant responses were overwhelmingly positive and included reports of feeling more positive, release from anxiety and worry, increased self-esteem and aiding in reducing the consumption of alcohol and methadone.

5.4.1.2 Egalitarianism

Another key impact of the hunter-gatherer foraging niche on social organisation is the absence of dominance hierarchies. Even the households with the best hunters rely heavily on food sharing to secure stable access to nutrition. This universal interdependence within foraging societies means that dominant behaviour is not a viable behavioural strategy. As such, hunter-gatherers are characterised by the *egalitarian syndrome*: consensus-based decision-making, no formal social ranks, an emphasis on autonomy, rejection of self-aggrandising behaviour and very weak notions of personal property (Woodburn, 1982). This ethos is enforced via *reverse hierarchy*, whereby any individual attempts at authoritarian behaviour are rebutted by a coalition of all other camp members via *levelling mechanisms* such as ridicule, ostracism and, in some cases, violence (Boehm et al., 1993). This value on social equality manifests in intriguing ways; for instance, if a hunter returns to camp with meat, they will speak in a self-deprecating manner about their kill or abilities. If they do not, others will do this for them: 'When a young man kills much meat, he comes to think of himself as a big man, and he thinks of the rest of us as his inferiors. We can't accept this. We refuse one who boasts, for someday his pride will make him kill somebody. So we always speak of his meat as worthless. In this way we cool his heart and make him gentle' (Lee, 1969: 4).

Interdependence and the absence of storage produce both economic and social equality within foraging communities. However, in post-Neolithic societies, once food storage mechanisms had developed, the risk and concomitant obligate cooperation encountered by foragers were eliminated. Kin groups differed in their ownership of land and livestock and accumulated heritable wealth, and the emerging dependence of the poor on the rich translated this economic inequality into social inequality. These remain rife in large-scale nation-states today: the income held by the richest 10% of a nation reaches 30.2% (USA) in the Western world and 51.8% (Namibia) elsewhere (Roser and Ortiz-Ospina, 2013). Social classes pervade the industrialised world, from those that are based purely on wealth to more culturally entrenched and inflexible institutions such as the Indian caste system. For the majority of society, having to accept an inferior economic and social status to the elite is a profound mismatch when contrasted with the egalitarianism of foraging communities.

Many public health scholars have highlighted the explanatory power of inequality for understanding variation in the prevalence of mental disorders across high-income countries, and there is a strong correlation (r = 0.73) between these two variables (Pickett and Wilkinson, 2008). It seems that one's relative social standing and wealth have much greater impacts on mental health than one's absolute economic circumstances. This comparison-based system of affect determination is intuitive from an evolutionary perspective since competition is the fundamental driver of natural selection: material wealth only translates into a competitive advantage in survival or reproduction if one has relatively more than other members of society. For instance, whilst gross domestic product (GDP) per capita is approximately 40% higher in the USA than Germany, the Gini index of inequality is also 30% higher (World Bank, 2020). Correspondingly, more than a quarter of residents living in the USA had experienced a mental health condition in the past year, while this proportion is less than 10% in Germany (Pickett and Wilkinson, 2008).

Associations with inequality are particularly high for anxiety and impulse control disorders (Pickett and Wilkinson, 2008). This is intuitive from the evolutionary perspective: those at the bottom of the economic and social ladder are likely to engage in risky and impulsive behaviours since they have much to gain and little to lose. They are also likely to experience stress in order to motivate such 'corrective' behaviours. Conversely, an evolved anxiety response is experienced by those at the top of the ladder, who must be hypervigilant towards others who threaten their position. Indeed, there is strong empirical evidence for the relationship between inequality, crime rates and violence across industrialised populations (Kelly, 2000). Stress responses to hierarchical positions are phylogenetically conserved, being suggestive of deep evolutionary roots. For instance, among male savannah baboons, an inverse relationship between hierarchical position and faecal glucocorticoid levels was found (Gesquiere et al., 2011). The exception to this trend was the alpha male, who had the highest glucocorticoid levels of all males in the group; his exceptionally high stress levels were likely induced by the constant threat and frequent attempts to usurp his position.

In contrast to non-human primate and post-Neolithic human societies, the absence of economic and social inequality among foragers, who do not accumulate wealth and are politically egalitarian, likely removes inequality as a potential driver of mental health problems. Accordingly, in a study of Hadza women, no relationship was found between 'social status' and chronic stress proxied by cortisol concentrations in hair (Fedurek et al., 2020). In fact, the authors highlighted their difficulty in identifying any proxies for social status due to the strong egalitarianism of the Hadza, and finally they used interviews to measure popularity and foraging reputation.

Some studies also point to a raised risk of psychotic disorders as inequality increases (Kirkbride et al., 2014). Paranoid schizophrenia and persecutory delusions may represent a phenotypic mismatch caused by overstimulation of a threat-detection response to resource competition and associated hostile local social environments, which were likely less prevalent in egalitarian ancestral communities. Similarly, a recent meta-analysis identified an association between inequality and depressive disorders (Ribeiro et al., 2017). One evolutionary hypothesis of depression is that it is an ancient adaptation to low status in dominance hierarchies. Symptoms such as social withdrawal, low self-esteem, feelings of shame, anhedonia and fatigue may have functioned to promote submission and discourage aggression towards more dominant individuals; some analogous behaviours such as avoidance of eye contact and social interaction with dominants occur in low-status baboons (Price, 1967). Price describes this hierarchy-driven behavioural syndrome as a 'vestigial and useless heirloom in man' (1967: 246). Indeed, among hunter-gatherers, this depressive psychology would not have been stimulated since hierarchies were absent altogether, and thus subordinate behaviour was never required. However, following the re-emergence of social status and class over the last 10,000 years, depression induced by low status may have returned as a novel risk factor for our species.

5.4.2 Childhood

Infancy and early childhood represent critical periods in which individual psychology is calibrated to prevailing socioecological conditions (Bowlby, 1969), and therefore they evolved as the periods of greatest neural plasticity (see also Chapters 14 and 15). Whilst increased stress reactivity may be an adaptive response to harsh environments, chronic exposure to psychosocial stressors in early life results in dysregulation of the hypothalamic–pituitary–adrenal axis and substantially increases the risk of an extensive range of mental disorders (McEwen, 2003).The childhood experiences of WEIRD and hunter-gatherer children differ markedly. The following sections describe these differences and consider their implications for mental health.

5.4.2.1 Autonomy, Exploration, Social Learning and Play

According to embodied capital theory, the long period of human childhood evolved to allow the necessary time to develop the complex skills required for our species' foraging niche (Kaplan et al., 2000). During childhood, foragers learn subsistence skills via exploration, practice and play.

Hunter-gatherer societies place heavy emphasis on individual autonomy (see Section 5.4.1.2), and this extends to children too. Parents rarely interfere with children's activities even when they play with machetes or burning embers (see Figure 5.3; see also www.youtube.com/watch?

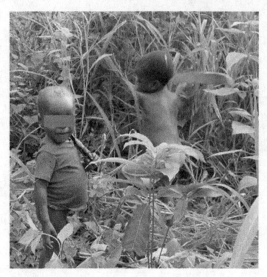

Figure 5.3 A BaYaka infant and child practicing using machetes (credit: Nikhil Chaudhary)

v=drJNIGOo0lI for footage from our field site). Our analysis of the ontogeny of BaYaka learning demonstrated that from infancy to early childhood learning occurs principally via imitation; after weaning, children are free to explore their surroundings and learning occurs in the context of playgroups and through practice (Salali et al., 2019).

The autonomous nature of childhood in hunter-gatherers contrasts with a WEIRD childhood, most of which is spent in formal education and supervised 'helicopter parenting'. In our observations, teaching accounted for only 6% of BaYaka learning events (Salali et al., 2019), and unlike in Western education, hunter-gatherers do not often give direct instructions when teaching. Instead, they create a learning opportunity, like providing a tool, and monitor the children's actions without interfering; children then adjust their behaviour according to the feedback they receive (Hewlett and Roulette, 2016; Salali et al., 2019). Therefore, teaching is more based on practice and feedback than in WEIRD cultures. For example, teaching via verbal explanation occurred only six times in the 10-hour videotapes of Aka (from the Central African Republic) caregiver–infant interactions (Hewlett and Roulette, 2016). Peer teaching is also common, and studies of Hadza and BaYaka children showed that child–child teaching represented 75% of observed teaching episodes (Lew-Levy et al., 2020).

Learning via play is much more common than teaching in the early childhoods of hunter-gatherers. After weaning, children start spending more time in mixed-aged playgroups, and field observations suggest that work-themed play facilitates the acquisition of subsistence skills based on gendered division of labour, social norms via supervision of younger members of the playgroup and cultural values during other forms of play (Boyette, 2016; Salali et al., 2019). Thus, in contrast to the dichotomous relationship of lesson time and play time in WEIRD schools, learning and play in hunter-gatherers are two sides of the same coin. Moreover, hunter-gatherer play is not competitive and fosters the collaborative interaction that is essential for successful subsistence (Boyette, 2016).

According to the Good Childhood Report (The Children's Society, 2020), declines in children's overall happiness with life and school are partially explained by increased fear of failure. WEIRD education is dominated by continuous grading, high-stakes concentrated examination periods, class separation based on abilities, teacher-led learning and punishment. This system, which encourages competition and is highly pressured, must negatively impact children's self-esteem and stimulate fear of failure. In contrast, hunter-gatherer learning does not include any of these ingredients, and learning via play is fun rather than pressured, 'assessed' incrementally and informally, peer to peer and, above all, inherently cooperative rather than competitive. It is therefore unsurprising that learning, which many argue has been the driving selective force for human brain expansion (Hermann et al., 2007), can generate phenotypic mismatch in children.

Given that an extended childhood likely evolved for developing and practicing subsistence skills (Kaplan et al., 2000), for most of our evolutionary history, a 'successful' childhood was characterised by high levels of physical activity and exploration. However, these learning styles are founded upon behaviours that are considered pathological in modern classroom environments and can result in ADHD diagnoses. Several of the Diagnostic and Statistical Manual of Mental Disorders, 5th Edition (DSM-5) diagnostic criteria explicitly refer to the disruptive effects of inattention in the context of schooling, and their associations with poor academic attainment are well established (Loe and Feldman, 2007). If ADHD is an environmental mismatch, improved outcomes may be possible via altering modern pedagogy. Clinicians have highlighted that young people with an ADHD diagnosis report the beneficial effects of physical activity intervals between academic classes (Swanepoel et al., 2017). Moreover, a recent meta-analysis of physical activity interventions ranging from swimming to climbing identified positive effects on all examined domains of executive function – inhibition, shifting, working memory and attention – among those with an ADHD diagnosis (Welsch et al., 2021).

5.4.2.2 Child-Rearing Practices

Although hunter-gatherer caregivers have a more laissez-faire approach to child-rearing, this does not mean that children are left alone. On the contrary, infants and young children are looked after by multiple caregivers, both parents and others (alloparents) (Apicella and Crittenden, 2015). Ethnographic observations have revealed common child-rearing features across several hunter-gatherer groups. These are on-demand breastfeeding, weaning between the ages of two and three, care from multiple individuals, close physical contact with caregivers and co-sleeping (Apicella and Crittenden, 2015).

Our focal sampling observations of BaYaka infants show that over the 12 daylight hours they are held for 4 hours, receive some form of direct care for 7 hours and are alone for less than half an hour, and crying is responded to promptly via singing, carrying and breastfeeding (Chaudhary, unpublished data, 2014). This indulgent and responsive caregiving likely aids in the development of secure attachment (Konner, 2016). 'Attachment' refers to the bond that develops between an infant and caregiver during the first years of life, and a secure attachment – where the infant seeks out the attachment figure in times of distress and feels comfortable to explore the environment in a caregiver's presence – is considered crucial for healthy development (Ainsworth, 1978).

In WEIRD societies where nuclear families prevail, infants usually form attachments with one or two principal caregivers. In contrast, hunter-gatherer children have extensive caregiver networks. For example, among the Efe of the Democratic Republic of the Congo, infants are in physical contact with an alloparent for 60% of the day, interact with 14 alloparents per day, are passed among caregivers 8 times per hour and are nursed by multiple women (Ivey, 2000; Tronick et al., 1987).

Mismatches in caregiving may affect the mental health of infants. Breastfeeding patterns in WEIRD societies are markedly different from those in hunter-gatherer societies. In the UK, only 23% of mothers continue breastfeeding until nine months (NHS Digital, 2012), whereas this is guaranteed among hunter-gatherers. Importantly, endocrine processes stimulated by breastfeeding relieve anxiety symptoms (Hahn-Holbrook and Haselton, 2014). Colic is less common among hunter-gatherers (Lummaa et al., 1998), indicative of lower psychosocial stress. It is hypothesised that given the constant physical proximity between hunter-gatherer and primate infants and their caregivers, infant crying literally functions as a 'cry for help' upon separation from caregivers. The substantially lower time in physical contact, especially skin-to-skin contact and co-sleeping, and higher frequency of being left alone among WEIRD infants represent pronounced mismatches that we believe are responsible for considerable infant distress.

The large alloparenting networks among foragers also permit constant physical proximity and continuous responsiveness to infants even when parents are occupied with other activities. Moreover, having multiple attachment figures buffers the negative impacts of having an insecure mother–infant relationship (van Ijzendoorn et al., 1992). Given the associations between unavailable or insensitive attachment figures in early life and a vast array of mental illnesses – depression, anxiety, post-traumatic stress disorder, obsessive-compulsive disorder, eating disorders, schizophrenia and suicidal tendencies (Mikulincer and Shaver, 2012) – we cannot overstate our expectation that hunter-gatherer childcare reduces psychiatric risk, or rather WEIRD childcare increases this risk. We strongly encourage further research into the long-term effects of alloparenting and highly sensitive caregiving on hunter-gatherer mental health. We expect that the benefits also extend to caregivers. For instance, breastfeeding and skin-to-skin contact are associated with lower incidence rates of maternal PPD (Hahn-Holbrook and Haselton, 2014; Mörelius et al., 2015). Moreover, alloparental support reduces the pressure and burden placed on parents; in our analysis of childcare in Agta and BaYaka foragers, only approximately 30% of infant and young children's close-proximity interactions were with their parents (Chaudhary, unpublished data, 2014).

5.4.3 Time Perspective and Future Orientation

Immediate-return (simple) hunter-gatherers acquire resources on a daily basis, consume them immediately and do not have food storage systems (Woodburn, 1982). Thus, long-term planning is largely redundant for foragers. For instance, we played a *future-discounting* game in which we asked the BaYaka and a neighbouring farmer population whether they would like one food item now or five tomorrow (Salali and Migliano, 2015). Approximately 80% of the BaYaka chose the one item today option compared with 40% of the farmers, who are presumably more accustomed to future planning seasons in advance. We expect that future orientation is largely determined by the timescales of resource acquisition and storage. WEIRD societies are at the extreme end of this spectrum: we frequently predict the impacts that our current choices will have on our lives decades later. Career trajectories are planned to optimise resource accumulation over a period of approximately 50 years, and considerable wealth is saved over similar timescales. Highly valued personal goals also tend to be realised over extended periods.

Emotions function as a behavioural motivation system; accordingly, our mood is heavily impacted by progress towards current goals rather than one's overall life situation (Nesse, 2004). When progress halts or reverses despite continued effort, low mood may be an adaptive driver of termination of this effort. However, in WEIRD societies, it can be very difficult to abort goals that have been planned for and worked on over extended periods. Continually attempting to achieve goals over extended periods without seeing any progress has been hypothesised as a major driver of depression in industrialised societies (Nesse, 2004). Similarly, anxiety is an emotional response that occurs in the anticipation of a future threat. Thus, the pronounced preoccupation with the future in WEIRD populations likely increases vulnerability to high levels of anxiety.

These differences between WEIRD and foraging societies in the timescales of resource acquisition and personal goals and, in turn, in time perspective represent a phenotypic mismatch, potentially contributing to mood disorders (Salali et al., 2021). In the West there has been growing interest in mindfulness practice, which encourages focusing on present experience rather than the future, which likely explains its well-established anxiety-reducing effects (Khourey et al., 2013). Increased mindfulness is also strongly associated with decreased intolerance of uncertainty, one of the largest predictors of anxiety (Salali et al., 2021). Priming experiments also suggest that time perspective may be highly flexible (Shevorykin et al., 2019); hence, therapies aiming to recalibrate it may be viable psychological treatments.

5.5 Future Directions and Conclusion

Here, we have outlined key mismatches in the domains of social organisation, child-rearing and timescales of goals and speculated about their impacts on mental health. Research testing these hypotheses is extremely scarce. We propose two key future directions for research: (1) epidemiological work testing whether the prevalence and severity of mental disorders are lower among hunter-gatherers; and (2) in such cases, identifying and quantifying the specific mismatches that may underpin this increased prevalence of mental disorders in WEIRD populations and trialling interventions that reduce these mismatches.

Epidemiological studies must consider cultural differences and the fact that most hunter-gatherers are illiterate with limited numeracy. Most psychological evaluations are done using established screening tools that often involve Likert scales or other forms of rating. From our own experience, asking the BaYaka to rate anything or about the frequency of a particular event is often met with confusion since these thinking styles are unfamiliar and unused in their culture. As such, tools from Western psychiatry must be adapted to ensure cultural appropriateness and comprehension. Balancing emic (culture-specific) with etic (universal) approaches is key; on the one hand, we aim to obtain comparable cross-cultural epidemiological data, while on the other, the expression and manifestation of emotions and mental illness (*idioms of distress*) vary across cultures (Littlewood, 1990). For instance, in India, depressed and anxious patients frequently present with pain in the extremities and other bodily symptoms, but this is uncommon in the West (Desai and Chaturvedi, 2017). Similarly, methods of identifying symptoms must be culturally calibrated. For example, social withdrawal is an important diagnostic criterion for many mental disorders; however, hunter-gatherers co-reside with many camp mates and live in open dwellings; thus, operationalising 'social withdrawal' is difficult. One solution we have considered is examining whether any camp members are not participating in *massana* rituals, which are usually camp-wide activities; this is a more culturally appropriate measure (emic) of a universal diagnostic criterion (etic). Moreover, given the complexity and subjectivity of emotion, it is difficult enough for individuals to effectively communicate inner mental states even when speaking the same language. Therefore, substantial time must be committed to harnessing a nuanced understanding of emotion-related vocabulary.

Identifying which mismatches are responsible for the higher prevalence rates of mental disorders among WEIRD populations must be hypothesis-driven. One technique would be detailed characterisation of the differences between WEIRD and hunter-gatherer populations and then implementing interventions to minimise any mismatch. For instance, the study of depression among the Tsimane found no association with old age, a relationship that is common in WEIRD contexts, which the authors speculated is caused by the elderly's productive redundancy (Stieglitz et al., 2015a). Future research could trial the impact of resident participation in productive activities such as gardening and cooking on mental well-being within elderly care homes, or foster a platform whereby the elderly can share their accumulated life experience and 'wisdom' with younger generations. Other promising avenues include examining how alternative education systems that foster exploration, peer learning and non-didactic teaching affect the educational attainment and distress of children with ADHD, as well as the prevalence of common mental health problems among students more generally. Data examining the long-term effects of replicating hunter-gatherer sensitive caregiving (i.e. breastfeeding on demand, co-sleeping, high responsiveness to crying and continuous proximity) would be invaluable. Additionally, studies examining the psychological well-being of individuals living in communes or 'intentional communities' will offer insight into the possibility of reducing mismatches in social organisation and support networks in modern society. Finally, engagement in synchrony-based community 'rituals' may be a particularly effective intervention for those experiencing chronic loneliness.

We hope that the descriptions of hunter-gatherer life and the speculations regarding their effects on mental health provided here will aid scholars in formulating and testing similar mismatch hypotheses. Like other fields of medicine, psychiatry has suffered somewhat from an emphasis on biochemical mechanisms and from neglect of upstream aetiology. Whilst the relationships between life circumstances and psychiatric health do receive some attention, expanding this approach to consider mismatches between industrialised and hunter-gatherer life will improve our understanding of *why* such relationships exist and will complement the heavy focus on the mechanistic *how*. Given the speed at which extant hunter-gatherer societies are becoming integrated into market economies, the window of opportunity to conduct this research is rapidly closing, and so this should be considered an urgent priority.

References

Abed, R., and Abbas, M. (2014). Can the new epidemiology of schizophrenia help elucidate its causation? *Irish Journal of Psychological Medicine*, 31, 1–5.

Ainsworth, M. (1978). The Bowlby–Ainsworth attachment theory. *Behavioral and Brain Sciences*, 1, 436–438.

Amir, D., and McAuliffe, K. (2020). Cross-cultural, developmental psychology: integrating approaches and key insights. *Evolution and Human Behavior*, 41, 430–444.

Apicella, C. L., and Crittenden, A. N. (2015). Hunter-gatherer families and parenting. In D. Buss (ed.), *The Handbook of Evolutionary Psychology*.

Hoboken, NJ: Wiley, pp. 797–827.

Arnold, J., Sunell, S., Nigra, B., et al. (2016). Entrenched disbelief: complex hunter-gatherers and the case for inclusive cultural evolutionary thinking. *Journal of Archaeological Method and Theory*, 23, 448–499.

Bailey, G., and Milner, N. (2002). Coastal hunter-gatherers and social evolution: marginal or central? *Before Farming*, 2002, 1–15.

Barkow, J., Cosmides, L., and Tooby, J. (eds.) (1992). *The Adapted Mind: Evolutionary Psychology and the Generation of Culture*. New York: Oxford University Press.

Beck, R., Cesario, T., Yousefi, A., et al. (2000). Choral singing, performance perception, and immune system changes in salivary immunoglobulin A and cortisol. *Music Perception*, 18, 87–106.

Biesele, M., and Barclay, S. (2001). Ju/'Hoan women's tracking knowledge and its contribution to their husbands' hunting success. *African Study Monographs, Supplement*, 26, 67–84.

Blurton-Jones, N., Smith, L., O'Connell, J., et al. (1992). Demography of the Hadza, an increasing and high density population of savanna foragers. *American Journal of Physical Anthropology*, 89, 159–181.

Bock, J., and Johnson, S. (2004). Subsistence ecology and play among the Okavango Delta peoples of Botswana. *Human Nature*, 15, 63–81.

Boehm, C., Barclay, H., Dentan, R., et al. (1993). Egalitarian behavior and reverse dominance hierarchy [and comments and reply]. *Current Anthropology*, 34, 227–254.

Bowlby, J. (1969). *Attachment and Loss, Vol. 1: Attachment*. New York: Basic Books.

Boyce, P (2003). Risk factors for postnatal depression: a review and risk factors in Australian populations. *Archives of Women's Mental Health*, 6, s43–s50.

Boyette, A. (2016). Children's play and culture learning in an egalitarian foraging society. *Child Development*, 87, 759–769.

Boyette, A., and Hewlett, B. (2017). Autonomy, equality, and teaching among Aka foragers and Ngandu farmers of the Congo Basin. *Human Nature*, 28, 289–322.

Chaudhary, N., Salali, G., Thompson, J. et al. (2016). Competition for cooperation: variability, benefits and heritability of relational wealth in hunter-gatherers. *Scientific Reports*, 6, 29120.

Church of England Research and Statistics (2019). *Statistics for Mission 2019*, 1–54. Retrieved from www.churchofengland.org/sites/default/files/2020-10/2019StatisticsForMission.pdf

Crittenden, A., and Schnorr, S. (2017). Current views on hunter-gatherer nutrition and the evolution of the human diet. *American Journal of Physical Anthropology*, 162, 84–109.

Desai, G., and Chaturvedi, S. (2017). Idioms of distress. *Journal of Neurosciences in Rural Practice*, 8, S094–S097.

Ding, Y.-C., Chi, H.-C., Grady, D., et al. (2002). Evidence of positive selection acting at the human dopamine receptor D4 gene locus. *Proceedings of the National Academy of Sciences of the United States of America*, 99, 309–314.

Dingle, G., Brander, C., Ballantyne, J., et al. (2004). Mental health benefits of choir singing for disadvantaged adults. *Psychology of Music*, 41, 405–421.

Duberstein, P., Conwell, Y., Conner, K., et al. (2004). Poor social integration and suicide: fact or artifact? A case–control study. *Psychological Medicine*, 34, 1331–1337.

Dunbar, R. (1998). The social brain hypothesis. *Evolutionary Anthropology*, 6, 178–190.

Dyble, M., Thompson, J., Smith, D., et al. (2016). Networks of food sharing reveal the functional significance of multilevel sociality in two hunter-gatherer groups. *Current Biology*, 26, 2017–2021.

Eisenberger, N. (2012). The neural bases of social pain: evidence for shared representations with physical pain. *Psychosomatic Medicine*, 74, 126–135.

Fedurek, P., Lacroix, L., Lehmann, J., et al. (2020). Status does not predict stress: women in an egalitarian hunter-gatherer society. *Evolutionary Human Sciences*, 2, E44.

Fischer, R., Callander, R., Reddish, P., et al. (2013). How do rituals affect cooperation? *Human Nature*, 24, 115–125.

Frackowiak, T., Oleszkiewicz, A., Butovskaya, M., et al. (2020). Subjective happiness among Polish and Hadza people. *Frontiers in Psychology*, 11, 1173.

Gesquiere, L., Learn, N., Simao, M., et al. (2011). Life at the top: rank and stress in wild male baboons. *Science*, 333, 357–360.

Gizer, I., Ficks, C., and Waldman, I. (2009). Candidate gene studies of ADHD: a meta-analytic review. *Human Genetics*, 126, 51–90.

Gray, P. (2013). Hunter-gatherer egalitarianism as a force for decline in sexual dimorphism. *Psychological Inquiry*, 24, 192–194.

Gurven, M., and Kaplan, H. (2007). Longevity among hunter-gatherers: a cross-cultural examination. *Population and Development Review*, 33, 321–365.

Gurven, M., and Lieberman, D. (2020). WEIRD bodies: mismatch, medicine and missing diversity. *Evolution and Human Behavior*, 41, 330–340.

Hahn-Holbrook, J., and Haselton, M. (2014). Is postpartum depression a disease of modern civilization? *Current Directions in Psychological Science*, 23, 395–400.

Hawkes, K. (2003). Grandmothers and the evolution of human longevity. *American Journal of Human Biology*, 15, 294–302.

Hawkley, L., and Cacioppo, J. (2010). A theoretical and empirical review of consequences and mechanisms. *Annals of Behavioral Medicine*, 40, 218–227.

Henrich, J., and McElreath, R. (2003). The evolution of cultural evolution. *Evolutionary Anthropology*, 12, 123–135.

Herlosky, K., Benyshek, D., Mabulla, I., et al. (2020). Postpartum maternal mood among Hadza foragers of Tanzania: a mixed methods approach. *Culture, Medicine and Psychiatry*, 44, 305–332.

Herrmann, E., Call, J., Hernàndez-Lloreda, M., et al. (2007) Humans have evolved specialized skills of social cognition: the cultural intelligence hypothesis. *Science*, 317, 1360–1366.

Hewlett, B. (1991). Demography and childcare in preindustrial societies. *Journal of Anthropological Research*, 47, 1–37.

Hewlett, B., and Roulette, C. (2016). Teaching in hunter-gatherer infancy. *Royal Society Open Science*, 3, 150403.

Hill, K., Walker, R., Božičević, M., et al. (2011). Co-residence patterns in hunter-gatherer societies show unique human social structure. *Science*, 331, 1286–1289.

Ivey, P. (2000) Cooperative reproduction in Ituri forest hunter-gatherers: who cares for Efe infants? *Current Anthropology*, 41, 856–866.

January, J., and Chimbari, M. (2018). Study protocol on criterion validation of Edinburgh Postnatal Depression Scale (EPDS), Patient Health Questionnaire (PHQ-9) and Centre for Epidemiological Studies-Depression (CES-D) screening tools among rural postnatal women; a cross-sectional study. *BMJ Open*, 8, e019085.

Kaplan, H., Hill, K., and Hurtado, M. (1990). Risk, foraging and food sharing among the Ache. In E. Cashdan (ed.), *Risk and Uncertainty in Tribal and Peasant Economies*. London: Routledge, pp. 107–143.

Kaplan, H., Hill, K., Lancaster, J., and Hurtado, M. (2000). A theory of human life history evolution: diet, intelligence, and longevity. *Evolutionary Anthropology*, 9, 156–185.

Kelly, M. (2000). Inequality and crime. *Review of Economics and Statistics*, 82, 530–539.

Kelly, R. (2013). *The Lifeways of Hunter-Gatherers: The Foraging Spectrum*. Cambridge: Cambridge University Press.

Khoury, B., Lecomte, T., Fortin, G., et al. (2013). Mindfulness-based therapy: a comprehensive meta-analysis. *Clinical Psychology Review*, 33, 763–771.

Kirkbride, J., Jones, P., Ullrich, S., et al. (2014). Social deprivation, inequality, and the neighborhood-level incidence of psychotic syndromes in East London. *Schizophrenia Bulletin*, 40, 169–180.

Konner, M. (2016). Hunter-gatherer infancy and childhood in the context of human evolution. In C. L. Meehan and A. N. Crittenden (eds.), *Childhood: Origins, Evolution, and Implications*. Santa Fe, NM: University of New Mexico Press, pp. 123–154.

Lee, R. (1969). Eating Christmas in the Kalahari. Retrieved from http://people.morrisville.edu/~reymers/readings/ANTH101/EatingChristmas-Lee.pdf

Lee, R., and Daly, R. (1999). *The Cambridge Encyclopedia of Hunters and Gatherers*. Cambridge: Cambridge University Press.

Lee, R., and DeVore, I. (1968). *Man the Hunter*. London: Aldine.

Leigh-Hunt, N., Bagguley, D., Bash, K., et al. (2017). An overview of systematic reviews on the public health consequences of social isolation and loneliness. *Public Health*, 152, 157–171.

Lew-Levy, S., Kissler, S., Boyette, A., et al. (2020). Who teaches children to forage? Exploring the primacy of child-to-child teaching among Hadza and BaYaka hunter-gatherers of Tanzania and Congo. *Evolution and Human Behavior*, 41, 12–22.

Liang, J., Krause, N., and Bennett, J. (2001). Social exchange and well-being: is giving better than receiving? *Psychology and Aging*, 16, 511–523.

Lim, G., Tam, W., Lu, Y., et al. (2018). Prevalence of depression in the community from 30 countries between 1994 and 2014. *Scientific Reports*, 8, 2861.

Littlewood, R. (1990) From categories to contexts: a decade of the 'new cross-cultural psychiatry'. *British Journal of Psychiatry*, 156, 308–327.

Loe, I., and Feldman, H. (2007). Academic and educational outcomes of children with ADHD. *Journal of Pediatric Psychology*, 32, 643–654.

Lummaa, V., Vuorisalo, T., Barr, R., et al. (1998) Why cry? Adaptive significance of intensive crying in human infants. *Evolution and Human Behavior*, 19, 193–202.

Marlowe, F. W. (2005). Hunter-gatherers and human evolution. *Evolutionary Anthropology*, 14, 54–67.

McEwen, B. (2003). Early life influences on life-long patterns of behavior and health. *Mental Retardation and Developmental Disabilities Research Reviews*, 9, 149–154.

McGee, R. (2015). Unemployment and depression among emerging adults in 12 states, behavioral risk factor surveillance system. *Preventing Chronic Disease*, 12, E38.

Mesoudi, A., Whiten, A., and Laland, K. (2004). Perspective: is human cultural evolution

Darwinian? Evidence reviewed from the perspective of the origin of species. *Evolution*, 58, 1–11.

Mikulincer, M., and Shaver, P. (2012). An attachment perspective on psychopathology. *World Psychiatry*, 11, 11–15.

Mörelius, E., Örtenstrand, A., Theodorsson, E., et al. (2015). A randomised trial of continuous skin-to-skin contact after preterm birth and the effects on salivary cortisol, parental stress, depression, and breastfeeding. *Early Human Development*, 91, 63–70.

Murphy, J. M. (1976). Psychiatric labelling in cross-cultural perspective. *Science*, 191, 1019–1028.

Nesse, R. M. (2004). Natural selection and the elusiveness of happiness. *Philosophical Transactions of the Royal Society B: Biological Sciences*, 359, 1333–1347.

Nesse, R. M. (2019). *Good Reasons for Bad Feelings: Insights from the Frontier of Evolutionary Psychiatry*. London: Allen Lane.

Nettle, D., Gibson, M., Lawson, D., et al. (2013). Human behavioral ecology: current research and future prospects. *Behavioral Ecology*, 24, 1031–1040.

NHS Digital (2012). Infant feeding survey – UK, 2010. London: NHS. Retrieved from https://digital.nhs.uk/data-and-information/publications/statistical/infant-feeding-survey/infant-feeding-survey-uk-2010

O'Keefe, J., and Cordain, L. (2004). Cardiovascular disease resulting from a diet and lifestyle at odds with our paleolithic genome: how to become a 21st-century hunter-gatherer. *Mayo Clinic Proceedings*, 79, 101–108.

Page, A., Viguier, S., Dyble, M., et al. (2016). Reproductive trade-offs in extant hunter-gatherers suggest adaptive mechanism for the Neolithic expansion. *Proceedings of the National Academy of Sciences of the United States of America*, 113, 4694–4699.

Pearce, E., Launay, J., and Dunbar, R. (2015). The ice-breaker effect: singing mediates fast social bonding. *Royal Society Open Science*, 2, 150221.

Pickett, K., and Wilkinson, R. (2008). People like us: ethnic group density effects on health. *Ethnicity & Health*, 4, 321–334.

Polimeni, J., and Reiss, J. (2002). How shamanism and group selection may reveal the origins of schizophrenia. *Medical Hypotheses*, 58, 244–248.

Pontzer, H., Wood, B., and Raichlen, D. (2018). Hunter-gatherers as models in public health. *Obesity Reviews*, 19, 24–35.

Porter, C., and Marlowe, F. (2007). How marginal are forager habitats? *Journal of Archaeological Science*, 34, 59–68.

Price, J. (1967). The dominance hierarchy and the evolution of mental illness. *Lancet*, 290, 243–246.

Raison, C., and Miller, A. (2012). The evolutionary significance of depression in pathogen host defense (PATHOS-D). *Molecular Psychiatry*, 18, 15–37.

Reyes-Garcia, V., Gallois, S., Pyhala, A., et al. (2021). Happy just because. A cross-cultural study on subjective wellbeing in three Indigenous societies. *PLoS ONE*, 16, e0251551.

Ribeiro, W., Bauer, A., Andrade, M., et al. (2017). Income inequality and mental illness-related morbidity and resilience: a systematic review and meta-analysis. *Lancet Psychiatry*, 4, 554–562.

Richardson, R. (2007). *Evolutionary Psychology as Maladapted Psychology*. Cambridge, MA: MIT Press.

Roser, M., and Ortiz-Ospina, E. (2013). *Income Inequality*. Our World in Data. Retrieved from https://ourworldindata.org/income-inequality

Salali, G. D., and Migliano, A. B. (2015). Future discounting in Congo Basin hunter-gatherers declines with socio-economic transitions. *PLoS ONE*, 10, e0137806.

Salali, G. D., Chaudhary, N., Bouer, J., et al. (2019). Development of social learning and play in BaYaka hunter-gatherers of Congo. *Scientific Reports*, 9, 11080.

Salali, G. D., Chaudhary, N., Thompson, J., et al. (2016). Knowledge-sharing networks in hunter-gatherers and the evolution of cumulative culture. *Current Biology*, 26, 2516–2521.

Salali, G. D., Uysal, M. S., and Bevan, A. (2021). Adaptive function and correlates of anxiety during a pandemic. *Evolution, Medicine, and Public Health*, 9, 393–405.

Shevorykin, A., Pittman, J., Bickel, W., et al. (2019). Primed for health: future thinking priming decreases delay discounting. *Health Behaviour and Policy Review*, 6, 363–377.

Shultziner, D., Stevens, T., Stevens, M., et al. (2010). The causes and scope of political egalitarianism during the Last Glacial: a multi-disciplinary perspective. *Biology and Philosophy*, 25, 319–346.

Small, R., Lumley, J., Yelland, J., et al. (2007). The performance of the Edinburgh Postnatal Depression Scale in English speaking and non-English speaking populations in Australia. *Social Psychiatry and Psychiatric Epidemiology*, 42, 70–78.

Smallwood, T., Giacomin, P., Loukas, A., et al. (2017). Helminth immunomodulation in autoimmune disease. *Frontiers in Immunology*, 8, 453.

Steptoe, A., Owen, N., Kunz-Ebrecht, S., et al. (2004). Loneliness and neuroendocrine, cardiovascular, and inflammatory stress responses in middle-aged men and women. *Psychoneuroendocrinology*, 29, 593–611.

Stieglitz, J., Schniter, E., von Rueden, C., et al. (2015a). Functional disability and social conflict increase risk of depression in older adulthood among Bolivian forager-farmers. *Journals of Gerontology, Series B: Psychological Sciences and Social Sciences*, 70, 948–956.

Stieglitz, J., Trumble, B., Thompson, M., et al. (2015b). Depression as sickness behavior? A test of the host defense hypothesis in a high pathogen population. *Brain, Behavior, and Immunity*, 49, 130–139.

Swanepoel, A., Music, G., Launer, J., et al. (2017). How evolutionary thinking can help us to understand ADHD. *BJPsych Advances*, 23, 410–418.

Tajfel, H., and Turner, J. C. (2019). The social identity theory of intergroup behavior. In J. T. Jost and J. Sidanius (eds.), *Political Psychology*. Hove: Psychology Press, pp. 276–293.

The Children's Society (2020). The Good Childhood Report. Retrieved from www.childrenssociety.org.uk/sites/default/files/2020-11/Good-Childhood-Report-2020.pdf

Tovo-Rodrigues, L., Callegari-Jacques, S., Petzl-Erler, M., et al. (2010). Dopamine receptor D4 allele distribution in Amerindians: a reflection of past behavior differences? *American Journal of Physical Anthropology*, 143, 458–464.

Tronick, E., Morelli, G., and Winn, S. (1987). Multiple caretaking of Efe (pygmy) infants. *New Series*, 89, 96–106.

United Nations (2015). *The United Nations Standard Minimum Rules for the Treatment of Prisoners (the Nelson Mandela Rules)*. Vienna: United Nations Office on Drugs and Crime.

van Ijzendoorn, M., Sagi, A., and Lambermon, M. (1992). The multiple caretaker paradox: data from Holland and Israel. *New Directions for Child and Adolescent Development*, 1992, 5–24.

van Schaik, C., and Burkart, J. (2011). Social learning and evolution: the cultural intelligence hypothesis. *Philosophical Transactions of the Royal Society B: Biological Sciences*, 366, 1008–1016.

Welsch, L., Alliott, O., Kelly, P., et al. (2021). The effect of physical activity interventions on executive functions in children with ADHD: a systematic review and meta-analysis. *Mental Health and Physical Activity*, 20, 100379.

Wilmsen, E., Denbow, J., Bicchieri, M., et al. (1990). Paradigmatic history of San-speaking peoples and current attempts at revision. *Current Anthropology*, 31, 489–524.

Woodburn, J. (1982). Egalitarian societies. *Man*, 17, 431–451.

Woody, C. A., Ferrari, A., Siskind, D., et al. (2017). A systematic review and meta-regression of the prevalence and incidence of perinatal depression. *Journal of Affective Disorders*, 29, 86–92.

World Bank (2020). World Bank Open Data. Retrieved from https://data.worldbank.org

Wrangham, R. W. (1980). An ecological model of female-bonded primate groups. *Behaviour*, 75, 262–300.

Chapter

6

Why Do Mental Disorders Persist?
Evolutionary Foundations for Psychiatry

Randolph M. Nesse*

Abstract

Discovering why natural selection has left humans vulnerable to mental disorders will make psychiatry more sensible and effective, but defining the appropriate objects and kinds of explanation remains challenging. Asking how a disorder increases fitness is a mistake; disorders are not adaptations and they do not have evolutionary explanations. The correct objects of explanation are the traits that make all members of a species vulnerable to a disorder. Task 1 is to describe the evolutionary origins and functions of the traits involved. Task 2 is to describe the proximate processes that result in the disorder. Task 3 is to discover why natural selection left the traits vulnerable to malfunction. Five main kinds of explanation need to be considered: stochasticity, path dependence, mismatch, trade-offs that benefit the individual and traits that benefit gene transmission at a cost to the individual. Depression, addiction, eating disorders, autism and schizophrenia are used to illustrate the opportunities and challenges of framing and testing hypotheses about vulnerability. Multiple explanations are often needed for a single disorder, frustrating the wish for simplicity. However, recognising the fundamental differences between organic and designed systems offers opportunities for resolving – or at least understanding – some enduring controversies in psychiatry.

Keywords

adaptationism, evolutionary biology, evolutionary medicine, evolutionary psychiatry, mental disorders, methodology, psychiatry

6.1 Introduction

Mental disorders don't have to exist. Natural selection could have eliminated the genetic variations that make us vulnerable to schizophrenia, autism and bipolar disorder. It could have shaped organisms that cooperate reliably without conflict. It could have made us capable of controlling our emotions and our impulses to eat and drink. But it didn't.

Genetic variations that cause mental disorders persist. Relationship conflicts arouse anger, jealousy, depression and wishes for spiteful revenge. And the belief that we can use willpower to reliably control our emotions, eating and drinking is an illusion. Mental disorders not only persist, they

are the greatest and least tractable health problems facing our species. Explaining why they persist in the face of natural selection will provide a missing scientific foundation that can make psychiatry more sensible, more effective and more like the rest of medicine.

Reaching agreement on the best evolutionary explanations for vulnerability to mental disorders will be challenging, however. Even for non-psychiatric diseases (see Chapter 2 for the differences between conditions, illness, disease and disorder, etc.), methods for framing and testing evolutionary hypotheses are still developing (Nesse, 2011). Applying those methods to mental disorders poses additional challenges. Observable tissue pathology is usually absent. Information-processing systems have failure modes that are different from those of physiological and anatomical systems. Behaviour and emotions are not shaped directly but via selection on genes that influence brain variations that interact with

* Thanks to Adam Hunt, Riadh Abed, Paul St John-Smith and Joon Yun for valuable comments and corrections.

84

environments to yield actions that vary in their effects on fitness. And selection forces emerge from and vary depending on culture. Challenges also arise from cognitive tendencies. Humans are fascinated by function and seduced by simplicity. These tendencies are major obstacles to progress in evolutionary psychiatry. It is tempting to view disorders as if they are adaptations and to look for possible benefits that could provide simple explanations. But disorders in themselves are not adaptations shaped by natural selection. They do not give net fitness benefits. They do not have evolutionary explanations. The correct objects of explanation are traits that make organisms vulnerable to disorders.

Considerations of function are, however, fundamental and of enormous value. Studying emotional disorders without knowing their evolutionary origins and functions encourages viewing symptoms as if they are diseases. The result is continual controversy about psychiatric diagnosis (see Chapter 2) and slow progress in research on emotional disorders. Looking for the brain abnormalities causing mental disorders without understanding normal function is like looking for the heart abnormalities causing heart failure without knowing what the heart is for.

Adding evolutionary considerations of function transformed ethology into the theoretical and experimental science of behavioural ecology (Westneat and Fox, 2010). Evolutionary psychology describes the evolutionary origins and fitness consequences of human behavioural and emotional traits (Buss, 2020; Lewis et al., 2017; Welling and Shackelford, 2019). Evolutionary medicine provides tools for framing and testing hypotheses about why natural selection has left us vulnerable to diseases (Gluckman et al., 2009; Nesse and Williams, 1994; Perlman, 2005; Stearns and Medzhitov, 2016; Williams and Nesse, 1991). Evolutionary psychiatry is now applying principles of evolutionary medicine to mental disorders (Abed and St. John Smith, 2016, 2022; Adriaens and De Block, 2011; Brüne, 2016; Crespi, 2020; Kennair, 2003; McGuire and Troisi, 1998; McGuire et al., 1992; Nesse, 1984, 2019; Wenegrat, 1990).

Conceptual confusions still obstruct progress, however. Some arise from a failure to grasp that proximate and evolutionary explanations are different and that both are essential (see Chapters 1 and 2). Controversy also continues about how best to frame and test hypotheses about behaviour (Buller, 2005; Buss and von Hippel, 2018). That evolutionary explanations are essential is now widely accepted, but controversies persist. Gould and Lewontin's critique of adaptationist explanations offered no guidance about how to actually go about testing evolutionary hypotheses (Gould and Lewontin, 1979). That omission and the article's clever rhetoric have left many scientists still thinking – decades later – that all hypotheses about function are untestable 'just-so stories'. Global debates about adaptation have now mostly been supplanted by the assessment of specific hypotheses with specific evidence (Pigliucci and Kaplan, 2000), but many scientists and doctors remain out of the loop.

Another obstacle is the tendency for simple, attractive explanations to persist because people pay attention only to confirming information (Staw, 1976). Conflicting views become the enemy, and the resulting debates are rarely resolved. The combination of commitment, confirmation bias, and preference for simplicity helps to explain the persistence of global debates about group selection, life history theory, adaptationism, nature versus nurture and genetic drift versus natural selection. Evolutionary psychiatry will progress faster if such global debates can be minimised by systematic consideration of all possible explanations for specific hypotheses. This makes it worthwhile to describe the proper objects and kinds of explanation in some detail.

6.2 The Objects of Explanation

Proposals abound for possible fitness benefits thought to explain depression, eating disorders, addiction, attention deficit hyperactivity disorder (ADHD), autism and even schizophrenia. One reason why this mistake is common is that some conditions frequently considered to be disorders or diseases are actually adaptations; pain, anxiety and low mood are examples. Another reason is that individuals at the tails of trait distributions where diseases become likely experience benefits as well as costs. A third reason is that explanations that propose a possible function for a disease often make good memes that spread fast irrespective of their veracity.

Mood disorders that reduce fitness are not adaptations, they are harmful products of dysfunctions in evolved mechanisms (Wakefield, 1992). They do not have evolutionary explanations in terms of their functions. However, the capacity for having and regulating mood is an adaptation. Understanding its evolutionary origins and functions is essential. Why the system is vulnerable to dysfunction is, however, a fundamentally different question.

Substance use and abuse have often been viewed as adaptive, but the appropriate objects of explanation are chemically mediated motivation and learning mechanisms. Understanding how those mechanisms give advantages is a different question from that of why they make us vulnerable to addiction. Why some individuals are more vulnerable than others is a third question. Discovering why the genetic differences that increase the risk of substance abuse persist will offer part of an answer. It will also be important to further test the hypothesis that natural selection shaped preferences for altered states or certain substances, especially alcohol and nicotine (Hagen et al., 2013; Slingerland, 2021). Such a confirmation would explain substance use but would not fully explain vulnerability to addiction and substance abuse that harms fitness.

Eating disorders have often been interpreted as adaptations, usually as extreme eating patterns that give advantages in special situations (Brüne, 2018; Mayhew et al., 2018). For instance, it has been proposed that when food sources are insufficient to sustain childbearing, restrictive dieting can stop reproductive cycling and prevent a useless pregnancy. However, starvation turns off cycling all by itself, and additional caloric restriction is likely to be fatal. The tendency of people with anorexia nervosa to engage in extreme exercise inspired the hypothesis that food scarcity may generate motivations to run that take starving people to places with more food. But anorexics exercise not to find food but to lose weight. The sexual competition hypothesis suggests that women are vulnerable to eating disorders because modern media augment the natural motivation for having a desirable body in order to get better mates (Abed, 1998). This explains why so many women use extreme caloric restriction in intense efforts to be attractive, but it does not by itself explain anorexia nervosa and bulimia (see Chapter 11 for a review and alternative perspective on eating disorders). That requires also

considering the adaptive response to starvation that induces gorging and increasing the body weight set point. Starvation from whatever cause in either sex sets off this response. The resulting out-of-control eating creates increasing fear of obesity and more intense efforts to restrict food intake in a vicious positive-feedback cycle that explains the connection between anorexia and bulimia (Nesse, 2017).

For autism, it is much harder to specify the trait that accounts for vulnerability, but the extremes of a dimension from systematising to empathising (Greenberg et al., 2018) and from autism to schizophrenia (Crespi and Dinsdale, 2019) may be important. Dysfunctions in capacities for social relationships that may reflect sex differences are involved, but pathology in autism ranges widely and can include excess sensitivity to stimuli, inability to inhibit repetitive behaviours, language and intellectual disabilities and epileptic seizures. The special abilities of some individuals with autism offer intriguing clues, but they are not universal traits shaped by selection and they do not increase Darwinian fitness. They may give clues to possible relevant modules and selection forces, but they cannot explain the persistence of the responsible genes.

After ascertaining that a condition is actually a disorder and not an adaptation, the search for an evolutionary explanation proceeds in three steps. Step 1 is to identify the trait(s) that make all individuals in a species vulnerable to the disorder. Step 2 is to understand the proximate mechanisms – genetic, physiological and psychological – that result in malfunction. Step 3 is to determine what combination of evolutionary explanations makes the trait vulnerable to failure. Five categories of potential explanation deserve detailed description.

6.3 Categories of Explanations for Vulnerability

Evolutionary questions about why natural selection left us vulnerable to mental disorders are specialised versions of evolutionary medicine questions about why we are vulnerable to disease in general (Gluckman et al., 2009; Nesse, 2005a; Nesse and Williams, 1994; Perlman, 2005; Stearns and Medzhitov, 2016). Table 6.1 provides a list of possible evolutionary explanations for vulnerability, a mapping to categories used previously in

Table 6.1. Evolutionary explanations for vulnerability

Categories	Previous categories	*Cui bono*
(0) Adaptations that can seem like disorders (Section 6.3.1)	Defences	The individual
(1) Stochasticity (Section 6.3.2.1)		No benefits
(2) Path dependence and major transitions (Section 6.3.2.2)	Constraints	No benefits
(3) Selection is slow/mismatch (Section 6.3.2.3)	Mismatch	No benefits now
	Fast pathogen evolution	No benefits
(4) Trade-offs and intrinsically vulnerable traits (Section 6.3.2.4)	Trade-offs	The individual
(5) Traits and trade-offs that benefit gene transmission at a cost to the individual (Section 6.3.2.5)	Traits that increase reproductive success at a cost to the individual	Genes

evolutionary medicine and information about who benefits (*cui bono*).

6.3.1 Adaptations That Can Seem Like Disorders: Negative Emotions

'Adaptations that can seem like disorders' is listed as item (0) in Table 6.1 because it is a crucial consideration that is not an explanation for vulnerability. Recognising negative emotions as adaptations is a major contribution of evolutionary psychiatry. They are usually symptoms, not diseases. Five major implications follow. First, recognition of emotions as symptoms encourages searching for life situations that might be arousing them. Second, determining whether an emotion is pathological depends on the presence or absence of the relevant situation. Third, normal emotions are often useless in the individual instance. Fourth, deficits of negative emotion and excesses of positive emotion are under-recognised disorders. Finally, an evolutionary perspective calls attention to the need to consider disorders of all emotions, not just anxiety and depression.

Specific functions have often been proposed for specific emotions. However, different emotions correspond not to different functions but to the different situations that have shaped them (Nesse, 1990; Plutchik, 1980; Wierzbicka, 1992). If one insists on defining an emotion in terms of its function, the function can be framed as: 'The function of Emotion E is to adjust physiology, expression, memory, cognition, facial expression and behaviour in ways that improve the ability to cope with the adaptive challenges in Situation S.' Sophisticated treatments for these issues are available (Al-Shawaf et al., 2016; Averill et al., 1994; Griffiths, 1997; Izard, 2010; Tooby and Cosmides, 1990; Wierzbicka, 1992).

The tendency to view different emotions as separate parts of a designed machine reflects a tacit creationism that is prevalent throughout biology (Nesse, 2020). Decades of debate about basic emotions continue because of trying to view emotions as distinct parts of a machine. However, emotions are suites of settings that evolved from precursor emotions with overlapping characteristics that were shaped to cope with somewhat overlapping situations. This explains why the symptoms of depression and anxiety disorders cannot be fully separated. Situations that threaten loss are highly associated with situations in which loss occurs, so anxiety and mood disorders have high comorbidity and many overlapping features.

The word 'depression' implies pathology to many people; the phrase 'low mood' allows description of symptoms that are usually – but not necessarily – products of intact mood-regulation systems. Most evolutionary explanations for low mood or depression describe possible functions. Those include soliciting aid, manipulating others, inhibiting effort in unpropitious times, conserving calories during winter or famine, avoiding attacks after losing a status competition, motivating contributions to a group when exclusion is a risk, inhibiting activity during infection and curtailing effort to free up time to solve a problem (Durisko et al., 2015; Hagen,

2011; Nesse, 2009; Rottenberg, 2014). Many authors advocate for the primacy of the function they think is most important. Unproductive debates ensue.

Progress will come by stepping back from attempts to pin a function on low mood and instead searching for the situations in which it is useful. In general terms, low mood is useful in unpropitious situations where efforts will be wasted or harmful (Nesse, 2000). The situation of failing efforts to make progress towards a goal is slightly less general (Carver and Scheier, 2014; Heckhausen, 2000; Klinger, 1975). However, these global situations do little to account for guilt, crying, low self-worth, rumination and hopelessness. More specific situations have shaped more specific kinds of low mood (Cheung et al., 2004; Gilbert, 2006; Monroe and Hadjiyannakis, 2002; Watson and Andrews, 2002). Loss of a status competition and being trapped in a subservient role seem especially salient in many cases of depression (Price and Sloman, 1987). Situations influencing status in a group also are especially potent influences on mood. However, non-social situations, such as inflammation, can also arouse appropriate low mood (Raison et al., 2006). Subtypes of low mood that arise in different situations are, however, not as distinct as we might like; they are overlapping states that evolved from common precursors. Investigating how different situations give rise to different symptom patterns is a crucial unfinished project (Keller and Nesse, 2006; see also Chapter 8 of this volume).

It will be essential to distinguish evolutionary explanations for the mood system from explanations for why it is vulnerable to dysfunction. Are cases of depression seen in psychiatric clinics mostly normal, useful low mood or mostly pathological depression? My impression after experience with thousands of depressed patients is about the same as that reported a century ago by Aubrey Lewis, the inaugural chair of the London Institute of Psychiatry: about a third of patients have low mood somewhat appropriate to their situation, about a third have grossly excessive responses to a life situation and about a third have fundamentally abnormal mood-regulation mechanisms (Lewis, 1934). However, studies using modern methods have yet to address the question systematically.

Why did natural selection leave mood-regulation mechanisms vulnerable to dysfunction? That question is fundamentally different from the question of why the capacity for normal low mood exists at all. All five evolutionary reasons are relevant. Before considering them, it is worthwhile to recognise that normal regulation mechanisms often give rise to useless emotions.

6.3.1.1 Why Most Experiences of Negative Emotion Are Useless but Normal

It seems obvious that normal emotions from normal mechanisms should be reliably useful and that useless emotions should be products of abnormal regulation mechanisms, but both statements are false. Many experiences of negative emotion are useless products of normal emotion regulation mechanisms. They are, in Wakefield's valuable nomenclature, harmful conditions that are not dysfunctions (Wakefield, 1992). Five different processes can result in normal mechanisms giving rise to useless or harmful emotions.

The smoke detector principle explains why false alarms and excessive defensive responses are normal and necessary (Nesse, 2005b). To ensure an early warning from every fire, smoke detectors are designed to go off when toast is burnt. The many annoying false alarms are worth it to ensure early warning about every real fire. Signal detection theory describes the optimal response threshold. The principle has been expanded to explain cognitive distortions as error management theory (Haselton and Nettle, 2006).

Adaptive sensitisation is a second reason why negative emotions are usually normal but useless. Repeated experiences of pain indicate that the mild cues of nociception have been insufficient to provide protection against tissue damage (Williams, 2016). Such experiences adaptively sensitise nociception and pain systems, so they go off more easily (Crook et al., 2014). Such self-sensitising systems are inherently vulnerable to runaway positive feedback, a possible evolutionary explanation for chronic pain that is equally relevant for anxiety disorders (Nesse and Schulkin, 2019).

A happenstance sequence of unlucky events is a third reason why normal mechanisms often give rise to useless experiences of negative emotion. One model considers an organism deciding, on each move, whether to forage or wait (Trimmer et al., 2015). Foraging brings rewards in 'good' environments but costs in 'bad' environments; the valence for the environment often reverses. Happenstance sequences of non-reward can result in giving up when rewards are available. A related model analyses the decision a fox must make about digging in holes that might contain tasty rabbits or dangerous badgers. When rabbits are more common than badgers, digging is worth it. But even when rabbits predominate, an unlucky sequence would cause a fox to give up on foraging. This illustrates how 'adaptive behaviour might lead to self-reinforcing pessimism' (Meacham and Bergstrom, 2016: 3). Depression researchers use the metaphor of 'kindling' to describe how previous episodes increase the risk of depression. Whether the phenomenon is pathology or an adaptive response remains uncertain.

Mismatch between ancient brains and modern environments is a fourth reason why normal mechanisms give rise to useless emotional responses (Griffiths and Bourrat, 2021). Mechanisms shaped to manage social life in small kin groups cause enormous problems when they are aroused by the exigencies of subservient roles in a modern bureaucracy. More details about this are given in Section 6.3.2.3 (also see Chapter 1).

Emotion regulation systems were shaped to maximise gene transmission, not individual health or happiness. We are inordinately distressed by our children's problems, even when there is nothing we can do to help, and emotions aroused in mating competitions often benefit our genes at a big cost to us. More details about this are given in Section 6.3.2.5.

6.3.1.2 Implications from Recognising That Some Apparent Disorders Are Adaptations

Recognising that negative emotions are often useless products of normal systems changes the approach for researchers, clinicians and patients. It encourages attending to the possible usefulness of symptoms, while also supporting the use of any safe means to dispatch useless suffering. It also suggests that most medications relieve negative emotions not by replacing deficient neurotransmitters but by blocking normal response systems, in the same way that analgesics block pain.

6.3.2 Things Natural Selection Cannot Do

Five reasons why natural selection leaves us vulnerable to disease are summarised briefly in this section. It would satisfy our wish for simplicity if vulnerability to each disorder could be attributed to just one reason, but most disorders require multiple explanations.

6.3.2.1 Stochasticity

Genetic drift is the null hypothesis for molecular evolution. Deleterious and advantageous genetic variants can be lost or go to fixation due to stochastic effects alone (Lynch et al., 2016). Fixation of mildly deleterious alleles is especially common in small populations, but their role in disease vulnerability is hard to assess because lack of variability makes them hard to identify. More obvious vulnerabilities arise from mutations that are generated constantly but selected out only slowly and from previously neutral alleles that become pathogenic in novel environments. Also, the process of brain development, while tightly canalised, is subject to unavoidable stochastic variations. Stochasticity is a powerful explanation for disease vulnerabilities.

Mutation–selection balance is the natural major candidate to explain disease-associated alleles (Keller and Miller, 2006; Kendler, 2013). The sequencing of the human genome brought hope that we would soon find the responsible alleles. Studies of candidate genes brought further hope, but almost none could be replicated. Genome-wide association studies (GWASs) expanded the data massively to discover that no common alleles have a substantial effect on the risk for major mental disorders (Kendler, 2013). Ever-larger studies have discovered that the effect size of an allele is inversely proportional to its prevalence, so each contributing allele explains about the same tiny proportion of variance. For schizophrenia, that amount is 0.04%, or 4 parts in 10,000 (Keller 2018). This is consistent with natural selection eliminating deleterious mutations with a speed proportional to their deleterious effect on fitness.

A third conclusion is also surprising: the responsible alleles are not specific to one disorder (Baselmans et al., 2021; Liu et al., 2020; Taylor et al., 2018). Also, the vast majority of relevant genetic variants are in non-coding regions. For simplicity, I use the word 'alleles' to describe all genetic variants. Massive overlap is found for alleles contributing to anxiety and depression, as well as for those contributing to bipolar disorder and schizophrenia. Polygenic risk scores use all data from all loci to predict risk. Polygenic risk scores for schizophrenia are significantly associated with autism, bipolar disorder and depression but are not associated with ADHD (Mistry et al., 2018). Intriguingly, the genetic risk for schizophrenia and autism have also been associated with creativity and educational attainment. This suggests a research strategy. If alleles that confer risk also confer benefits, then individuals in the decile with the *lowest* risk for a major mental disorder should have deficits in some areas. This is the most interesting research idea that emerged from my review of psychiatric genetics in preparation for this chapter.

6.3.2.2 Path Dependence/Major Transitions

The inability to redesign a trait from scratch makes organic systems fundamentally different from machines. The nerves and vessels in the eye come between the light and the retina, but they can never be rerouted because the transition would require thousands of generations in a fitness valley. Path dependence also imposes substantial constraints on robustness at the genetic level. We tend to think about the fitness effects of new alleles in isolation, but they enter networks of massively pleiotropic genes that each interact with thousands of others (Haig, 2020).

Major transitions to a new niche leave organisms vulnerable because of path dependence and the slowness of natural selection. For instance, the transition to an upright posture has left us vulnerable to hernias, haemorrhoids, foot pain, back pain, pregnancy problems and varicose veins. Our ancestors must have suffered terribly during the transition to bipedalism 4 million years ago. The transition to the social-cognitive niche is more recent but at least as wrenching (Hrdy and Burkart, 2020; Whiten and Erdal, 2012; also see Chapters 1, 3 and 4 of this volume). In just the past few hundred thousand years, our ancestors became capable of trade and complex society. Language capabilities may have developed within the past 50,000 years (see Chapter 4 for a discussion on the evolution of language). Settled living and agricultural surpluses in just the past 20,000 years made possible new means of social control, new kinds of hierarchies, new social roles, changed mating and parenting patterns, and cities. Our brains are evolving to cope with these changes but not fast enough to ensure robustness. The development of language has been cited as a

specific explanation for vulnerability to schizophrenia (Crow, 1997), but many other factors are likely involved (Brüne, 2016; Del Giudice, 2018).

Our limited ability to inhibit impulses is another example. Getting long-term gains in a complex social context often requires inhibiting impulses to take short-term rewards. Inhibiting self-interested behaviour is crucial for social success, but this ability is limited in many people. Capacities for empathy and intuiting others' motives are also crucial to maximising social benefits, but they too still remain crude.

6.3.2.3 Mismatch and the Slowness of Natural Selection

Natural selection is slow compared to rates of environmental change, and it is far slower than the evolution of pathogens and the arrival of new mutations. Vulnerabilities result.

The slow pace of purging deleterious mutations is an obvious cause of disease. Selection is also slow to control selfish genetic elements that insert and replicate themselves in the genome despite the costs to individuals (Ågren and Clark, 2018). It is amazing that selection has managed to sufficiently reduce mutation rates and control selfish elements to maintain a stable genome – if, indeed, it has.

Mismatch of phenotypes with modern environments is inevitable given the slowness of natural selection (Gluckman and Hanson, 2006; Griffiths and Bourrat, 2021). Everyone knows that the environments we have created to satisfy our wishes for sweets, salt, fat and leisure have resulted in epidemics of chronic disease. Obesity and eating disorders are prime examples, but alcoholism and drug addiction are also made possible by ready access to substances and means of administration that have only recently become available. Lack of selection until recent times against these often fatal disorders is an essential part of any evolutionary explanation.

What about emotional and relationship problems? Are they far more common now than a few decades ago? How about compared to a few hundred years ago? What about before the rise of agriculture? Every generation thinks that things were better for previous generations, but that is mostly an illusion resulting from the saliency of problems now and the fading of painful memories with time.

Epidemiological studies using randomly chosen subjects do not show major increases in mental disorders in recent decades (Bebbington and McManus, 2020), although there is some evidence for increases in depression across longer intervals (Hidaka, 2012). However, social media now seem poised to harm our mental health as much as fast food harms our physical health. We can't resist its pull despite the anxiety, depression and feelings of social inadequacy that are aroused by unprecedented social comparisons (Vogel et al., 2014). While apparently rapid increases in rates of autism and ADHD could reflect changing diagnostic patterns, it remains possible that these rates are being increased by environmental factors or assortative mating of individuals who carry vulnerability alleles.

Discovering the prevalence of mental disorders in hunter-gatherers is an important opportunity that is fading fast. There are good reasons why it has not been done. Samples of thousands are required for accurate epidemiological studies, but most hunter-gatherer groups contain only scores of people. Diagnostic instruments have limited reliability even in modern societies; their performance in other settings would be questionable. Nonetheless, we should gather as much data as we can from as many populations as possible before it is too late (Konner, 2002).

Valuable generalisations can be extracted from the cross-cultural data collected by the International Consortium for Psychiatric Epidemiology using standardised diagnostic criteria and random sampling methods (Kessler et al., 2014). Rates of schizophrenia, autism and obsessive-compulsive disorder (OCD) vary somewhat between countries but not dramatically. Behavioural disorders such as eating disorders and addiction have long been present at low rates, but they are increased and show moderate variations in developed societies. Rates of emotional disorders, by contrast, vary by more than eightfold in different countries (Kessler and Bromet, 2013). This does not implicate modern environments specifically, but it indicates that rates are strongly influenced by factors that differ between countries.

The role of mismatch is important for ADHD (Swanepoel et al., 2017; also see Chapter 14 of this volume). The simplest proposal is that a short attention span imposed no costs for ancestral humans, so it should not be considered a disorder, but we don't know if it imposes costs in other cultures. Some authors ask how ADHD gives advantages; this illustrates the mistake of viewing the extreme of a trait as an adaptation. Fitness in ancestral environments should peak near the population average value of a trait. The strongly male-skewed sex ratio of ADHD is consistent worldwide (Fayyad et al., 2017). This encourages asking whether higher levels of activity and faster task switching give advantages for males or if their increased vulnerability reflects a system more prone to dysfunction. Low Apgar scores are the single best predictor of ADHD, being present in twice as many boys with ADHD as controls (Hanć et al., 2018). However, a recent review failed to confirm the role of most prenatal factors (Sciberras et al., 2017), increasing uncertainty about the possibility that some cases of ADHD are, as it was previously called, minimal brain dysfunction.

Extensive research on the developmental origins of health and disease has examined how capacities for plasticity can yield maladaptive outcomes in modern environments (Nettle et al., 2013). For instance, the tendency for low-birth-weight infants to later become obese, diabetic and hypertensive has been attributed to a mechanism that could have evolved to adjust metabolism to cope with harsh environments predicted by experience *in utero* (Gluckman et al., 2019). Primate studies have not confirmed fitness benefits from such plasticity (Tung et al., 2016), but the genomic imprinting mechanism that mediates the effect is quite specific and powerful. A related mechanism increases the responsiveness of the stress system to early adversity (Meaney and Szyf, 2005). These changes could be epiphenomena, but even if they are adaptations they might well impose costs greater than benefits in relatively safe and well-provisioned modern environments.

The slowness of natural selection relative to pathogen evolution is less relevant for psychiatry than in the rest of medicine, but caudate damage induced by antibodies to streptococci accounts for some cases of OCD (Swedo et al., 2004). Also, some cases of schizophrenia are caused by *Toxoplasma gondii*, parasites with the clever strategy of inducing fearlessness in mice that that gets the parasite reliably into its cat host (Burgdorf et al., 2019). More generally, inflammation is responsible for some depression (Miller and Raison, 2016), and it is central to the pathophysiology of Alzheimer's disease (Heneka et al., 2015). The pathognomonic plaques in Alzheimer's disease are composed of amyloid beta. This has often been assumed to be a toxic by-product of brain metabolism; however, drugs that disrupt amyloid beta do not slow progression. A different approach might have been pursued if the antimicrobial function of amyloid beta had been recognised earlier (Soscia et al., 2010). Similarly, the *APOE e4* allele, which is strongly associated with Alzheimer's disease, is viewed as pathological, but it helps to defend against pathogens; this is likely why it slows cognitive decline in horticulturalists (Trumble et al., 2017; see also Chapter 17 of this volume). Alzheimer's disease research may offer an unfortunate case study of how the lack of an evolutionary perspective can slow progress.

Considering mismatch and the slowness of natural selection is useful. Knowing that natural selection has not protected us from addiction helps patients to feel less defective and more respectful of their foe. It could also help young people to recognise the risks of drug experimentation. Understanding the starvation protection response helps eating disorder patients understand why restrictive dieting doesn't work. Understanding the trade-offs in mechanisms that protect against brain infection can advance our understanding of Alzheimer's disease. And discovering the factors that account for the eightfold national differences in rates of depression could do more to relieve depression than all current treatment efforts. The difficulty, of course, is in finding the responsible causes in the midst of massive variations in media exposure, diet, exercise, workplaces, religion and family structure and the likelihood that multiple factors are responsible. Getting comparison data from hunter-gatherer communities should be a high priority.

6.3.2.4 Trade-Offs That Benefit the Individual

Trade-offs are inherent to every system, whether evolved or designed. Cars that get better gas mileage have reduced acceleration and vice versa, so most cars have acceleration and gas mileage in the middle range. Those at the extremes reveal the costs of the trade-offs. Slow, efficient cars sometimes get into accidents because they can't merge easily into fast traffic; fast cars sometimes get into accidents because they are fast.

Trade-offs are also illustrated by the problems experienced by individuals at diametric extremes (Badcock, 2019; Crespi and Dinsdale, 2019; Crespi and Go, 2015; Del Giudice and Crespi, 2018). Individuals with heavier body weight are more likely to survive a famine but less likely to escape from a predator. Greater than average anxiety increases safety at the cost of lost opportunities. Greater than average low mood reduces useless efforts at the cost of lost opportunities. A tendency to persist increases success at some tasks, but rapidly shifting attention is superior for others. A tendency to make causal connections readily results in more theories that can predict events but more superstitions and false beliefs. Gregariousness increases the number of social connections, but introversion increases their depth. The reduced fitness experienced by individuals with trait values at the tails creates stabilising selection; it narrows the distribution but rarely enough to protect everyone.

Some trade-offs are more likely than others to result in vulnerability to disorders. Much depends on the shape of the fitness function. If it is flat and broader than the trait distribution, the trait value should not strongly influence fitness and few individuals should experience vulnerability. However, narrow fitness functions with steep slopes cause problems for individuals whose values diverge only modestly from the mean and even for those at the mean. Steep, narrow fitness functions are often products of arms races. The possibility of death from infection selects strongly against even moderate deficiencies in immune response, while the risks of autoimmune disease and faster ageing select against stronger immune responses. Even at the optimum trait value, vulnerabilities from infection and excess immune responses persist (Graham, 2013).

Selection that maximises performance can also result in vulnerability, especially when winner-take-all competitions shape cliff-edged fitness functions. Race cars are stripped down to a lean edge where a high risk of catastrophic failure is the price for having a chance to win. Breeding horses for speed results in long, thin leg bones that are vulnerable to fracture. Selection for high cognitive performance may have shaped cliff-edged fitness functions that make humans vulnerable to major disorders such as schizophrenia (Nesse, 2004).

Legacies of the major transition to the human socio-cognitive niche (Hrdy and Burkart, 2020; Pinker, 2010; Whiten and Erdal, 2012) may account for vulnerabilities more generally. Strong selection on path-dependent systems could account for some mental disorders. The challenge will be knowing where to look. It could be that trade-offs at the trait level are a good place to start. For instance, abilities to create theories of causation could overshoot and result in vulnerability to paranoia and delusions. However, problems can arise from lower levels. If neuronal pruning in childhood (Sellgren et al., 2019) maximises some cognitive ability, overshooting in some individuals could have implications for schizophrenia. If the advantages of a large brain are associated with fast brain growth in the first year of life, this could outpace the control capacity of canalisation mechanisms with implications for autism, where exceptionally fast early brain growth is typical. In summary, 'Many psychotic symptoms and syndromes may be considered trade-offs, primarily manifesting themselves in domains related to the evolution of our "social brain"' (Brüne, 2004: 49). Variations in brain development or neuronal pruning could, of course, cause disorders even if they are not associated with performance advantages.

The socio-cognitive niche creates and is created by the social selection that has made humans wonderfully cooperative at the cost of much distress and vulnerability. Partner choices are selection forces. Tendencies to choose sexual partners with certain characteristics shape extreme traits like peacock tails that maximise reproduction at the expense of the individual's health and longevity. Tendencies to choose the best possible social partners can also shape extreme traits with major benefits and costs to individuals (Frank, 2006; Hrdy and Burkart, 2020; Nesse, 2007; West-Eberhard, 1979). People prefer social partners who are honest, empathic, wealthy and generous, so individuals with those characteristics get the best partners and associated fitness benefits. This creates strong selection for prosocial traits and for preferences for partners with those traits. The result is a species with unparalleled capacities for cooperation, commitment, relationships and morality that come at the cost of vast distress from guilt, social anxiety, low self-esteem and extreme concern about reputation. Prosocial traits benefit groups, but

they are shaped because they increase the inclusive fitness of individuals who are preferred as partners.

Cybernetic analysis of control systems also suggests a source of special vulnerability (DeYoung and Krueger, 2018; Nesse, 2021). Positive feedback is ubiquitous in optimal control systems. It switches a process all the way on or off. Many actions, once begun, are best continued. For instance, starting to eat initiates a positive-feedback loop that motivates continuing until satiation or until the food is gone. If the off mechanism fails, an eating binge results. Mood systems are especially vulnerable to positive feedback. Failure lowers motivation, encouraging more failure. Success in pursuing a goal, especially a status goal, indicates a propitious situation in which additional investments will likely pay off. This can initiate runaway increases in mood of the sort seen in a manic episode. Most people experience a decline in mood shortly after a major success. This apparently senseless mood reduction may well be an adaptation that protects against a positive-feedback cycle of escalating mood (Nesse, 2019). Or it may just be an epiphenomenon of neurochemical systems recovering after recent strong activity.

6.3.2.5 Trade-Offs That Benefit Genes at a Fitness Cost to Individuals

Natural selection doesn't give a fig about our happiness; it just maximises gene transmission, often at the expense of health, welfare and longevity. Several kinds of selection shape traits that benefit genes at our expense.

Sexual selection shapes traits that increase reproductive success at a cost to the individual. Men get a larger fitness pay off than women for abilities to compete for mates, and they pay the price of threefold higher mortality rate in early adulthood and a much shorter lifespan (Kruger and Nesse, 2006; Lemaître et al., 2020). The costs of traits that increase mating success for women are harder to identify because of the lack of a comparison group. An extraordinary proportion of life problems and resulting mental disorders arise from mating conflicts (Buss, 1988). Unrequited love, the pain of being rejected, the fear of being left, being stalked, being harassed, jealousy and being trapped in an abusive relationship are common precipitants of mental disorders. In stable relationships, infertility causes much distress.

Sexual selection also shapes traits that impose risks related to childbearing and parenting (Hrdy, 1999; Strassmann, 1981). The costs and risks of pregnancy are borne mainly by women, but both partners can be consumed by the travails of parenting, and concern for the welfare of grown children wreaks havoc on many lives. These problems result from traits shaped to benefit gene transmission even at the cost of individual health.

Kin selection shapes tendencies to make sacrifices that benefit family members who share genes identical by descent (Griffin and West, 2003). The costs of such sacrifices are highest and most satisfying for children and siblings, but problems experienced by extended family members can nonetheless cause great distress. Traits costly to individuals were once thought to evolve because of their benefits to groups, but this works only if group members are kin who share genes identical by descent. Alleles that result in an individual having lower inclusive fitness than other group members will be selected out even if they benefit the group (West et al., 2021). While selection for benefits to the group is not a viable explanation, selection by the group is powerful. Social selection shapes prosocial traits whose benefits to the group are wonderful side effects of their benefits for maximising the transmission of an individual's genes. These prosocial traits make culture possible, and culture creates emergent selection forces that further advance the process.

Cultural group selection describes how groups with stronger norms succeed at the expense of other groups. Those norms also create emergent forces of natural selection that shape human emotional and behavioural tendencies (Richerson et al., 2015). They promote cooperation but at the cost of neurosis and social anxiety. And while cooperation that benefits the group sounds nice, it can also be a product of ruthless punishment imposed by a despot to control and exploit subordinates.

Competitions between paternal and maternal genomes are also implicated. As David Haig has pointed out, alleles from the paternal line get advantages from inducing more maternal investment in a pregnancy, while those from the maternal line benefit more from reserving resources for future reproduction (Haig, 2020). Subtle mechanisms that imprint genes from the father differently from those of the mother seem well suited to advancing the interests of each genome and causing problems (Haig, 2008).

Sexually antagonistic selection offers yet another example of how selection can benefit genes at the expense of individuals. Alleles with different benefits and costs to males and females can be maintained despite increasing the vulnerability of one sex. Wonderful complexity ensues (Frank and Crespi, 2011).

Antagonistic pleiotropy can explain the persistence of genes that increase the individual's Darwinian fitness at one life phase or situation with costs later or in other situations. The classic example is a gene that causes ageing but is selected for because it offers benefits early in life when selection is stronger (Williams, 1957). When such alleles are fixed, their effects will not show up in genetic studies. Other fixed alleles can persist because their costs are outweighed by benefits that are manifest only in certain environments. A hypothetical example is a tendency to carry extra fat stores that imposes costs in most generations but might be life-saving in a generation that faces starvation.

Balancing selection maintains polymorphisms because different alleles give benefits in different environments (Power et al., 2015). Sometimes the benefits are to the individual, but sometimes benefits are to gene transmission at a cost to the individual. The sickle cell allele (Hb-S) is the classic example. Heterozygotes do better than homozygous individuals in environments where malaria is present. However, frequency-dependent selection also influences the polymorphism prevalence: Hb-S gives advantages when rare, but as it becomes common the proportion of homozygous individuals with sickle cell disease increases, so selection turns against the allele. Heterozygote advantage has often been suggested as a possible mechanism maintaining polymorphisms for mental disorders, but it is viable only for alleles with large effects and therefore is unlikely to account for mental disorders.

The more general possibility that alleles causing mental disorders persist in the genome because they give fitness benefits remains under consideration. For instance, some studies find schizophrenia to be associated with creativity (Nettle and Clegg, 2006), and others find indicators of positive selection on autism single-nucleotide polymorphisms (SNPs) (Polimanti and Gelernter, 2017). However, increasingly large

GWASs find no evidence for positive selection for SNPs associated with schizophrenia and good evidence for strong background selection eliminating deleterious variants in areas enriched with schizophrenia-associated SNPs (Smeland et al., 2020). Plain old mutation-selection balance looks increasingly like the main explanation for highly heritable serious mental disorders (Keller, 2018).

The unanswered question is why syndromes like autism and schizophrenia have relatively consistent characteristics. Why are these the failure modes? Why are they influenced by so many variants with tiny effects? I think we will eventually discover that some systems have been shaped to performance peaks adjacent to fitness cliffs that make them intrinsically vulnerable to certain kinds of failure, and that the genetic variants that influence these risks include mutations being selected out and alleles that are beneficial, harmful or neutral depending on the genetic background and the environment.

6.4 Conclusion

Mental disorders need evolutionary explanations, but viewing disorders as adaptations is a mistake. The correct objects of explanation are traits that leave all members of a species vulnerable to a disorder. Most explanations are based on a combination of five main reasons why natural selection has left us vulnerable:

- *The inherent stochasticity of natural selection and development* that limits optimality is responsible for much vulnerability, especially for serious, highly heritable disorders.
- *Path dependence* is also responsible for vulnerability, especially after major transitions such as the human shift to the socio-cognitive niche.
- *The slowness of natural selection* results in mismatch with fast-changing environments that contributes to the vulnerability to some disorders, especially addiction and eating disorders, but mismatch does not offer a global explanation for all mental disorders.
- *Trade-offs* combine with stochasticity to leave some individuals at maladaptive trait extremes, but the risk depends on the shape and spread of the fitness function.
- Finally, vulnerability can result from *traits that maximise gene transmission at a cost to health.*

The fact that more than one factor influences our vulnerability to a single disorder frustrates our natural wish for simplicity. However, considering all factors systematically will eventually provide solid evolutionary answers to the question of why natural selection left us so vulnerable to so many mental disorders, and those answers will provide a new foundation that will make psychiatry more sensible, more effective and much more like the rest of medicine.

References

Abed, R. T. (1998). The sexual competition hypothesis for eating disorders. *British Journal of Medical Psychology*, **71**, 525–547.

Abed, R. T., and St John-Smith, P. (2016). Evolutionary psychiatry: a new College special interest group. *BJPsych Bulletin*, **40**, 233–236.

Abed, R. T., and St. John Smith, P. (eds.) (2022). *Evolutionary Psychiatry: Current Perspectives on Evolution and Mental Health*. Cambridge: Cambridge University Press.

Adriaens, P. R., and De Block, A. (2011). *Maladapting Minds: Philosophy, Psychiatry, and Evolutionary Theory*. Oxford; New York: Oxford University Press.

Ågren, J. A., and Clark, A. G. (2018). Selfish genetic elements. *PLoS Genetics*, **14**, e1007700.

Al-Shawaf, L., Conroy-Beam, D., Asao, K., and Buss, D. M. (2016). Human emotions: an evolutionary psychological perspective. *Emotion Review*, **8**, 173–186.

Averill, J. R., Clore, G. L., Frijda, N. H., ... Davidson, R. J. (1994). What is the function of emotions? In P. Ekman and R. J. Davidson (eds.), *The Nature of Emotion: Fundamental Questions*. New York: Oxford University Press, pp. 97–136.

Badcock, C. (2019). *The Diametric Mind: New Insights into AI, IQ, the Self, and Society*. Tallinn: TLU Press.

Baselmans, B. M. L., Yengo, L., van Rheenen, W., and Wray, N. R. (2021). Risk in relatives, heritability, SNP-based heritability, and genetic correlations in psychiatric disorders: a review. *Biological Psychiatry*, **89**, 11–19.

Bebbington, P. E., and McManus, S. (2020). Revisiting the one in four: the prevalence of psychiatric disorder in the population of England 2000–2014. *British Journal of Psychiatry*, **216**, 55–57.

Brüne, M. (2004). Schizophrenia – an evolutionary enigma?

Neuroscience & Biobehavioral Reviews, **28**, 41–53.

Brüne, M. (2016). *Textbook of Evolutionary Psychiatry and Psychosomatic Medicine*, Vol. **1**. Oxford: Oxford University Press.

Brüne, M. (2018). Evolutionary psychology of eating disorders: an explorative study in patients with anorexia nervosa and bulimia nervosa. *Frontiers in Psychology*, **9**, 12.

Buller, D. J. (2005). *Adapting Minds: Evolutionary Psychology and the Persistent Quest for Human Nature*. Cambridge, MA: MIT Press.

Burgdorf, K. S., Trabjerg, B. B., Pedersen, M. G., ... Ullum, H. (2019). Large-scale study of *Toxoplasma* and cytomegalovirus shows an association between infection and serious psychiatric disorders. *Brain, Behavior, and Immunity*, **79**, 152–158.

Buss, D. M. (1988). The evolution of human intrasexual competition: tactics of mate attraction. *Journal of Personality and Social Psychology*, **54**, 616–628.

Buss, D. M. (2020). Evolutionary psychology is a scientific revolution. *Evolutionary Behavioral Sciences*, **14**, 316–323.

Buss, D. M., and von Hippel, W. (2018). Psychological barriers to evolutionary psychology: ideological bias and coalitional adaptations. *Archives of Scientific Psychology*, **6**, 148.

Carver, C. S., and Scheier, M. F. (2014). The experience of emotions during goal pursuit. In R. Pekrun and L. Linnenbrink-Garcia (eds.), *International Handbook of Emotions in Education*. London: Routledge, pp. 56–72.

Cheung, M.-P., Gilbert, P., and Irons, C. (2004). An exploration of shame, social rank and rumination in relation to depression. *Personality and Individual Differences*, **36**, 1143–1153.

Crespi, B. J. (2020). Evolutionary and genetic insights for clinical psychology. *Clinical Psychology Review*, **78**, 101857.

Crespi, B. J., and Dinsdale, N. (2019). Autism and psychosis as diametrical disorders of embodiment. *Evolution, Medicine, and Public Health*, **2019**, 121–138.

Crespi, B. J., and Go, M. C. (2015). Diametrical diseases reflect evolutionary–genetic trade-offs: evidence from psychiatry, neurology, rheumatology, oncology and immunology. *Evolution, Medicine, and Public Health*, **2015**, 216–253.

Crook, R. J., Dickson, K., Hanlon, R. T., and Walters, E. T. (2014). Nociceptive sensitization reduces predation risk. *Current Biology*, **24**, 1121–1125.

Crow, T. J. (1997). Is schizophrenia the price that *Homo sapiens* pays for language? *Schizophrenia Research*, **28**, 127–141.

Del Giudice, M. (2018). *Evolutionary Psychopathology*, Vol. **1**. Oxford: Oxford University Press.

Del Giudice, M., and Crespi, B. J. (2018). Basic functional trade-offs in cognition: an integrative framework. *Cognition*, **179**, 56–70.

DeYoung, C. G., and Krueger, R. F. (2018). A cybernetic theory of psychopathology. *Psychological Inquiry*, **29**, 117–138.

Durisko, Z., Mulsant, B. H., and Andrews, P. W. (2015). An adaptationist perspective on the etiology of depression. *Journal of Affective Disorders*, **172**, 315–323.

Fayyad, J., Sampson, N. A., Hwang, I., ... on behalf of the WHO World Mental Health Survey Collaborators (2017). The descriptive epidemiology of DSM-IV Adult ADHD in the World Health Organization World Mental Health Surveys. *ADHD Attention Deficit and Hyperactivity Disorders*, **9**, 47–65.

Frank, S. A. (2006). Social selection. In C. W. Fox and J. B. Wolf (eds.), *Evolutionary Genetics: Concepts and Case Studies*. New York: Oxford University Press, pp. 350–363.

Frank, S. A., and Crespi, B. J. (2011). Pathology from evolutionary conflict, with a theory of X chromosome versus autosome conflict over sexually antagonistic traits. *Proceedings of the National Academy of Sciences of the United States of America*, **108**, 10886–10893.

Gilbert, P. (2006). Evolution and depression: issues and implications. *Psychological Medicine*, **36**, 287–297.

Gluckman, P. D., and Hanson, M. (2006). *Mismatch: Why Our World No Longer Fits Our Bodies*. New York: Oxford University Press.

Gluckman, P. D., Beedle, A., and Hanson, M. (2009). *Principles of Evolutionary Medicine*. Oxford: Oxford University Press.

Gluckman, P. D., Low, F. M., and Hanson, M. A. (2019). Evolutionary medicine, pregnancy, and the mismatch pathways to increased disease risk. In J. Schulkin and M. Powe (eds.), *Integrating Evolutionary Biology into Medical Education: For Maternal and Child Healthcare Students, Clinicians, and Scientists*. New York: Oxford University Press, pp. 13–26.

Gould, S. J., and Lewontin, R. C. (1979). The spandrels of San Marco and the Panglossian paradigm: a critique of the adaptationist programme. *Proceedings of the Royal Society London*, **205**, 581–598.

Graham, A. L. (2013). Optimal immunity meets natural variation: the evolutionary biology of host defence. *Parasite Immunology*, **35**, 315–317.

Greenberg, D. M., Warrier, V., Allison, C., and Baron-Cohen, S. (2018). Testing the Empathizing–Systemizing theory of sex differences and the Extreme Male Brain theory of autism in half a million people. *Proceedings of the National Academy of Sciences of the United States of America*, **115**, 12152–12157.

Griffin, A. S., and West, S. A. (2003). Kin discrimination and the benefit of helping in cooperatively breeding vertebrates. *Science*, **302**, 634–636.

Griffiths, P. E. (1997). *What Emotions Really Are: The Problem of Psychological Categories*. Chicago, IL: University of Chicago Press.

Griffiths, P. E., and Bourrat, P. (2021). The Idea of Mismatch in Evolutionary Medicine. *PhilSci Archives*. Retrieved from http://philsci-archive.pitt.edu/19349/

Hagen, E. H. (2011). Evolutionary theories of depression: a critical review. *Canadian Journal of Psychiatry*, **56**, 716–726.

Hagen, E. H., Roulette, C. J., and Sullivan, R. J. (2013). Explaining human recreational use of 'pesticides': the neurotoxin regulation model of substance use vs. the hijack model and implications for age and sex differences in drug consumption. *Frontiers in Psychiatry*, **4**, 142.

Haig, D. A. (2020). *From Darwin to Derrida: Selfish Genes, Social Selves, and the Meanings of Life*. Cambridge, MA: MIT Press.

Haig, D. A. (2008). Kinship asymmetries and the divided self. *Behavioral and Brain Sciences*, **31**, 271–272.

Hanć, T., Szwed, A., Słopień, A., Wolańczyk, T., Dmitrzak-Węglarz, M., and Ratajczak, J. (2018). Perinatal risk factors and ADHD in children and adolescents: a hierarchical structure of disorder predictors. *Journal of Attention Disorders*, **22**, 855–863.

Haselton, M. G., and Nettle, D. (2006). The paranoid optimist: an integrative evolutionary model of cognitive biases. *Personality and Social Psychology Review*, **10**, 47–66.

Heckhausen, J. (2000). Evolutionary perspectives on human motivation. *American Behavioral Scientist*, **43**, 1015–1029.

Heneka, M. T., Carson, M. J., Khoury, J. E., . . . Kummer, M. P. (2015). Neuroinflammation in Alzheimer's disease. *Lancet Neurology*, **14**, 388–405.

Hidaka, B. H. (2012). Depression as a disease of modernity: explanations for increasing prevalence. *Journal of Affective Disorders*, **140**, 205–214.

Hrdy, S. B. (1999). *Mother Nature: A History of Mothers, Infants, and Natural Selection*, 1st ed. New York: Pantheon Books.

Hrdy, S. B., and Burkart, J. M. (2020). The emergence of emotionally modern humans: implications for language and learning. *Philosophical Transactions of the Royal Society B: Biological Sciences*, **375**, 20190499.

Izard, C. E. (2010). The many meanings/aspects of emotion: definitions, functions, activation, and regulation. *Emotion Review*, **2**, 363–370.

Keller, M. C. (2018). Evolutionary perspectives on genetic and environmental risk factors for psychiatric disorders. *Annual Review of Clinical Psychology*, **14**, 471–493.

Keller, M. C., and Miller, G. (2006). Resolving the paradox of common, harmful, heritable mental disorders: which evolutionary genetic models work best? *Behavioral and Brain Sciences*, **29**, 385–404.

Keller, M. C., and Nesse, R. M. (2006). The evolutionary significance of depressive symptoms: different adverse situations lead to different depressive symptom patterns. *Journal of Personality and Social Psychology*, **91**, 316–330.

Kendler, K. S. (2013). What psychiatric genetics has taught us about the nature of psychiatric illness and what is left to learn. *Molecular Psychiatry*, **18**, 1058–1066.

Kennair, L. E. O. (2003). Evolutionary psychology and psychopathology. *Current Opinion in Psychiatry*, **16**, 691–699.

Kessler, R. C., and Bromet, E. J. (2013). The epidemiology of depression across cultures. *Annual Review of Public Health*, **34**, 119–138.

Kessler, R. C., Aguilar-Gaxiola, S., Alegria, M., . . . Vega, W. A. (2014). The International Consortium in Psychiatric Epidemiology. Retrieved from www.tigis.cz/images/stories/psychiatrie/2000/01/03kess.pdf

Klinger, E. (1975). Consequences of commitment to and disengagement from incentives. *Psychological Review*, **82**, 1–25.

Konner, M. (2002). *The Tangled Wing: Biological Constraints on the Human Spirit*, 2nd ed., rev. and updated. New York: Times Books.

Kruger, D. J., and Nesse, R. M. (2006). An evolutionary life-history framework for understanding sex differences in human mortality rates. *Human Nature*, **17**, 74–97.

Lemaître, J.-F., Ronget, V., Tidière, M., . . . Gaillard, J.-M. (2020). Sex differences in adult lifespan and aging rates of mortality across wild mammals. *Proceedings of the National Academy of Sciences of the United States of America*, **117**, 8546–8553.

Lewis, A. J. (1934). Melancholia: a clinical survey of depressive states. *Journal of Mental Science*, **80**, 1–43.

Lewis, D. M., Al-Shawaf, L., Conroy-Beam, D., Asao, K., and Buss, D. M. (2017). Evolutionary psychology: a how-to guide. *American Psychologist*, **72**, 353.

Liu, S., Rao, S., Xu, Y., ... Zhang, F. (2020). Identifying common genome-wide risk genes for major psychiatric traits. *Human Genetics*, **139**, 185–198.

Lynch, M., Ackerman, M. S., Gout, J.-F., ... Foster, P. L. (2016). Genetic drift, selection and the evolution of the mutation rate. *Nature Reviews Genetics*, **17**, 704–714.

Mayhew, A. J., Pigeyre, M., Couturier, J., and Meyre, D. (2018). An evolutionary genetic perspective of eating disorders. *Neuroendocrinology*, **106**, 292–306.

McGuire, M. T., and Troisi, A. (1998). *Darwinian Psychiatry*. New York: Oxford University Press.

McGuire, M. T., Marks, I. M., Nesse, R. M., and Troisi, A. (1992). Evolutionary biology: a basic science for psychiatry. *Acta Psychiatrica Scandinavica*, **86**, 89–96.

Meacham, F., and Bergstrom, C. T. (2016). Adaptive behavior can produce maladaptive anxiety due to individual differences in experience. *Evolution, Medicine, and Public Health*, **2016**, 270–285.

Meaney, M. J., and Szyf, M. (2005). Environmental programming of stress responses through DNA methylation: life at the interface between a dynamic environment and a fixed genome. *Dialogues in Clinical Neuroscience*, **7**, 103–23.

Miller, A. H., and Raison, C. L. (2016). The role of inflammation in depression: from evolutionary imperative to modern treatment target. *Nature Reviews Immunology*, **16**, 22–34.

Mistry, S., Harrison, J. R., Smith, D. J., Escott-Price, V., and Zammit, S. (2018). The use of polygenic risk scores to identify phenotypes associated with genetic risk of schizophrenia: systematic

review. *Schizophrenia Research*, **197**, 2–8.

Monroe, S. M., and Hadjiyannakis, K. (2002). The social environment and depression: the role of awareness. In I. Gotlib and C. Hammen (eds.), *Handbook of Depression*. New York: Guilford Press, pp. 314–340.

Nesse, R. M. (1984). An evolutionary perspective on psychiatry. *Comprehensive Psychiatry*, **25**, 575–580.

Nesse, R. M. (1990). Evolutionary explanations of emotions. *Human Nature*, **1**, 261–289.

Nesse, R. M. (2000). Is depression an adaptation? *Archives of General Psychiatry*, **57**, 14–20.

Nesse, R. M. (2004). Cliff-edged fitness functions and the persistence of schizophrenia (commentary). *Behavioral and Brain Sciences*, **27**, 862–863.

Nesse, R. M. (2005a). Maladaptation and natural selection. *Quarterly Review of Biology*, **80**, 62–70.

Nesse, R. M. (2005b). Natural selection and the regulation of defenses. *Evolution and Human Behavior*, **26**, 88–105.

Nesse, R. M. (2007). Runaway social selection for displays of partner value and altruism. *Biological Theory*, **2**, 143–155.

Nesse, R. M. (2009). Explaining depression: neuroscience is not enough, evolution is essential. In C. M. Pariente, R. M. Nesse, D. J. Nutt, ... L. Wolpert (eds.), *Understanding Depression: A Translational Approach*. Oxford: Oxford University Press, pp. 17–35.

Nesse, R. M. (2011). Ten questions for evolutionary studies of disease vulnerability. *Evolutionary Applications*, **4**, 264–277.

Nesse, R. M. (2017). Anorexia: a perverse effect of attempting to control the starvation response. *Behavioral and Brain Sciences*, **40**, e125.

Nesse, R. M. (2019). *Good Reasons for Bad Feelings: Insights from the Frontier of Evolutionary Psychiatry*. New York: Dutton.

Nesse, R. M. (2020). Tacit Creationism in Emotions Research. *Emotion Researcher, ISRE's Sourcebook for Research on Emotion and Affect*. Retrieved from http://emotionresearcher .com/tacit-creationism-in-emotion-research

Nesse, R. M. (2021). Evolutionary Medicine Needs Engineering Expertise. National Academy of Engineering Perspectives. Retrieved from www .nationalacademies.org/news/ 2021/10/evolutionary-medicine-needs-engineering-expertise

Nesse, R. M., and Schulkin, J. (2019). An evolutionary medicine perspective on pain and its disorders. *Philosophical Transactions of the Royal Society B: Biological Sciences*, **374**, 20190288.

Nesse, R. M., and Williams, G. C. (1994). *Why We Get Sick: The New Science of Darwinian Medicine*. New York: Vintage Books.

Nettle, D., and Clegg, H. (2006). Schizotypy, creativity and mating success in humans. *Proceedings of the Royal Society of London B: Biological Sciences*, **273**, 611–615.

Nettle, D., Frankenhuis, W. E., and Rickard, I. J. (2013). The evolution of predictive adaptive responses in human life history. *Proceedings of the Royal Society of London B: Biological Sciences*, **280**, 20131343.

Perlman, R. L. (2005). Why disease persists: an evolutionary nosology. *Medicine, Health Care and Philosophy*, **8**, 343–350.

Pigliucci, M., and Kaplan, J. (2000). The fall and rise of Dr Pangloss: adaptationism and the Spandrels paper 20 years later. *Trends in Ecology & Evolution*, **15**, 66–70.

Pinker, S. (2010). The cognitive niche: coevolution of intelligence, sociality, and language. *Proceedings of the National Academy of Sciences of the United States of America*, 107, 8993–8999.

Plutchik, R. (1980). *Emotion: A Psychoevolutionary Synthesis.* New York: Harper and Row.

Polimanti, R., and Gelernter, J. (2017). Widespread signatures of positive selection in common risk alleles associated to autism spectrum disorder. *PLoS Genetics*, 13, e1006618.

Power, R. A., Steinberg, S., Bjornsdottir, G., ... Stefansson, K. (2015). Polygenic risk scores for schizophrenia and bipolar disorder predict creativity. *Nature Neuroscience*, 18, 953–955.

Price, J. S., and Sloman, L. (1987). Depression as yielding behavior: an animal model based on Schyelderup-Ebbe's pecking order. *Ethology and Sociobiology*, 8, 85s–98s.

Raison, C. L., Capuron, L., and Miller, A. H. (2006). Cytokines sing the blues: inflammation and the pathogenesis of depression. *Trends in Immunology*, 27, 24–31.

Richerson, P., Baldini, R., Bell, A., ... Zefferman, M. (2015). Cultural group selection plays an essential role in explaining human cooperation: a sketch of the evidence. *Behavioral and Brain Sciences*, 39, E30.

Rottenberg, J. (2014). *The Depths: The Evolutionary Origins of the Depression Epidemic.* New York: Basic Books.

Sciberras, E., Mulraney, M., Silva, D., and Coghill, D. (2017). Prenatal risk factors and the etiology of ADHD – review of existing evidence. *Current Psychiatry Reports*, 19, 1.

Sellgren, C. M., Gracias, J., Watmuff, B., ... Wang, J. (2019). Increased synapse elimination by microglia in schizophrenia patient-derived models of synaptic pruning. *Nature Neuroscience*, 22, 374–385.

Slingerland, E. (2021). *Drunk: How We Sipped, Danced, and Stumbled Our Way to Civilization.* New York: Little, Brown Spark.

Smeland, O. B., Bahrami, S., Frei, O., ... Andreassen, O. A. (2020). Genome-wide analysis reveals extensive genetic overlap between schizophrenia, bipolar disorder, and intelligence. *Molecular Psychiatry*, 25, 844–853.

Soscia, S. J., Kirby, J. E., Washicosky, K. J., ... Tanzi, R. E. (2010). The Alzheimer's disease-associated amyloid β-protein is an antimicrobial peptide. *PLoS ONE*, 5, e9505.

Staw, B. M. (1976). Knee-deep in the big muddy: a study of escalating commitment to a chosen course of action. *Organizational Behavior and Human Performance*, 16, 27–44.

Stearns, S. C., and Medzhitov, R. (2016). *Evolutionary Medicine.* Sunderland, MA: Sinauer Associates, Inc.

Strassmann, B. I. (1981). Sexual selection, paternal care, and concealed ovulation in humans. *Ethology and Sociobiology*, 2, 31–40.

Swanepoel, A., Music, G., Launer, J., and Reiss, M. J. (2017). How evolutionary thinking can help us to understand ADHD. *BJPsych Advances*, 23, 410–418.

Swedo, S. E., Leonard, H. L., and Rapoport, J. L. (2004). The pediatric autoimmune neuropsychiatric disorders associated with streptococcal infection (PANDAS) subgroup: separating fact from fiction. *Pediatrics*, 113, 907–911.

Taylor, M. J., Martin, J., Lu, Y., ... Lichtenstein, P. (2018). Association of genetic risk factors for psychiatric disorders and traits of these disorders in a Swedish population twin sample. *JAMA Psychiatry*, 76, 280–289.

Tooby, J., and Cosmides, L. (1990). The past explains the present:

emotional adaptations and the structure of ancestral environments. *Ethology and Sociobiology*, 11, 375–424.

Trimmer, P. C., Higginson, A. D., Fawcett, T. W., McNamara, J. M., and Houston, A. I. (2015). Adaptive learning can result in a failure to profit from good conditions: implications for understanding depression. *Evolution, Medicine, and Public Health*, 2015, 123–135.

Trumble, B. C., Stieglitz, J., Blackwell, A. D., ... Kaplan, H. (2017). Apolipoprotein E4 is associated with improved cognitive function in Amazonian forager-horticulturalists with a high parasite burden. *FASEB Journal*, 31, 1508–1515.

Tung, J., Archie, E. A., Altmann, J., and Alberts, S. C. (2016). Cumulative early life adversity predicts longevity in wild baboons. *Nature Communications*, 7, 11181.

Vogel, E. A., Rose, J. P., Roberts, L. R., and Eckles, K. (2014). Social comparison, social media, and self-esteem. *Psychology of Popular Media Culture*, 3, 206–222.

Wakefield, J. C. (1992). Disorder as harmful dysfunction: a conceptual critique of DSM-III-R's definition of mental disorder. *Psychological Review*, 99, 232–247.

Watson, P. J., and Andrews, P. W. (2002). Toward a revised evolutionary adaptationist analysis of depression: the social navigation hypothesis. *Journal of Affective Disorders*, 72, 1–14.

Welling, L. L. M., and Shackelford, T. K. (eds.) (2019). *The Oxford Handbook of Evolutionary Psychology and Behavioral Endocrinology.* New York: Oxford University Press.

Wenegrat, B. (1990). *Sociobiological Psychiatry: Normal Behavior and Psychopathology.* Lexington, MA: Lexington Books.

West, S. A., Cooper, G. A., Ghoul, M. B., and Griffin, A. S. (2021).

Ten recent insights for our understanding of cooperation. *Nature Ecology & Evolution*, 5, 419–430.

West-Eberhard, M. J. (1979). Sexual selection, social competition, and evolution. *Proceedings of the American Philosophical Society*, **123**, 222–234.

Westneat, D. F., and Fox, C. W. (eds.) (2010). *Evolutionary Behavioral Ecology*. Oxford;

New York: Oxford University Press.

Whiten, A., and Erdal, D. (2012). The human socio-cognitive niche and its evolutionary origins. *Philosophical Transactions of the Royal Society B: Biological Sciences*, **367**, 2119–2129.

Wierzbicka, A. (1992). Defining emotion concepts. *Cognitive Science: A Multidisciplinary Journal*, **16**, 539–581.

Williams, A. C. de C. (2016). What can evolutionary theory tell us about chronic pain? *Pain*, **157**, 788–790.

Williams, G. C. (1957). Pleiotropy, natural selection, and the evolution of senescence. *Evolution*, **11**, 398–411.

Williams, G. C., and Nesse, R. M. (1991). The dawn of Darwinian medicine. *Quarterly Review of Biology*, **66**, 1–22.

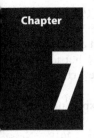

Chapter

7

Anxiety Disorders in Evolutionary Perspective

Randolph M. Nesse

Abstract

Anxiety disorders make sense only in the evolutionary context of the origins and functions of normal anxiety. Anxiety is an adaptation that adjusts diverse aspects of individuals in ways that increase fitness in dangerous situations. Subtypes were partially differentiated by different dangers. Anxiety is not fully differentiated from other aversive emotions, especially low mood. Anxiety disorders result when regulation systems fail. Explaining them requires considering five possible reasons for vulnerability. However, much harmful anxiety arises from normal mechanisms. These insights are valuable in the clinic, and they suggest new research initiatives.

Keywords

anxiety disorders, emotions, evolutionary medicine, evolutionary psychiatry, fear, panic

Key Points

- Natural selection partially differentiated subtypes of anxiety that increase the ability to cope with different kinds of dangers.
- Useless or harmful anxiety often arises from normal mechanisms.
- Explaining the utility of anxiety and the role of vicious cycles is often very helpful for patients engaged in behaviour therapy.

7.1 What Evolution Offers

It is possible to provide effective treatment for anxiety disorders without an evolutionary perspective. I did that full-time for a decade, before I finally recognised how useful evolutionary principles could be for psychiatry (Nesse, 1984). Understanding the origins and function of normal anxiety transformed my treatment of anxiety disorders and improved clinical outcomes. The improvement didn't come from doing some special evolutionary kind of therapy; it came from a fundamental reframing of what anxiety is and what anxiety disorders are. Instead of asking only what is wrong with people who have disorders, I began asking the two evolutionary questions that need answers to understand any disorder. The first is the origins and adaptive significance of the traits

that causes the vulnerability. For anxiety disorders that is easy: the capacity for the anxiety and the system that regulates its expression increase fitness in dangerous situations. The second question is why the systems are vulnerable to malfunction. It was soon obvious that this question needed to be answered for all diseases, and that evolutionary medicine more generally needed to be developed before the subfield of evolutionary psychiatry (Williams and Nesse, 1991).

Much of my interest in evolutionary approaches came about because I was appalled by the vast prevalence of anxiety and depression. It seemed to me that whoever designed the organism must have been incompetent or malevolent. However, working with George Williams soon made it clear that there are several reasons why natural selection leaves us vulnerable to so many medical problems (Nesse, 2005a; Nesse and Williams, 1994). It is severely constrained by stochasticity, which limits the ability to find solutions, steadily degrades the genome and limits canalisation. Natural selection cannot start over to correct a suboptimal design. It is too slow to keep up with fast-changing environments and fast-evolving pathogens. It cannot create traits free from the trade-offs that leave them vulnerable. And natural selection maximises gene transmission, often at the expense of health (see Chapter 6). These categories have proved valuable for understanding why some traits leave us vulnerable to diseases.

Despite George's reluctance, we added one more category: defences that often seem like diseases. Pain, fever and cough are exemplars. They are protective responses expressed in situations where they are useful: tissue damage, infection and foreign matter in the respiratory tree, respectively. Only gradually have I come to understand George's reluctance. Defences are fundamentally different from the other categories: they are adaptations, not explanations for why natural selection has left us vulnerable. Their aversiveness and their associated costs can make even normal defensive responses seem like diseases. Also, they are prone to dysregulation, which can make them become real diseases (e.g. chronic pain). Most significant of all, defensive responses that arise from normal regulation mechanisms are often useless or harmful. An evolutionary analysis of anxiety and its disorders seems simple but turns out to illustrate the challenges as well as the opportunities for evolutionary psychiatry.

7.2 Normal Anxiety

Anxiety and fear are emotions. Emotions exist only because they have given selective advantages. This makes it tempting to try to define different emotions in terms of their functions. Fear protects against present danger, anxiety against possible dangers. However, defining emotions in terms of their functions risks tacit creationism: the tendency to view bodies as if they are machines (Nesse, 2020). Machines have distinct parts with specific functions connected in sensible ways by an engineer with a plan. Bodies are very different. Functions are often carried out by multiple interacting parts with blurry boundaries and infernally complex connections that defy our wishes for simplicity. Fear and anxiety are not completely separate so I will use the term 'anxiety' to describe both.

An explicitly evolutionary approach looks for the structure of emotions in the evolutionary history that shaped them. Instead of sharply distinct basic emotions envisioned by an engineer, natural selection has shaped overlapping suites of changes that increase fitness in situations that have recurred often over evolutionary time (Al-Shawaf et al., 2016; Del Giudice, 2021; Keltner,

2019; Ketelaar, 2015; Nesse, 1990; Nesse and Ellsworth, 2009; Plutchik, 1970; Tooby and Cosmides, 2000). Thus, different emotions correspond not to different functions, but to different situations and the adaptive challenges of those situations.

A complete evolutionary explanation of any trait requires answers to all of Tinbergen's four questions (Natterson-Horowitz, 2019; Nesse, 2013; Pfaff et al., 2019; Tinbergen, 1963). What is the mechanism? What is its ontogeny? What is its phylogeny? What is its adaptive significance? Answers to the first two questions provide proximate explanation (see Chapters 1 and 2). Answers to the latter two questions provide an evolutionary explanation.

The *mechanisms* of anxiety have been the focus of intense study for decades. Psychological mechanisms for learning and generalisation of anxiety are well described. Brain mechanisms that mediate these responses are increasingly well understood (Kalin et al., 2005). Many sources are available, so mechanisms will not be further elaborated here except to note that there is partial but not complete differentiation of the brain loci, neurotransmitters and pathways that mediate anxiety. Also of special significance is the discovery that an older neural pathway for fast transmission of signals about danger has been overlaid with a second slower pathway that incorporates more knowledge about context and prior experience (LeDoux, 2000).

The *ontogeny* of anxiety has likewise been well studied (Barlow, 2000; Costello et al., 2005). The pioneer of evolutionary psychiatry, John Bowlby, observed the fear infants experience on separation from their mothers (Bowlby, 1973). The field of attachment research is based on the functional significance of fears that help individuals cope with a particular situation at a particular time of life (Simpson, 1999; Troisi, 2020). Infants across different cultures develop a fear of strangers that is likely to be adaptive (Konner, 1972). Nightmares concerning animals under the bed are very common and easy to interpret in an evolutionary context where there were many wild animals but no houses. When children begin social life in groups, fears of being rejected or abandoned emerge in a process that elaborates into the extraordinary richness and complexity of social life (Brosnan et al., 2017). This sequence of different fears appearing at different times in development matches the phases in which they would be useful.

The *phylogeny* of anxiety goes back as far as behaviour (LeDoux, 2012). Even bacteria detect risky situations and swim away from them (Lyon et al., 2021; Tagkopoulos et al., 2008). Direct escape from a present danger is usually thought of as fear, while anxiety is the associated emotion that facilitates avoidance of dangerous situations. Anxiety is akin to the nociceptive responses that prevent tissue damage, while fear is akin to immediate anticipation of damage, and sadness is akin to pain that occurs when tissue is being damaged.

Anxiety is often equated with stress. Walter Cannon gave the name 'stress' to the emergency system associated with the adrenal medulla response (Cannon, 1929), but it was Hans Selye who recognised the role of the adrenal cortex in the 'general adaptation syndrome' (Selye, 1936); Selye resisted calling it 'stress' until 1946. The common view that the hypothalamic–pituitary–adrenal system is activated mostly by danger is incorrect. It is aroused by situations that require vigorous activity for effective coping – especially threats, but also opportunities. It is not aroused reliably by situations that cause psychological anxiety. The stress response allocates extra metabolic and behavioural resources in situations where the benefits are greater than the costs (McEwen, 2019; Nesse et al., 2016; Sapolsky, 2000). The sympathetic nervous system accomplishes the same ends on a shorter timescale. The parasympathetic nervous system shifts resources to storage and repair when situations permit.

Adaptive significance, the focus of Tinbergen's fourth question, is more subtle than it seems. Anxiety adjusts many different parameters that increase fitness when expressed in situations associated with danger. Different adjustments are useful for different kinds of danger. This has differentiated generic anxiety into partially differentiated subtypes, each of which corresponds to a different danger and, interestingly, a different corresponding anxiety disorder (Nesse and Marks, 1994). The human wish for simplicity encourages thinking about them as different essentialised diseases, but they evolved from common precursor emotions to cope with situations that are not entirely distinct. The resulting anxiety subtypes are not crisply differentiated, and path dependence and mismatch result in characteristics that can be poorly suited to the situation. For instance, muscle tension is useful in preparation for flight, but in social anxiety it causes useless or harmful trembling.

Each anxiety subtype induces changes in physiology, attention, motivation, behaviour, facial expression, posture and vocal characteristics. Those suites of responses evolve in conjunction with mechanisms that monitor for the presence of the relevant situation and regulate anxiety expression accordingly. But how do organisms detect the relevant situation? Are anxiety responses innate or learned? The answer to the latter question is 'both', of course, but a full answer is much more interesting.

The cues that arouse anxiety innately differ from species to species, but for mammals there is moderate consistency in unconditioned fear being aroused by sudden loud noises, rapidly moving looming objects, pain, screams and being alone in a strange place. For humans, being the object of unsmiling attention from a group of strangers may also qualify.

What about fear of snakes? Is it innate? A wonderful series of experiments conducted by Susan Mineka and colleagues showed that lab-reared infant monkeys are quite happy to reach across a toy snake to get a piece of banana. However, a single viewing of a video in which another monkey express fear of snakes suffices to establish an enduring fear response (Mineka et al., 1984). Watching a similar video of another monkey expressing fear of a flower does not create a comparable response. This is a classic example of prepared learning (Seligman, 1971).

We need to revisit tacit creationism. Imagine for a moment how natural selection shaped anxiety-regulation mechanisms. There is no essentialised image of a snake in the system, nor is there a specific circuit to anxiety centres. Selection acted on tiny heritable variations in brain structure that influence connections between cues and anxiety-regulation mechanisms. Any cue that has been associated with a danger across evolutionary time can be recruited to connect readily to anxiety. Connections that increase fitness become more frequent; those that don't are selected out. The result is nothing like perfection. Irrelevant cues may be incorporated, and cues that might be useful might never get incorporated. Responses that are not useful may persist as part of a network of responding. Nonetheless, the system does a reasonable job of arousing appropriate anxiety responses in situations where they could be useful.

So far, we have covered only normal anxiety. What about anxiety disorders? Individuals that we see in anxiety disorder clinics all are characterised by anxiety excessive for the situation. Whether an anxiety response is excessive or not depends entirely on the situation, and understanding the relevant situations requires an evolutionary perspective. That perspective immediately calls attention to a class of unrecognised anxiety disorders. Individuals with deficient anxiety responses (i.e. hypophobia) have a disorder at least as serious as those who have excessive anxiety (Marks and Nesse, 1994). People with hypophobia do not request treatment, however, and their disorders are not treated or even recognised.

Even with knowledge of the situations that arouse anxiety normally it is hard to distinguish normal from abnormal responses. Diagnostic criteria rely on the frequency, severity and inappropriateness of responses, but the line they draw between normal and abnormal anxiety is artificially sharp. Therefore, some people who don't reach diagnostic criteria nonetheless want and would benefit from treatment, while some who do reach diagnostic criteria have anxiety that seems to arise from normal regulation mechanisms. An evolutionary perspective does not solve the dilemma of diagnostic criteria for anxiety disorders, but it can explain why the problem has been impossible to resolve.

7.3 Explaining Vulnerability to Anxiety Disorders

Anxiety-regulation mechanisms are prone to dysfunction. It is tempting to try to explain disorders by looking for associated selective advantages, but that is a mistake. Disorders are not adaptations. They do not have net fitness benefits. They are not products of natural selection. They are not appropriate objects of evolutionary explanation. Instead, the appropriate objects of explanation are traits that leave us vulnerable to disorders. In this case, the traits are the evolved mechanisms that regulate anxiety. There are five main kinds of possible explanation for why a trait might be vulnerable to malfunction (see Chapter 6 for details).

Stochasticity, which is inherent to natural selection, is the main explanation for vulnerability

to anxiety disorders. Genetic variations leave some individuals with excessive anxiety responses and others with deficient responses. Developmental stochasticity and differences in life experiences further increase the variance. The breadth of anxiety sensitivity is remarkably wide, ranging from vastly too much to vastly too little. This suggests that stabilising selection has been limited because the fitness function is relatively flat or because prior environments have varied substantially in the degree of risk. The distribution seems to skew towards excessive anxiety, but the lack of data correlating the degree of anxiety with fitness in ancestral environments makes it hard to tell what would be optimal.

Path dependence makes it impossible for natural selection to start afresh to correct a suboptimal design. In the case of anxiety disorders, this is reflected in the somewhat separate fast and slow pathways to arousing anxiety and the lack of integration of information from higher centres. This is why logical explanations about the lack of danger posed by a snake or a spider do nothing to reduce anxiety. Path dependence also accounts for the shared characteristics of anxiety that are unhelpful in a particular situation, such as sweating while giving a public presentation.

Mismatch between bodies and modern environments accounts better for deficient anxiety responses than excessive ones. We would be better off with more fear of guns, dirty needles, driving fast and electrical wires. Perhaps another 10,000 years of natural selection will provide us with better such protection. Mismatch can also help to explain some anxiety excesses.

Trade-offs are inherent to all responses. People with a great tendency to anxiety get protection at the expense of missed opportunities. People with deficient anxiety can take risks that bring benefits at the cost of damage and loss.

Traits that benefit genes at the expense of the individual are not as relevant to anxiety as they are to some other disorders, although parents sometimes are consumed by fears about their children's welfare – a perfectly natural response that nonetheless benefits genes more than the individuals experiencing the anxiety.

Each of these five reasons for vulnerability needs consideration for each anxiety disorder. However, it is difficult to tell where normal ends and where disorder begins (Faucher and Forest, 2021; Horwitz and Wakefield, 2012; Stein, 2013;

Wakefield, 1992). With that in mind, it is useful to recognise that bad feelings are often useless or harmful products of normal mechanisms.

7.4 Why Bad Feelings Are Often Useless but Normal

It seems obvious that anxiety produced by normal regulation mechanisms should be reliably useful and that useless anxiety should be a product of abnormal regulation mechanisms. Neither assumption is correct. The assumption that useless anxiety usually arises from defective regulation mechanisms has spurred enormous efforts to find brain abnormalities that don't exist. The assumption that all expressions of normal emotion should be useful has spurred wild speculations about the possible fitness benefits of disorders. Debates about the disease status of 'harmful dysfunctions' continue to be intense (Faucher and Forest, 2021; Wakefield, 2020). An evolutionary framework helps by calling attention to five reasons why useless or harmful anxiety is produced by intact regulation mechanisms. These are different from the five reasons for vulnerability to disorder, but there is some overlap.

The smoke detector principal is the most important explanation for useless anxiety (Nesse, 2005b; Nesse and Williams, 1994; also see Chapters 1 and 6 of this volume). The presence of a danger is often uncertain. Whether or not a defensive response should be expressed depends on the likelihood that the danger is actually present, the cost of a protective response and the average cost if no response is expressed but the danger turns out to be actually present. The optimal response threshold is illustrated by considering the costs of expressing or not expressing a panic attack when a predator might be present. The utility of the panic response was recognised by Walter Cannon in his description of the fight-or-flight response (Cannon, 1939). In the face of life-threatening danger, massive physiological arousal, muscle tension and a strong motivation to flee are all potentially life-saving. If a false alarm in that system costs 100 calories but failing to express the response when a predator is actually present costs 100,000 calories, then it is optimal to express a response whenever the probability of the predator being present is greater than 1 in 1,000. This means – and I couldn't believe it when I first did this calculation – that 999 panic episodes out of 1,000 will be false alarms that are perfectly normal

products of an optimal regulation system. Signal detection theory provides more sophisticated analyses of such trade-offs (Bateson et al., 2011; Green and Swets, 1966). But the brain does not need to do calculus; it simply expresses, on average across many people in many situations, responses that maximise fitness.

The capacity for adjusting the anxiety threshold as a function of experience is a secondary anxiety-regulation mechanism with great benefits and substantial risks. For tissue damage, proprioception provides protection. Only when that fails does tissue damage occur, arousing pain. Repeated arousal of pain means that dangers have not been adequately protected against and that increased sensitivity of the proprioception and pain systems will be beneficial. This runs the risk of initiating a positive-feedback loop that creates chronic pain (Nesse and Schulkin, 2019; Williams, 2016). For other dangers and losses, anxiety mediates avoidance of the danger, but if it fails, fear and possible loss result. Repeated experiences of fear indicate a dangerous environment where increased anxiety can be beneficial despite its costs. Here, too, the system comes with an inherent risk of initiating a vicious cycle. More on this is discussed in Section 7.5.3.

Mismatch results in normal mechanisms expressing useless anxiety. We have far too much fear of harmless snakes and insects. In cultures where experiences with such organisms are common, social transmission provides individuals with knowledge about which snakes, spiders and insects are dangerous and which are harmless. In modern environments, most people never have experiences that allow such learning. Thus, most of my patients with snake phobias had never encountered a snake in the wild and I don't recall even one who had experienced a snake bite. I am feeling slightly apprehensive at this very moment. A webcam mounted on a gooseneck stand is bent in an arc, bringing it close to my face and causing a tiny bit of anxiety that is relieved by bending it into an upright, less snake-like position.

However, mismatch mostly accounts for deficient anxiety responses. People have nowhere near enough fear of guns, dirty needles, driving, drugs and electrical wires. Perhaps we will in 10,000 years. For now, hypophobia is rampant.

Happenstance unfortunate sequences of events can interact with normal mechanisms to give maladaptive responses. Modelling demonstrates how such maladaptations can persist (Greggor et al., 2019; Meacham and Bergstrom, 2016; Trimmer et al., 2015)

Benefits to genes at a cost to the individual can cause anxiety that is useless for the individual but useful for the individual's genes in children and other kin. Many parents twist themselves in knots with worries about the dangers faced by their children; this completely natural anxiety benefits genes at a cost to the individual.

7.5 Anxiety Disorders

7.5.1 Epidemiology

Anxiety disorders are the most common mental disorders; epidemiological data describe the details (Kessler et al., 2010; Michael et al., 2007). In Western countries, lifetime prevalence rates of any anxiety disorder range from 14% to 29%. Panic disorder, agoraphobia, generalised anxiety disorder (GAD) and obsessive-compulsive disorder (OCD) have lifetime prevalence rates mostly in the range of 1–4%, while simple phobias and social phobias are more common, with estimates in the range of 2–14%. Specific and social phobias usually have their onsets in childhood, while GAD, panic disorder and agoraphobia tend to begin in late adolescence or early adulthood. Comorbidity among anxiety disorders is high; 74% of individuals with one anxiety disorder also have another. The rate is over 90% for those with GAD or panic disorder, and individuals with GAD are 12.3 times more likely to have panic disorder than individuals without GAD. The average odds ratio for an individual with one anxiety disorder having a second anxiety disorder is 6.6. Rates of anxiety disorders in non-Western countries tend to be substantially lower, with 12-month prevalence rates being about half of those in Western countries and with substantially lower rates for specific phobias, social phobias and GAD (Michael et al., 2007).

Anxiety disorders have major overlaps with other mental disorders, especially depression. Data from the National Comorbidity Study Replication show that the lifetime risk of any mood disorder is increased by factors ranging from 3.45 for phobias to 5.83 for GAD (Merikangas and Swanson, 2010). Interestingly, the genetic variations that predispose individuals to major depression are mostly the same as those that predispose individuals to GAD (Kendler et al., 1992; Middeldorp et al., 2005; Taylor et al., 2019).

Anxiety disorders have moderate heritabilities, in the range of 30–40%. Women have twice the risk for most anxiety disorders as men, with the exception being OCD where differences are small. The risk is lower for married individuals and those who have higher levels of education, employment and income. A history of physical, emotional or sexual abuse was found in 35% of subjects with major depression and panic disorder (Young et al., 1997); most likely these are the lasting effects of family conflict, but it is hard to control for genetic factors. Children with three or more early stressful experiences are considerably more likely to develop depression or GAD in response to military training (Bandoli et al., 2017).

The disorders recognised by clinicians and described in official diagnostic nomenclatures map remarkably well to different subtypes of normal anxiety and the dangers they map onto (see Table 7.1).

7.5.2 Phobias

In Western countries, about 12% of people have had a specific phobia severe enough to reach diagnostic criteria at sometime in their life, and in any given year the rate is about 9%. Many are phobias of insects and small animals. The brain shows responses to such images even before they reach consciousness (Ohman et al., 2007). Most people with simple phobias cannot recall a precipitating incident and many say they have had the problem for as long as they can remember (Poulton and Menzies, 2002). Also, individuals who fear heights as teenagers were *less* likely than others to have been injured in a childhood fall, presumably because those who were injured had – and still have – hypophobia (Poulton et al., 1998). However, such studies have severe methodological limitations (Mineka and Öhman, 2002). A model that incorporates innate tendencies and preparedness to learn anxiety offers an explanation for why some things are much more likely to cause phobias than others (Mineka and Zinbarg, 2006).

Generalisations do not do justice to the diversity one sees in the clinic. One of my patients recalled, while being treated for a fear of small insects, being suddenly whisked out the back door

Table 7.1. Anxiety disorders and corresponding dangers

Disorder	Danger
Small animal phobia	Harm from small animals
Height phobia	Falling
Blood, illness, injury phobia	Bleeding, tissue damage
Agoraphobia	Vulnerability in open places
Claustrophobia	Vulnerability in closed places
Post-traumatic stress disorder	Life-threatening danger
Panic disorder	Predators and dire dangers
Illness anxiety disorder	Undiagnosed disease
Somatic symptoms disorder	Undiagnosed disease
Separation anxiety disorder	Isolation from kin and friends
Social anxiety disorder	Rejection or attack by a social group
Body dysmorphic disorder	Being viewed as unattractive
Obsessive-compulsive disorder	Dire consequences from an oversight
Hoarding disorder	Shortages of vital resources
Generalised anxiety disorder	Dangers of all kinds

of a paediatrician's office at age 7 to a polio ward, where she lay alone and paralysed watching insects crawl up the wall next to her. A woman with a snake phobia recalled stopping with her father on a rural road where he chopped a snake into pieces, put them in a Mason jar and had her hold it between her legs for the rest of the journey. My psychoanalytic supervisors were delighted, but they were astounded to learn that an hour of exposure therapy cured her. Most patients with phobias, however, have no idea what caused their disorders.

Treatment for phobias is reliably effective if it's possible to get the phobic person to maintain close contact with the phobic object for an extended period (Eaton et al., 2018). The challenge is often great, given that such therapy fights the natural urge to escape from danger. What works best is to have the patient stay close to the phobic object until the anxiety reduces somewhat, even from 90 to 80 on a 100-point scale. Once patients realise that progress is possible, they are motivated to continue with treatment that is usually effective. The benefit seems not to be from unlearning; instead, new inhibitory impulses are created.

The traits that account for vulnerability to phobias are the preparedness of some cues to be associated with anxiety and the capacity for learning. The main evolutionary explanation for vulnerability to phobias is the stochasticity of brain variations – inherited and acquired – that result in some people developing phobias. They are genuine disorders, not adaptations. Mismatch may also contribute, especially because of a lack of experience and a lack of cultural knowledge.

Discussing the evolutionary reasons for vulnerability to phobias helps patients to realise that their symptoms are simply an exaggeration of a useful response, not a disease that means that they have an abnormal brain. Furthermore, explaining that natural selection shaped a mechanism to reduce anxiety after extended exposures helps many to complete behaviour therapy.

7.5.3 Panic Disorder and Agoraphobia

Panic disorder offers a good example of how evolutionary thinking can be helpful in the clinic. For the first decade of practice in an anxiety clinic, I explained to patients that their panic attacks were a product of a mental disorder and that a combination of medication and behaviour therapy could help. Many said they knew their condition was not mental because they could feel their heart pounding. When I mentioned genetic predispositions, many interpreted this to mean they could not be helped. When I shifted to explaining that panic attacks are a normal, useful response to extreme danger and that panic disorder results from false alarms in that system, patients immediately appreciated the evolutionary context even without hearing the 'e-word'. This explanation made sense of their symptoms, so they no longer needed to attribute them to cardiac or neurological disease. In particular, the overwhelming mental focus on escape and the wish to flee became coherent, allowing them to complete behaviour therapy exercises that otherwise would have been impossible.

An evolutionary perspective also revealed a clinical phenomenon I had not previously recognised. I knew that freezing is an essential part of the panic response for other animals, but I had never heard about this response from any of the scores of patients with panic disorder I had seen. When I began asking, I found – to my amazement – that about half of patients reported feeling unable to move for a moment at the onset of panic.

About half of patients with panic attacks have agoraphobia, and most patients with agoraphobia have experienced panic attacks or some similar sudden episodes associated with fear. The nature of this connection has been explored with neurological and psychodynamic theories. However, from an evolutionary point of view the connection is straightforward. If you have repeatedly encountered a predator or other life-threatening danger on recent forays away from camp, it is smart to stay home if possible, to venture out only with comrades and to be ready to flee at the merest hint of danger. This explanation is enormously helpful to patients. They still need to follow through with often distressing exposure exercises, but the protocol now makes more sense to them. They realise that wide open spaces were indeed a situation of vulnerability for our ancestors. Patients with claustrophobia realise that enclosed spaces were also especially dangerous. The setting where humans in general feel most at peace is an open park-like setting with little underbrush and small, climbable trees (Kaplan, 1987). This is no surprise.

Why does natural selection leave us vulnerable to panic disorder and agoraphobia? The smoke detector principal offers part of an explanation, but panic disorder is not a normal adaptive response – it is a crippling disease. Like other anxiety disorders, it is heritable, and it is influenced by early adverse experiences and current stressors. Repeated exposure to big risks adaptively adjusts the system to greater sensitivity. However, the crucial pathological process involves a positive-feedback cycle that is set in motion when symptoms of panic are themselves viewed as dangerous, as they often are after patients hear from an emergency room physician, 'It does not seem to be your heart, but you should be very careful and come back immediately if your symptoms return.' Patients begin monitoring for rapid heartbeat and shortness of breath, which inevitably occur, spurring mounting fear, whose symptoms soon spiral into

another attack. Patients find this explanation helpful.

They also find an evolutionary explanation helpful for grasping how medications work. Learning that benzodiazepines and alcohol offer only temporary relief at the price of more fear later is helpful for reducing their use. Antidepressants, however, block full-blown panic attacks quite nicely in most patients. Patients often ask if the drug is simply covering over symptoms. They appreciate learning that using medication for some months to stop panic attacks helps the system to become less sensitive, thus making long-term improvement likely even after the medication is discontinued. Telling patients that they likely will continue to have 'mini-attacks' for some weeks helps to alleviate concern about such experiences.

Vulnerability to panic attacks and agoraphobia runs strongly in families, members of which presumably have superior protection from dangers at the cost of a higher risk of experiencing panic disorder. Panic attacks are also more common in individuals who have experienced early adversity, which is no surprise because this often reflects a dangerous environment. Initial attacks are often set off by being in a strange town, being jet-lagged, drinking in the evening and having several cups of coffee in the morning. Interpreting the resulting panic attack as a possible heart attack initiates a vicious cycle. However, physicians who understand this can effectively prevent the creation of an iatrogenic disorder.

7.5.4 Post-traumatic Stress Disorder

A single experience of life-threatening danger is enough to set off an acute stress disorder and, in many people, post-traumatic stress disorder (PTSD) (Breslau et al., 1995; Yehuda et al., 2015). Watching someone else be killed can have equal or greater repercussions. Patients with PTSD ruminate about the danger and become hypersensitive to cues that indicate even the merest possibility that it may be recurring. Several authors have considered the possibility that such responses are an evolved adaptation, with even a minuscule chance of life-threatening danger justifying an intense protective response (Cantor, 2009). If this was an adaptation, however, most people would have such a response to a traumatic event, and these responses would increase their fitness. Neither seems to be correct. Epidemiological studies show that a majority of people have had an intensely traumatic experience, but only a minority develop PTSD. Vulnerability factors include genetics, sex and previous experiences of trauma, anxiety or depression (Breslau et al., 1995). New data from the Turkana in Africa show that symptoms of arousal are associated with the experience of danger, but symptoms of depression are more closely associated with the 'moral injury' of moral violations (Zefferman and Mathew, 2020). The meaning of warfare and social support for warriors in the Turkana may explain why they experience less depression than soldiers in Western countries.

The utility of a short-term response to trauma seems obvious, especially if the danger may still be present. However, the enduring symptoms of PTSD are more likely to be pathological manifestations of a system pushed beyond its normal range of functioning (Liberzon and Abelson, 2016). PTSD is an example of a disorder that is more likely for people at the tail end of a distribution. What that distribution is remains uncertain. Does the risk of PTSD mainly result from a low threshold for responding or a high intensity of response, or from failure to moderate the responses in the weeks after the trauma? These are good questions.

7.5.5 Hypochondria

Excess concern about health is now diagnosed as 'illness anxiety disorder' for those with general concerns and 'somatic symptoms disorder' for those who cannot be reassured about specific symptoms (Furer et al., 2007). The relevant danger is, of course, disease. The fear arises from a conviction that something dire is wrong and an inability to accept medical reassurance. Specifying the traits responsible for vulnerability is difficult, but confirmation bias is prominent in sustaining the belief despite contrary evidence. The origins of beliefs that one has an undiagnosed disease are products of social learning and sometimes psychodynamic mechanisms. It is tempting to attribute vulnerability mainly to novel technological environments in which sophisticated tests can reveal hidden illnesses and treatments can sometimes cure serious diseases. But preoccupation with symptoms and the desire to find explanations seem to be prevalent everywhere. It has been suggested that symptoms of illness have evolved to serve signalling functions and that this opens up opportunities for communication and manipulation (Tiokhin, 2016) that can result in positive attention that encourages additional experience or communication of symptoms (Wenegrat, 1995).

7.5.6 Separation Anxiety Disorder

The utility of separation anxiety early in life is now obvious thanks to John Bowlby's pioneering work (Bowlby, 1973). Our clinic saw many newly arrived university students who could not function because of separation anxiety disorder, although they called it homesickness (Silove et al., 2010). Being separated from parents for the first time and exposed to new sorts of social and academic competition, as well as new opportunities for drug use and sexual adventures, can set the scene for intense separation anxiety. Most such patients reported previous difficulties going to summer camps and other childhood activities away from family. If the student can be integrated into campus life with friends and successful activities and studies, the problem usually fades quickly. Sometimes, however, it escalates and interferes with social life and academic performance, requiring a move home that can be devastating. Intense treatment is appropriate to prevent such a feedback cycle from developing.

Separation anxiety disorder is a classic example of a disorder resulting from the failure of anxiety to fade after its normal expression early in development. It is probably best attributed to being at the tail end of the distribution of separation fear, but it could also represent a defect in the system that usually tempers such fear in the process of maturation.

7.5.7 Body Dysmorphic Disorder

The belief that one is unattractive can be as intractable as the belief that one has an undiagnosed disease (Stein, 2017; Veale and Gilbert, 2014). It's often present in people who are, to other people's perceptions, very attractive indeed. However, once the belief in one's unattractiveness gets established it can be used to account for all manner of experiences, such as being rejected by a date. The normal trait related to this disorder is wanting to be attractive. In the usual range, this is almost certainly useful. In a modern society with extraordinarily attractive images on billboards and screens and the availability of enhancing surgery, intense competition can lead to morbid preoccupation. Plastic surgeons often sent prospective patients to our clinic to ask if we thought psychological treatment might be more helpful than surgery. We often said yes, but we rarely convinced the patients. A different version of the same problem is experienced by patients who believe – despite all reassurance – that they smell bad. These syndromes all reflect the extraordinary degree to which people care about what other people think about them, a tendency that is deeply ingrained for good evolutionary reasons.

7.5.8 Social Anxiety Disorder

Social anxiety is so overwhelmingly common it is hard to say what is normal and what is pathological. The criteria defining social anxiety disorder are set so that only about 5% of people qualify for a lifetime diagnosis (Stein et al., 2017); however, most people feel considerable discomfort when in front of a crowd in an evaluative situation, and 13% of young adults report strong social fears (Fehm et al., 2008). The risks in such situations are many and considerable. Saying something that appears stupid can harm one's reputation. Revealing covert hostile feelings can ruin relationships. Even success can prove problematic if it threatens the status of others in the group who are likely to retaliate. Worst of all, simply appearing nervous in front of a group can reduce social status, causing fears that one will appear nervous – a perfect set-up for a nasty positive-feedback cycle.

While being the centre of social attention does involve risks, they are not nearly as great as most people assume – a finding possibly explained by the smoke detector principle. Treatments that try to help people avoid errors in public presentations can help, but reducing the fear of making mistakes requires making mistakes. Doing and saying silly things are difficult at first, but soon most patients realise that most people don't notice, and if they do notice they don't care very much, and even if they do care they generally forget them by the next day.

Social fears can be extremely intense. Some of our patients had no social contacts whatsoever and were incapable of writing a cheque at the grocery store or of going to a bank. Some dropped out of school and some were unemployed, while one man stayed alone in his trailer at the end of a dead-end road. These are serious disorders, but they are responsive to treatment. Such treatment goes better if the several routes to social anxiety can be investigated carefully and discussions with the patient can consider the role of positive-feedback cycles in perpetuating the disorder.

The trait that makes us vulnerable to social anxiety disorders is caring a lot about what others think about us. This almost certainly has been shaped by natural selection (Brosnan et al., 2017; Gilbert, 2014; Leary and Kowalski, 1995; Stein and Vythilingum, 2007; Tone et al., 2019). Maintaining a good reputation is essential for maximising benefits in exchange relationships. However, capacities for extreme prosocial tendencies including guilt and embarrassment seem likely to have been shaped by social selection (Frank, 2006; Hammerstein and Noë, 2016; Nesse, 2007; West-Eberhard, 1975; Westneat, 2012). Sexual selection is the familiar process in which competition to be chosen as a mate results in extreme traits. Social selection is the more general category in which social choices shape traits. Choices of social partners influence fitness strongly. Having partners with resources and tendencies to share them gives big advantages. To get such partners, people must demonstrate those traits themselves. This results in intense competition – possibly even runaway competition – to have and display desirable social traits such as honesty, generosity and the ability to sense what others want. The pairing process creates a hierarchy, with substantial benefits going to those who are – and who have – the best partners. Those who are perceived as poor partners do badly. This creates strong selection to avoid being perceived as lacking in resources, generosity, trustworthiness or loyalty to partners. It also creates constant monitoring of how others respond to every word and gesture. The miracle is that we can at times relax with friends.

7.5.9 Obsessive-Compulsive Disorder

Most of the repeated thoughts and behaviours of people with OCD are attempts to prevent possible dire outcomes from a minor misstep (Brüne, 2006; Robbins et al., 2019; Stein, 2002). The concern is more often about fear of accidentally harming others than it is about being harmed oneself. In this sense, it is the converse of paranoid fears of being harmed by others. So people with OCD wash their hands until they are raw, clean surfaces until they are burnished and ruminate for hours about whether the door was locked to protect others as well as themselves.

What trait makes us vulnerable to OCD? It does not seem to be carefulness in general, which is more characteristic of obsessive-compulsive personality, an entirely different condition that mostly involves conscientiousness and contempt for those who are careless. The anxiety associated with OCD escalates as the person considers stopping some protective behaviour such as washing or cleaning. What if some toxin or pathogen is still on the doorknob? My child could touch it and get sick and die. What if I left the hair-curling iron turned on? It could start a fire that burns down the house and kills my dog. What if I hit someone while driving and didn't notice? I should circle around the block and check. But what if the person I hit was already taken to the hospital? I should circle the block again and call the hospital to check.

One could make a case that a system for keeping hostile impulses unconscious has failed and the obsessions are a secondary defence. But after seeing hundreds of patients with OCD, I think they are aware of many impulses that other people don't notice, but their levels of hostility only rarely struck me as excessive.

The trait that accounts for vulnerability to repeated checking is the mechanism that normally turns off protective behaviours when they have been completed sufficiently. Most of us wash our hands cursorily; if we know our hands are contaminated, we wash until they seem clean, then concern is swept out of mind. This is a variant of the mechanism that makes decisions possible. We weigh options, decide and then convince ourselves that we made the right decision – a tendency that makes it possible to move on. Psychological tendencies towards confirmation bias and dissonance reduction are useful in this respect. People with schizophrenia often lack this useful cognitive distortion, so every decision is wracked by interminable ambivalence and second-guessing. For people with OCD, the inability to reach a comfortable decision is mainly due to concerns about how much safety behaviour is enough.

Neurological findings associated with OCD further suggest that OCD is not just the extreme of a trait but a pattern of symptoms that can result

from damage to the head of the caudate nucleus. Evidence for this includes precipitation of OCD by stroke in the basal ganglia or by autoimmune responses to streptococcal infection in childhood, as well as symptom relief from surgical disruption of adjacent circuits (Robbins et al., 2019). Further evidence is provided by OCD's comorbidity with Tourette's syndrome, which involves an inability to inhibit movements and gesticulations that is associated with caudate nucleus damage (Hirschtritt et al., 2015). OCD can also be an enduring complication of taking atypical antipsychotic drugs (Lykouras et al., 2003).

Taken together, these findings suggest that OCD may not result from the extreme of any trait; it may instead be a pattern of symptoms that results from damage to the caudate nucleus, very much like the syndrome of hyperextension of the lower extremities and contraction of the arm muscles that results from spinal cord transection. In this model, no evolutionary explanation is needed, except perhaps for the reasons why the caudate is especially vulnerable to damage. Of course, OCD vulnerability could result from anatomical damage in some individuals and from being at the extreme end of harm avoidance for others.

7.5.10 General Anxiety Disorder

GAD is characterised by preoccupation with worries of all sorts (Brown et al., 1994; Wittchen and Hoyer, 2001). Will my spouse have an accident on the way home? Will my children catch Lyme disease from playing in the yard? Will my medical insurance be cancelled because I didn't pay my doctor's bill on time? Such concerns may seem minor, but when I ask GAD patients, 'What percentage of your time and effort goes to preventing bad things from happening?' the answer is usually over 80%, and often over 95%.

Psychologists identify two motivational global states: promotion and prevention (Higgins and Spiegel, 2007). Individuals in a promotion state put efforts towards getting something or accomplishing something. Individuals in a prevention state put efforts towards preventing loss, harm or damage. From this perspective, patients with GAD are at the prevention end of the promotion–prevention distribution. The most likely explanation for vulnerability is simply stochasticity. Stabilising selection has not sufficiently narrowed the distribution to protect people at the extremes. But could local anatomical or physiological abnormalities like those that cause OCD be responsible? Yes, but the evidence for such lesions is sparse, while the evidence for a dimension ranging from promotion to prevention is strong.

As is the case for other disorders arising from trait extremes, GAD calls attention to the other extreme: hypophobia. People who spend 95% of their efforts on promotion and 5% on prevention should be prone to accidents and mistakes of all causes, but their condition has not yet been recognised as a mental disorder.

The genetics of GAD are of especial interest. The responsible loci seem to be the same as those that predispose individuals to major depression (Kendler et al., 1992). This suggests that both traits may have evolved from common precursor states that protect against loss. Low mood protects against wasted effort, while anxiety protects against other losses. It's possible that modern societies initiate enough new worries to shift many people into the pathological category. As for trade-offs, those at either end of the distribution do badly.

7.6 Conclusions

Anxiety and its disorders illustrate the value of systematically considering all possible explanations for vulnerability. Recognising that the capacity for anxiety is an adaptation is the place to start, but this does not justify viewing disorders as adaptations. Instead, it suggests that stochasticity limits the ability of stabilising selection to narrow the distribution sufficiently to protect everyone in a population from disorder. Mismatch is relevant for some anxiety disorders, but additional data are needed to assess its role. Trade-offs are inherent for any dimensional trait, but the advantages for individuals with high levels of anxiety are not sufficient to compensate for the disadvantages. Individuals with low levels of anxiety have different advantages and disadvantages. Individuals in the middle range are assumed to do best, or at least to have done so in ancestral environments. Some syndromes, however, such as OCD, may not be extremes of any adaptive trait, but instead may reflect patterns of dysfunction that result from neural damage.

While an evolutionary perspective does not constitute a new kind of therapy, it does fundamentally transform the schema for understanding anxiety disorders. In particular, it challenges the assumption that useless anxiety arises mainly from defective brain mechanisms; normal mechanisms seem more often to be responsible. This should shift the neuroscientific approach to anxiety disorders from searching only for specific abnormalities to instead searching for the many factors likely to influence an individual's trait value on the distribution. It also should encourage much more attention being paid to systems thinking and the prominent role of positive feedback in creating and maintaining severe anxiety disorders.

As noted already, patients often deeply appreciate recognising that their symptoms are not simply manifestations of pathology, but instead are useful responses that have overshot the mark. They also especially value recognising how runaway systems can maintain their symptoms. This often makes it possible for them to complete behaviour therapy exercises that would otherwise have been even more difficult for them.

References

Al-Shawaf, L., Conroy-Beam, D., Asao, K., and Buss, D. M. (2016). Human emotions: an evolutionary psychological perspective. *Emotion Review*, **8**, 173–186.

Bandoli, G., Campbell-Sills, L., Kessler, R. C., ... Stein, M. B. (2017). Childhood adversity, adult stress, and the risk of major depression or generalized anxiety disorder in US soldiers: a test of the stress sensitization hypothesis. *Psychological Medicine*, **47**, 2379–2392.

Barlow, D. H. (2000). Unraveling the mysteries of anxiety and its disorders from the perspective of emotion theory. *American Psychologist*, **55**, 1247–1263.

Bateson, M., Brilot, B., and Nettle, D. (2011). Anxiety: an evolutionary approach. *Canadian Journal of Psychiatry*, **56**, 707–715.

Bowlby, J. (1973). *Separation: Vol. 2: Anxiety and Anger*. New York: Basic Books, Inc.

Breslau, N., Davis, G. C., and Andreski, P. (1995). Risk factors for PTSD-related traumatic events: a prospective analysis. *American Journal of Psychiatry*, **152**, 529–35.

Brosnan, S. F., Tone, E. B., and Williams, L. (2017). The evolution of social anxiety. In T. K. Shackelford and V. Zeigler-Hill (eds.), *The Evolution of*

Psychopathology. Cham: Springer International Publishing, pp. 93–116.

Brown, T. A., Barlow, D. H., and Liebowitz, M. R. (1994). The empirical basis of generalized anxiety disorder. *American Journal of Psychiatry*, **151**, 1272–1280.

Brüne, M. (2006). The evolutionary psychology of obsessive-compulsive disorder: the role of cognitive metarepresentation. *Perspectives in Biology and Medicine*, **49**, 317–329.

Cannon, W. B. (1929). *Bodily Changes in Pain, Hunger, Fear, and Rage. Researches into the Function of Emotional Excitement*. New York: Harper and Row.

Cannon, W. B. (1939). *The Wisdom of the Body*. New York: Norton.

Cantor, C. (2009). Post-traumatic stress disorder: evolutionary perspectives. *Australian & New Zealand Journal of Psychiatry*, **43**, 1038–1048.

Costello, E. J., Egger, H. L., and Angold, A. (2005). The developmental epidemiology of anxiety disorders: phenomenology, prevalence, and comorbidity. *Child and Adolescent Psychiatric Clinics*, **14**, 631–648.

Del Giudice, M. (2021). The motivational architecture of emotions. In L. Al-Shawaf and T. K. Shackelford (eds.), *The Oxford Handbook of Evolution and the Emotions*. Oxford; New York: Oxford University Press, p. 39.

Eaton, W. W., Bienvenu, O. J., and Miloyan, B. (2018). Specific phobias. *Lancet Psychiatry*, **5**, 678–686.

Faucher, L., and Forest, D. (2021). Defining mental disorder: Jerome Wakefield and his critics. Retrieved from http://mitpress.mit.edu/9780262045643

Fehm, L., Beesdo, K., Jacobi, F., and Fiedler, A. (2008). Social anxiety disorder above and below the diagnostic threshold: prevalence, comorbidity and impairment in the general population. *Social Psychiatry and Psychiatric Epidemiology*, **43**, 257–265.

Frank, S. A. (2006). Social selection. In C. W. Fox and J. B. Wolf (eds.), *Evolutionary Genetics: Concepts and Case Studies*. Oxford; New York: Oxford University Press, pp. 350–363.

Furer, P., Walker, J. R., and Stein, M. B. (2007). *Treating Health Anxiety and Fear of Death: A Practitioner's Guide*. Cham: Springer Science+Business Media.

Gilbert, P. (2014). Evolutionary models: practical and conceptual utility for the treatment and study of social anxiety disorder. In J. W. Weeks (ed.), *The Wiley Blackwell Handbook of Social Anxiety Disorder*. Hoboken, NJ: Wiley Blackwell, pp. 24–52.

Green, D. M., and Swets, J. A. (1966). *Signal Detection Theory and Psycho-physics*. New York: Wiley.

Greggor, A. L., Trimmer, P. C., Barrett, B. J., and Sih, A. (2019). Challenges of learning to escape evolutionary traps. *Frontiers in Ecology and Evolution*, 7, 408.

Hammerstein, P., and Noë, R. (2016). Biological trade and markets. *Philosophical Transactions of the Royal Society B: Biological Sciences*, **371**, 20150101.

Higgins, E. T., and Spiegel, S. (2007). Promotion and prevention strategies for self-regulation. In R. F. Baumeister and K. D. Vohs (eds.), *Handbook of Self-Regulation: Research, Theory, and Applications*. New York: Guilford Press, pp. 171–187.

Hirschtritt, M. E., Lee, P. C., Pauls, D. L., . . . for the Tourette Syndrome Association International Consortium for Genetics (2015). Lifetime prevalence, age of risk, and genetic relationships of comorbid psychiatric disorders in Tourette syndrome. *JAMA Psychiatry*, **72**, 325–333.

Horwitz, A. V., and Wakefield, J. C. (2012). *All We Have to Fear: Psychiatry's Transformation of Natural Anxieties into Mental Disorders*. New York: Oxford University Press.

Kalin, N. H., Shelton, S. E., Fox, A. S., Oakes, T. R., and Davidson, R. J. (2005). Brain regions associated with the expression and contextual regulation of anxiety in primates. *Biological Psychiatry*, 58, 796–804.

Kaplan, S. (1987). Aesthetics, affect, and cognition: environmental preference from an evolutionary perspective. *Environment and Behavior*, **19**, 3–32.

Keltner, D. (2019). Toward a consensual taxonomy of emotions. *Cognition and Emotion*, 33, 14–19.

Kendler, K. S., Neale, M. C., Kessler, R. C., Heath, A. C., and Eaves, L. J. (1992). Major depression and generalized anxiety disorder. Same genes, (partly) different environments? *Archives of General Psychiatry*, **49**, 716–722.

Kessler, R. C., Ruscio, A. M., Shear, K., and Wittchen, H.-U. (2010). Epidemiology of anxiety disorders. In M. B. Stein and T. Steckler (eds.), *Behavioral Neurobiology of Anxiety and Its Treatment*. Berlin: Springer, pp. 21–35.

Ketelaar, T. (2015). Evolutionary psychology and emotion: a brief history. In V. Zeigler-Hill, L. M. Welling, and T. K. Shackelford (eds.), *Evolutionary Perspectives on Social Psychology*. Cham: Springer International Publishing, pp. 51–67.

Konner, M. J. (1972). Aspects of the developmental ethology of a foraging people. In N. B. Jones (ed.), *Ethological Studies of Child Behaviour*. Cambridge: Cambridge University Press, pp. 285–304.

Leary, M. R., and Kowalski, R. M. (1995). *Social Anxiety*. New York: Guilford Press.

LeDoux, J. E. (2000). Emotion circuits in the brain. *Annual Review of Neuroscience*, **23**, 155–184.

LeDoux, J. E. (2012). Evolution of human emotion. *Progress in Brain Research*, **195**, 431–442.

Liberzon, I., and Abelson, J. L. (2016). context processing and the neurobiology of post-traumatic stress disorder. *Neuron*, **92**, 14–30.

Lykouras, L., Alevizos, B., Michalopoulou, P., and Rabavilas, A. (2003). Obsessive-compulsive symptoms induced by atypical antipsychotics. A review of the reported cases. *Progress in Neuro-Psychopharmacology and Biological Psychiatry*, **27**, 333–346.

Lyon, P., Keijzer, F., Arendt, D., and Levin, M. (2021). *Reframing Cognition: Getting Down to Biological Basics*. London: The Royal Society.

Marks, I., M., and Nesse, R. M. (1994). Fear and fitness: an evolutionary analysis of anxiety disorders. *Ethology and Sociobiology*, **15**, 247–261.

McEwen, B. S. (2019). The good side of 'stress'. *Stress*, **22**, 524–525.

Meacham, F., and Bergstrom, C. T. (2016). Adaptive behavior can produce maladaptive anxiety due to individual differences in experience. *Evolution, Medicine, and Public Health*, **2016**, 270–285.

Merikangas, K. R., and Swanson, S. A. (2010). Comorbidity in anxiety disorders. *Current Topics in Behavioral Neurosciences*, **2**, 37–59.

Michael, T., Zetsche, U., and Margraf, J. (2007). Epidemiology of anxiety disorders. *Psychiatry*, **6**, 136–142.

Middeldorp, C. M., Cath, D. C., Van Dyck, R., and Boomsma, D. I. (2005). The co-morbidity of anxiety and depression in the perspective of genetic epidemiology. A review of twin and family studies. *Psychological Medicine*, **35**, 611–624.

Mineka, S., and Öhman, A. (2002). Born to fear: non-associative vs associative factors in the etiology of phobias. *Behaviour Research and Therapy*, **40**, 173–184.

Mineka, S., and Zinbarg, R. (2006). A contemporary learning theory perspective on the etiology of anxiety disorders: it's not what you thought it was. *American Psychologist*, **61**, 10–26.

Mineka, S., Davidson, M., Cook, M., and Keir, R. (1984). Observational conditioning of snake fear in rhesus monkeys. *Journal of Abnormal Psychology*, **93**, 355–372.

Natterson-Horowitz, B. (2019). Tinbergean approach to clinical medicine. In J. Schulkin and M. Power (eds.), *Integrating Evolutionary Biology into Medical Education: For Maternal and Child Healthcare Students, Clinicians, and Scientists*. Oxford: Oxford University Press, pp. 187–197.

Nesse, R. M. (1984). An evolutionary perspective on psychiatry. *Comprehensive Psychiatry*, **25**, 575–580.

Nesse, R. M. (1990). Evolutionary explanations of emotions. *Human Nature*, **1**, 261–289.

Nesse, R. M. (2005a). Maladaptation and natural selection. *Quarterly Review of Biology*, **80**, 62–70.

Nesse, R. M. (2005b). Natural selection and the regulation of defenses. *Evolution and Human Behavior*, **26**, 88–105.

Nesse, R. M. (2007). Runaway social selection for displays of partner value and altruism. *Biological Theory*, **2**, 143–155.

Nesse, R. M. (2013). Tinbergen's four questions, organized: a response to Bateson and Laland. *Trends in Ecology & Evolution*, **28**, 681–682.

Nesse, R. M. (2020). Tacit Creationism in Emotions Research. *Emotion Researcher, ISRE's Sourcebook for Research on Emotion and Affect*. Retrieved from http://emotionresearcher.com/tacit-creationism-in-emotion-research

Nesse, R. M., and Ellsworth, P. C. (2009). Evolution, emotions, and emotional disorders. *American Psychologist*, **64**, 129–139.

Nesse, R. M., and Schulkin, J. (2019). An evolutionary medicine perspective on pain and its disorders. *Philosophical Transactions of the Royal Society B: Biological Sciences*, **374**, 20190288.

Nesse, R. M., and Williams, G. C. (1994). *Why We Get Sick: The New Science of Darwinian Medicine*. New York: Vintage Books.

Nesse, R. M., Bhatnagar, S., and Ellis, B. (2016). Evolutionary origins and functions of the stress response system. In G. Fink (ed.), *Stress: Concepts, Cognition, Emotion, and Behavior*. Amsterdam: Elsevier, pp. 95–101.

Ohman, A., Carlsson, K., Lundqvist, D., and Ingvar, M. (2007). On the unconscious subcortical origin of human fear. *Physiology & Behavior*, **92**, 180–185.

Pfaff, D., Tabansky, I., and Haubensak, W. (2019). Tinbergen's challenge for the neuroscience of behavior. *Proceedings of the National Academy of Sciences*, **116**, 9704–9710.

Plutchik, R. (1970). Emotions, evolution, and adaptive processes. In M. Arnold (ed.), *Feelings and Emotions*. Amsterdam: Elsevier, pp. 3–24.

Poulton, R., and Menzies, R. G. (2002). Non-associative fear acquisition: a review of the evidence from retrospective and longitudinal research. *Behaviour Research and Therapy*, **40**, 127–149.

Poulton, R., Davies, S., Menzies, R. G., Langley, J. D., and Silva, P. A. (1998). Evidence for a non-associative model of the acquisition of a fear of heights. *Behavioural Research and Therapy*, **36**, 537–44.

Robbins, T. W., Vaghi, M. M., and Banca, P. (2019). Obsessive-compulsive disorder: puzzles and prospects. *Neuron*, **102**, 27–47.

Sapolsky, R. M. (2000). Stress hormones: good and bad. *Neurobiology of Disease*, **7**, 540–542.

Seligman, M. E. (1971). Phobias and preparedness. *Behavior Therapy*, **2**, 307–320.

Selye, H. (1936). A syndrome produced by diverse nocuous agents. *Nature*, **148**, 84–85.

Silove, D. M., Marnane, C. L., Wagner, R., Manicavasagar, V. L., and Rees, S. (2010). The prevalence and correlates of adult separation anxiety disorder in an anxiety clinic. *BMC Psychiatry*, **10**, 21.

Simpson, J. A. (1999). Attachment theory in modern evolutionary perspective. In J. Cassidy, P. R. Shaver, J. Cassidy, and P. R. Shaver, eds., *Handbook of Attachment: Theory, Research, and Clinical Applications*. New York: Guildford Press, pp. 115–140.

Stein, D. J. (2002). Obsessive-compulsive disorder. *Lancet*, **360**, 397–405.

Stein, D. J. (2013). What is a mental disorder? A perspective from cognitive-affective science. *Canadian Journal of Psychiatry*, **58**, 656–662.

Stein, D. J. (2017). Evolutionary psychiatry and body dysmorphic disorder. In K. A. Phillips (ed.), *Body Dysmorphic Disorder: Advances in Research and Clinical Practice*. Oxford:

Oxford University Press, pp. 243–252.

Stein, D. J., and Vythilingum, B. (2007). Social anxiety disorder: psychobiological and evolutionary underpinnings. *CNS Spectrums*, **12**, 806–809.

Stein, D. J., Lim, C. C. W., Roest, A. M., … WHO World Mental Health Survey Collaborators (2017). The cross-national epidemiology of social anxiety disorder: data from the World Mental Health Survey Initiative. *BMC Medicine*, **15**, 143.

Tagkopoulos, I., Liu, Y.-C., and Tavazoie, S. (2008). Predictive behavior within microbial genetic networks. *Science*, **320**, 1313–1317.

Taylor, M. J., Martin, J., Lu, Y., … Lichtenstein, P. (2019). Association of genetic risk factors for psychiatric disorders and traits of these disorders in a Swedish population twin sample. *JAMA Psychiatry*, **76**, 280–289.

Tinbergen, N. (1963). On the aims and methods of ethology. *Zeitschrift Für Tierpsychologie*, **20**, 410–463.

Tiokhin, L. (2016). Do symptoms of illness serve signaling functions? (Hint: yes). *Quarterly Review of Biology*, **91**, 177–195.

Tone, E. B., Nahmias, E., Bakeman, R., … Schroth, E. A. (2019). Social anxiety and social behavior: a test of predictions from an evolutionary model. *Clinical Psychological Science*, **7**, 110–126.

Tooby, J., and Cosmides, L. (2000). Evolutionary psychology and the emotions. In M. Lewis and J. Haviland-Jones (eds.), *Handbook of Emotions*, 2nd ed. New York: Guilford Press, pp. 91–115.

Trimmer, P. C., Higginson, A. D., Fawcett, T. W., McNamara, J. M., and Houston, A. I. (2015). Adaptive learning can result in a failure to profit from good

conditions: implications for understanding depression. *Evolution, Medicine, and Public Health*, **2015**, 123–135.

Troisi, A. (2020). Childhood trauma, attachment patterns, and psychopathology: an evolutionary analysis. In G. Spalletta, D. Janiri, F. Piras, and G. Sani (eds.), *Childhood Trauma in Mental Disorders: A Comprehensive Approach*. Cham: Springer International Publishing, pp. 125–142.

Veale, D., and Gilbert, P. (2014). Body dysmorphic disorder: the functional and evolutionary context in phenomenology and a compassionate mind. *Journal of Obsessive-Compulsive and Related Disorders*, **3**, 150–160.

Wakefield, J. C. (1992). The concept of mental disorder: on the boundary between biological facts and social values. *American Psychologist*, **47**, 373–388.

Wakefield, J. C. (2020). Addiction from the harmful dysfunction perspective: how there can be a mental disorder in a normal brain. *Behavioural Brain Research*, **389**, 112665.

Wenegrat, B. (1995). *Illness and Power*. New York: New York University Press.

West-Eberhard, M. J. (1975). The evolution of social behavior by kin selection. *Quarterly Review of Biology*, **50**, 1–33.

Westneat, D. F. (2012). Evolution in response to social selection: the importance of interactive effects of traits on fitness. *Evolution*, **66**, 890–895.

Williams, A. C. de C. (2016). What can evolutionary theory tell us about chronic pain? *Pain*, **157**, 788–790.

Williams, G. C., and Nesse, R. M. (1991). The dawn of Darwinian medicine. *Quarterly Review of Biology*, **66**, 1–22.

Wittchen, H.-U., and Hoyer, J. (2001). Generalized anxiety disorder: nature and course. *Journal of Clinical Psychiatry*, **62**, 15–21.

Yehuda, R., Hoge, C. W., McFarlane, A. C., ... Hyman, S. E. (2015). Post-traumatic stress disorder. *Nature Reviews Disease Primers*, **1**, 1–22.

Young, E. A., Abelson, J. L., Curtis, G. C., and Nesse, R. M. (1997). Childhood adversity and vulnerability to mood and anxiety disorders. *Depression*, **5**, 66–72.

Zefferman, M. R., and Mathew, S. (2020). An evolutionary theory of moral injury with insight from Turkana warriors. *Evolution and Human Behavior*, 41, 341–353.

Evolutionary Perspectives on Depression

8

Markus J. Rantala and Severi Luoto

Abstract

We propose that major depressive disorder is not a unitary disease. Instead, different triggering factors causing periods of low mood can give rise to different and sometimes even opposite symptom patterns. Some of the symptoms of depression are maladaptive; others may be psychobehavioural adaptions to solve the adaptive problem that triggered the depressive episode. It is therefore logical to subtype depressive episodes according to their triggering factors. In evolutionary psychiatry, depressive episodes can be classified into discrete subtypes that are induced by infection, long-term stress, loneliness, traumatic experience, hierarchy conflict, grief, romantic relationship dissolution, post-partum events, season, chemicals, somatic diseases and starvation. In hunter-gatherers and in people who have traditional lifestyles, periods of low mood only rarely turn into episodes that fulfil the diagnostic criteria of major depressive disorder. Modern lifestyles cause low-grade inflammation and an increased susceptibility to chronic stress, which introduce symptoms of sickness behaviour into reactive short-term mood changes. Therefore, features of contemporary environments may prevent the normalisation of mood after adverse life events, resulting in major depressive disorder. An evolutionary approach to depression helps to identify the factors in our environments and lifestyles that contribute to greater susceptibility to this debilitating disorder, which can inform both prevention and treatment of depression. We further propose that the treatment of major depressive disorder should be tailored according to the patient's depression subtype, focusing on the root causes of the disorder rather than alleviating symptoms with drugs.

Keywords

chronic stress, evolutionary psychiatry, evolutionary psychology, gut microbiota, major depressive disorder, MDD, mismatch hypothesis, mood change, neuroinflammation, stress responsivity

Key Points

- We classify depression into 12 subtypes.
- Different adverse life events lead to different patterns of symptoms, suggesting that different subtypes of depression arise based on the triggering factors.
- Major depressive disorder is a disease caused by features of the contemporary Western lifestyle: social isolation, limited physical activity, chronic stress and unhealthy food.
- Major depressive disorder is associated with neuroinflammation.

8.1 Introduction

Major depressive disorder (MDD) is the most prevalent psychiatric disorder. With recent developments in evolutionary psychiatry, multiple evolutionary explanations have been proposed to explain the evolutionary origins of MDD and the possible adaptive functions of its symptoms (e.g., Andrews and Thomson, 2009; Badcock et al., 2017; Nesse, 2019; Nettle, 2004). However, none of the explanations have received full acceptance nor provided improvements in the efficacy of treatments. For example, 30–60% of patients with MDD are not responsive to available pharmacotherapeutic interventions, the remission rate is often below 50% and the recurrence rate is more than 85% within 10 years of a depressive episode (Sim et al., 2016).

In our view, the main reason why previous evolutionary explanations have failed to provide good explanations for MDD and why pharmacological treatments have had such low efficacy is because MDD is not a single disorder (Rantala et al., 2018). Another reason why it is difficult to provide convincing evolutionary explanations for the symptoms of depression by studying the behaviour of depressed people is that because the environment has changed from the environment in which our psychobehavioural adaptations evolved, previously adaptive behaviours might have become maladaptive (see Chapter 1). If we want to understand the evolutionary functions of depression symptoms, we should understand what were their functions in ancestral humans in ancestral environments, which constitute the main selective landscapes underlying the psychobehavioural predispositions that characterise contemporary humans.

In this chapter, we argue that MDD is a disease of modern lifestyles. We also provide evolutionary explanations for each symptom that is used in the diagnostic criteria of MDD. Finally, we propose a subtyping of depressive episodes according to the proximate factors that triggered the mood changes and their possible ultimate (i.e. evolutionary) functions.

8.1.1 MDD as a Disease of Modern Lifestyle

The prevalence of MDD varies greatly between countries. For example, a World Health Organization survey found that the lifetime prevalence of MDD varies from 19.2% observed in the USA to 3.3% observed in Romania (Merikangas et al., 2011). The prevalence of MDD has also increased over time. Chinese people born after 1966, for instance, were 22.4 times more likely to suffer from a depressive episode than Chinese people born before 1937 (Lee et al., 2007). A meta-analysis of Minnesota Multiphasic Personality Inventory data of American college (n = 63,706) and high school (n = 13,870) students found that young adults were six to eight times more likely to meet the diagnostic criteria of MDD in 2007 compared to their peers in 1938 (Twenge et al., 2010). A population study in Lundby, Sweden, found that the point prevalence of depression in 1957 was 0.8%, while in 1972 it was 2.6% (Hagnell et al., 1993) and in 2009 it was 10.8% in Sweden overall (Johansson et al., 2013). It has been estimated that the total number of people

living with MDD worldwide increased by 49.86% between 1990 and 2017 (Liu et al., 2020).

Anthropologists who examined hunter-gatherer societies that have lifestyles closer to those of our ancestors have reported that MDD (which fulfils the diagnostic criteria of the Diagnostic and Statistical Manual of Mental Disorders (DSM)) is very rare compared to people who have a modern lifestyle. For example, a study of the Kaluli people of New Guinea found that only 1 in 2000 people interviewed met the criteria for being clinically depressed (Schieffelin, 1986). Similar findings have been reported for the Thai-Lao of Thailand (Keyes, 1986), the Toraja of Indonesia (Hollan and Wellenkamp, 1994, 1996) and the Bushmen of the Kalahari (Thomas, 2006). Cross-cultural analyses have found that the degree of modernisation correlates with higher prevalence of MDD in a dose-dependent manner (Colla et al., 2006).

The best evidence indicating that the prevalence of depression is associated with modern lifestyle comes from the Old Order Amish, who still have a lifestyle resembling that of the eighteenth century. Egeland and Hostetter (1983) studied the prevalence of MDD for five years and found that only 41 out of 8186 adult Amish individuals met the diagnostic criteria, suggesting that the prevalence of MDD is only 0.5% in the Amish. The one-year prevalence of MDD among other Americans is 10.4% (Hasin et al., 2018). Therefore, this difference in the prevalence of major MDD is at least 20-fold. However, this may be an underestimate because among other US citizens the estimate is given as a one-year prevalence, while Egeland and Hostetter (1983) gave the five-year prevalence among the Amish. Naturally, the low prevalence of MDD does not mean that hunter-gatherers or the Old Order Amish do not experience periods of low mood, sadness or grief. However, it seems that in hunter-gatherers or the Old Order Amish such periods just do not transform into episodes of MDD that would fulfil the diagnostic criteria of the DSM-5 or the International Classification of Diseases, 10th revision (ICD-10).

8.1.2 Why Does Modern Lifestyle Increase the Risk of MDD?

One evolutionary psychological explanation for the current 'epidemic' of MDD in developed countries is that our bodies and minds have simply not evolved in line with the Western way of life (Rantala et al., 2018). In modern societies, there are many lifestyle factors that may increase the risk that an episode of low mood or sadness exacerbates into an episode of MDD. We don't exercise enough, we eat too much, we get too much energy from food but too few nutrients, we don't spend enough time in nature, we sleep too little, our community is reduced, large families are rarer and many suffer from loneliness even when surrounded by millions of people in big cities (Hidaka, 2012; see also Chapters 1 and 2 of this volume). In addition, the modern lifestyle has led to reduced diversity in our gut microbiomes (Schnorr et al., 2014). These changes have brought such diseases of modern lifestyle as cardiovascular disease, adult-onset diabetes, osteoporosis, gastrointestinal cancers, autoimmune diseases, allergies and many more diseases that do not exist among peoples with a hunter-gatherer lifestyle (Lindeberg, 2010). Common to these diseases is that they are all associated with low-grade inflammation (Furman et al., 2019).

Low-grade inflammation not only causes diseases of modern lifestyle, but also increases the likelihood of developing MDD. The depressant effect of low-grade inflammation is particularly pronounced in autoimmune diseases in which the amount of proinflammatory cytokines is constantly elevated. For example, up to 70% of people with rheumatoid arthritis develop clinical depression at some point in their lives (Matcham et al., 2013). Many studies and meta-analyses have found that the concentrations of circulating C-reactive protein (a biomarker of inflammation) and proinflammatory cytokines are higher in patients with MDD than in controls (Goldsmith et al., 2016; Osimo et al., 2019). Follow-up studies have suggested that inflammation is a cause rather than simply a consequence of the illness (Khandaker et al., 2014; Zalli et al., 2016).

Experimental evidence supports the hypothesis that proinflammatory cytokines cause mood changes. For example, the typhoid vaccine substantially increases the amount of proinflammatory cytokines in blood and lowers mood as soon as three hours after vaccination (Harrison et al., 2009). Symptoms of depression have also been observed in experiments in which non-depressed patients have been given proinflammatory cytokines against hepatitis C virus (Bonaccorso et al., 2001). In addition, experiments in which healthy subjects have been administered endotoxins produced by *Escherichia coli* have shown an elevated amount of proinflammatory cytokines in the blood and an emergence of depressive symptoms (Eisenberger et al., 2010).

Further support for the hypothesis that low-grade inflammation plays a role in MDD comes from numerous studies and meta-analyses that have found that anti-inflammatory agents alleviate symptoms of depression (Kappelmann et al., 2017; Kohler-Forsberg et al., 2019). Low-grade systemic inflammation causes neuroinflammation (i.e., the inflammatory response of microglial cells), which is a key factor that interacts with the three neurobiological correlates of MDD: dysregulation of the serotonergic system, dysregulation of the hypothalamic–pituitary–adrenal axis and alteration of the continuous production of adult-generated neurons in the dentate gyrus of the hippocampus (Troubat et al., 2021). This neuroinflammatory hypothesis of depression is supported by brain imaging studies that have found signs of neuroinflammation in depressed patients (Holmes et al., 2018; Richards et al., 2018; Setiawan et al., 2015).

It appears that as neuroinflammation affects neurotransmitters that influence mood, especially serotonin (Rantala et al., 2019), neuroinflammation prevents the normalisation of mood after an individual has experienced an adverse life situation, and it may also exacerbate the symptoms of depression (Rantala et al., 2018). In addition, the increase in the amount of proinflammatory cytokines associated with low-grade inflammation may cause the body to begin to respond to it as it does to infection – that is, to produce sickness behaviours that help save energy so that the immune system can defeat the 'infection' (Rantala et al., 2018).

If we want to understand why inflammation increases the risk that normal mood changes turn into MDD, we must first understand, at the ultimate level, why certain symptoms associated with depression exist in the first place.

8.2 The Function of Depression Symptoms

8.2.1 Emotional Pain

Natural selection has equipped us with the ability to sense physical pain so that we do not harm our bodies. It teaches us to avoid doing the painful thing again (Williams, 2016). Pharmacologically reducing pain can be detrimental to an individual's long-term health (Rantala et al., 2017). As with physical pain, the purpose of mental pain is to make an individual avoid future activities that have led to mental pain or decreased mood in the past. Thus, mental pain, like physical pain, can be adaptive.

8.2.2 Rumination

Rumination about events that triggered depression is more common in situations where the same event can be expected to recur (Keller and Nesse, 2006). Continuous rumination about the events that led to depression helps the depressed person to avoid similar situations in the future and to solve related social and psychological problems (Andrews and Thomson, 2009). However, this does not mean that rumination about negative things is adaptive in all situations, and excessive rumination can be detrimental to the person's ability to move on with their life.

8.2.3 Lack of Concentration

Depressed people tend to perform poorly in tests that measure the ability to concentrate. They also often find it difficult to study and work because they do not know how to focus on what they are reading. Difficulty concentrating can manifest as indecision and frustration. Lack of concentration is the result of depressed people thinking about things other than what they should be focusing on (Andrews and Thomson, 2009). The things that constantly come to mind are normally related to the factors that triggered the depressive episode. Lack of concentration is a by-product of rumination about the things that triggered the depression and can thus be adaptive (Watson and Andrews, 2002).

8.2.4 Changes in Weight

Appetite can either increase or decrease depending on which factor has triggered the depressive episode. The most likely explanation for the weight gain associated with depression is related to 'comfort eating'. Many depressed people experience increased cravings, especially for carbohydrate-rich and fatty foods, as eating them stimulates dopamine secretion in the brain's reward system and causes momentary mood rise (Macht and Simons, 2000). In addition, sleep problems, which are often associated with depression, increase appetite and cause weight gain (Magee et al., 2009).

Loss of appetite in depression may result from an increase in the levels of proinflammatory cytokines caused by prolonged stress, infection or low-grade inflammation. Proinflammatory cytokines increase the body's production of leptin (Andreasson et al., 2007). Leptin is a satiety hormone that is released into the blood by adipose tissue. It reduces appetite and hunger. Cytokine-induced loss of appetite may be an adaptation to overcome diseases. Many animals also lose their appetite after becoming ill or injuring themselves (Exton, 1997), which reduces activity and saves energy. The reduction in appetite and fasting can enhance the functioning of the immune system in a number of ways (Wilhelm et al., 2021).

8.2.5 Anhedonia

Anhedonia refers to the inability to feel pleasure. Feelings of pleasure and joy are adaptations produced by natural selection: they motivate individuals to behave in ways that helped our ancestors pass on their genes to future generations (Barron et al., 2010). Depressed people typically lose interest in doing things that used to produce joy and pleasure, such as partaking in hobbies, attending social events or having sex. A person's appetite may decrease when eating no longer causes the same pleasure as before. Experimental studies in humans and many other animals have shown that injecting proinflammatory cytokines causes anhedonia (Rantala et al., 2018). The anhedonia caused by an infection is adaptive as it reduces activity and so conserves energy for the immune system. Anhedonia caused by neuroinflammation rather than infection, however, is often maladaptive (Rantala et al., 2018).

8.2.6 Sleep Problems

The presentation of sleep problems may differ depending on the triggering factor of MDD. A depressed person might have problems falling asleep, waking up at night, suffering from early-morning wakening or sleeping too much. An increased need for sleep may occur in the types of depression where saving energy has been beneficial. For example, after losing or failing to achieve an important goal in a hierarchy conflict, it is sometimes better to sleep and save energy for a new attempt. In addition, the increased need for sleep in a disease state caused by an infection helps save energy. Winter depression is character-ised by an increased need for sleep, which seems to be a maladaptive by-product of the reduced amount of light and low-grade inflammation that cause disruption to the circadian clock (Rantala et al., 2018).

A stressed person has lighter sleep, wakes up often and may wake up to the slightest sound. When sleeping, a person is at their most vulnerable and is unable to defend themselves. A stressed person's amygdala is overactive, raising stress hor-mone levels and alerting the body to danger. This is reflected in the quality of sleep. In contemporary developed societies, sources of sound at night are mostly harmless, but in our evolutionary history this was not always the case, and nocturnal sounds could have come from an approaching predator or a hostile person, making it beneficial for a stressed person to have light sleep.

Rumination about the things that triggered the depression causes insomnia because it keeps the mind overactive and makes it difficult to fall asleep (Watson and Andrews, 2002). For example, after a relationship ends, a person may ruminate at night about the reasons why the relationship went wrong and what should have been done differently. In these cases, the brain prioritises rumination over sleep.

8.2.7 Exhaustion

In the context of infection, exhaustion helps to conserve the body's energy resources for use by the immune system. High proinflammatory cyto-kine levels resulting from peripheral low-grade inflammation or neuroinflammation may cause exhaustion because the brain responds to them in a similar way as to an infection. Exhaustion may also result from chronic fatigue arising from the sleep problems caused by stress or rumin-ation, and as such it is maladaptive (Rantala et al., 2018).

8.2.8 Psychomotor Agitation or Slowness

Some depressed people also experience psycho-motor agitation or retardation. Agitation refers to anxiety accompanied by severe restlessness. It can manifest as inadvertent movements, walking back and forth, wringing of hands, constantly putting on and taking off clothes or other similar activities. In the context of depression, psycho-motor restlessness often appears to be a by-product of the associated anxiety, having no adap-tive function (Rantala et al., 2018), and it is often a side effect of antipsychotics (Gillies et al., 2013).

Psychomotor retardation manifests as a slowing down of thoughts and movements. This may be a by-product of sleep problems and/or a person concentrating their cognitive resources on rumination about the matters that led to the depression. Psychomotor retardation is one symptom of sickness behaviour, but it can also be the pathological consequence of peripheral low-grade inflammation and/or neuroinflamma-tion (Rantala et al., 2018)

8.2.9 Pessimism

Pessimism leads to a gloomy and negative world view. Studies show that people are normally over-optimistic about future prospects and their own abilities, and failures and depression dissolve this delusion of optimism. Pessimism reduces the pur-suit of achievements in situations where failure is likely. It is adaptive in situations where past fail-ures predict future ones (Rantala et al., 2018).

8.2.10 Excessive Guilt

An individual may feel guilty about the event(s) that triggered their depression. Feelings of guilt make one reflect upon how their actions led to that outcome and thus help minimise the likeli-hood of the same thing happening again. The greater the role played by one's own actions in the situations that led to the event that triggered the depression, the greater the sense of guilt (Keller and Nesse, 2006).

8.2.11 Loss of Self-Confidence

Because self-confidence regulates progress in social hierarchies, the loss of self-esteem that occurs as a result of a hierarchy conflict prevents one from challenging those higher in the social hierarchy and thus protects one from new prob-lems. Traditionally, psychologists have thought that good self-esteem leads to success. However, research suggests that good self-esteem is the result rather than the cause of success in a social hierarchy (Baumeister et al., 2003). Successes enhance self-esteem and failures lower it.

8.2.12 Recurrent Thoughts of Death

Thoughts of death and suicide are common in depressed people. Although suicide sounds like an eminently maladaptive solution, suicide may have increased inclusive fitness in our ancestors as a result of kin selection (see Chapter 1). Suicide can help pass on an individual's genes to the next generation in a situation where that individual is a burden to their close relatives and their own reproductive potential is weak. By taking their own life, an individual may contribute to the reproductive success of their close relatives and thus to the proliferation of their own genes. In such a case, that individual's close relatives would have one mouth less to feed and no sick individual to look after (Decatanzaro, 1986). Indeed, several studies have shown that suicidal thoughts and suicides are more common in those who have poor chances of reproduction and who feel they are merely a burden to their loved ones (Rantala et al., 2018; see also Chapter 9 of this volume for an alternative perspective on suicide).

In experimental studies in humans, it has been found that simply injecting proinflammatory cytokines into the bloodstream causes suicidal thoughts in some healthy subjects (Capuron et al., 2002). It is highly likely that the increase in the levels of proinflammatory cytokines associated with clinical depression as well as bipolar disorder produces maladaptive suicidal ideation. The brain seems to respond in the same way to acute infection and neuroinflammation. Indeed, the intensity of low-grade inflammation is directly related to suicidal ideation (O'Donovan et al., 2013; Holmes et al., 2018).

The threat of suicide is also an effective way to get attention and help from close relatives and community members who benefit from the existence of the individual (e.g., a former spouse if the couple has children together). For a threat to be credible, a person must be serious about it, as a result of which some people may end up killing themselves (Rantala et al., 2018).

8.3 Subtypes of Depression

A peculiar aspect of MDD is that two people diagnosed with this disorder may have completely opposite patterns of symptoms. For example, a person with depression can gain or lose weight, as well as suffer from excessive sleepiness, insomnia or poor sleep quality. Speech and movement, in turn, can slow down or speed up. Different depressive episodes may have different symptom profiles even for the same person. Evolutionary psychologists think that the symptoms of depression have evolved to solve the adaptive problem(s) that caused the depressive episode and that different adverse life events may lead to different patterns of depressive symptoms (Keller and Nesse, 2005; Keller et al., 2007). It is probable that different adverse life events trigger different psychological adaptations that were crafted by natural selection as responses to the adaptive problems in question. Thus, from an evolutionary psychological viewpoint, it is logical to subtype depression episodes according to the triggering factor(s). We therefore present a classification of depressive episodes into 12 subtypes based on the proximate mechanisms and ultimate functions that trigger the mood change that leads to the depression (Rantala et al., 2018) (Figure 8.1).

8.3.1 Infection-Induced Depression

Owing to selective pressures caused by parasites and pathogens, natural selection has equipped us with an immune system and many other adaptations to combat parasites and pathogens (Schmid-Hempel, 2011), including the behavioural immune system (Schaller and Park, 2011). One of these adaptations is sickness behaviour, which includes somatic, cognitive and behavioural changes that help individuals overcome infection by conserving metabolic resources for the use of the immune system, thus avoiding further infections (Anders et al., 2013). Symptoms of sickness behaviour include anorexia, psychomotor retardation, sleep disturbances, anergia, anhedonia, weakness, malaise, listlessness, hyperalgesia and impaired concentration (Dantzer, 2001). All of these symptoms seem to be adaptations against infection, helping the immune system function more effectively (Anders et al., 2013). If the infection is contagious, the social withdrawal caused by sickness behaviour may reduce the likelihood that an individual will infect their kin – a behavioural feature that increases an individual's inclusive fitness (cf. Gardner and West, 2014). Social withdrawal caused by anhedonia, fatigue, hypersomnia and psychomotor retardation reduces

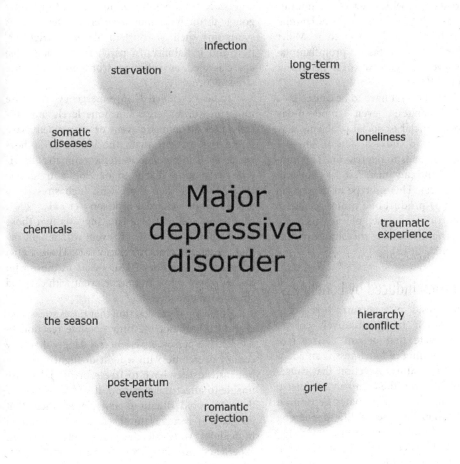

starvation

infection

long-term
stress

somatic
diseases

loneliness

Major
depressive
disorder

chemicals

traumatic
experience

the season

hierarchy
conflict

post-partum
events

grief

romantic
rejection

Figure 8.1 Subtypes of depression based on evolutionary psychiatry (Rantala et al., 2018)

mobility and helps to conserve energy for immune defence (Anders et al., 2013). It is important to note that, in contemporary humans, the elevated low-grade inflammation in the body that is caused by an unhealthy lifestyle can lead to similar psychopathological consequences as infections do.

8.3.2 Depression Induced by Long-Term Stress

Short-term stress can be beneficial due to its performance-boosting effect, but if it becomes chronic it may cause numerous health problems, including depression (Yang et al., 2015). In our evolutionary history, stress was statistically associated with a higher probability of being wounded, and thus some parts of our immune system are designed to become upregulated as a response to stress while some parts become

downregulated (Slavich and Irwin, 2014). Chronic stress causes endocrine and immune system dysfunctions that contribute to sustained low-grade inflammation, causing neuroinflammation, which influences neurotransmitter levels and mood (Berk et al., 2013). The symptoms of depression induced by chronic stress include reduced mood, fatigue, self-blame, appetite problems, concentration problems, suicidal ideation, sleep problems, psychomotor problems and anhedonia. Psychomotor problems (289%) and interest loss (217%) showed the largest increases and suicidal ideation (146%) and sleep problems (52%) showed the smallest increases with stress, suggesting that stress affects depressive symptoms differentially (Fried et al., 2015).

Prolonged stress is also known to upregulate the immune system by causing the gut to leak non-pathogenic commensal microbes into the peripheral circulation, which activates immune defence and causes an increase in proinflammatory cytokines in the blood (reviewed in Miller and Raison, 2016). This increase in proinflammatory cytokine levels triggers sickness behaviour and may lead to MDD.

Chronic stress does not have to be caused by a life-threatening danger; even modern-day working life or financial or social problems may be stressful enough to cause a state of chronic stress response that leads to depression. This subtype of depression can manifest as burnout (Bianchi et al., 2021). This subtype of depression is a maladaptive by-product of a prolonged stress response, occurring because of a mismatch between the current and the ancestral environment (Rantala et al., 2018).

8.3.3 Depression Induced by Loneliness

Loneliness is the result of a person's social contacts not qualitatively or quantitatively corresponding to the state that person desires (see Chapter 13). The feeling of loneliness is an adaptation produced by natural selection that causes an individual to seek out the company of others.

Humans are highly social primates. Separation from a social group has been a life-threatening danger in our evolutionary environment, as surviving alone at the mercy of nature has been difficult and often impossible. An evolutionarily salient facet of loneliness is that it is impossible to reproduce alone. As a consequence, a person unknowingly perceives loneliness as a threat, which is reflected in the activation of the amygdala and increased stress hormone levels. If the stress reaction caused by loneliness persists for a long time, it causes neuroinflammation, which leads to MDD, and this does not help a person to seek the company of others (Rantala et al., 2018).

8.3.4 Depression Induced by Traumatic Events

Most people experience some traumatic events in their lifetime. For some, the traumatic memories of the event come back as flashbacks or nightmares and cause anxiety and fear. Such people may begin to avoid objects, places and people that remind them of the traumatic event. They may also begin to isolate themselves from other people

and suffer from emotional numbness. Constantly going through traumatic events often causes symptoms such as constant alertness, frightfulness and irritability. In psychiatry, such people are classified as suffering from post-traumatic stress disorder (PTSD).

Studies conducted in emergency response units measuring stress hormone levels immediately after a traumatic event or an accident have found that patients with the lowest stress hormone levels immediately after a traumatic experience were more likely to develop a traumatic stress disorder than those with high stress hormone levels (Aardal-Eriksson et al., 2001; Mouthaan et al., 2014). This suggests that those who respond to a traumatic event with a fight-or-flight reaction do not develop PTSD. The essential question is: why does PTSD occur in those who do not respond to a traumatic event with elevated stress hormone levels?

A fight-or-flight reaction that raises stress hormone levels is not the only possible reaction to danger. If a person experiences a danger that they cannot overcome with a fight-or-flight response but instead they have to freeze or are otherwise unable to affect the situation, it will be better for them to avoid situations and places where that danger may recur. Natural selection has favoured individuals who effectively remember such an experience and thus avoid being in similar situations again. Thus, PTSD appears to be an evolved adaptation to avoid situations that have traumatic qualia associated with them (Rantala et al., 2018).

In people with contemporary Western lifestyle (s), PTSD is often associated with symptoms of depression. For example, a large meta-analysis composed of 57 studies reported a MDD comorbidity rate of 52% among both military personnel and civilians suffering from PTSD (Rytwinski et al., 2013). Although PTSD is associated with hypocortisolism (Bicanic et al., 2013), PTSD patients have elevated concentrations of proinflammatory cytokines (Gill et al., 2009), which explains why PTSD often takes on features of sickness behaviour and leads to depression. It seems that contemporary Western lifestyles and low-grade inflammation change previously adaptive PTSD into a non-adaptive state of MDD by incorporating symptoms of sickness behaviour with PTSD, probably aggravating PTSD symptoms (Rantala et al., 2018). This hypothesis is supported by a study on Turkana warriors from Kenya, which found that in Turkana warriors traumatic events led to fewer PTSD symptoms associated with depression than in Western soldiers (Zefferman and Mathew, 2021). The important point to note is that Turkana warriors practice nomadic pastorialism, a lifestyle that is very different from that of contemporary Western people. In contrast to people with contemporary Western lifestyles, Turkana warriors have excellent cardiometabolic health (Lea et al., 2020), suggesting that they do not suffer from low-grade inflammation. This hypothesis is also supported by findings showing that smoking, obesity and low physical activity increase the risk of chronic PTSD (Buckley et al., 2004; Olff et al., 2006), while micronutrient intake may decrease it (Rucklidge et al., 2012). Thus, although PTSD per se seems to be an adaptation caused by natural selection to avoid the cause of the trauma, it seems that the depression triggered by PTSD is a pathological consequence caused by modern Western lifestyles (Rantala et al., 2018).

8.3.5 Depression Induced by Hierarchy Conflict

In many social species, defeat in a hierarchy conflict causes depressive-like behaviour and physical responses that are similar to those seen in depressed humans (Rygula et al., 2005; Shively et al., 1997). In a defeated person, depression works as a sign of forfeit and as an honest signal that the defeated individual is no longer a threat to the winner. This submissive status may prevent the defeated person's expulsion from the group. Decreased self-esteem prevents the defeated individual from re-challenging the winner, thus helping the individual to conserve their bioenergetic resources (and possibly save their lives) in a situation where winning is unlikely. While clear physical hierarchy conflicts are rare in contemporary societies, conflicts still occur in the form of bullying at school or the workplace and may lead to this type of depression (Rantala et al., 2018).

In this subtype, a person does not react to conflict in the social hierarchy with a fight-or-flight response; instead, they give up. This subtype is therefore characterised by adrenocortical hyporesponsiveness and hypocortisolism, which indicate a downregulated stress response. This has been demonstrated in mice, where social defeat leads to elevated stress hormone levels in most individuals, but a subset give up and become depressed after repeated social defeats and show adrenocortical hyporesponsiveness and hypocortisolism (Bowens et al., 2012). Although depression induced by hierarchy conflict is an adaptation, this does not mean that it is always adaptive in contemporary societies; instead, it is possible that low-grade inflammation may change this into a maladaptive state of MDD (Rantala et al., 2018).

8.3.6 Depression Induced by Grief

Animals generally grieve after the death of their pups, parents or reproductive partners. They may also mourn the death of a member of their social group with whom they have spent a lot of time. The grief triggered by the loss of loved ones does not appear to be an adaptation produced by natural selection as it does not appear to increase an individual's fitness in any way – at least not in non-social species. Depression caused by loss is more likely to be a by-product of the ability to form long-term attachment relationships. Grief is the price we have to pay when the attachment relationship is finally broken. This assumption is supported by the fact that a person may also experience symptoms of depression as a result of the death of their beloved dog, horse or other pet. The stronger the attachment, the longer the symptoms of depression last. On the other hand, the knowledge of the pain caused by the loss of an important person or pet makes us take more care of the people or pets that are important to us (Rantala et al., 2018).

In humans, losing a partner causes a sharp increase in stress hormone levels (Buckley et al., 2012). The increase in stress hormone levels and the resulting increase in proinflammatory cytokines in the blood may explain why grief can lead to MDD. A study on individuals whose spouses had recently passed away found that those with the highest levels of proinflammatory cytokines in their blood (suggesting severe low-grade inflammation) had the strongest symptoms of grief and the highest probability that grief and low mood would turn into MDD (Fagundes et al., 2019). This suggests that contemporary Western lifestyles and the resulting increase in chronic stress and low-grade inflammation increase the likelihood that normal grief and the associated decline in mood will turn into MDD (Luoto et al., 2018).

8.3.7 Depression Induced by Romantic Relationship Dissolution

A brain imaging study on recently dumped individuals found that they showed the same areas of activity as are activated in people with cocaine withdrawal symptoms (Fisher et al., 2010). Because romantic love is a form of addiction where love causes dopamine bursts in the brain, its withdrawal symptoms are also similar to those of drug addiction (Bode and Kushnick, 2021). Although some of the symptoms associated with romantic relationship dissolution may be withdrawal symptoms, some of the other symptoms seem to be adaptations caused by natural selection. For example, ruminating on the cause of the relationship dissolution can help an individual to avoid repeating the same mistakes in future relationships (Andrews and Thomson, 2009). On the other hand, decreased self-esteem causes a person to lower the aspirations they have for potential mates to better correspond with their own market value. Depression can also serve as a signal for the abandoner that the relationship was important to the abandoned person. It may arouse so much empathy in the abandoner that they return to the relationship (Rantala et al., 2018). It is possible that unhealthy factors inherent in Western lifestyles or traumatic childhood experiences that are known to be associated with increased stress responsiveness may contribute to the chronic stress caused by romantic relationship dissolution, leading to MDD in the most vulnerable individuals (Rantala et al., 2018). Inflammation also plays a role in relationship problems: troubled marriages are linked with heightened inflammation, and hostile marital behaviour increases inflammation in couples (Kiecolt-Glaser, 2018).

8.3.8 Post-partum Depression

Post-partum depression occurs in 10–15% of women in the six months following childbirth (Brummelte and Galea, 2010). In addition to regular depressive symptoms, mothers who suffer from post-partum depression typically feel a loss of interest in their baby and may even develop harmful intentions towards them. Other symptoms include crying, suicidal ideation, bouts of anger and hopelessness (Brummelte and Galea, 2016).

Post-partum depression is linked to the mother feeling that she is receiving inadequate support from the father or from kin. This can lead to the feeling that she cannot cope with her parental duties (Myers and Emmott, 2021). In our evolutionary past, it would have been catastrophic for a lone mother to be left to care for a child on her own. If a woman continued investing in a child whose survival was unlikely, she would have had fewer offspring than a woman who ceased her investment and postponed reproduction. As a healthier child has a higher likelihood of survival, it is not surprising that poor health in the child predicts post-partum depression in the mother (Rantala et al., 2018).

It appears that the primary function of post-partum depression is not deserting the child. Rather, post-partum depression may function as a signal to kin and the spouse that the mother needs more support. It seems that post-partum depression is an adaptation that might not be adaptive in all cases due to the environmental mismatch between our evolutionary environment and modern conditions (Rantala et al., 2018).

8.3.9 Season-Related Depressions
8.3.9.1 Winter Depression

In temperate and northern latitudes, winter depression is the most common seasonal affective disorder (SAD). In winter depression, symptoms often begin in autumn and abate in spring and summer, during which mild hypomania may occur. In SAD, symptoms typically intensify in the afternoon. Features of SAD include general fatigue, decreased libido, increased need to sleep and increased appetite, especially for carbohydrates and starchy foods (Rantala et al., 2018).

It appears that winter depression is a maladaptive by-product of the failure of a person's circadian rhythm to match the reduced daytime length (Rantala et al., 2018). Since inflammation and chronic stress may disrupt the circadian rhythm (Mavroudis et al., 2013), it seems that Western lifestyles may increase the risk of winter depression (Rantala et al., 2018). This hypothesis is supported by the finding that winter depression is much lower among the Old Order Amish than in other populations in the same latitudes, despite the lack of electric lighting in the Old Order Amish (Raheja et al., 2013).

8.3.9.2 Spring Depression

In contrast to winter depression, some individuals feel more depressed during spring and early summer. They sleep less and wake up earlier, and their mood is worst in the morning; they also have a decreased appetite and lose weight (Boyce and Parker, 1988). In a temperate climate, the prevalence of suicides peaks in spring/early summer, and the suicide rate is lowest during the period of winter depression (Reutfors et al., 2009). The possible proximate mechanisms underlying spring depression are allergenic reactions to pollen that increase low-grade inflammation and the increase of sunlight in spring that elevates the brain's serotonin levels to an excessive degree, exacerbating depressive and anxious symptoms in individuals who have an upregulated serotonergic system due to chronic stress (Rantala et al., 2018). Thus, spring depression seems to be a maladaptive by-product of seasonal changes in the amount of daylight and/or allergens.

8.3.10 Chemically Induced Depression

Depression may be caused by substance abuse or it can be a side effect of medication (American Psychiatric Association, 2013). Over 40% of alcoholics meet the criteria for MDD, and as many as 70% of these are classified as substance-induced depression in DSM-5 (Schuckit, 2006). Unlike in many other subtypes of depression, alcoholics suffering from depression are not depressed all day, every day (Schuckit, 2006). They therefore may not fulfil the DSM-5 criteria for MDD. Unlike with other depression subtypes, the symptoms of substance-induced depression decrease or disappear with abstinence (Schuckit, 2006), making it easier to identify this subtype. In addition to changing neurotransmitter functioning, one way in which alcohol may bring about depression is by causing the leak of non-pathogenic commensal bacteria from the gut into the peripheral circulation, which triggers the production of proinflammatory cytokines and leads to the symptoms of sickness behaviour (Rantala et al., 2018).

Depressed individuals often self-medicate their low mood and anxiety with alcohol and other drugs – even if alcohol per se did not induce the depressive episode. Substance use typically does not help to address the adaptive problem that led to the original mood change, although alcohol and other drugs may temporarily improve mood and reduce anxiety. Substance use can instead have hazardous long-term consequences for mental health (Leeies et al., 2010). Consuming alcohol may alter the previously adaptive mood change to a maladaptive state of MDD as it increases the production of the proinflammatory cytokines that cause the symptoms of sickness behaviour (Rantala et al., 2018).

8.3.11 Depression Induced by Somatic Diseases

Many somatic diseases are commonly comorbid with MDD. For example, neurological conditions like Alzheimer's disease, Parkinson's disease, migraine, epilepsy, stroke and traumatic brain injury, as well as several neuroendocrine conditions such as Cushing's disease and hypothyroidism, are associated with an increased risk of MDD (Bulloch et al., 2015; Kim et al., 2015). A particularly salient example is multiple sclerosis – an inflammatory, demyelinating disease of the central nervous system – in which the lifetime prevalence of depression may exceed 50% (Beal et al., 2007).

MDD is commonly comorbid with cancer. The risk of MDD is 5.4 times higher in cancer patients than in the general population (Hartung et al., 2017). There are three main reasons why cancer may induce depression: (1) receiving a cancer diagnosis may lead to a state of chronic stress and anxiety that can trigger MDD; (2) chemotherapy, radiotherapy and surgery can result in depression induced by sickness behaviour; and (3) cancer itself can raise proinflammatory cytokine levels, triggering sickness behaviour. There is substantial evidence for all of these causes (Rantala et al., 2018). In many cases, depression induced by somatic diseases appears to be a maladaptive state as it impairs recovery from illness and increases mortality (Pinquart and Duberstein, 2010).

8.3.12 Starvation-Induced Depression

Starvation-induced depression can be seen as a psychological adaptation that helps an individual overcome famine. During starvation, the body begins to save energy by reducing its investment in bodily functions and behaviours that are not necessary for immediate survival, like growth, immune function and reproduction. At the beginning of starvation, physical activity increases, leading to a higher probability of finding food (Exner et al., 2000). However, prolonged starvation leads to apathy and social withdrawal in order to save energy. Starvation lowers mood, causes irritation and anhedonia, diminishes sexual interest and reduces the ability to concentrate on tasks that require major cognitive processing because the starved individual is obsessed with finding food (Keys, 1950).

8.4 Problems with the Current Diagnostic Criteria of Depression

The current way of diagnosing MDD based on the number and duration of symptoms is problematic when viewed from an evolutionary psychological perspective. The current distinction between a person with MDD and a healthy person is based on the *number* of symptoms and as such is completely arbitrary. In addition, the current diagnostic criteria automatically assume that all symptoms of depression are bad for the patient and should be eliminated. Whether depression causes harm to an individual's normal life does not in itself, from the perspective of evolutionary psychiatry, justify classifying depression as a disorder that should be pharmacologically treated. For example, fever caused by the flu is harmful to everyday life, although it is a naturally produced adaptation that helps an individual overcome the disease and as such is beneficial (Williams and Nesse, 1991). From an evolutionary psychological perspective, a reactive short-term mood change turns into a maladaptive period of depression that requires intervention when a patient's symptoms no longer serve the purpose for which natural selection has shaped them or when the symptoms are more intense than those that would serve the adaptive function (Rantala et al., 2018).

It is an even more complicated situation when a person experiences many different negative life events, triggering more than one subtype of depression, as a result of which the future combination of symptoms may no longer be a helpful response to any factor that led to the decline in mood. The symptoms can become too severe as a result of several different negative events, chronic stress or the low-grade inflammation caused by the novel conditions of contemporary Western lifestyles; therefore, they no longer serve their adaptive purpose. In such cases, the symptoms may produce a condition that can be classified as pathological depression (Luoto et al., 2018).

8.5 Conclusions

The prevailing artificial classification of MDD should be radically reviewed and efforts should be made to assess on an individual basis whether a state of depression is a reactive response to an adverse life event or a consequence of neuroinflammation (Erjavec et al., 2021; Luoto et al., 2018; Rantala et al., 2018; Troubat et al., 2021). In order to provide the best treatment, efforts should also be made to assess whether the state of depression has become maladaptive. On the other hand, it is worth remembering that even if a certain behavioural response to adversity has been adaptive in our evolutionary environment (s), it may be maladaptive in contemporary life (also see Chapters 1, 2 and 5).

In diagnosing a patient's depression, it is essential to consider: what is the adaptive benefit, if any, of the patient's depressive symptoms in the patient's life context? If the symptoms help to solve the adaptive problem that triggered the depressive episode, pharmacologically treating the symptoms may not be beneficial for the patient. From the point of view of evolutionary psychiatry, a more effective approach might be to counsel the patient on how to overcome the adaptive problem and to encourage lifestyle changes so that the reactive depression does not turn into a maladaptive depression (Luoto et al., 2018; Rantala et al., 2018).

Since stress and low-grade inflammation may cause neuroinflammation and symptoms of sickness behaviour and since they may increase the adaptive symptoms of reactive short-term mood change to maladaptive levels, it is also important to alleviate stress and low-grade inflammation. Thus, we propose that rather than trying to alleviate all of the symptoms of depression simply with drugs, the treatment of depression should also be based on various forms of psychotherapy and lifestyle interventions that are targeted at alleviating the stress, inflammation and other proximate mechanisms behind depression (Luoto et al., 2018).

References

Aardal-Eriksson, E., Eriksson, T. E., Thorell, L. H., 2001. Salivary cortisol, posttraumatic stress symptoms, and general health in the acute phase and during 9-month follow-up. *Biological Psychiatry* 50, 986–993.

American Psychiatric Association, 2013. *Diagnostic and Statistical Manual of Mental Disorders: DSM-5.* American Psychiatric Publishing, Washington, DC.

Anders, S., Tanaka, M., Kinney, D. K., 2013. Depression as an evolutionary strategy for defense against infection. *Brain, Behavior, and Immunity* 31, 9–22.

Andreasson, A., Arborelius, L., Erlanson-Albertsson, C., Lekander, M., 2007. A putative role for cytokines in the impaired appetite in depression. *Brain, Behavior, and Immunity* 21, 147–152.

Andrews, P. W., Thomson, J. A., Jr, 2009. The bright side of being blue: depression as an adaptation for analyzing complex problems. *Psychological Review* 116, 620–654.

Badcock, P., Davey, C., Whittle, S., Allen, N., Friston, K., 2017. The depressed brain: an evolutionary system theory. *Trends in Cognitive Science* 21, 182–194.

Barron, A. B., Sovik, E., Cornish, J. L., 2010. The roles of dopamine and related compounds in reward-seeking behavior across animal phyla. *Frontiers in Behavioral Neuroscience* 4, 163.

Baumeister, R. F., Campbell, J. D., Krueger, J. I., Vohs, K. D., 2003. Does high self-esteem cause better performance, interpersonal success, happiness, or healthier lifestyles? *Psychological Science* 4, 1–44.

Beal, C. C., Stuifbergen, A. K., Brown, A., 2007. Depression in multiple sclerosis: a longitudinal analysis. *Archives of Psychiatric Nursing* 21, 181–191.

Berk, M., Williams, L. J., Jacka, F. N., O'Neil, A., Pasco, J. A., Moylan, S., Allen, N. B., Stuart, A. L., Hayley, A. C., Byrne, M. L., Maes, M., 2013. So depression is an inflammatory disease, but where does the inflammation come from? *BMC Medicine* 11, 200.

Bianchi, R., Verkuilen, J., Schonfeld, I. S., Hakanen, J. J., Jansson-Frojmark, M., Manzano-Garcia, G., Laurent, E., Meier, L. L., 2021. Is burnout a depressive condition? A 14-sample meta-analytic and bifactor analytic study. *Clinical Psychological Science* 9, 579–597.

Bicanic, I. A. E., Postma, R. M., Sinnema, G., De Roos, C., Olff, M., Van Wesel, F., Van de Putte, E. M., 2013. Salivary cortisol and dehydroepiandrosterone sulfate in adolescent rape victims with post traumatic stress disorder. *Psychoneuroendocrinology* 38, 408–415.

Bode, A., Kushnick, G., 2021. Proximate and ultimate perspectives on romantic love. *Frontiers in Psychology* 12, 573123.

Bonaccorso, S., Puzella, A., Marino, V., Pasquini, M., Biondi, M., Artini, M., Almerighi, C., Levrero, M., Egyed, B., Bosmans, E., Meltzer, H. Y., Maes, M., 2001. Immunotherapy with interferon-alpha in patients affected by chronic hepatitis C induces an intercorrelated stimulation of the cytokine network and an increase in depressive and anxiety symptoms. *Psychiatry Research* 105, 45–55.

Bowens, N., Heydendael, W., Bhatnagar, S., Jacobson, L., 2012. Lack of elevations in glucocorticoids correlates with dysphoria-like behavior after repeated social defeat. *Physiology & Behavior* 105, 958–965.

Boyce, P., Parker, G., 1988. Seasonal affective-disorder in the southern-hemisphere. *American Journal of Psychiatry* 145, 96–99.

Brummelte, S., Galea, L. A. M., 2010. Depression during pregnancy and postpartum: contribution of stress and ovarian hormones. *Progress in Neuro-Psychopharmacology & Biological Psychiatry* 34, 766–776.

Brummelte, S., Galea, L. A. M., 2016. Postpartum depression: etiology, treatment and consequences for maternal care. *Hormones and Behavior* 77, 153–166.

Buckley, T. C., Mozley, S. L., Bedard, M. A., Dewulf, A. C., Greif, J., 2004. Preventive health behaviors, health-risk behaviors, physical morbidity, and health-related role functioning impairment in veterans with post-traumatic stress disorder. *Military Medicine* 169, 536–540.

Buckley, T. C., Sunari, D., Marshall, A., Bartrop, R., McKinley, S., Tofler, G., 2012. Physiological correlates of bereavement and the impact of bereavement interventions. *Dialogues in Clinical Neuroscience* 14, 129–139.

Bulloch, A. G. M., Fiest, K. M., Williams, J. V. A., Lavorato, D. H., Berzins, S. A., Jette, N., Pringsheim, T. M., Patten, S. B., 2015. Depression – a common disorder across a broad spectrum of neurological conditions: a cross-sectional nationally representative survey. *General Hospital Psychiatry* 37, 507–512.

Capuron, L., Gumnick, J. F., Musselman, D. L., Lawson, D. H., Reemsnyder, A., Nemeroff, C. B., Miller, A. H., 2002. Neurobehavioral effects of interferon-alpha in cancer patients: phenomenology and paroxetine responsiveness of symptom dimensions. *Neuropsychopharmacology* 26, 643–652.

Colla, J., Buka, S., Harrington, D., Murphy, J. M., 2006. Depression and modernization: a cross-cultural study of women. *Social Psychiatry and Psychiatric Epidemiology* 41, 271–279.

Dantzer, R., 2001. Cytokine-induced sickness behavior: mechanisms and implications. *Annals of the New York Academy of Sciences* 933, 222–234.

Decatanzaro, D., 1986. A mathematical-model of evolutionary pressures regulating self-preservation and self-destruction. *Suicide and Life-Threatening Behavior* 16, 166–181.

Egeland, J. A., Hostetter, A. M., 1983. Amish Study, I: affective disorders among the Amish, 1976–1980. *American Journal of Psychiatry* 140, 56–61.

Eisenberger, N. I., Inagaki, T. K., Mashal, N. M., Irvin, M. R., 2010. Inflammation and social experience: an inflammatory challenge induces feelings of social disconnection in addition to depressed mood. *Brain, Behavior, and Immunity* 24, 558–563.

Erjavec, G. N., Sagud, M., Perkovic, M. N., Strac, D. S., Konjevod, M., Tudor, L., Uzun, S., Pivac, N., 2021. Depression: biological markers and treatment. *Progress in Neuro-Psychopharmacology & Biological Psychiatry* 105, 110139.

Exner, C., Hebebrand, J., Remschmidt, H., Wewetzer, C., Ziegler, A., Herpertz, S., Schweiger, U., Blum, W. F., Preibisch, G., Heldmaier, G., Klingenspor, M., 2000. Leptin suppresses semi-starvation induced hyperactivity in rats: implications for anorexia nervosa. *Molecular Psychiatry* 5, 476–481.

Exton, M. S., 1997. Infection-induced anorexia: active host defence strategy. *Appetite* 29, 369–383.

Fagundes, C., Brown, R., Chen, M., Murdock, K., Saucedo, L., LeRoy, A., Wu, E., Garcini, L., Shanane, A., Baameur, F., Heijnen, C., 2019. Grief, depressive symptoms, and inflammation in the spousally bereaved.

Psychoneuroendocrinology 100, 190–197.

Fisher, H. E., Brown, L. L., Aron, A., Strong, G., Mashek, D., 2010. Reward, addiction, and emotion regulation systems associated with rejection in love. *Journal of Neurophysiology* 104, 51–60.

Fried, E. I., Nesse, R. M., Guille, C., Sen, S., 2015. The differential influence of life stress on individual symptoms of depression. *Acta Psychiatrica Scandinavica* 131, 465–471.

Furman, D., Campisi, J., Verdin, E., Carrera-Bastos, P., Targ, S., Franceschi, C., Ferrucci, L., Gilroy, D. W., Fasano, A., Miller, G. W., Miller, A. H., Mantovani, A., Weyand, C. M., Barzilai, N., Goronzy, J. J., Rando, T. A., Effros, R. B., Lucia, A., Kleinstreuer, N., Slavich, G. M., 2019. Chronic inflammation in the etiology of disease across the life span. *Nature Medicine* 25, 1822–1832.

Gardner, A., West, S. A., 2014. Inclusive fitness: 50 years on. *Philosophical Transactions of the Royal Society B: Biological Sciences* 369, 20130356.

Gill, J. M., Saligan, L., Woods, S., Page, G., 2009. PTSD is associated with an excess of inflammatory immune activities. *Perspectives in Psychiatric Care* 45, 262–277.

Gillies, D., Sampson, S., Beck, A., Rathbone, J., 2013. Benzodiazepines for psychosis-induced aggression or agitation. *Cochrane Database of Systematic Reviews* 12, CD003079.

Goldsmith, D. R., Rapaport, M. H., Miller, B. J., 2016. A meta-analysis of blood cytokine network alterations in psychiatric patients: comparisons between schizophrenia, bipolar disorder and depression. *Molecular Psychiatry* 21, 1696–1709.

Hagnell, O., Ojesjo, L., Otterbeck, L., Rorsman, B., 1993. Prevalence of mental disorders, personality traits and mental complaints in

the Lundby Study. A point prevalence study of the 1957 Lundby cohort of 2,612 inhabitants of a geographically defined area who were re-examined in 1972 regardless of domicile. *Scandinavian Journal of Social Medicine* 50, 1–75.

Harrison, N. A., Brydon, L., Walker, C., Gray, M. A., Steptoe, A., Critchley, H. D., 2009. Inflammation causes mood changes through alterations in subgenual cingulate activity and mesolimbic connectivity. *Biological Psychiatry* 66, 407–414.

Hartung, T. J., Brahler, E., Faller, H., Harter, M., Hinz, A., Johansen, C., Keller, M., Koch, U., Schulz, H., Weis, J., Mehnert, A., 2017. The risk of being depressed is significantly higher in cancer patients than in the general population: prevalence and severity of depressive symptoms across major cancer types. *European Journal of Cancer* 72, 46–53.

Hasin, D. S., Sarvet, A. L., Meyers, J. L., Saha, T. D., Ruan, W. J., Stohl, M., Grant, B. F., 2018. Epidemiology of adult DSM-5 major depressive disorder and its specifiers in the United States. *JAMA Psychiatry* 75, 336–346.

Hidaka, B. H., 2012. Depression as a disease of modernity: explanations for increasing prevalence. *Journal of Affective Disorders* 140, 205–214.

Hollan, D. W., Wellenkamp, J. C., 1994. *Contentment and Suffering: Culture and Experience in Toraja.* Columbia University Press, New York.

Hollan, D. W., Wellenkamp, J. C., 1996. *The Thread of Life: Toraja Reflections on the Life Cycle.* University of Hawaii Press, Honolulu, HI.

Holmes, S. E., Hinz, R., Conen, S., Gregory, C. J., Matthews, J. C., Anton-Rodriguez, J. M., Gerhard, A., Talbot, P. S., 2018. Elevated translocator protein in anterior cingulate in major depression and a role for inflammation in suicidal thinking: a positron emission tomography study. *Biological Psychiatry* 83, 61–69.

Johansson, R., Carlbring, P., Heedman, A., Paxling, B., Andersson, G., 2013. Depression, anxiety and their comorbidity in the Swedish general population: point prevalence and the effect on health-related quality of life. *PeerJ* 1, e98.

Kappelmann, N., Lewis, G., Dantzer, R., Jones, P., Khandaker, G., 2017. Antidepressant activity of anti-cytokine treatment: a systematic review and meta-analysis of clinical trials of chronic inflammatory conditions. *Molecular Psychiatry* 23, 335–343.

Keller, M. C., Nesse, R. M., 2005. Is low mood an adaptation? Evidence for subtypes with symptoms that match precipitants. *Journal of Affective Disorders* 86, 27–35.

Keller, M. C., Nesse, R. M., 2006. The evolutionary significance of depressive symptoms: different adverse situations lead to different depressive symptom patterns. *Journal of Personality and Social Psychology* 91, 316–330.

Keller, M. C., Neale, M. C., Kendler, K. S., 2007. Association of different adverse life events with distinct patterns of depressive symptoms. *American Journal of Psychiatry* 164, 1521–1529.

Keyes, C., 1986. The interpretive basis of depression. In: A. Kleinman, B. J. Good (eds.), *Culture and Depression: Studies in the Anthropology and Cross-Cultural Psychiatry of Affect and Disorder*. University of California Press, pp. 153–174.

Keys, A., 1950. *The Biology of Human Starvation*. University of Minnesota Press, Minneapolis, MN.

Khandaker, G. M., Pearson, R. M., Zammit, S., Lewis, G., Jones, P. B., 2014. Association of serum interleukin 6 and C-reactive protein in childhood with depression and psychosis in young adult life: a population-based longitudinal study. *JAMA Psychiatry* 71, 1121–1128.

Kiecolt-Glaser, J. K., 2018. Marriage, divorce, and the immune system. *American Psychologist* 73, 1098–1108.

Kim, E. Y., Kim, S. H., Rhee, S. J., Huh, L., Ha, K., Kim, J., Chang, J. S., Yoon, D. H., Park, T., Ahn, Y. M., 2015. Relationship between thyroid-stimulating hormone levels and risk of depression among the general population with normal free T4 levels. *Psychoneuroendocrinology* 58, 114–119.

Kohler-Forsberg, O., Lydholm, C. N., Hjorthoj, C., Nordentoft, M., Mors, O., Benros, M.E., 2019. Efficacy of anti-inflammatory treatment on major depressive disorder or depressive symptoms: meta-analysis of clinical trials. *Acta Psychiatrica Scandinavica* 139, 404–419.

Lea, A. J., Martins, D., Kamau, J., Gurven, M., Ayroles, J. F., 2020. Urbanization and market integration have strong, nonlinear effects on cardiometabolic health in the Turkana. *Science Advances* 6, eabb1430.

Lee, S., Tsang, A., Zhang, M. Y., Huang, Y. Q., He, Y. L., Liu, Z. R., Shen, Y. C., Kessler, R. C., 2007. Lifetime prevalence and inter-cohort variation in DSM-IV disorders in metropolitan China. *Psychological Medicine* 37, 61–71.

Leeies, M., Pagura, J., Sareen, J., Bolton, J. M., 2010. The use of alcohol and drugs to self-medicate symptoms of posttraumatic stress disorder. *Depression and Anxiety* 27, 731–736.

Lindeberg, S., 2010. *Food and Western Disease: Health and Nutrition from an Evolutionary Perspective*. Wiley-Blackwell, Oxford.

Liu, Q. Q., He, H. R., Yang, J., Feng, X. J., Zhao, F. F., Lyu, J., 2020.

Changes in the global burden of depression from 1990 to 2017: findings from the Global Burden of Disease study. *Journal of Psychiatric Research* 126, 134–140.

Luoto, S., Karlsson, H., Krams, I., Rantala, M., 2018. Depression subtyping based on evolutionary psychiatry: from reactive short-term mood change to depression. *Brain, Behavior, and Immunity* 69, 630.

Macht, M., Simons, G., 2000. Emotions and eating in everyday life. *Appetite* 35, 65–71.

Magee, C. A., Huang, X. F., Iverson, D. C., Caputi, P., 2009. Acute sleep restriction alters neuroendocrine hormones and appetite in healthy male adults. *Sleep and Biological Rhythms* 7, 125–127.

Matcham, F., Rayner, L., Steer, S., Hotopf, M., 2013. The prevalence of depression in rheumatoid arthritis: a systematic review and meta-analysis. *Rheumatology* 52, 2136–2148.

Mavroudis, P. D., Scheff, J. D., Calvano, S. E., Androulakis, I. P., 2013. Systems biology of circadian-immune interactions. *Journal of Innate Immunity* 5, 153–162.

Merikangas, K. R., Jin, R., He, J.-P., Kessler, R. C., Lee, S., Sampson, N. A., Viana, M. C., Andrade, L. H., Hu, C., Karam, E. G., Ladea, M., Medina-Mora, M. E., Ono, Y., Posada-Villa, J., Sagar, R., Wells, J. E., Zarkov, Z., 2011. Prevalence and correlates of bipolar spectrum disorder in the World Mental Health Survey Initiative. *Archives of General Psychiatry* 68, 241–251.

Miller, A. H., Raison, C. L., 2016. The role of inflammation in depression: from evolutionary imperative to modern treatment target. *Nature Reviews Immunology* 16, 22–34.

Mouthaan, J., Sijbrandij, M., Luitse, J. S. K., Goslings, J. C., Gersons, B. P. R., Olff, M., 2014. The role of acute cortisol and DHEAS in predicting acute and chronic

PTSD symptoms. *Psychoneuroendocrinology* 45, 179–186.

Myers, S., Emmott, E., 2021. Communication across maternal social networks during the UK's national lockdown and its association with postnatal depressive symptoms. *Frontiers in Psychology* 12, 648002.

Nesse, R. M., 2019. *Good Reasons for Bad Feelings.* Allen Lane, London.

Nettle, D., 2004. Evolutionary origins of depression: a review and reformulation. *Journal of Affective Disorders* 81, 91–102.

O'Donovan, A., Rush, G., Hoatam, G., Hughes, B. M., McCrohan, A., Kelleher, C., O'Farrelly, C., Malone, K. M., 2013. Suicidal ideation is associated with elevated inflammation in patients with major depressive disorder. *Depression and Anxiety* 30, 307–314.

Olff, M., Meewisse, M. L., Kleber, R. J., van der Velden, P. G., Drogendijk, A. N., van Amsterdam, J. G. C., Opperhuizen, A., Gersons, B. P. R., 2006. Tobacco usage interacts with postdisaster psychopathology on circadian salivary cortisol. *International Journal of Psychophysiology* 59, 251–258.

Osimo, E. F., Baxter, L. J., Lewis, G., Jones, P. B., Khandaker, G. M., 2019. Prevalence of low-grade inflammation in depression: a systematic review and meta-analysis of CRP levels. *Psychological Medicine* 49, 1958–1970.

Pinquart, M., Duberstein, P. R., 2010. Depression and cancer mortality: a meta-analysis. *Psychological Medicine* 40, 1797–1810.

Raheja, U. K., Stephens, S. H., Mitchell, B. D., Rohan, K. J., Vaswani, D., Balis, T. G., Nijjar, G. V., Sleemi, A., Pollin, T. I., Ryan, K., Reeves, G. M., Weitzel, N., Morrissey, M., Yousufi, H., Langenberg, P., Shuldiner, A. R., Postolache, T. T., 2013. Seasonality of mood and behavior in the Old Order Amish. *Journal of Affective Disorders* 147, 112–117.

Rantala, M. J., Luoto, S., Krama, T., Krams, I., 2019. Eating disorders: an evolutionary psychoneuroimmunological approach. *Frontiers in Psychology* 10, 2200.

Rantala, M. J., Luoto, S., Krams, I., 2017. An evolutionary approach to clinical pharmacopsychology. *Psychotherapy and Psychosomatics* 86, 370–371.

Rantala, M. J., Luoto, S., Krams, I., Karlsson, H., 2018. Depression subtyping based on evolutionary psychiatry: proximate mechanisms and ultimate functions. *Brain, Behaviour, and Immunity* 69, 603–617.

Reutfors, J., Osby, U., Ekbom, A., Nordstrom, P., Jokinen, J., Papadopoulos, F. C., 2009. Seasonality of suicide in Sweden: relationship with psychiatric disorder. *Journal of Affective Disorders* 119, 59–65.

Richards, E. M., Zanotti-Fregonara, P., Fujita, M., Newman, L., Farmer, C., Ballard, E. D., Machado-Vieira, R., Yuan, P. X., Niciu, M. J., Lyoo, C. H., Henter, I. D., Salvadore, G., Drevets, W. C., Kolb, H., Innis, R. B., Zarate, C. A., 2018. PET radioligand binding to translocator protein (TSPO) is increased in unmedicated depressed subjects. *EJNMMI Research* 8, 57.

Rucklidge, J. J., Andridge, R., Gorman, B., Blampied, N., Gordon, H., Boggis, A., 2012. Shaken but unstirred? Effects of micronutrients on stress and trauma after an earthquake: RCT evidence comparing formulas and doses. *Human Psychopharmacology – Clinical and Experimental* 27, 440–454.

Rygula, R., Abumaria, N., Flugge, G., Fuchs, E., Ruther, E., Havemann-Reinecke, U., 2005. Anhedonia and motivational deficits in rats: impact of chronic social stress. *Behavioural Brain Research* 162, 127–134.

Rytwinski, N. K., Scur, M. D., Feeny, N. C., Youngstrom, E. A., 2013. The co-occurrence of major depressive disorder among individuals with posttraumatic stress disorder: a meta-analysis. *Journal of Traumatic Stress* 26, 299–309.

Schaller, M., Park, J. H., 2011. The behavioral immune system (and why it matters). *Current Directions in Psychological Science* 20, 99–103.

Schieffelin, E., 1986. The cultural analysis of depressive affect: an example from New Guinea. In: A. M. Kleinman, B. Good (eds.), *Culture and Depression: Studies in the Anthropology and Cross-Cultural Psychiatry of Affect and Disorder.* University of California Press, pp. 101–133.

Schmid-Hempel, P., 2011. *Evolutionary Parasitology: The Integrated Study of Infections, Immunology, Ecology, and Genetics.* Oxford University Press, Oxford.

Schnorr, S. L., Candela, M., Rampelli, S., Centanni, M., Consolandi, C., Basaglia, G., Turroni, S., Biagi, E., Peano, C., Severgnini, M., Fiori, J., Gotti, R., De Bellis, G., Luiselli, D., Brigidi, P., Mabulla, A., Marlowe, F., Henry, A. G., Crittenden, A. N., 2014. Gut microbiome of the Hadza hunter-gatherers. *Nature Communications* 5, 3654.

Schuckit, M. A., 2006. Comorbidity between substance use disorders and psychiatric conditions. *Addiction* 101, 76–88.

Setiawan, E., Wilson, A. A., Mizrahi, R., Rusjan, P. M., Miler, L., Rajkowska, G., Suridjan, I., Kennedy, J. L., Rekkas, V., Houle, S., Meyer, J. H., 2015. Role of translocator protein density, a marker of neuroinflammation, in the brain during major depressive episodes. *JAMA Psychiatry* 72, 268–275.

Shively, C. A., LaberLaird, K., Anton, R. F., 1997. Behavior and physiology of social stress and depression in female cynomolgus monkeys. *Biological Psychiatry* 41, 871–882.

Sim, K., Lau, W. K., Sim, J., Sum, M. Y., Baldessarini, R. J., 2016. Prevention of relapse and recurrence in adults with major depressive disorder: systematic review and meta-analyses of controlled trials. *International Journal of Neuropsychopharmacology* 19, pyv076.

Slavich, G. M., Irwin, M. R., 2014. From stress to inflammation and major depressive disorder: a social signal transduction theory of depression. *Psychological Bulletin* 140, 774–815.

Thomas, E., 2006. *The Old Way: A Story of the First People.* Farrar, Straus and Giroux, New York.

Troubat, R., Barone, P., Leman, S., Desmidt, T., Cressant, A., Atanasova, B., Brizard, B., El Hage, W., Surget, A., Belzung, C., Camus, V., 2021. Neuroinflammation and depression: a review. *European Journal of Neuroscience* 53, 151–171.

Twenge, J. M., Gentile, B., DeWall, C. N., Ma, D., Lacefield, K., Schurtz, D. R., 2010. Birth cohort increases in psychopathology among young Americans, 1938–2007: a cross-temporal meta-analysis of the MMPI. *Clinical Psychology Review* 30, 145–154.

Watson, P. J., Andrews, P. W., 2002. Toward a revised evolutionary adaptationist analysis of depression: the social navigation hypothesis. *Journal of Affective Disorders* 72, 1–14.

Wilhelm, C., Jayagopi Surendar, J., Karagiannis, F., 2021. Enemy or ally? Fasting as an essential regulator of immune responses. *Trends in Immunology* 42, 389–400.

Williams, A. C. D., 2016. What can evolutionary theory tell us about chronic pain? *Pain* 157, 788–790.

Williams, G. C., Nesse, R. M., 1991. The dawn of Darwinian medicine. *Quarterly Review of Biology* 66, 1–22.

Yang, L. F., Zhao, Y. H., Wang, Y. C., Liu, L., Zhang, X. Y., Li, B. J., Cui, R. J., 2015. The effects of psychological stress on depression. *Current Neuropharmacology* 13, 494–504.

Zalli, A., Jovanova, O., Hoogendijk, W. J. G., Tiemeier, H., Carvalho, L. A., 2016. Low-grade inflammation predicts persistence of depressive symptoms. *Psychopharmacology* 233, 1669–1678.

Zefferman, M., Mathew, S., 2021. Combat stress in a small-scale society suggests divergent evolutionary roots for posttraumatic stress disorder symptoms. *Proceedings of the National Academy of Sciences* 118, e2020430118.

On the Randomness of Suicide
An Evolutionary, Clinical Call to Transcend Suicide Risk Assessment

C. A. Soper, Pablo Malo Ocejo and Matthew M. Large

Abstract

Converging theoretical and empirical evidence points to suicide being a fundamentally aleatory event – that risk of suicide is opaque to useful assessment at the level of the individual. This chapter presents an integrated evolutionary and clinical argument that the time has come to transcend efforts to categorise peoples' risk of taking their own lives. A brighter future awaits mental healthcare if the behaviour's essential non-predictability is understood and accepted. The pain-brain evolutionary theory of suicide predicts *inter alia* that all intellectually competent humans carry the potential for suicide, and that suicides will occur largely at random. The randomness arises because, over an evolutionary timescale, selection of adaptive defences will have sought out and exploited all operative correlates of suicide and will thus have exhausted those correlates' predictive power. Completed suicides are therefore statistical residuals – events intrinsically devoid of informational cues by which the organism could have avoided self-destruction. Empirical evidence supports this theoretical expectation. Suicide resists useful prediction at the level of the individual. Regardless of the means by which the assessment is made, people rated 'high risk' seldom take their own lives, even over extended periods. Consequently, if a prevention treatment is sufficiently safe and effective to be worth allotting to the 'high-risk' subset of a cohort of patients, it will be just as worthwhile for the rest. Prevention measures will offer the greatest prospects for success where the aleatory nature of suicide is accepted, acknowledging that 'fault' for rare, near-random, self-induced death resides not within the individual but as a universal human potentiality. A realistic, evolution-informed, clinical approach is proposed that focuses on *risk communication* in place of risk assessment. All normally sapient humans carry a vanishingly small daily risk of taking their own lives but are very well adapted to avoiding that outcome. Almost all of us nearly always find other solutions to the stresses of living.

Keywords

evolution, pain-brain, positive psychology, risk assessment, suicide

Key Points

- The pain-brain model of suicide offers the greatest explanatory power of the theories in the current evolutionary literature. It proposes that, notwithstanding population-level patterns, suicide will occur essentially at random among normal adolescent and adult individuals.
- Individual suicide risk cannot be usefully gauged by any known method. Suicide is probably not amenable to prediction even in principle.

- Treatment decisions decided purely on the basis of a risk assessment (safety plans, psychopharmacology, hospital admission, etc.) can be presumed to be misdirected. Individuals judged to be 'at risk' are probably in no greater danger of taking their own lives than are other vulnerable service users. All patients need suitable care and compassion with current situations managed accordingly.
- Someone troubled by suicidal thoughts needs to be listened to, empathically and

without judgement. They can be reassured that while all normally intelligent adolescents and adults are at some risk, suicide is an extremely unlikely outcome despite such thoughts.

- A review of a person's strengths, goals and psychological resources may be useful. Patients may benefit from the advice that they have inherited psychological defences that enabled their ancestors successfully to handle life's challenges.

Workers in mental health are often expected to take a view on whether a patient is a danger to themselves (APA, 2003; Graney et al., 2020; NICE, 2011; WHO, 2014). For psychiatrists, suicide risk assessment has become a routine activity, a professional responsibility and a core competency requirement (Rudd and Roberts, 2019; Silverman and Berman, 2014). However, as this chapter will explain, multiple lines of evidence are now pointing to the impotence of risk assessment in suicide prevention, and indeed to its potential harms. Both theory and epidemiology indicate that suicide – the act of deliberately killing oneself (WHO, 2014) – is a fundamentally random event. While patterns can be seen at the group level, virtually every intellectually competent human being carries a small risk of wilful self-destruction. This risk cannot, even in principle, be usefully assessed at the level of the individual.

We first set out the theoretical evidence of suicide's aleatoriness, drawing on Soper's (2018, 2021) pain-and-brain (henceforth 'pain-brain') evolutionary model, and then we show how the empirical evidence supports this theoretical position. In view of strong clinical benefits that would be expected to arise from accepting suicide's randomness, we recommend an alternative strategy for helping patients in distress – one that focuses on *risk communication*, transcending risk assessment.

9.1 Evolutionary Theory Points to Suicide's Randomness

The pain-brain theory holds that suicide evolved as a noxious by-product of two primary adaptations that, when combined, would logically result in deliberate self-killing. They come together in our species and ours alone (Soper, 2018, 2021).

The first, pain, is an ancient self-protective signal that enables animals to navigate fitness hazards in their external and internal environments. The aversiveness of pain is designed precisely to induce action to end or escape it. The second suicidogenic adaptation is the exceptional intellect of the mature human brain, which is able to obey the imperative to escape pain, effectively but maladaptively, by terminating its own consciousness. These dual 'pain' and 'brain' conditions – motivation and means, respectively – are not only necessary for deliberate self-killing but sufficient. Any animal aware that it could relieve its suffering by ending its own life would be expected to seize the opportunity. By this light, suicide can be understood as the default human response to intolerable distress.

Pain-brain is not the only evolutionary model of suicide: alternatives have been advanced by Syme and Hagen (2018; Syme et al., 2016), deCatanzaro (1981) and others (see reviews in Bering, 2018; Gunn, 2017). However, it arguably offers the greatest explanatory power, predicting diverse patterns in suicidality, psychopathology and other psychological phenomena that are otherwise, as a set, unaccounted for (Gunn et al., 2021; Lester, 2019b; Soper, 2022).

9.1.1 Suicide Is an Adaptive Problem

The pain-brain evolutionary analysis suggests that suicide has existed as an ambient survival hazard from a time, deep in human prehistory, when a population of ancestral humans encephalised to the extent of being able to grasp the idea of their own personal mortality. A developmental counterpart of that ancient phylogenetic Rubicon can be seen being crossed today in the age pattern of suicide's first onset. Virtually non-existent in early childhood, suicidality emerges suddenly in adolescence and remains endemic thereafter (Borges et al., 2012). Potential for suicidal behaviour arrives during normal cognitive maturation, alongside heightened self-awareness and executive functions (Cuddy-Casey and Orvaschel, 1997; Shaffer and Fisher, 1981; Soper, 2018). The existence of a threshold of intellectual competence parsimoniously explains not only young children's immunity and suicide's ontogenesis, but also the absence of suicide among non-human animals (Preti, 2011) and the rarity of completed suicides among human adults with severe intellectual disability (Baechler, 1975/1979; Tromans et al., 2020).

By a process of random mutation with selective retention, suicide, as a recurring fitness threat, drove the evolution of special-purpose anti-suicide adaptations. Indeed, so extreme is the threat that the task of avoiding suicide has likely posed a superordinate biological challenge for our species. Many important features have been hypothesised to contribute to our success in colonising and dominating the planet: bipedalism, tool-making, theory of mind, language, culture and so on. But as Soper (2019a, 2021) points out, none of these assets will have much of an impact on reproductive success if a hominid so endowed, on reaching reproductive age, kills itself. For these other attributes to shape human evolution, special-purpose adaptations had, in our ancestral past, to manage the fitness cost of suicidality.

9.1.2 Evolved Defences against Suicide: 'Fenders' and 'Keepers'

Figure 9.1 shows conceptually how these cost-managing adaptations are thought to work. At the top of the diagram, suicide's 'pain' and 'brain' precursors combine to generate very many potential suicidal trajectories, marked by a dense mass of dots. Virtually all of these are filtered out by successive lines of anti-suicide defences, arranged below, so that only very few instantiate as suicidal acts, marked by scattered dots near the bottom of Figure 9.1.

Blocking the way are, first, front-line defences, labelled *fenders*. These take two forms, pain-type and brain-type, respectively addressing suicide's 'pain' and 'brain' evolutionary authors. Various *pain-type fenders* seek to neutralise the motivation for suicide by limiting the experiencing of emotional distress. They manifest in diverse, uniquely human phenomena of positive psychology (Hirsch et al., 2018). Affective well-being is managed homeostatically, so that we are kept fairly happy most of the time and are able to deal with shocks without too much disruption. This warmer-than-neutral state is maintained by two levers: on one side, the negative impact of bad news is suppressed by psychodynamic defences and other forms of self-serving self-deception, while on the other side, recreational behaviours are promoted, for no adaptive

purpose other than to induce pleasure. The whole affect-managing system is coordinated by an optimistic worldview, often involving religious or spiritual belief.

A separate set of encultured *brain-type fenders* denies access to the intellectual means of suicide, seeking to put the idea of self-killing beyond cognitive reach. By propagating an anti-suicide taboo, fear of what may come in an afterlife, and stigmatising punishments for loved ones left behind, brain-type fenders make suicide feel awkward to think or talk about, doubtfully effective as way to escape pain, and self-evidently wrong.

Towards the bottom of Figure 9.1 is an array of last-line defences, labelled *keepers*. These are emergency measures. They activate among post-pubescents at times of chronic and intense distress, aiming to stop suicidal ideas from escalating into actions. As with fenders, keepers also instantiate in pain-type and brain-type forms. *Pain-type keepers* make suicide unnecessary; they numb, divert or otherwise attenuate the power of emotional pain to motivate suicide, but at a cost of disrupting motivational systems generally. *Brain-type keepers* meanwhile downgrade intellectual functions sufficiently to make suicide difficult to organise, but at a cost of making any other equivalently complex task difficult too.

Keepers are thought to manifest in a variety of symptoms of common mental disorders, including addictions, non-suicidal self-harm and major depression, (Soper, 2018, 2021). This idea may feel counterintuitive, but it is not new or outlandish; it was advanced decades ago from within mainstream psychiatry. Himmelhoch (1988), in the *Journal of Clinical Psychiatry*, argued that diverse psychopathologies may demonstrate evolved anti-suicide defences in action. Hundert (1992), of Harvard Medical School, similarly proposed that psychotic delusions may perform an evolved anti-suicide function. Although not usually discussed in evolutionary terms, some depressive symptoms are thought to suppress the motivation to act on suicidal thoughts (Hendin, 1975; Rogers et al., 2018), to the extent that psychiatrists have long been trained to beware of patients' risk intensifying when depression starts to lift (Meehl, 1973). More detailed discussions of hypothesised evolved anti-suicide machinery can be found elsewhere (Gunn et al., 2021; Humphrey, 2018; Soper, 2018, 2021).

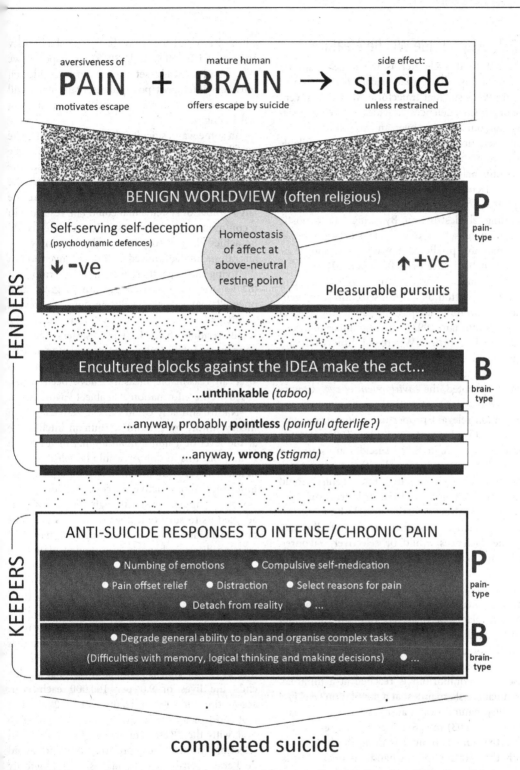

Figure 9.1 Schematic of evolved anti-suicide defences. See text for commentary (adapted from Soper (2018), with permission)

9.1.3 Why Suicide Will Be Aleatory

Relevant to this chapter is the largely random nature of any filtrate that reaches the bottom of Figure 9.1 – suicidal trajectories that circumvent the organism's defences. Suicides will be intrinsically random because, over an evolutionary time-scale, selection will have sought out all available cues from the organism's internal and external environment that usefully presage this fatal outcome.[1] Detectable correlates will have been fully exploited for the purpose of pre-empting and avoiding self-destruction. By acting on prognostic information, selection will have exhausted that information's predictive power. There should be no actionable indicators left (Soper, 2019b).

This randomising dynamic is not peculiar to suicide. Evolution by natural selection tends generally to promote adaptations up to the *edge of chaos* (Kauffman, 1993) – the boundary between order and disorder. Where all fitness-relevant regularities have been subsumed, what remains is noise, devoid of predictive utility. As Chapter 1 noted, the *environment of evolutionary adaptedness* is a statistical composite of the adaptation-relevant properties of ancestral environments (Tooby and Cosmides, 1990). By the same principle, completed suicides are statistical residuals – scenarios tagged with no adaptation-relevant markers with which the organism could have predicted and avoided self-destruction.

While evolved defences would eliminate suicide's predictive cues, they would not eliminate suicide. Defences would be selectively favoured only up to a least-bad compromise position, where the fitness benefit of responding to additional actuarial information is cancelled out by the incremental cost. The human brain has to strike a balance between blocking self-killing and impairing the emotional and cognitive functions that the organism needs to compete successfully against other mature adults for mates and other resources. Equilibrium is reached at a minimal, irreducible risk, manifest at a population level in a so-called natural (Yang and Lester, 2021) or base (Goldney, 2003) rate. Suicides are the residue left after the human brain has done the best it can with the information to hand. In other words,

while 'Zero Suicide' may be a laudable policy aspiration (Brodsky et al., 2018), as a species we are not biologically set up for zero suicide; all normally intelligent post-pubescent humans will carry a low, but above-zero, risk of near-random self-killing.

In some ways, suicide is like a plane crash. The possibility of a crash is unfortunately in the nature of heavier-than-air flight because the default position of an aeroplane is not in the sky; planes have to work to stay aloft. There are any number of systems that could fail, resulting in a common outcome: a crash. Zero crashes could be achieved, in theory, simply by keeping every aircraft grounded. Indeed, before the invention of the flying machine, there were none to crash. But the benefits of modern flight are so great that, once all that *can* practically be done to prevent accidents *has* been done, we fly, and we accept the small residual hazard. The disasters that do happen are intrinsically unpredictable (or at least they should be) because they are what remains after all reasonable measures have been taken, based on the information available, to avoid them.

Nature similarly could achieve zero suicide in theory simply by 'grounding' human intelligence at the level of a non-human animal or a human infant. But this immunity would be self-defeating because mature humans need species-typical cognition for reproductive success. Suicides occasionally happen even though evolution has adapted us to survive in the continuous presence of the suicide hazard, in the same way that freak aviation disasters happen even though planes are designed specifically not to crash (Soper, 2019a). Our defences are very good, but they cannot be failsafe given the extraordinary engineering challenge that the human psyche has to meet: to have continuously to hand elective death as a way to relieve suffering, while not actually exercising that option. From this perspective, the remarkable feature of *Homo sapiens* is not so much that suicide ends the lives of 9.0 per 100,000 each year, accounting for 1.3% of deaths (WHO, 2021), but that most of us nearly always find other ways to deal with the stresses of living. As products of selection, humans are precisely built to avoid deliberate self-killing as far as is biologically practicable.

This evolutionary perspective is relevant because it means that for clinicians to forecast suicide accurately at the individual level they would

---

[1] No teleological meaning is intended by the use of metaphors such 'sought out' and 'exploited'. Natural selection operates, of course, by a 'blind' process.

have to outperform the patient's own organismic anti-suicide machinery. If the process of selection has done the expected thing, consuming all utilis- able cues of danger, then the behaviour should be an aleatory phenomenon. Although there may be observable patterns at a macro level, individual sui- cides can be understood as outputs of a chaotic system (Lester, 2019a), or *mental accidents* (Ajdacic-Gross et al., 2019). They ought to be 'pre- dictably unpredictable' (Soper, 2019b: 37).

9.2 Empirical Evidence of Suicide's Randomness

The empirical record agrees with the theoretical expectation: suicide does indeed appear to be an essentially random event. Despite decades of research, no mix of risk factors, alleged warning signs, so-called red flags or other supposed cues has been found that comes close to predicting suicidal behaviour with useful accuracy (Belsher et al., 2019; Carter et al., 2017; Chan et al., 2016; Corke et al., 2021; Fosse et al., 2017; Franklin et al., 2017; Large et al., 2016; Mulder et al., 2016). Regardless of the assessment method, the great majority (95.0–97.5%) of people assessed as 'high risk' do not take their own lives even over an extended period. That is to say, a judgement that a patient is at 'high risk' is likely to be a false positive, with a $\geq 95\%$ chance of being wrong (Large et al., 2016). The most accurate assessment on a case-by-case basis is one where everyone is designated 'low risk'. Meanwhile, many – and in some studies most – suicides will occur among people who were not thought to be in particular danger (Large, 2017; NCISH, 2017; Wyder et al., 2021). Even though assessment tends to produce an exaggerated perception of the risk, where an individual's risk is declared, it is almost always 'low' prior to suicide (Rahman and Kapur, 2014). Most incidents occur among people who appeared normal to the extent that they remained outside of the mental healthcare system (NCISH, 2017; Stone et al., 2018); presumably, then, most cases are not associated with enough *prima facie* evidence of danger even to invite assessment.

These statistical realities put health workers in a corner. When confronted with an individual who has tried to take their own life, we naturally worry about what is to come, and some form of risk assessment is almost universally recom- mended. However, this is precisely the situation when predictive tools – anyway weak – are weakest: when all patients carry the prominent risk factor of self-harm, these tools cannot be used to discriminate between them (Corke et al., 2021). And we understandably have sometimes strong ideas about the future safety or vulnerability of our patients, but the science is challenging these preconceptions. It is telling us to be little more confident about suicidal outcomes than if we were shooting dice. A recent review makes the point unequivocally: 'Our ability to predict future sui- cidal behaviour is no better than chance' (Zortea et al., 2020: 73).

9.2.1 Multiple Lines of Empirical Evidence Converge on Suicide's Randomness

The virtually absolute erroneousness of suicide risk assessment, its predictive accuracy 'near 0' (Belsher et al., 2019: E1), is more than just a technical issue. It is not the kind of problem that can be finessed with more data or a cleverer methodology. Several strands of evidence from recent meta-analyses converge on suicide being opaque to prediction even in principle. One is the lack of progress in science's search for predict- ors. Although research in this field has grown exponentially over half a century, more recent studies achieve no better results than earlier ones (Carter et al., 2017; Franklin et al., 2017). Another is that no category of risk factor – mood disorder, suicidal ideation, past suicide attempt and so on – predicts significantly more accurately than any other (Franklin et al., 2017). That is to say, there is no detectable target for the research effort to home in on, no basis for narrowing the search space. Another is that no research methodology performs better than any other; for example, stud- ies using larger samples produce greater statistical validity than those with smaller samples but no greater predictive power (Franklin et al., 2017).

Most tellingly, there is no advantage in com- bining risk factors or otherwise adding complex- ity to assessment techniques. Methods that take into account many input variables perform as poorly as those using only a few (Corke et al., 2021; Taylor et al., 2021). This finding points to the source of uncertainty as aleatory rather than epistemic. More knowledge doesn't help. Assessing suicide risk is like trying to forecast the behaviour of dice: knowing more about the dice's weight, constituent materials, centre of gravity, etc., might allow finer calculation of actuarial probabilities but will be useless for determining which throw will produce a double six. Greater methodological sophistication does not overcome the essential randomness of the outcome.

This point deserves closer attention. Various professional bodies now explicitly recommend against simplistic assessments based on checklists of risk factors, score cards, risk scales and the like – instruments that remain in widespread use despite being uselessly inaccurate (APA, 2003; Belsher et al., 2019; Graney et al., 2020; NICE, 2012; Royal College of Psychiatrists, 2020). But the discommendation is curiously selective. It proscribes a particular *approach* to the endeavour, rather than the endeavour itself. It skips over the problem that more complex 'holistic' approaches that are put forward for use instead – 'comprehensive review' (Royal College of Psychiatrists, 2020), 'psychosocial assessment' (Steeg et al., 2018) and the like – are no more empirically supported than the formulaic tools they are meant to replace. Suicide risk assessment by clinical intuition is as unreliable as any other method (Carter et al., 2017; Corke et al., 2021; Franklin et al., 2017). Success is unlikely to be found in blending techniques either: adding a hunch, even an expert one, to actuarial prediction in this situation is as likely to introduce bias as to reduce error.

The aleatory uncertainty that thwarts a personalised psychosocial approach equally foils its mechanised opposite: artificial intelligence (AI), computerised algorithms and 'big data'. Whether the extra complexity is handled by medics or machines, more information does not produce better results (Corke et al., 2021). Notwithstanding the proleptic discourse surrounding AI in suicide prevention – 'the sense that we are on the cusp of a medical/scientific breakthrough' that pervades more than a century of literature in suicide research (Marsh, 2016: 28) – results so far indicate no easy progress in this direction (McHugh and Large, 2020). From an evolutionary perspective it is easy to see why: the human organism's own anti-suicide algorithm has had an immense head start. Success would require not only a recurring cue to be found that thousands of generations of intense selection

missed, but also the available prognostic data would need to be processed and actioned more effectively than is already achieved by 'the most sophisticated computer in the known universe' (Lieberman, 2013: 200) – the human brain.

As a final line of evidence, commonplace experience accords with the epidemiology. Suicide strikes like a bolt from the blue. For the actors themselves, those who survive often report that their attempts were impulsive, passing from first thought to would-be final act within a matter of minutes (Deisenhammer et al., 2009). As for bereaved loved ones, shock, confusion and disbelief characterise their immediate reactions to the news (Dyregrov et al., 2012); that is to say, they had no forewarning. Mental health workers are similarly taken aback by suicides of patients, despite presumably knowing more than most about supposed 'red flags' (Castelli Dransart et al., 2017). Jaworski and Scott (2016: 216) capture the bewilderment of those left behind: 'Despite all the signs we are told to look for, suicide is like a bracket that arrives as a closing without any opening.'

9.2.2 The Gap between Evidence and Belief

In view of the above tessellating theoretical and empirical evidence, it is safe to deduce that suicides happen largely at random. A case for the behaviour's intrinsic non-predictability can be confidently argued.

In legal settings it *is* so argued, and to a judicial standard of proof. Psychiatrists can and do explain in court – empathically but with assurance – that an individual suicide is virtually never predictable (Ryan et al., 2015a; St John-Smith et al., 2009). Attorneys experienced in defending malpractice suits, when it is alleged that a clinician 'should have seen it coming', are ready to brief juries on the distorting effect of viewing suicide through the lens of hindsight (Schultz, 2000). After the event, the act can take on the appearance of predictability, almost of inevitability; but however the assessment is made, an assessor who rates an individual as being at 'high risk' before the event will almost certainly be wrong. It should not be a contentious point that no-one, physicians included, can be prescient or omnipotent in a scenario governed by aleatory uncertainty. As observed in a recent interview, 'psychiatrists are doctors, not soothsayers' (Sanati, 2021: 192).

Psychiatry has made a litigious rod for its own back in this regard because an expectation of liability arises in part from medicine's own counterfactual orthodoxy (Large et al., 2012). Despite the lack of an evidential substrate, there is a persistent assumption in medical science, implicit or explicit, that suicides can be foreseen with meaningful accuracy, and therefore in principle can be forestalled by personally targeted interventions. Thus, pages of the medical press list risk factors (Turecki and Brent, 2016), 'red flags' (Cole-King and Platt, 2017) and 'danger signals' (Campbell and Hale, 2017), while offering no empirical reason to believe that any combination thereof usefully distinguishes future suicides from non-suicides in clinical settings. Even the World Health Organisation (WHO, 2014: 29), in a poster-like graphic, declares as 'Fact' that '[t]he majority of suicides have been preceded by warning signs, whether verbal or behavioural' – while leaving the grounds for this assertion signally unexplained.

The zeitgeist rests on a fallacy. It assumes that suicide's correlates, weak and usually measured after the event, can be taken as portents. While it is invidious to spotlight examples, a meta-analysis by Pompili et al. (2016: 12–13) illustrates the error. Dismissing as 'myth' the idea that people who talk about suicide rarely do take their own lives, the authors claim that 'suicidal communication' is a clinically robust predictor:

> Our data shows that SC [suicidal communication] seems to have a good positive predictive value, at least among adults. Therefore it is critical that any explicit SC be followed by a referral to a mental health professional and the arrangement of an adequate prevention plan.

But the studies included in the meta-analysis do not support this recommendation. Being retrospective, they testify rather that fishing trips often yield fish. When tasked with finding plausible 'suicidal communication' with the benefit of hindsight, psychological autopsies frequently deliver. There is no evidence that talk of suicide reliably predicts self-killing and considerable evidence that it doesn't. A longitudinal community study (n = 3481) found that most suicide attempts (74%) happened among people who had not reported suicidal ideas, while few of those who had disclosed such ideas made an attempt even over a follow-up period of more than

a decade (9%) (Kuo et al., 2001; see also ten Have et al., 2009). Vanishingly few completed suicide, it can be presumed, since attempters outnumber completers by some 30 times (CDC, 2021). A great many people admit to thinking about ending it all: one in five Europeans (Castillejos et al., 2021) and half of American college students (Drum et al., 2009) at some stage in their lives, and a quarter of young American adults in one stressful month alone (Czeisler et al., 2020). Nowhere close to this number go on to take their own lives, or try. Notwithstanding 'suicidal communication', the pooled 4.66 odds ratio calculated by Pompili et al. (2016) themselves from case–control studies points to suicide being extremely unlikely. Applying this multiple to a global baseline of about 1 suicide per 10,000 population per annum (WHO, 2021), the day-to-day odds against a particular individual dying in this way remain in the order of a million to one.

Pompili et al.'s (2016) article is widely cited and far from alone in misreading the epidemiology in this way. Another recent review, Mann et al. (2021), similarly cites post-mortem reports to argue that suicide is presaged by untreated depression, although there are equally no grounds to believe that depressive symptoms – or any other psychopathology – usefully indicate prospective risk (Carter et al., 2017; Franklin et al., 2017). The editor of a leading suicidology journal likewise insists, apparently on the strength of *post hoc* observation alone, 'It is important to reiterate that warning signs for suicide do clearly exist' (Joiner, 2010: 86). And so on.

There is a gulf between data and doctrine. We should in theory expect suicide to be a largely random outcome, and the empirical record agrees, but medicine's prevailing belief holds otherwise. Suicide's predictability constitutes a 'myth in search of facts' (Chiles et al., 2019: 8).

9.2.3 Why Do We Expect Suicide Risk to Be Assessable?

Faith in suicide risk assessment, despite clear evidence of its inutility, is a phenomenon worthy of study in its own right (Carter et al., 2017). Solving the puzzle as to why it endures is beyond the scope of this chapter, but we can point to suggestive clues.

There is no doubt much well-intentioned wishful thinking. We suspect that some clinicians, confident in their powers of foresight (Gale et al., 2016), act on what they *feel* to be true, and certainly what we would *want* to be true – that suicide is somehow predictable and therefore preventable at the individual level. These feelings and desires are natural and understandable. But the science is telling us otherwise; it says that suicide's alleged precedents are simply not specific enough to be taken as actionable indicators.

For some mental health professionals, the futility of trying to measure suicide risk is an elephant in the room: the anomaly is in plain sight, but few want to discuss or acknowledge it (Chiles et al., 2019; Espeland et al., 2021). For others, the activity may be a reassuring routine, affirmed by the non-suicides both of those judged 'low risk' and of those judged, and treated, as 'high risk'. There is the ascendant issue of reputational risk management to consider, both professional (Groth and Boccio, 2019; Jacobson, 2017; Ross et al., 2020) and corporate (Power, 2004). Perhaps even pharmaceutical marketing interests may be involved (Jacobson, 2015). More alibi than rationale, incidental benefits might arguably arise where risk assessment leads to a wider and more useful therapeutic discussion between patient and carer (Draper, 2012). There is an operational issue: if not by this means, then some other way would have to be found to triage mental health patients (Lester, 2019b). More broadly, health workers and managers must work within organisational constraints – a pressure to conform not only to conventional practices but perhaps, psychologically, to conventional beliefs as well (Williams, 2021).

Motivated misbelief may arise also because we health workers, being human, have demons of our own. The very idea of suicide risk assessment helps to keep our finger reassuringly pointing the other way. As long as we view suicide as something that happens to *other* people, belonging to *them* and arising from *their* problems, we can imagine ourselves exempt. It is not easy to take on board the full implications of suicide's universality and randomness. Although extremely unlikely, it could happen to virtually any post-pubescent, ourselves included. Indeed, healthcare professionals have a higher rate of suicide than the general population (Milner et al., 2013). It may be higher still among psychiatrists (Dutheil et al., 2019). Defensive denial seems to be ubiquitous in this terrain, displayed in a near-universal conviction that self-killings can be pinned to some cause (residing in *others*) that is, in principle, identifiable. We need a specific reason, an acceptable answer to the question, 'Why?' (Campbell, 2001; Franklin, 2018). Selecting one is a secondary business, guided along encultured lines. Around the world and in different historical eras, different traditions rationalise suicide in different ways, usually from a judgemental, stigmatising (or *othering*; Zou et al., 2021) position. Popular explanations include bad luck, evil spirits, stupidity, vengeance, immorality and criminality (Bohannan, 1960;; Solano et al., 2018), as well as the psychosocial, pathology-focused paradigm that currently holds sway in the West (Hjelmeland and Knizek, 2019; Soper, 2021). This latter style of explanation, manifested in suicide risk assessment, may feel self-evidently 'right' to modern Western sensibilities, but it is no more objective than any other, no less socially constructed (Atkinson, 1978; Marsh 2010) and just as unevidenced. It has been dubbed by Kral (1998: 221) the 'great origin myth', and by Soper (2019b) *suigiston*, highlighting parallels with another ill-founded paradigm: early chemists' belief in the fiery element *phlogiston*. Non-existent as we now know, phlogiston was never found despite its intuitive appeal and a century-long scientific search. The same can be said of the special contingencies that supposedly lead people to take their own lives.

Besides such motley forces, there is also a feeling that to accept the full implications of suicide's randomness would be a nihilistic position, a counsel of despair. As Lester (2019b: 154) notes, there is a sense that 'poor prediction is better than no prediction'. To counter this sentiment, we devote the rest of this chapter to a positive vision: how mental healthcare might look, for the better, if we transcended the old notion of trying to assess suicide risk.

9.3 A Brighter Future: Mental Health beyond Suicide Risk Assessment

Suicide risk assessment is not cost-free. Consider the burdens that could be lifted by not doing it. They begin with the opportunity cost of time and other healthcare resources wasted in carrying out the procedure, of itself an intrusive, complex and time-consuming intervention (Cole-King et al., 2013). They extend into diverse unintended consequences for the healthcare organisation, patient and clinician.

9.3.1 Costs to Be Saved for the Organisation, Patient and Clinician

For the organisation, any treatment decision made on the basis of a 'high-risk' designation – including so-called safety plans (House, 2020), psychopharmacology (Braun et al., 2016) and hospitalisation (Large and Kapur, 2018) – may be presumed to misallocate resources given that the deciding assessment was almost certainly wrong. Although a hypothetical economic case may be argued (Ross et al., 2021), there is no clinical logic in rationing treatments in this manner. If an intervention is effective and benign enough for those (mis)judged to be 'at risk', it would be virtually as worthwhile (or, indeed, as unhelpful, or even harmful) for the rest of the patient cohort.

With regard to patients, an ethical issue to be addressed is to what extent it is acceptable to label as 'high risk' and impose onerous costs – disruptive interventions and potential stigma – on large numbers of people who were never going to take their own lives, in the hope of stopping the suicides of an unidentifiable few. This question is all the more pressing given that the countervailing benefit, measured in suicides prevented, is at best weak (Fox et al., 2020; Paris, 2021). It is doubtful, notably, whether lives are saved by administering antidepressants (Hengartner et al., 2021) or by hospitalisation (Chung et al., 2019; Large and Kapur, 2018).

For the clinician, suicide risk assessment creates avoidable stress and conflict (Elzinga et al., 2020; Espeland et al., 2021; Groth and Boccio, 2019). Clinicians face problems because the procedure brings with it the potential for blame and potential liability, especially if a patient is declared 'low risk' but does take their own life. Clinicians are thus called to manage an emergent secondary risk to themselves and their organisation, rather than focusing on the needs of the patient. Undrill (2007: 296) makes the point tersely: 'When a doctor constructs a patient as a source of threat to their professional integrity, they have stopped acting as a doctor to that patient.' As a form of insurance – as in 'cover yourself' (Espeland et al., 2021) – assessment would be expected to incentivise the assessor to err on the side of caution, to overrate the hazard. The low positive predictive value of risk assessments suggests that this is indeed what happens (Pokorny, 1983).

The assessment process raises conflict for patients too, because it may be in their interest not to be candid. Being defined as 'high risk' might lead to treatments they do not need, and being defined as 'low risk' might deprive them of treatments they needed and/or wanted (Large et al., 2011a). As already noted, the treatment given to those declared 'high risk' may be disruptive to their personal lives. Interventions may entail the prescribing of drugs with significant side effects, and/or protracted therapy, and possibly hospitalisation, with or without compulsion. There may also be psychological consequences: a person judged to be a threat to themselves may have to deal with resulting feelings of fear, deficiency and inadequacy, and a stigmatising social reaction (Mayer et al., 2020). In this light, it is understandable that many patients choose not to disclose their suicidal thoughts in clinical interviews (Blanchard and Farber, 2020; Obegi, 2021), and it is questionable whether an informed person would even consent to being assessed.

Thus, while the psychiatrist risk-assesses the patient, the patient might reasonably be risk-assessing the psychiatrist – as someone who can potentially harm them either by enforcing treatment that is not of value or by denying treatment that they want (Sanati, 2021). None of this gaming is conducive to a therapeutic relationship based on authenticity and trust (Michel and Jobes, 2011). The kind of reception that distressed patients find most helpful is one in which they feel heard and accepted, without judgement (Nicholas et al., 2020). This desired mode of relating is undermined by risk assessment, which can hardly but place the assessor in a judgemental position (Szmukler and Rose, 2013).

9.3.2 Benefits of Transcending Suicide Risk Assessment

We envision a different approach: one based on evolutionary understanding, acceptance of the empirical facts, and an embracement of suicide's aleatoric nature. Such a stance could form the basis of a more fruitful connection between health professional and patient because it relocates 'fault' for suicide outside of the individual (Ajdacic-Gross et al., 2019; Silverman and Maris, 1995). With the potential for suicide being understood as a dreadful but universal feature of the human condition, rather than a personal defect or deficiency, clinician and client can meet each other as fellows. Neither is in especially exigent danger, and both face about as much risk as does any other post-pubescent human. Identifying as a peer, the health worker may more easily empathise. This is a big ask. Facing the patient on the same plane in this way implies, as noted earlier, that we health workers accept our own vulnerability. It also implies waiver of a power asymmetry that has privileged medicine for centuries (Weinberg, 2015). But such levelling does stand to make us more collaborative and effective therapists (Michel and Jobes, 2011).

Properly informed, the clinician can more helpfully focus on *risk communication* instead of risk assessment (Chiles et al., 2019; Ryan et al., 2015b; Sanati, 2021). We can offer genuine reassurance. This is not to dismiss a patient's concerns about their self-destructive ideas and behaviours: suicidality should be discussed fearlessly and with understanding (Large et al., 2017). It is not to ignore a current situation that needs to be managed with common sense. Nor is it to dismiss the clinician's understandable concern for the future of their patient. It is, rather, to present the actuarial fact that, over a foreseeable future, and however desperate the patient feels now, suicide remains an extremely unlikely outcome (Mammen et al., 2020). Suicidal crises and episodes of self-harm almost always resolve themselves in time (Fox et al., 2020; Moran et al., 2012). In Box 9.1, we offer suggestions on how suicidality may usefully be explained, its fearfulness de-stung and the danger put into realistic perspective.

In place of a process that 'others' distressed people, we can look for ways to 'belong' them (Reynolds, 2016). For sure they do belong, and the belonging begins on a vast scale. As a regular human being, having inherited protections that kept every one of their ancestors alive at least long enough to start a family, the patient can consider themselves well equipped to handle, in their own time and in their own way, whatever lies ahead. They possess a genius for survival that has accumulated over countless generations; in this real sense, all of their fore-fathers and -mothers are on their side.

Relieved of the need to dwell on the negatives of risk and disorder, the meeting can concentrate on the patient's strengths (Hirsch et al., 2018; Michaud et al., 2021; White et al., 2016).

Clinicians can help patients to explore, appreciate and build on their own resources. They have, after all, survived thus far. It may be useful to review religious or spiritual beliefs; nourishing family, social and pet relations; and competences, projects, aspirations and so on. A focus on risk assessment has a magnifying effect on the perception of danger. By the same token, focusing on the patient's connections and capabilities can foster a vision of hope (Magyary, 2002; Wand, 2011).

Expectable benefits ripple out beyond the patient. Acceptance of suicide's essential randomness – as an unforeseeable biological accident – would help to ease the irrational guilt that often besets people bereaved in this way, health workers included (Greenberg and Shefler, 2014; Hendin et al., 2004). At a time of trauma, confusion and vulnerability, they need the facts stated unambiguously. *There were no signs.* There may be lessons to be learnt, but no one could have seen it coming. To insinuate otherwise, as an ethos of risk assessment does, is to add cruel and gratuitous torment to survivors' grief.

Wider benefits would arise from an implied shift in the burden of prevention from clinicians to public health policymakers. With there being no effective way to pick 'at-risk' individuals out for special treatment, effective interventions must necessarily take place at the level of populations. This is true even in mental healthcare settings: the most effective way to stop suicides in hospitals is by restricting access to lethal means, such as by the removal of ligature points, or by whole-cohort care programmes, rather than through treatment plans based on personal risk assessment (Chung et al., 2019; Large et al., 2011b; Tishler and Reiss, 2009). But as most suicides happen among people who have not accessed mental health services, the greatest scope for prevention lies in community-wide initiatives (Blanco et al., 2021; Davidson et al., 2018). In this regard, there is good evidence of the efficacy of means restriction (Chen et al., 2016; Westers, 2020). Indeed, the most likely explanation for the fall in the global suicide rate in recent decades is the reduced access to pesticides commonly used for self-poisoning in China, India and elsewhere (Mew et al., 2017). Wider still, acknowledgement that the real levers of suicide prevention operate more in the community than in the individual could help to refocus policymakers' attention on moderating the

Box 9.1   **Risk communication: how to transcend suicide risk assessment**

1 Be Sceptical of Simplistic Solutions

An interested reader can easily find guidelines as to how to assess and manage people who are judged to be 'suicidal'. These guidelines focus on people with suicidal ideation and behaviour, list numerous suicide risk factors and recommend various pathways based on suicide risk assessment. This approach is flawed because many, if not most, people who die by suicide have no known history of being 'suicidal' or have had little or no contact with mental health services. The guidelines fail both because many potential suicides are missed by the focus on those who are 'suicidal' and because suicide risk assessment is least effective among groups defined by self-harm or suicide attempts. Our first recommendation is to ignore simplistic or overly proscriptive guides to suicide risk management and instead to rely more on your humanity, clinical skills and global clinical judgement.

2 Be Alert for Distress

Focus on a broader group of people who might be loosely described as 'distressed' and do not arbitrarily exclude those judged not to be suicidal. To this end, you can use a very broad definition of 'distressed'. Common forms of distress are anxiety, depression and anger. Common causes of distress are perceived threats, losses, insult, injury and frustration. This is not an exhaustive list.

3 Be an Active Listener

With the aim of reducing suicide outcomes, listen carefully to any distressed person you meet. Be human, honest and as helpful as is appropriate. This does not mean you should be overwhelming; any interaction should be calm, nuanced and open. You can assume that almost all distressed people have some suicidal thinking. This thinking might be obvious, revealed by quiet questioning, or concealed. Learning about a person's suicidal thinking might help you understanding their distress, but it is rarely its cause. Many people with suicidal ideas rightly consider them to be products of their situation and experiences, but they may also view them as a potential way to stay in control. Focusing on suicidal thoughts can overshadow the distressed person's actual and perceived problems. An excessive focus on suicidal thoughts and behaviours can also be interpreted as a threat to the person's autonomy and agency. On the other hand, trying to understand why the person is distressed is likely to be intrinsically helpful.

4 Be Respectful

It is best to assume – just like yourself – that a distressed person has agency for decision-making and an ability to consider the thinking of others. Any consideration of future self-inflicted harm needs to acknowledge this fundamental human element; suicide risk assessment is not analogous to an insurer considering the fate of a house or a car, or an aviation engineer looking for cracks in an aircraft wing. Refrain from tick-box approaches and lists of risk factors.

5 Be Calm, Don't Panic

If you want to assist a distressed person, do not panic yourself. Suicidal thoughts and behaviours can be frightening, but deregulation of your feelings will heighten the patient's anxiety and emotions. Some patients will make choices you would not make yourself or that you think are too risky. Remember that suicide is a rare outcome even among the most overtly suicidal people and that each person is the product of both thousands of generations of selection and a lifetime of personal survival.

6 Tread Softly

Many distressed people will have difficulty trusting and communicating with you. While it might be better to have a more complete picture of the distressed person, knowing less should not cause you more anxiety. There is no evidence that more information improves judgements about future suicide. Don't interrogate; if you face a choice between maintaining or developing rapport and getting a more complete picture, tolerate a degree of uncertainty.

Box 9.1 *(cont.)*

7 Be Humble

Be realistic about your abilities and endeavour to empower the person. Every person has strengths that have kept them alive, and there is scant evidence that you can do much to improve on this. Don't exaggerate the effectiveness of suicide-preventing interventions or underestimate the side effects of any treatment.

8 Use Hospitalisation Sparingly

Make judgements that a distressed person needs to be contained in a hospital very carefully. No suicide risk factor or combination of risk factors can bring sufficient certainty about future suicide to detain a person against their will. Remember: psychiatric hospitalisation can be traumatic, stigmatising and isolating, and suicide rates in psychiatric hospitals are relatively high. The person's views need to be first and foremost in any decision about hospital care and, when the there is a clear lack of reasoning, the views of those who know the person best should be given weight.

9 Use the Medical Evidence Base

While the outcome of any assessment must suit and be helpful to the distressed person, advice about specific suicide-prevention measures should be based on evidence. It might be rational, for example, to take steps to limit access to lethal means of suicide (e.g. firearms) because of the evidence of the efficacy of such restrictions on lowering the suicide risk. But the role of hospitalisation, medications or psychotherapies should not be overstated and, conversely, the strength of the patient's own protective mechanisms should not be underestimated.

10 Be an Educated Educator

You will need to reduce the anxiety experienced by friends and relatives. This is a difficult but not impossible task, and it helps if you know the science. Educating colleagues steeped in psychiatric orthodoxy might be more challenging still, but it is essential because it can help them to help the distressed people they meet. In your educational role, also listen and explain, trust the intelligence of others and be persistently friendly, honest and knowledgeable.

socioeconomic root causes of mental ill health, not least poverty, injustice and displacement (Patel, 2015).

9.4 A New Direction for Suicide Research

Perhaps the largest gap in our understanding of suicidality, and certainly a neglected area of research, concerns the evolved psychological devices that usually keep suicide at bay (Gunn et al., 2021; Himmelhoch, 1988; Humphrey, 2018; Soper, 2021). We can be confident these exist – if they didn't, our species would not have come this far and we would not be here to discuss the matter – but little thought has been given as to what they are and how they operate.

We need this knowledge. It is likely that once we have an idea of how the organism's anti-suicide defences work, and in good part only then, we will be able to intervene in a manner cognisant of the human psyche's capacity for self-restoration. The prize here is that professionals in mental health may work according to a principle that is well known to their colleagues in physiological medicine. All wise medics know that it is the organism that does much of the healing. The physician expertly sets a fracture, but it is the organism that repairs the bone. Thus, the best prospects for success should be found in interventions that promote and capitalise upon the organism's own homeostatic mechanisms. There remains very little such understanding in psychopathology. It is known that most common mental disorders ease spontaneously given time and favourable psychosocial conditions, with or without medical intervention (Goldberg and Goodyer, 2005), but how and why this happens is unclear, and rarely even discussed. Perhaps it is by a related mechanism that suicidal crises tend to be ephemeral, coming and going often within minutes (Drum et al., 2009). This rapid progression into and out of danger could offer important opportunities for preventative interventions, especially in the field of means restriction, because it suggests that obstructions that cause only a brief delay in a suicidal endeavour, or add only slightly to its complexity, would be expected to deliver disproportionately strong results.

9.5 Conclusion

Both evolutionary theory (Soper, 2018, 2021) and the empirical record (Corke et al., 2021) point to suicide being an essentially random event. It resists meaningful risk assessment at the level of the individual. An evolutionary view of the behaviour, as an unfortunate feature of our species from which no normal adolescent or adult is immune, offers a constructive reframing of suicidology's public health, clinical and research agenda. The stance emphasises that the primary onus for prevention rests at a public health level in population-wide measures. In clinical settings, it could help to accelerate the de-implementation of risk assessment; provide a coherent conceptual basis on which clinicians can explain suicidality to their patients and reassure them about the real nature of the hazard; and guide decisions about helpful interventions. An informed therapeutic encounter can arm the patient with a justified sense of empowerment, adequacy and self-confidence.

As for research priorities, suicidology's decades-long search for a usefully accurate method of risk assessment now looks to us to be misplaced. Better prospects for progress lie in seeking to identify, understand and exploit the evolved defences that keep most humans safe from self-killing. The focus could profitably shift from making arbitrary and unhelpful judgements of individual risk to asking more positively why, almost always, we choose to live.

References

Ajdacic-Gross, V., Hepp, U., Seifritz, E. and Bopp, M. 2019. Rethinking suicides as mental accidents: towards a new paradigm. *Journal of Affective Disorders*, 252, 141–151.

APA 2003. *Practice Guideline for the Assessment and Treatment of Patients with Suicidal Behaviors*. New York: American Psychiatric Association.

Atkinson, J. M. 1978. *Discovering Suicide: Studies in the Social Organization of Sudden Death*. London: Macmillan.

Baechler, J. 1975/1979. *Les Suicides*. New York: Basic Books.

Bartley, B. A., Kim, K., Medley, J. K. and Sauro, H. M. 2017. Synthetic biology: engineering living systems from biophysical principles. *Biophysical Journal*, 112, 1050–1058.

Belsher, B. E., Smolenski, D. J., Pruitt, L. D., Bush, N. E., Beech, E. H., Workman, D. E., Morgan, R. L., Evatt, D. P., Tucker, J. and Skopp, N. A. 2019. Prediction models for suicide attempts and deaths: a systematic review and simulation. *JAMA Psychiatry*, 76, 642–651.

Bering, J. M. 2018. *A Very Human Ending: How Suicide Haunts Our Species*. London: Transworld.

Blanchard, M. and Farber, B. A. 2020. 'It is never okay to talk about suicide': patients' reasons for concealing suicidal ideation in psychotherapy. *Psychotherapy Research*, 30, 124–136.

Blanco, C., Wall, M. M. and Olfson, M. 2021. A population-level approach to suicide prevention. *JAMA*, 325, 2339–2340.

Bohannan, P. (ed.) 1960. *African Homicide and Suicide*. Princeton, NJ: Princeton University Press.

Borges, G., Chiu, W. T., Hwang, I., Panchal, B. N., Ono, Y., Sampson, N., Kessler, R. C. and Nock, M. K. 2012. Prevalence, onset, and transitions among suicidal behaviors. In: M. K. Nock, G. Borges and Y. Ono (eds.), *Suicide: Global Perspectives from the WHO World Mental Health Surveys*. Cambridge: Cambridge University Press, pp. 65–74.

Braun, C., Bschor, T., Franklin, J. and Baethge, C. 2016. Suicides and suicide attempts during long-term treatment with antidepressants: a meta-analysis of 29 placebo-controlled studies including 6,934 patients with major depressive disorder. *Psychotherapy and Psychosomatics*, 85, 171–179.

Brodsky, B. S., Spruch-Feiner, A. and Stanley, B. 2018. The Zero Suicide Model: applying evidence-based suicide prevention practices to clinical care. *Frontiers in Psychiatry*, 9, 33.

Campbell, D. and Hale, R. 2017. *Working in the Dark: Understanding the Pre-Suicide State of Mind*. London: Routledge.

Campbell, F. 2001. Living and working in the Canyon of Why. *Proceedings of the Irish Association of Suicidology*, 6, 96–97.

Carter, G., Milner, A., Mcgill, K., Pirkis, J., Kapur, N. and Spittal, M. J. 2017. Predicting suicidal behaviours using clinical instruments: systematic review and meta-analysis of positive predictive values for risk scales. *British Journal of Psychiatry*, 210, 387–395.

Castelli Dransart, D. A., Treven, M., Grad, O. T. and Andriessen, K. 2017. Impact of client suicide on health and mental health professionals. In: K. Andriessen, K. Krysinska and O. T. Grad (eds.), *Postvention in Action: The International Handbook of Suicide Bereavement Support*. Boston, MA: Hogrefe, pp. 245–254.

Castillejos, M. C., Huertas, P., Martín, P. and Küstner, B. 2021. Prevalence of suicidality in the European general population: a systematic review and meta-analysis. *Archives of Suicide Research*, 24, 810–828.

CDC 2021. *Preventing Suicide*. Atlanta, GA: Centers for Disease Control and Prevention, National Center for Injury Prevention and Control.

Chan, M. K., Bhatti, H., Meader, N., Stockton, S., Evans, J., O'Connor, R. C., Kapur, N. and Kendall, T. 2016. Predicting suicide following self-harm: systematic review of risk factors and risk scales. *British Journal of Psychiatry*, 209, 277–283.

Chen, Y.-Y., Chien-Chang Wu, K., Wang, Y. and Yip, P. 2016. Suicide prevention through restricting access to suicide means and hotspots. In: R. C. O'Connor and J. Pirkis (eds.), *International Handbook of Suicide Prevention*, 2nd ed. Chichester: John Wiley and Sons, pp. 545–560.

Chiles, J. A., Strosahl, K. D. and Roberts, L. W. 2019. *Clinical Manual for Assessment and Treatment of Suicidal Patients*. Washington, DC: American Psychiatric Association.

Chung, D., Hadzi-Pavlovic, D., Wang, M., Swaraj, S., Olfson, M. and Large, M. M. 2019. Meta-analysis of suicide rates in the first week and the first month after psychiatric hospitalisation. *BMJ Open*, 9, e023883.

Cole-King, A. and Platt, S. 2017. Suicide prevention for physicians: identification, intervention and mitigation of risk. *Medicine*, 45, 131–134.

Cole-King, A., Green, G., Gask, L., Hines, K. and Platt, S. 2013. Suicide mitigation: a compassionate approach to suicide prevention. *Advances in Psychiatric Treatment*, 19, 276–283.

Corke, M., Mullin, K., Angel-Scott, H., Xia, S. and Large, M. M. 2021. Meta-analysis of the strength of exploratory suicide prediction models; from clinicians to computers. *BJPsych Open*, 7, 1–11.

Cuddy-Casey, M. and Orvaschel, H. 1997. Children's understanding of death in relation to child suicidality and homicidality. *Clinical Psychology Review*, 17, 33–45.

Czeisler, M. É., Lane, R. I., Petrosky, E., Wiley, J. F., Christensen, A., Njai, R., Weaver, M. D., Robbins, R. C., Facer-Childs, E. R., Barger, L. K., Czeisler, C. A., Howard, M. E. and Rajaratnam, S. M. W. 2020. *Substance Use, and Suicidal Ideation during the COVID-19 Pandemic*. Washington, DC: US Department of Health and Human Services/Centers for Disease Control and Prevention.

Davidson, C. L., Slish, M. L., Rhoades-Kerswill, S., O'Keefe, V. M. and Tucker, R. P. 2018. Encouraging health-promoting behaviors in primary care to reduce suicide rates. In: J. K. Hirsch, E. C. Chang and J. Kelliher Rabon (eds.), *A Positive Psychological Approach to Suicide: Theory, Research, and Prevention*. Cham: Springer, pp. 161–181.

DeCatanzaro, D. 1981. *Suicide and Self-Damaging Behavior:* *A Sociobiological Perspective*. New York: Academic Press.

Deisenhammer, E. A., Ing, C.-M., Strauss, R., Kemmler, G., Hinterhuber, H. and Weiss, E. M. 2009. The duration of the suicidal process: how much time is left for intervention between consideration and accomplishment of a suicide attempt? *Journal of Clinical Psychiatry*, 70, 19–24.

Draper, B. 2012. Isn't it a bit risky to dismiss suicide risk assessment? *Australian and New Zealand Journal of Psychiatry*, 46, 385–386.

Drum, D. J., Brownson, C., Denmark, A. B. and Smith, S. E. 2009. New data on the nature of suicidal crises in college students: shifting the paradigm. *Professional Psychology: Research and Practice*, 40, 213–222.

Dutheil, F., Aubert, C., Pereira, B., Dambrun, M., Moustafa, F., Mermillod, M., Trousselard, M., Lesage, F.-X. and Navel, V. 2019. Suicide among physicians and health-care workers: a systematic review and meta-analysis. *PLoS ONE*, 14, e0226361.

Dyregrov, K., Plyhn, E. and Dieserud, G. 2012. *After the Suicide: Helping the Bereaved to Find a Path from Grief to Recovery*. London: Jessica Kingsley.

Elzinga, E., De Kruif, A. J., De Beurs, D. P., Beekman, A. T., Franx, G. and Gilissen, R. 2020. Engaging primary care professionals in suicide prevention: a qualitative study. *PLoS ONE*, 15, e0242540.

Espeland, K., Hjelmeland, H. and Knizek, B. L. 2021. A call for change from impersonal risk assessment to a relational approach: professionals' reflections on the national guidelines for suicide prevention in mental health care in Norway. *International Journal of Qualitative Studies on Health and Well-Being*, 16, 1868737.

Forte, A., Sarli, G., Polidori, L., Lester, D. and Pompili, M. 2021. The role of new technologies to prevent suicide in adolescence: a systematic review of the literature. *Medicina*, 57, 109.

Fosse, R., Ryberg, W., Carlsson, M. K. and Hammer, J. 2017. Predictors of suicide in the patient population admitted to a locked-door psychiatric acute ward. *PLoS ONE*, 12, e0173958.

Fox, K. R., Huang, X., GuzmÁN, E. M., Funsch, K. M., Cha, C. B., Ribeiro, J. D. and Franklin, J. C. 2020. Interventions for suicide and self-injury: a meta-analysis of randomized controlled trials across nearly 50 years of research. *Psychological Bulletin*, 146, 1117–1145.

Franklin, J. C. 2018. Suicide prediction remains difficult despite decades of research. Scientific American. Retrieved from www.scientificamerican.com/article/suicide-prediction-remains-difficult-despite-decades-of-research/

Franklin, J. C., Ribeiro, J. D., Fox, K. R., Bentley, K. H., Kleiman, E. M., Huang, X., Musacchio, K. M., Jaroszewski, A. C., Chang, B. P. and Nock, M. K. 2017. Risk factors for suicidal thoughts and behaviors: a meta-analysis of 50 years of research. *Psychological Bulletin*, 143, 187–232.

Gale, T. M., Hawley, C. J., Butler, J., Morton, A. and Singhal, A. 2016. Perception of suicide risk in mental health professionals. *PLoS ONE*, 11, e0149791.

Goldberg, D. and Goodyer, I. 2005. *The Origins and Course of Common Mental Disorders*. Hove: Routledge.

Goldney, R. D. 2003. A novel integrated knowledge explanation of factors leading to suicide. *New Ideas in Psychology*, 21, 141–146.

Graney, J., Hunt, I. M., Quinlivan, L., Rodway, C., Turnbull, P.,

Gianatsi, M., Appleby, L. and Kapur, N. 2020. Suicide risk assessment in UK mental health services: a national mixed-methods study. *Lancet Psychiatry*, 7, 1046–1053.

Greenberg, D. and Shefler, G. 2014. Patient suicide. *Israel Journal of Psychiatry and Related Sciences*, 51, 193–198.

Groth, T. and Boccio, D. E. 2019. Psychologists' willingness to provide services to individuals at risk of suicide. *Suicide and Life-Threatening Behavior*, 49, 1241–1254.

Gunn, J. F. 2017. The Social Pain Model. *Crisis*, 38, 281–286.

Gunn, J. F., Malo Ocejo, P. and Soper, C. A. 2021. Evolutionary psychology and suicidology. In: T. K. Shackelford (ed.), *The SAGE Handbook of Evolutionary Psychology*, Vol. 3. London: SAGE, pp. 51–93.

Hagström, A. S. 2020. Based theater and 'stigmatized trauma': the case of suicide bereavement. *Frontiers in Psychology*, 11, 1129.

Hendin, H. 1975. Growing up dead: student suicide. *American Journal of Psychotherapy*, 29, 327–338.

Hendin, H., Haas, A. P., Maltsberger, J. T., Szanto, K. and Rabinowicz, H. 2004. Factors contributing to therapists' distress after the suicide of a patient. *American Journal of Psychiatry*, 161, 1442–1446.

Hengartner, M. P., Amendola, S., Kaminski, J. A., Kindler, S., Bschor, T. and Ploderl, M. 2021. Suicide risk with selective serotonin reuptake inhibitors and new-generation serotonergic-noradrenergic antidepressants in adults: a systematic review and meta-analysis of observational studies. *Journal of Epidemiology and Community Health*. DOI: 10.1136/jech-2020-214611.

Himmelhoch, J. M. 1988. What destroys our restraints against

suicide? *Journal of Clinical Psychiatry*, 49, 46–52.

Hirsch, J. K., Chang, E. C. and Kelliher Rabon, J. (eds.) 2018. *A Positive Psychological Approach to Suicide*. Cham: Springer.

Hjelmeland, H. and Knizek, B. L. 2019. The emperor's new clothes? A critical look at the interpersonal theory of suicide. *Death Studies*, 44, 168–178.

House, A. 2020. Self-harm and suicide in adults: will safety plans keep people safe after self-harm? *BJPsych Bulletin*, 46, 1–3.

Humphrey, N. 2018. The lure of death: suicide and human evolution. *Philosophical Transactions of the Royal Society of London. Series B, Biological Sciences*, 373, 20170269.

Hundert, E. M. 1992. The brain's capacity to form delusions as an evolutionary strategy for survival. In: M., Spitzer, F., Uehlein, M. A. Schwartz and C. Mundt (eds.), *Phenomenology, Language & Schizophrenia*. New York: Springer, pp. 346–354.

Jacobson, G. 2017. Practice and malpractice in the evaluation of suicidal patients. In: R. Schouten (ed.), *Mental Health Practice and the Law*. New York: Oxford University Press, pp. 61–92.

Jacobson, R. 2015. Many antidepressant studies found tainted by pharma company influence. *Scientific American*, 29, 26. Retrieved from www.scientificamerican.com/article/many-antidepressant-studies-found-tainted-by-pharma-company-influence/

Jacobucci, R., Littlefield, A. K., Millner, A. J., Kleiman, E. M. and Steinley, D. 2021. Evidence of inflated prediction performance: a commentary on machine learning and suicide research. *Clinical Psychological Science*, 9, 129–134.

Jaworski, K. and Scott, D. G. 2016. Understanding the unfathomable in suicide: poetry, absence, and the corporeal body. In: J. C. White, I. Marsh, M. J. Kral and J. S. Morris (eds.), *Critical Suicidology: Re-thinking Suicide Research and Prevention for the 21st Century*. Vancouver, BC: UBC Press, pp. 209–228.

Joiner, T. E. 2010. *Myths about Suicide*. Cambridge, MA: Harvard University Press.

Kahne, M. J. 1966. Suicide research: a critical review of strategies and potentialities in mental hospitals (part II). *International Journal of Social Psychiatry*, 12, 177–186.

Kauffman, S. A. 1993. *The Origins of Order: Self Organization and Selection in Evolution*. Oxford: Oxford University Press.

Kral, M. J. 1998. Suicide and the internalization of culture: three questions. *Transcultural Psychiatry*, 35, 221–233.

Kuo, W.-H., Gallo, J. J. and Tien, A. Y. 2001. Incidence of suicide ideation and attempts in adults: the 13-year follow-up of a community sample in Baltimore, Maryland. *Psychological Medicine*, 31, 1181–1191.

Large, M. M. 2017. Emerging consensus on the positive predictive (and clinical) value of suicide risk assessment. *British Journal of Psychiatry*, Letter, 21 March.

Large, M. M. and Kapur, N. 2018. Psychiatric hospitalisation and the risk of suicide. *British Journal of Psychiatry*, 212, 269–273.

Large, M. M., Kaneson, M., Myles, N., Myles, H., Gunaratne, P. and Ryan, C. J. 2016. Meta-analysis of longitudinal cohort studies of suicide risk assessment among psychiatric patients: heterogeneity in results and lack of improvement over time. *PLoS ONE*, 11, e0156322.

Large, M. M., Ryan, C. J. and Callaghan, S. 2012. Hindsight bias and the overestimation of suicide risk in expert testimony. *The Psychiatrist*, 36, 236–237.

Large, M. M., Ryan, C. J., Carter, G. and Kapur, N. 2017. Can we usefully stratify patients according to suicide risk? *BMJ*, 359, j4627.

Large, M. M., Ryan, C. J., Singh, S. P., Paton, M. B. and Nielssen, O. B. 2011a. The predictive value of risk categorization in schizophrenia. *Harvard Review of Psychiatry*, 19, 25–33.

Large, M. M., Smith, G., Sharma, S., Nielssen, O. and Singh, S. 2011b. Systematic review and meta-analysis of the clinical factors associated with the suicide of psychiatric in-patients. *Acta Psychiatrica Scandinavica*, 124, 18–19.

Lester, D. 2019a. Suicide, chaos theory, non-linearity, and the tipping point. In: D. Lester (ed.), *The End of Suicidology: Can We Ever Understand Suicide?* New York: Nova Science Publishers, pp. 89–96.

Lester, D. (ed.) 2019b. *The End of Suicidology: Can We Ever Understand Suicide?* New York: Nova Science Publishers.

Lieberman, M. D. 2013. *Social: Why Our Brains Are Wired to Connect*. Oxford: Oxford University Press.

Magyary, D. 2002. Positive mental health: a turn of the century perspective. *Issues in Mental Health Nursing*, 23, 331–349.

Mammen, O., Tew, J., Painter, T., Bettinelli, E. and Beckjord, J. 2020. Communicating suicide risk to families of chronically suicidal borderline personality disorder patients to mitigate malpractice risk. *General Hospital Psychiatry*, 67, 51–57.

Mann, J. J., Michel, C. A. and Auerbach, R. P. 2021. Improving suicide prevention through evidence-based strategies: a systematic review. *American Journal of Psychiatry*, 178, 611–624.

Marsh, I. 2016. Critiquing contemporary suicidology. In: J. C. White, I. Marsh, M. J. Kral and J. S. Morris, (eds.), *Critical Suicidology: Re-thinking Suicide Research and Prevention for the 21st Century*. Vancouver, BC: UBC Press, pp. 15–30.

Mayer, L., RÜSch, N., Frey, L. M., Nadorff, M. R., Drapeau, C. W., Sheehan, L. and Oexle, N. 2020. Anticipated suicide stigma, secrecy, and suicidality among suicide attempt survivors. *Suicide and Life-Threatening Behavior*, 50, 706–713.

McHugh, C. M. and Large, M. M. 2020. Can machine-learning methods really help predict suicide? *Current Opinion in Psychiatry*, 33, 369–374.

Meehl, P. E. 1973. Why I do not attend case conferences. In: *Psychodiagnosis: Selected Papers*. Minneapolis: University of Minnesota Press, pp. 225–302.

Mew, E. J., Padmanathan, P., Konradsen, F., Eddleston, M., Chang, S.-S., Phillips, M. R. and Gunnell, D. 2017. The global burden of fatal self-poisoning with pesticides 2006–15: systematic review. *Journal of Affective Disorders*, 219, 93–104.

Michaud, L., Dorogi, Y., Gilbert, S. and Bourquin, C. 2021. Patient perspectives on an intervention after suicide attempt: the need for patient centred and individualized care. *PLoS ONE*, 16, e0247393.

Michel, K. and Jobes, D. A. 2011. *Building a Therapeutic Alliance with the Suicidal Patient*. Washington, DC: American Psychological Association.

Milner, A., Spittal, M. J., Pirkis, J. and Lamontagne, A. D. 2013. Suicide by occupation: systematic review and meta-analysis. *British Journal of Psychiatry*, 203, 409–416.

Moran, P., Coffey, C., Romaniuk, H., Olsson, C., Borschmann, R., Carlin, J. B. and Patton, G. C. 2012. The natural history of self-harm from adolescence to young adulthood: a population-based cohort study. *Lancet*, 379, 236–243.

Mulder, R., Newton-Howes, G. and Coid, J. W. 2016. The futility of risk prediction in psychiatry. *British Journal of Psychiatry*, 209, 271–272.

NCISH 2017. *The National Confidential Inquiry into Suicide and Homicide by People with Mental Illness. Annual Report: England, Northern Ireland, Scotland and Wales.* Manchester: University of Manchester.

NICE 2011. *Self-Harm in Over 8s: Long-Term Management (CG133).* London: National Institute for Health and Care Excellence.

NICE 2012. *Self-Harm: The NICE Guideline on Longer-Term Management.* London: The British Psychological Society and The Royal College of Psychiatrists.

Nicholas, A., Pirkis, J. and Reavley, N. 2020. What responses do people at risk of suicide find most helpful and unhelpful from professionals and non-professionals? *Journal of Mental Health.* DOI: 10.1080/ 09638237.2020.1818701.

Obegi, J. H. 2021. How common is the denial of suicidal ideation? A literature review. *General Hospital Psychiatry*, 72, 92–95.

Paris, J. 2021. Can we predict or prevent suicide? An update. *Preventive Medicine*, 152, 1–5.

Patel, V. 2015. Addressing social injustice: a key public mental health strategy. *World Psychiatry*, 14, 43–44.

Pokorny, A. D. 1983. Prediction of suicide in psychiatric patients: report of a prospective study. *Archives of General Psychiatry*, 40, 249–257.

Pompili, M., Murri, M. B., Patti, S., Innamorati, M., Lester, D., Girardi, P. and Amore, M. 2016. The communication of suicidal intentions: a meta-analysis.

Psychological Medicine, 46, 2239–2253.

Power, M. 2004. *The Nature of Risk: The Risk Management of Everything.* London: Demos.

Preti, A. 2011. Do animals commit suicide? Does it matter? *Crisis*, 32, 1–4.

Rahman, M. S. and Kapur, N. 2014. Quality of risk assessment prior to suicide and homicide (letter). *Psychiatric Bulletin*, 38, 46–47.

Reynolds, V. 2016. Hate kills: a social justice response to 'suicide'. In: J. C. White, I. Marsh, M. J. Kral and J. S. Morris (eds.), *Critical Suicidology: Re-thinking Suicide Research and Prevention for the 21st Century.* Vancouver, BC: UBC Press, pp. 169–187.

Rogers, M. L., Ringer, F. B. and Joiner, T. E. 2018. The association between suicidal ideation and lifetime suicide attempts is strongest at low levels of depression. *Psychiatry Research*, 270, 324–328.

Ross, E. L., Zuromski, K. L., Reis, B. Y., Nock, M. K., Kessler, R. C. and Smoller, J. W. 2021. Accuracy requirements for cost-effective suicide risk prediction among primary care patients in the US. *JAMA Psychiatry*, 78, 642–650.

Ross, N. E., Ciuffetelli, G. and Rozel, J. S. 2020. Legal concerns after a patient suicide. *Current Psychiatry*, 19, 22–23.

Royal College of Psychiatrists 2020. *Self-Harm and Suicide in Adults: Final Report of the Patient Safety Group (College Report CG229).* London: RCPsych.

Rudd, M. D. and Roberts, L. W. 2019. Assessment of suicide risk. In: L. W. Roberts (ed.), *Textbook of Psychiatry*, 7th ed. Washington, DC: American Psychiatric Association Publishing, pp. 91–110.

Ryan, C. J., Callaghan, S. and Large, M. 2015a. The importance of

least restrictive care: the clinical implications of a recent High Court decision on negligence. *Australasian Psychiatry*, 23, 415–417.

Ryan, C. J., Large, M., Gribble, R., Macfarlane, M., Ilchef, R. and Tietze, T. 2015b. Assessing and managing suicidal patients in the emergency department. *Australasian Psychiatry*, 23, 513–516.

Sanati, A. 2021. Interview, Matthew Large. *BJPsych Bulletin*, 45, 190–192.

Schultz, D. T. 2000. Defending suicide-related malpractice cases: a lawyer's perspective. *Journal of Psychiatric Practice*, 6, 345–348.

Shaffer, D. and Fisher, P. 1981. The epidemiology of suicide in children and young adolescents. *Journal of the American Academy of Child Psychiatry*, 20, 545–565.

Silverman, M. M. and Berman, A. L. 2014. Training for suicide risk assessment and suicide risk formulation. *Academic Psychiatry*, 38, 526–537.

Silverman, M. M. and Maris, R. W. 1995. The prevention of suicidal behaviors: an overview. *Suicide and Life-Threatening Behavior*, 25, 10–21.

Solano, P., Pizzorno, E., Pompili, M., Serafini, G. and Amore, M. 2018. Conceptualizations of suicide through time and socio-economic factors: a historical mini-review. *Irish Journal of Psychological Medicine*, 35, 75–86.

Soper, C. A. 2018. *The Evolution of Suicide.* Cham: Springer.

Soper, C. A. 2019a. Adaptation to the suicidal niche. *Evolutionary Psychological Science*, 5, 454–471.

Soper, C. A. 2019b. Beyond the search for *suigiston*: how evolution offers oxygen for suicidology. In: V. Zeigler-Hill and T. K. Shackelford (eds.), *Evolutionary Perspectives on Death.* Cham: Springer, pp. 37–61.

Soper, C. A. 2021. *The Evolution of Life Worth Living: Why We Choose to Live*. Cambridge, UK: Author.

Soper, C. A. 2022. Ethological problems with the interpersonal theory of suicide. *OMEGA – Journal of Death and Dying*. DOI: 10.1177/00302228211073010

St John-Smith, P., Michael, A. and Davies, T. 2009. Coping with a coroner's inquest: a psychiatrist's guide. *Advances in Psychiatric Treatment*, 15, 7–16.

Steeg, S., Quinlivan, L., Nowland, R., Carroll, R., Casey, D., Clements, C., Cooper, J., Davies, L., Knipe, D. and Ness, J. 2018. Accuracy of risk scales for predicting repeat self-harm and suicide: a multicentre, population-level cohort study using routine clinical data. *BMC Psychiatry*, 18, 113.

Stone, D. M., Simon, T. R., Fowler, K. A., Kegler, S. R., Yuan, K., Holland, K. M., Ivey-Stephenson, A. Z. and Crosby, A. E. 2018. Vital signs: trends in state suicide rates – United States, 1999–2016 and circumstances contributing to suicide – 27 states, 2015. *Morbidity and Mortality Weekly Report*, 67, 617–624.

Syme, K. L. and Hagen, E. H. 2018. When saying 'sorry' isn't enough: is some suicidal behavior a costly signal of apology? A cross-cultural test. *Human Nature*, 30, 117–141.

Syme, K. L., Garfield, Z. H. and Hagen, E. H. 2016. Testing the bargaining vs. inclusive fitness models of suicidal behavior against the ethnographic record. *Evolution and Human Behavior*, 37, 179–192.

Szmukler, G. and Rose, N. 2013. Risk assessment in mental health care: values and costs. *Behavioral Sciences & the Law*, 31, 125–140.

Taylor, A. K., Steeg, S., Quinlivan, L., Gunnell, D., Hawton, K. and Kapur, N. 2021. Accuracy of individual and combined risk-scale items in the prediction of repetition of self-harm: multicentre prospective cohort study. *BJPsych Open*, 7, E2.

Ten Have, M., De Graaf, R., Van Dorsselaer, S., Verdurmen, J., Van'T Land, H., Vollebergh, W. and Beekman, A. 2009. Incidence and course of suicidal ideation and suicide attempts in the general population. *Canadian Journal of Psychiatry*, 54, 824–833.

Tishler, C. L. and Reiss, N. S. 2009. Inpatient suicide: preventing a common sentinel event. *General Hospital Psychiatry*, 31, 103–109.

Tooby, J. and Cosmides, L. 1990. The past explains the present: emotional adaptations and the structure of ancestral environments. *Ethology and Sociobiology*, 11, 375–424.

Tromans, S., Umar, A., Torr, J., Alexander, R. and Bhaumik, S. 2020. Depressive disorders in people with intellectual disability. In: R. Alexander and S. Bhaumik (eds.), *Oxford Textbook of the Psychiatry of Intellectual Disability*. Oxford: Oxford University Press, pp. 105–116.

Turecki, G. and Brent, D. A. 2016. Suicide and suicidal behaviour. *Lancet*, 387, 1227–1239.

Undrill, G. 2007. The risks of risk assessment. *Advances in Psychiatric Treatment*, 13, 291–297.

Wand, T. 2011. Investigating the evidence for the effectiveness of risk assessment in mental health care. *Issues in Mental Health Nursing*, 33, 2–7.

Weinberg, S. 2015. *To Explain the World: The Discovery of Modern Science*. New York: Harper Collins.

Westers, N. J. 2020. 25 years of suicide research and prevention: how much has changed? *Clinical Child Psychology and Psychiatry*, 25, 729–733.

White, J. C., Marsh, I., Kral, M. J. and Morris, J. S. 2016. Rethinking suicide. In: J. C. White, I. Marsh, M. J. Kral and J. S. Morris (eds.), *Critical Suicidology: Re-thinking Suicide Research and Prevention for the 21st Century*. Vancouver, BC: UBC Press, pp. 2–11.

WHO 2014. *Preventing Suicide: A Global Imperative*. Geneva: World Health Organization.

WHO 2014. *Suicide Worldwide in 2019: Global Health Estimates*. Geneva: World Health Organization.

Williams, D. 2021. Socially adaptive belief. *Mind & Language*, 36, 333–354.

Wyder, M., Ray, M. K., Russell, S., Kinsella, K., Crompton, D. and Van Den Akker, J. 2021. Suicide risk assessment in a large public mental health service: do suicide risk classifications identify those at risk? *Australasian Psychiatry*, 29, 322–325.

Yang, B. and Lester, D. 2021. Is there a natural suicide rate? An update and review. *Suicide Studies*, 2, 5–12.

Zortea, T. C., Cleare, S., Melson, A. J., Wetherall, K. and O'Connor, R. C. 2020. Understanding and managing suicide risk. *British Medical Bulletin*, 134, 73–84.

Zou, W., Tang, L. and Bie, B. 2021. The stigmatization of suicide: a study of stories told by college students in China. *Death Studies*. DOI: 10.1080/07481187.2021.1958396

Evolutionary Perspectives on Schizophrenia Spectrum Disorders

Martin Brüne

Abstract

The term 'schizophrenia' refers to a group of disorders that seem to occur worldwide, with clinical pictures being strikingly similar across cultures. Evolutionary explanations of these disorders are warranted for at least two reasons: the first concerns their prevalence in all known ethnicities; the second relates to the need to explain the paradox as to why the conditions are maintained despite the greatly decreased fecundity of the affected individuals. Accordingly, a plethora of heterogeneous hypotheses – unparalleled among other psychiatric disorders – have been put forth, some of which deal with genetic considerations, others with environmental risk factors, and a few consider the adaptive advantages associated with the genes that predispose to schizophrenia. None of the evolutionary scenarios has the potential to account for the diversity of the symptomatology or to cover all of the biological and non-biological aspects of schizophrenia or schizophrenia spectrum disorders. This chapter aims at discussing the most relevant evolutionary hypotheses of schizophrenia, arguing that a symptom-based approach to psychotic disorders from an evolutionary perspective may improve upon the existing models of schizophrenia.

Keywords

dysconnectivity, genetics, human evolution, immunology, schizophrenia, social cognition, symptom-related approach, trade-off

Key Points

- Schizophrenia is a severe mental illness that occurs worldwide and is associated with a reduction in life expectancy and reproductive success.
- The evolutionary questions as to why genes predisposing to or associated with schizophrenia are maintained in human gene pools remain unresolved.
- Among the most plausible scenarios, genes conferring increased risk for schizophrenia are preserved because they have been sexually selected or are relevant for immune function.
- Another hypothetical scenario links the signs and symptoms associated with schizophrenia to the manipulatory action of intracellular parasites such as *Toxoplasma gondii*.
- Finally, due to its clinical heterogeneity, a symptom-based approach to elucidate the

evolutionary history of schizophrenia may be more informative than the attempt to search for holistic explanations.

10.1 Introduction

The term 'schizophrenia' (literally: 'split mind') was coined by the Swiss psychiatrist Eugen Bleuler in opposition to the accepted expression 'dementia praecox' ('premature dementia'). Bleuler considered ambivalence, autism (not to be confused with childhood autism, which was introduced several decades later), affective flattening and disordered thinking (loosening of associations) as the core symptoms of the schizophrenias (note the plural that Bleuler always emphasised; Bleuler, 1911). Current diagnostic manuals such as the Diagnostic and Statistical Manual, Version 5 (DSM-5; American Psychiatric Association, 2013) define schizophrenia by (1) the presence of delusions, (2) hallucinations, (3) disorganised thinking, (4) disorganised or abnormal motor behaviour, including catatonic features, and (5) negative symptoms such as affective flattening or inappropriate affect. A diagnosis can be made if at least two of these five main domains are fulfilled, of which one must be (1), (2) or (3). The symptoms must have been present for at least six months, including a one-month active phase during which delusions, hallucinations or disorganisation must have been prominent. DSM-5 has dropped the distinction between different subtypes of schizophrenia and has introduced instead a dimensional rating of the primary symptoms (American Psychiatric Association, 2013).

Schizophreniform disorder applies to psychotic states that do not fulfil the time criterion for schizophrenia but are otherwise identical to schizophrenia. However, a diagnosis of schizophreniform disorder also does not require impaired social or occupational functioning (prodromal states may fall into this category). The debate over the relationship of schizoaffective disorder and delusional disorder with schizophrenia has still not been settled, though both still belong to the broader phenotypic spectrum of schizophrenia. Delusional disorder is rare (at least in clinical settings) and has some commonalities with schizophrenia (abnormal content of thought), but it also overlaps to some extent with obsessive-compulsive disorder (preoccupation with improbable beliefs). Finally, cycloid psychoses (brief psychotic disorders) are associated with symptoms of the schizophrenia spectrum but differ in terms of their episodic course and good prognosis.

The heterogeneity of the clinical pictures of schizophrenia and schizophrenia spectrum disorders is underscored by the fact that none of the symptoms mentioned above is pathognomonic or specific to schizophrenia. This is critical to keep in mind, specifically when discussing evolutionary hypotheses of schizophrenia. Attempts to define endophenotypes of schizophrenia on the basis of biological or behavioural markers (Jablensky, 2006) have largely failed, even though there is some evidence for a neurodevelopmental subtype of schizophrenia characterised by motor abnormalities such as clumsy movements and other neurological soft signs since early childhood (Murray, 1994).

Most traditional textbooks of psychiatry still reiterate the false dogma of a stable 1% prevalence

of schizophrenia across populations, despite mounting evidence that there is much more variation in prevalence rates (McGrath, 2006). Schizophrenia usually becomes manifest in late adolescence or young adulthood (Jennen-Steinmetz et al., 1997), with sex differences in onset and a male to female ratio of about 1.2 to 1.0 (DeLisi et al., 1997). Even in developed countries, the life expectancy of people with schizophrenia is reduced by about 14.5 years compared to the general population (Hjorthøj et al., 2017). In addition, a puzzling finding is that fecundity, particularly in men with schizophrenia, is reduced by at least 50%.

These largely undisputed facts about schizophrenia call for evolutionary explanations because the prevalence of schizophrenia is far higher than can be explained by random mutation. Moreover, the grossly reduced reproductive success of individuals with schizophrenia would predict that, over time, genes predisposing to schizophrenia would be eliminated from the gene pool, but no such evidence exists. Further questions from an evolutionary point of view refer to the age of manifestation and environmental risk factors, which do not seem to be adequately appreciated by mainstream psychiatry in terms of possible causality. Accordingly, this chapter highlights the most relevant evolutionary enquiries into the aetiology and pathogenesis of schizophrenia, structured along Tinbergen's four levels of explanations (for details, see Chapter 1).

10.2 Proximate Factors Involved in Schizophrenia

10.2.1 Ontogeny

Several non-evolutionary hypotheses about environmental risk factors for schizophrenia concern childhood adversity (Khashan et al., 2008; Wahlbeck et al., 2001) or use of illicit drugs (Patel et al., 2020) and are not explicitly discussed here. It is worth recognising that wild, unguarded speculations about a familial causation of schizophrenia can potentially be harmful. The 'schizophrenogenic mother' is perhaps the most infamous example (discussed in Parker, 1982).

Evolutionary developmental hypotheses of schizophrenia have focused on 'developmental instability' models, suggesting that schizophrenia may result from an incapacity to 'buffer' the negative effects of multiple mutations, pathogens and toxins. In line with this proposition, 'fluctuating asymmetry' (FA), defined as the degree of asymmetry of bilateral characters that are, on average, symmetrical in the population, has been found to be larger in twin pairs concordant for schizophrenia than in discordant pairs. This could suggest that genetic or environmental factors lead to an imprecise expression of the developmental design (i.e. greater FA; Yeo et al., 1999). Consistent with the FA hypothesis, individuals with schizophrenia seem to display a greater number of minor physical abnormalities, including hypertelorism, greater homozygosity of blood alleles, lower premorbid intelligence, reduced cortical volume and instability of functional and anatomical lateralisation of brain functions.

Other evolutionarily based developmental hypotheses have highlighted the possibility that a delay in brain maturation could cause abnormal brain lateralisation, a finding that has been discussed intensely in the case of schizophrenia (Crow, 1999; Saugstad, 1999). According to this hypothesis, attenuated brain development may be associated with reduced dendritic branching, dysfunctional intra- and interhemispheric connectivity and connectivity and a diminished number of neurons due to a prolonged pruning process (reviewed in Burns, 2004). Indeed, as Burns (2004) has argued, schizophrenia may be considered as a trade-off for the evolution of social intelligence in primates, associated with an increase in cortical connectivity among frontotemporal pathways emerging some 5–6 million years ago. A relatively recent, hitherto unknown mutation during human evolution may have caused greater vulnerability to disruption of brain connectivity (Burns, 2004).

The developmental considerations are consistent with the typical time of onset of schizophrenia, whereby developmental insults during foetal cell migration become clinically manifest in adolescence or early adulthood when myelination is due to complete. Moreover, sexual dimorphism in myelination (with boys maturing later) may account for sex differences in the onset of psychosis due to a prolonged period of enhanced susceptibility in males compared to females (Randall, 1998).

However, none of these evolutionary developmental hypotheses are entirely consistent with clinical phenotypes and genetics, although they offer plausible and testable ways to study the neurodevelopmental subtypes of schizophrenia (reviewed in Mittal et al., 2007).

10.2.2 Mechanisms

10.2.2.1 Genetic and Epigenetic Hypotheses

It remains undisputed that schizophrenia is highly heritable, with concordance rates in monozygotic twins of about 48% (Owen et al., 2007). In addition, adoption studies suggest that shared genetics are more relevant than shared environments (Karlsson, 1968; Kety et al., 1994; Tienari et al., 2000), whereby individuals with a higher genetic risk are also more vulnerable to adverse life events (Tienari et al., 2004).

Genetic linkage studies have found susceptibility loci for schizophrenia on almost every single chromosome, including the sex chromosomes, but replication of findings in different populations has proven difficult (Badner and Gershon, 2002; Bailer et al., 2002; Hung et al., 2001; Kim et al., 1999; Laval et al., 1998; Sanders et al., 2008). A large genome-wide association study (GWAS) identified 108 independent loci putatively conveying genetic risk for schizophrenia (Schizophrenia Working Group of the Psychiatric Genomics Consortium, 2014). The search for candidate genes has produced a plethora of findings that are too numerous to clearly grasp. Genes involved in dopamine and glutamate turnover seem to play a role (Schizophrenia Working Group of the Psychiatric Genomics Consortium, 2014), as well as polymorphic variations of genes encoding neurotrophins and DISC1 (which is disrupted in schizophrenia; McGlashan and Hoffman, 2000; Sei et al., 2007). In addition, a functional genomics approach proposes that genes encoding DISC1, transcription factor 4 (TCF4), myelin basic protein (MBP) and a heat-shock protein (HSPA1B) are important candidate genes involved in schizophrenia (Ayalew et al., 2012). DISC1 plays a role in neurodevelopment and MBP in myelination, whereas TCF4 is expressed in the immune system as well as in neurons, and HSPA1B is involved in stress-response mechanisms. Another GWAS has identified a locus on chromosome 6 near a region coding for the major histocompatibility complex, emphasising the role of the immune system in the pathogenesis of schizophrenia (Flint and Munafò, 2014).

The search for genetic factors involved in schizophrenia is interesting from an evolutionary point of view because researchers have long believed that they could identify single genes with large effect sizes. Indeed, the idea was that some genetic factor would convey a survival and reproductive advantage in individuals who are heterozygous carriers of such vulnerability genes, whereas the homozygous carriers would express the phenotype of schizophrenia (Huxley et al., 1964). This model, known as 'balanced polymorphism', is well established for a few monogenetic recessive diseases such as sickle cell-associated anaemia, where heterozygous carriers of the allele are better protected against malaria infection than non-carriers, but with fatal consequences for individuals who are homozygous (i.e. having two copies of the gene; Alison, 1954). As regards schizophrenia, studies suggesting higher survival rates of offspring from families with one parent with schizophrenia, greater resistance to infectious diseases or diminished risk for accidents in relatives of people with the condition have not been replicated (reviewed in Brüne, 2004).

One intensely discussed evolutionary hypothesis, put forth by T. J. Crow in the 1990s, is worth summarising because it tried to cover many clinical aspects as well as biological markers associated with schizophrenia. In a nutshell, Crow's idea was that a single gene was involved in the evolution of human language by regulating the establishment of hemispheric dominance. Accordingly, schizophrenia could be a by-product of the 'speciation event', implying that *Homo sapiens* appeared due to a sudden (saltatorial) genetic event rather than by gradual evolution (Crow, 1990, 1995). Empirical support for Crow's hypothesis comprises findings in children who later develop psychosis disorders. They are more often ambidextrous and have more language disorders and behavioural disturbances than children who as adults do not become psychotic. In addition, pre-psychotic children more frequently have poorer reading abilities and perform more poorly in tasks requiring lateralised hand skills relative to control subjects, suggesting that psychosis-related developmental disturbances may be associated with a delayed or incomplete establishment of hemispheric dominance (Crow et al., 1996). Other anatomical findings concern reduced cerebral asymmetry in schizophrenia patients compared with controls (Goldstein et al., 2002).

Crow proposed that, given that the genomes of chimpanzees and humans differ only in around 1.5% of base pairs, a crucial incident must have happened since the time that these two species split from a common ancestor some 5 million years ago. Provided that the incidence rates of 'core' schizophrenia were cross-culturally similar, the mutation in question must have occurred before *Homo sapiens* left Africa, perhaps 150,000 years ago. As regards the locus of this gene, Crow argued that if such a gene allows the hemispheres to develop independently from one another to a certain degree, and if males and females differ with respect to their cerebral asymmetry (which they actually do), then sexual selection may be involved in hemispheric specialisation, suggesting that the gene would sit on a homologous X–Y locus (Kim et al., 1999). Indeed, there is evidence to suggest that a chromosomal region was transposed at some point during hominid evolution from the X to the Y chromosome after the splitting of the human and the chimpanzee lines, with subsequent deletions and inversions at this locus. Crow therefore speculated that a gene called '*Protocadherin XY*' could be involved in establishing hemispheric dominance (Laval et al., 1998), but an association of schizophrenia with this chromosomal region has not been confirmed (DeLisi et al., 2000). In summary, Crow's hypothesis (updated by Crow to include epigenetic regulation of the *Protocadherin XY* gene; Crow, 2012) has largely been refuted on genetic as well as clinical grounds, even though it has some merits as it rigorously applies evolutionary thinking to a psychiatric condition. However, the search for the oligogenetic underpinnings of schizophrenia have proven unsuccessful.

From an evolutionary genetics point of view, findings from large GWASs are more compatible with the idea that the genetic risk for schizophrenia arises from the accumulation of alleles each of which is infrequent in the population but that are collectively very common across loci. Thus, according to this 'watershed model', if a certain number of such unfavourable alleles is surpassed, brain dysfunction may be more likely to occur as a functional correlate of this genetic risk situation (Keller and Miller, 2006).

While again speculative and not specific for schizophrenia, evolutionarily guided genetic studies have revealed that positive selection may play a role. Indeed, the genes coding for DISC1, dysbindin and neuregulin may have been positively selected for during human evolution (Bord, 2006; Crespi et al., 2007). Likewise, genes involved in brain metabolism that are also associated with an increased risk for schizophrenia seem to have undergone positive selection (Khaitovich et al., 2008). More recent studies based on GWASs have concluded, however, that positive selection or adaptive introgression of Neanderthal genes does not play a major role in the genetic risk for schizophrenia. Instead, it has been shown that common variants associated with schizophrenia largely occur in chromosomal regions under strong background selection. In fact, in regions under strong selection pressure, genes with large deleterious effects are removed by negative selection. This reduces genetic diversity in these regions, such that genes with small deleterious effects can prevail via genetic drift (Pardiñas et al., 2018). Similarly, Liu et al. (2019) observed strong negative selection of genes associated with a risk for schizophrenia in anatomically modern humans compared to archaic human species (Neanderthals and Denisovans), which has recently been corroborated by Yao et al. (2020), who observed positive selection only in a minority of genes associated with schizophrenia.

Whatever the precise evolutionary mechanism underlying the risk for schizophrenia may be, at present no convincing model exists, which is not entirely unexpected in light of the vast variation of the clinical phenotype.

Aside from genetic studies, an intriguing epigenetic hypothesis concerning schizophrenia suggests that genomic imprinting may account for clinical aspects of the syndrome, especially when viewed in contrast to autism. Genomic imprinting results from differential methylation of male or female DNA. Indeed, from an evolutionary point of view, there is conflict between the maternal and paternal genes of the embryo over the amount of maternal investment. More specifically, it seems to be in the interest of paternally inherited genes to extract a greater amount of resources than is optimal for the mother. Maternally inherited genes, in contrast, may be selected to allow the embryo to extract resources at a rate closer to the mother's optimum. While genomic imprinting pertains to perhaps 1% of the genome, it is often involved in the regulation of somatic growth, mainly targeting

the placenta, but also affecting the brain. Imbalanced expression of imprinted genes in the brain has been demonstrated for Prader–Willi syndrome and Angelman syndrome, where a deletion of a particular part of the DNA located on the long arm of chromosome 15 in one parent may lead to the expression of only maternal or paternal genes. While maternally inherited genes cause Prader–Willi syndrome, characterised by poor sucking and weak crying in infants, paternal imprinting causes Angelman syndrome, which shows some opposite features compared to Prader–Willi syndrome. Akin to the case of these syndromes, Crespi and Badcock (2008) have argued that genomic imprinting may cause autism (associated with brain overgrowth) when paternally imprinted genes prevail, whereas schizophrenia could arise from maternally imprinted genes leading to undergrowth of certain brain areas. This hypothesis has some charm, as it is compatible with some biological features of autism and schizophrenia and also with studies indicating a common genetic vulnerability of these syndromes (e.g. van Os and Kapur, 2009; also see Chapter 15 of this volume), but it is still far from being generally accepted.

10.2.2.2 Social Stress

A substantial proportion of the risk factors for schizophrenia is non-genetic. Specifically, the observation that changes in social environments caused by migration, isolation, loss in social rank or the break-up of a romantic relationship can contribute to the manifestation of schizophrenia is not new (Cantor-Graae and Selten, 2005; Odegaard, 1932; Zelt, 1981). There is also evidence to suggest that schizophrenia is more frequent in urban compared with rural environments (Krabbendam and van Os, 2005), and the impact of migration increases the risk for schizophrenia in at least the first and second generations (Cantor-Graae and Selten, 2005). This has strikingly been shown in the indigenous population of Papua New Guinea, where the incidence of schizophrenia sharply increased with greater intensity of contact with Western civilisation and migration to Western settlements (Torrey et al., 1974). These non-genetic risk factors for schizophrenia make perfect sense from an evolutionary point of view, considering the divergence of modern from ancestral environments (see Chapter 1). Indeed, the anthropological record indicates that humans lived in small-scale communities for most of their evolutionary history and that xenophobic attitudes towards strangers were common. Following up on this thread, Abed and Abbas (2011) have argued that schizophrenia could reflect an extreme of variation of 'out-group intolerance'; that is, (genetically) vulnerable individuals exposed to novel (or adverse) social-environmental conditions brought about by migration, urbanicity, poverty or ostracism may be at risk of developing schizophrenia (Abed and Abbas, 2011, 2014). Testable predictions deriving from this hypothesis comprise higher rates of schizophrenia in males (due to greater exposure to groups of other males), migration to a different cultural background, social exclusion and changing role models during adolescence. Concerning the first prediction, the content of persecutory delusions has been found to differ between men and women regarding the number and sex of persecutors, as well as regarding the degree of familiarity with the perceived persecutors. Specifically, in a study involving a German and a Russian sample of patients with schizophrenia, men more often felt threatened by groups of strange males, whereas women more often felt persecuted by individuals from their personal environment (Zolotova and Brüne, 2006). Abed and Abbas' (2011, 2014) out-group intolerance hypothesis is also compatible with ethological studies of schizophrenia. Studies into the non-verbal behaviour of patients with schizophrenia have revealed signs of heightened vigilance towards potential threats from others and a desire for greater interpersonal distance. Moreover, analyses of patients' non-verbal behaviour indicate more frequent 'cut-off' behaviours, submissive gestures, flight and motivational ambivalence, suggestive of social defeat or entrapment, whereas paranoid patients tend to display signals of social threat such as 'staring' (Annen et al., 2012; Brüne et al., 2008; Krause et al., 1989; McGuire and Polsky, 1979; Pitman et al., 1987; Troisi et al., 1998, 2007).

Together, evolutionary hypotheses concerning non-genetic risk factors for schizophrenia are consistent with the idea that social stress features among the most relevant issues, whereby the specificity of these factors for schizophrenia needs to be carved out in greater detail.

10.2.2.3 Immunological Hypotheses

A large number of studies have examined the hypothesis of an association between intrauterine exposure to infectious agents and the risk of developing neuropsychiatric disorders, including schizophrenia – an approach that has recently received greater attention in relation to the SARS-CoV-2 pandemic (recently summarised in Zimmer et al., 2021). In fact, Menninger (1926) was among the first to propose that the influenza pandemic in the first decades of the twentieth century was causally involved in the risk of schizophrenia, among other neuropsychiatric diseases. A reformulation considering the prenatal exposure to infectious material and postnatal risk for schizophrenia has become known as the 'two-hit' hypothesis (Bayer et al., 1999). Accordingly, a 'first hit' would be a prenatal insult (infectious or nutritional; as regards the latter, see, for instance, the literature on the aftermath of the 'Dutch Hunger Winter'; Susser and Lin, 1992), whereas a 'second hit' would affect a developmentally vulnerable brain (for a recent critique, see Davis et al., 2016). Similarly, it has been suggested that many cases of schizophrenia may arise from chronic ('mild') encephalitis (Bechter, 2013).

Aside from viral hypotheses, another intriguing infectious model of schizophrenia concerns the idea that a latent infection with *Toxoplasma gondii* may account for a large number of cases worldwide (Delgado García and García Landa, 1979). It is estimated that about 2 billion people worldwide are infected with *T. gondii*. In most cases the infection is clinically silent; however, risk of infection with *T. gondii* is heavily impacted by the genetic make-up of one's major histocompatibility complex (Blanchard et al., 2015), a factor to be considered in the case of schizophrenia (Flint and Munafò, 2014).

T. gondii is a protozoic agent that infects warm-blooded animals. The protozoon has a complex life cycle, with cats (Felidae) being the definitive host for its sexual reproduction. Through defecation, oocysts in cat faeces can infect intermediate hosts by oral ingestion of contaminated soil or water, but intake of raw or undercooked meat and sexual intercourse can also lead to infection. In intermediate hosts, *T. gondii* reproduces asexually. The then-developing bradyzoites travel to the brain, heart, muscle tissue and other organs, where they build cysts and remain for the host's lifetime. The reproductive cycle of *T. gondii* closes when felines feed on infected animals through predation.

The most interesting aspect that makes this model highly interesting in terms of its possible role in schizophrenia, at least from a theoretical perspective, relates to *T. gondii*'s potential to actively manipulate the intermediate host's behaviour for its own reproductive benefit. Rodents infected with *T. gondii*, for example, show increased levels of activity and strikingly 'careless' behaviour. They lose their innate avoidance of the odour of cat urine and instead seem to approach locations containing cat (urine) odour in a nearly 'suicidal' manner, thus increasing their risk of predation (for an overview, see Flegr, 2007).

As regards schizophrenia, at least 40 studies have demonstrated significantly elevated immunoglobulin G antibody serum levels against *T. gondii*. Conversely, individuals who possess *T. gondii* antibodies have a 2.7-fold elevated risk for schizophrenia compared to antibody-naïve subjects (Torrey et al., 2007). How the risk for schizophrenia interacts with genetics is unknown, but the association seems plausible in light of the role of immunologically relevant genes that are considered crucial to the pathogenesis of schizophrenia (Flint and Munafò, 2014). In any event, the risk for schizophrenia associated with *T. gondii* infection exceeds the risk conveyed by any single gene putatively involved in schizophrenia (Webster et al., 2013).

Animal studies suggest that *T. gondii* impacts the host's dopamine turnover and glutamatergic pathways, another facet that is consistent with the prevailing neurotransmitter models of schizophrenia (Howes et al., 2015). Even the behavioural phenotype of schizophrenia is reconcilable with the idea that manipulation by *T. gondii* could be involved. Most researchers have proposed that human *T. gondii* infection is 'accidental' (Flegr, 2007; Kano et al., 2020; Webster et al., 2013). However, this is not so certain when viewed from an evolutionary point of view, especially in light of reports suggesting that chimpanzees – our closest extant relatives – lose their fear of leopard urine when infected with *T. gondii* (Poirette et al., 2016). In the case of humans as targets, the primary manipulatory goal of *T. gondii* may not be the loss of fear of cat odour (though coincidentally olfaction is compromised in humans infected with *T. gondii*); rather, the manipulatory action of *T. gondii* in humans may aim at exclusion from the social community. This seems plausible because in highly social species like *Homo sapiens* individuals may have borne the greatest risk of predation in ancestral environments when isolated from the social group. Indeed, it is generally accepted that the survival of early humans was only possible through the formation of cooperative social groups (Tomasello, 2014). Accordingly, I have proposed elsewhere that a significant number of cases of schizophrenia could be the phenotypic correlate of parasitic manipulation by *T. gondii* that ultimately promotes social exclusion (Brüne, 2019). In fact, many 'core' symptoms associated with schizophrenia support this idea. For example, the conviction of being manipulated by some unknown agent is clinically deemed as 'delusional', while doctors seldom take into consideration that there might be a kernel of truth in the patients' perceptions. Along similar lines, schizophrenia-associated cognitive, particularly social-cognitive impairments lead patients to believe that others have malevolent intentions, thus giving way to paranoid ideation and causing social withdrawal or aggression against the perceived perpetrator, which ultimately promotes active or passive marginalisation of the individual. With regards to negative symptoms, affective flattening, apathy and abulia cause rejection from others, and many patients fail to experience social interaction as rewarding (Lee et al., 2018). Moreover, catatonia resembles disrupted fight-or-flight mechanisms (such as stupor being akin to tonic immobility; Moskowitz, 2004). Together, the typical signs and symptoms associated with schizophrenia can be interpreted in ways supporting the idea that they serve the parasite's biological interests (i.e. to increase the risk of predation for its host by forcing the individual to leave or be expelled from their social community). Even though speculative, the hypothesis that manipulative parasites may play a role in the origin of schizophrenia is in stark contrast to other evolutionary views suggesting that there might be a hitherto undiscovered selective advantage of the schizophrenia phenotype itself that explains the maintenance of 'risk genes' in the human gene pool, which is discussed in the next section.

10.3 Evolutionary Factors Involved in Schizophrenia

10.3.1 Phylogeny

As far as is known to date, there is no evidence to suggest that schizophrenia or anything similar exists in non-human animals. This is entirely different from mood disorders, obsessive-compulsive disorder or post-traumatic stress disorder, of which homologous syndromes have been described in non-human primates, although mainly in captivity rather than in natural surroundings (e.g. Brüne et al., 2006; Ferdowsian et al., 2012, 2013). There is also a body of literature on animal models of schizophrenia (e.g. Juckel et al., 2011) that largely seek to mimic the 'two-hit' model by producing inflammatory reactions in the offspring of pregnant rodents. While this approach has produced some insights into inflammatory signals and behavioural correlates of impaired neurodevelopment, it does not have the potential to account for the entire (heterogeneous) phenotype that we refer to as schizophrenia(s). Put another way, the cognitive, emotional and behavioural requisites for the full picture of schizophrenia to develop seem to rely on quite uniquely human brain functions. An intriguing hypothesis about schizophrenia-associated symptoms – foremost auditory hallucinations – was put forth by the psychologist Julian Jaynes some 45 years ago (Jaynes, 1976). According to the hypothesis of the 'bicameral mind', consciousness and self-reflectivity emerged late in human evolution – just a few thousand years ago. Prior to that, the right and the left hemispheres acted more independently from one another ('bicameral'), whereby the right hemisphere produced command hallucinations upon which behaviour was enacted, whereas the left hemisphere was necessary for language production. In the state of the 'bicameral mind', hallucinated voices were necessarily perceived as 'alien'. With the advent of written language, the distribution of labour between the two hemispheres was no longer required, such that the 'breakdown' of the 'bicameral mind' initiated the ability for conscious reflection and self-awareness. Schizophrenia, by analogy, was hypothesised to resemble more closely a state of 'bicameral' brain activity (Jaynes, 1976). While there is no room for an extensive discussion of Jaynes' hypothesis, it seems very unlikely that a cultural event (the invention of written language) had such an impact on biological (brain) evolution. There is also little evidence to suggest that language evolved slowly with commands arising 40,000 years ago, nouns some 25,000 years ago and names not until 10,000 years before present, as suggested by Jaynes (1976).

Tracing back the first case of schizophrenia in evolutionary history is a futile endeavour simply because the heterogeneity of the syndrome precludes simple mono-causal explanations. It is nevertheless worth exploring the question of the possible adaptive value of selected features of schizophrenia.

10.3.2 Adaptive Value

As already pointed out in the introductory paragraphs to this section, there is unequivocal evidence that individuals with schizophrenia have a reduced life expectancy and fewer offspring compared to the general population. However, these may be the by-products of traits that are adaptive. As regards the first issue, in most countries the difference in longevity in comparison to the population mean is about 14.5 years, with men facing a greater loss of years than women (Hjorthøj et al., 2017). If this would be compensated for by a larger number of offspring, one could argue that there was a trade-off between early reproduction and longevity, but this is not the case. Instead, the fecundity of individuals with schizophrenia is greatly reduced (Power et al., 2013), and there is evidence to suggest that infant mortality among children of mothers or fathers with schizophrenia is twice that of the general population (Nilsson et al., 2008). In addition, brothers of individuals with schizophrenia also have fewer offspring compared to the general population (Power et al., 2013), and the same is true for the offspring of individuals with schizophrenia (Svensson et al., 2007), suggesting that there is probably no indirect adaptive value or 'heterozygosity advantage' (as discussed in Section 10.2.2.1). Indeed, this possibility has been debated for some time. For example, Kellett (1973) speculated that schizotypy may be associated with a reproductive advantage by establishing territoriality, in which more prosocial individuals would often fail. Along similar lines, other evolutionarily informed hypotheses have argued for the adaptive advantages of 'diluted' phenotypes of the schizophrenia spectrum, including greater selfishness (Allen and Sarich, 1998), shamanism and religious leadership (Polimeni and Reiss, 2002, 2003), 'Odyssean' personality (Jarvik and Deckard, 1977) or group-splitting behaviour (Stevens and Price, 2000). Specifically, Stevens and Price (2000) suggested that the genetic susceptibility to developing schizophrenia emerged as an adaptation to facilitate group splitting. This hypothesis is based on the assumption that, under ancestral conditions, human social groups inevitably tended to split up at some point, whereby the capacity to replace old belief systems with new ones would be characteristic of cult leaders and people with schizophrenia. Together, these hypotheses emphasised an adaptive value of 'asocial' behaviour. Indirect evidence comes from more recent accounts suggesting that schizophrenia could reflect 'low-fitness variants' of sexually selected traits (Shaner et al., 2004). Del Giudice (2010) has presented a mathematical model according to which the neutral or even positive selection of the schizoptypical traits that may be associated with greater mating success through superior verbal creativity could compensate for the reduced fertility rate of individuals with schizophrenia. This approach is interesting as it links the idea of an adaptive advantage for individuals with 'diluted' phenotypes of schizophrenia with the long-debated issue of creativity. Indeed, data from Iceland, which is supposed to have had a fairly stable gene pool over centuries, suggest an exceptional creative potential in relatives of psychotic individuals (Karlsson, 1968), although this is stronger for relatives of individuals with bipolar affective disorder than schizophrenia (Post, 1994). Isaac Newton and John Nash are two famous examples of such, and a son of Albert Einstein was affected by schizophrenia (for an overview, see Polimeni and Reiss, 2003). Recent research suggests that women seem to prefer creative over wealthy men as short-term partners, whereby creativity may serve as a fitness indicator (Haselton and Miller, 2006), though this finding is based on a relatively small sample size. Moreover, Lawn et al. (2019) report that genetic liability to schizophrenia may confer greater mating success (i.e. number of sexual partners) but not greater fitness in terms of number of offspring. Together, these studies seem to support the role of sexual selection in traits associated with schizophrenia and potentially explain why this group of disorders is maintained in populations (Del Giudice, 2017).

10.4 Discussion

A large number of articles have explored the evolutionary 'enigma' of schizophrenia (Brüne,

2004). The key question is why the condition has prevailed in humans in spite of the low fecundity and premature deaths of affected individuals. Put another way, natural selection should have eliminated the genetic liability to schizophrenia if the reproductive disadvantage was not compensated for by anything else that directly or indirectly affects the survival or reproduction of individuals carrying these genes, which, theoretically, embraces people with schizophrenia themselves and their genetically close relatives.

This chapter has sought to summarise the most important evolutionary hypotheses of schizophrenia (Table 10.1). At present, none of these evolutionary hypotheses sufficiently accounts for the preservation of genes predisposing to schizophrenia, sex differences in the age at its onset and its multifaceted symptomatology. Indeed, one of the most difficult problems is that there is no sign, symptom or biochemical or structural marker that is pathognomonic (i.e. specific) to schizophrenia. This fact alone makes it extremely unlikely that any one evolutionary hypothesis has the potential to explain all of the possible phenotypes subsumed under the term 'schizophrenia(s)'.

Whether this entails abandoning the clinical concept of schizophrenia altogether, as suggested by Bentall et al. (1988), is open to debate. In any event, the loss of the diagnostic differentiation promoted by DSM-5 may not be the best solution. Conversely, subtyping schizophrenia could be a fruitful approach specifically within an evolutionary perspective. As Beckmann and Franzek (2000) have pointed out, when looking at Leonhard's classification of schizophrenia (Leonhard, 2003), systematic catatonia is rather sporadic, whereas periodic catatonia runs in families and is largely genetically determined. Moreover, cycloid psychoses and systematic schizophrenias emerge largely due to environmental insults, whereas unsystematic schizophrenias are predominantly inherited. However, this classification is almost unknown outside of German-speaking psychiatry and has not succeeded; it is a classic example of the problem associated with 'splitting' (i.e. Leonhard) versus 'lumping' (DSM-5).

An alternative to the evolutionary analyses of complex phenotypes could be the examination of individual signs and symptoms, such as paranoia, catatonia, etc. Such an approach would not only endorse the concept of continua rather than

Table 10.1. Evolutionary hypotheses about schizophrenia organised according to Tinbergen's four questions

Four areas of biology		Two objects of explanation	
Two kinds of explanation	*Proximate* Explains how organisms work by describing mechanisms and their ontogeny	*Ontogeny* Developmental instability (Yeo et al., 1999) Slow maturation (Saugstad, 1999)	*Mechanism* Genetic morphism (Huxley et al., 1964) 'Watershed' model (Keller and Miller, 2006) Negative selection (Liu et al., 2019; Yao et al., 2020) Genomic imprinting (Crespi and Badcock, 2008) Price for language (Crow, 1995) Dysconnectivity (Burns, 2004) Parasitic manipulation (Flegr, 2007)
	Evolutionary Explains how a trait came to its current form and how variations were influenced by selection and other evolutionary factors	*Phylogeny* Bicameral mind (Jaynes, 1976)	*Adaptive significance* Sexually selected trait, including creativity (Del Giudice, 2017; Haselton and Miller, 2006; Karlsson, 1968; Shaner et al., 2004) Positive selection of genes associated with schizophrenia (Bord, 2006; Crespi et al., 2007; Khaitovich et al., 2008) Out-group intolerance (Abed and Abbas, 2011, 2014) Eccentricity/shamanism (Polimeni and Reiss, 2002, 2003; Stevens and Price, 2000) Reduced cancer risk (Preti and Wilson, 2011)

Modified after Medicus (2015) and Nesse (2013).

disease entities in psychiatry but also be compatible with more observation-driven, evolutionary, 'bottom-up' analyses, but at the cost of difficulties in associating individual symptoms or clusters of signs and symptoms (i.e. syndromes) with genetics (Brüne, 2002). Evolutionary approaches recognise that many psychological (and somatic) dysfunctions may arise due to a mismatch of modern environmental conditions with the ancestral world to which our human mind once adapted (Nesse, 2005). Other signs and symptoms may be regarded as trade-offs (or design flaws) because 'optimality' in nature is non-existent (otherwise evolution would not happen). As such, many psychotic symptoms and syndromes may be considered trade-offs, primarily manifesting themselves in domains related to the evolution of our 'social brain' (Abed and Abbas, 2011; Burns, 2004).

For instance, 'out-group intolerance' (Abed and Abbas, 2011, 2014) may be associated with

heightened vigilance for potential social threat, misinterpretation of social signals as malicious, jumping to conclusions and a bias against disconfirmatory evidence (Moritz and Woodward, 2006). Aside from formal thought disorders and cognitive distortions, many aspects pertaining to the content of delusional beliefs appear to be tightly linked to scenarios that were selectively important in humanity's evolutionary past. The uniformity of delusional content across cultures suggests that universal patterns relating to survival and reproduction are mirrored in delusions. As already noted in Section 10.2.2.2, the content of persecutory delusions has been found to differ between men and women regarding the number and sex of persecutors, as well as regarding the degree of familiarity with the perceived persecutor. Specifically, men seem to more often feel threatened by groups of strange males, whereas women more often identify potential persecutors from within their personal environment as potential persecutors. Paranoid men and women both primarily report fears of being physically injured or assaulted. The rationale for these sex differences in persecutory delusional content could be that the main sources of ancestral threats for men in the environment of evolutionary adaptedness (see Chapter 1) were indeed strange males from other tribes; by contrast, women who under ancestral conditions formed the nucleus of cooperative social groups were perhaps more threatened by ostracism and social exclusion (Zolotova and Brüne, 2006). From a phylogenetic point of view, territorial competition and warfare between troops of rivalling male chimpanzees have been reported to be highly prevalent, perhaps partly corresponding to the competitive struggle for existence in ancestral human societies (Wrangham, 1999). In addition, in extant hunter-gatherer or horticultural societies, up to 25% of males and some 13% of females die in combat or through other violent interactions (Radcliffe-Brown, 1948; Schiefenhövel, 1995).

Along the same lines, delusions relating to mating effort and reproduction differ markedly between men and women, with remarkable similarities across cultures. These differences, in part, are based on sex differences in parental investment. Since women invest more than men in potential offspring, females are usually choosier in terms of mate choice. Conversely, as paternity is less certain than maternity, male vigilance towards female infidelity was strongly selected. Regarding delusional disorders, these divergent selection pressures are strikingly mirrored in erotomania, the delusional conviction of being loved by another person, which typically occurs in women, and delusional jealousy, typically a male delusion (Brüne, 2003). In cases of erotomania, women typically choose socially high-ranking men (politicians, physicians, actors, sportsmen, etc.) onto whom they project their romantic beliefs. In contrast, delusional jealousy in men aims at retaining partners and securing their sexual fidelity.

Catatonia is equally interesting from an evolutionary point of view because it seems to reflect, in part, ancient mechanisms associated with fight-or-flight responses. For example, catatonic stupor resembles primitive fear reactions akin to the tonic immobility ('playing dead') observed in many animal species (Abrams et al., 2009; Kretschmer, 1926/1960; Moskowitz, 2004). Tonic immobility occurs in animals upon impending predatory threat, particularly in situations in which flight is precluded. The animal stops moving and shows heightened vigilance and analgesia, followed by a ferocious struggle to escape. The latter resembles catatonic agitation. With regards to the autonomic nervous system, tonic immobility can be associated with an initial increase in heart rate that can suddenly drop below baseline. Such autonomic instability can also accompany catatonic stupor (Ostermann et al., 2013). Other catatonic signs including waxy flexibility, automatic obedience, *mitgehen* and *mitmachen*, which can be interpreted as contextually abnormal submissive behaviours. Catatonic stupor is often indistinguishable from dissociative states, which may occur in situations that trigger the re-experience of traumatic insults or other situations associated with unbearably intense fear (Shilo et al., 1995).

10.5 Conclusions

Evolutionary hypotheses about schizophrenia are abundant, but many are difficult to test. Problems relate to the heterogeneity of the phenotypic picture (Pearlson and Folley, 2008), the vague boundaries between psychosis and 'normalcy' (van Os et al., 1999) and the uncertain diagnostic validity of the 'core' symptoms, as reflected in recent changes from DSM-IV to DSM-5. It may be more appropriate to study individual symptoms, symptom clusters or endophenotypes rather than choosing a broad phenotypic concept for evolutionary enquiries (Brüne, 2004). On the other hand, there is a need for addressing 'open' genetic questions in order to resolve the 'Devil's triangle' of high heritability, high prevalence and low reproductive fitness (Doi et al., 2009). There is also the possibility that up to a third of cases of schizophrenia are aetiologically related to immunological processes, including parasitic manipulation by *T. gondii* (Flegr, 2007).

Evolutionary approaches to psychiatric disorders show great promise, first due to their theoretical empirical testability and second because, currently, evolutionary theory provides the only credible meta-theory and scientific framework that has the potential to integrate diverse findings from studies into the genetics, brain imaging, biochemistry and psychotherapeutic aspects of schizophrenia.

References

Abed, R. T. and Abbas, M. J. (2011). A reformulation of the social brain theory for schizophrenia: the case for out-group intolerance. *Perspectives in Biology and Medicine*, 54, 132–151.

Abed, R. T. and Abbas, M. J. (2014). Can the new epidemiology of schizophrenia help elucidate its causation? *Irish Journal of Psychological Medicine*, 31, 1–5.

Abrams, M. P., Carleton, R. N., Taylor, S. and Asmundson, G. J. (2009). Human tonic immobility: measurement and correlates. *Depression and Anxiety*, 26, 550–556.

Allen, J. S. and Sarich, V. M. (1998). Schizophrenia in an evolutionary perspective. *Perspectives in Biology and Medicine*, 32, 132–153.

Allison, A. C. (1954). Protection afforded by the sickle cell trait against subtertian malarial infection. *British Medical Journal*, 1, 290–294.

American Psychiatric Association (2013). *Diagnostic and Statistical Manual of Mental Disorders – DSM-5 Handbook of Differential Diagnosis*. Arlington, VA: American Psychiatric Association.

Annen, S., Roser, P. and Brüne, M. (2012). Non-verbal behavior during clinical interviews: similarities and dissimilarities between schizophrenia, mania, and depression. *Journal of Nervous and Mental Disease*, 200, 26–32.

Ayalew, M., Le-Niculescu, H., Levey, D. F. et al. (2012). Convergent functional genomics of schizophrenia: from comprehensive understanding to genetic risk prediction. *Molecular Psychiatry*, 17, 887–905.

Badner, J. A. and Gershon, E. S. (2002). Meta-analysis of whole-genome linkage scans of bipolar disorder and schizophrenia. *Molecular Psychiatry*, 7, 405–411.

Bailer, U., Leisch, F., Meszaros, K. et al. (2002). Genome scan for susceptibility loci for schizophrenia and bipolar disorder. *Biological Psychiatry*, 52, 40–52.

Bayer, T. A., Falkai, P. and Maier, W. (1999). Genetic and nongenetic vulnerability factors in schizophrenia: the basis of the 'two hit hypothesis'. *Journal of Psychiatric Research*, 33, 543–554.

Bechter, K. (2013). Updating the mild encephalitis hypothesis of schizophrenia. *Progress in Neuropsychopharmacology & Biological Psychiatry*, 42, 71–91.

Beckmann, H. and Franzek, E. (2000). The genetic heterogeneity of 'schizophrenia'. *World Journal of Biological Psychiatry*, 1, 35–41.

Bentall, R. P., Jackson, H. F. and Pilgrim, D. (1988). Abandoning the concept of 'schizophrenia': some implications of validity arguments for psychological research into psychotic phenomena. *British Journal of Clinical Psychology*, 27, 303–324.

Blanchard, N., Dunay, I. R. and Schlüter, D. (2015). Persistence of *Toxoplasma gondii* in the central nervous system: a fine-tuned balance between the parasite, the brain and the immune system. *Parasite Immunology*, 37, 150–158.

Bleuler, E. (1911). *Dementia praecox oder die Gruppe der Schizophrenien*. Leipzig: Deutike.

Bord, L., Wheeler, J., Paek, M. et al. (2006). Primate disrupted-in-schizophrenia-1 (DISC1): high divergence of a gene for major mental illnesses in recent evolutionary history. *Neuroscience Research*, 56, 286–293.

Brüne, M. (2002). Towards an integration of interpersonal and biological processes: evolutionary psychiatry as an empirically testable framework for psychiatric research. *Psychiatry*, 65, 48–57.

Brüne M. (2003). Social cognition and behaviour in schizophrenia. In *The Social Brain: Evolution and Pathology*, M. Brüne, H. Ribbert and W. Schiefenhövel (eds.). Chichester: John Wiley and Sons, pp. 277–313.

Brüne, M. (2004). Schizophrenia – an evolutionary enigma? *Neuroscience and Biobehavioral Reviews*, 28, 41–53.

Brüne, M. (2019). Latent toxoplasmosis: host–parasite interaction and psychopathology. *Evolution Medicine and Public Health*, 2019, 212–213.

Brüne, M. and Schiefenhövel, W. (eds.) (2019). *Oxford Handbook of Evolutionary Medicine*. Oxford: Oxford University Press.

Brüne, M., Brüne-Cohrs, U., McGrew, W. C. and Preuschoft, S. (2006). Psychopathology in great apes: concepts, treatment options and possible homologies to human psychiatric disorders. *Neuroscience and Biobehavioral Reviews*, 30, 1246–1259.

Brüne, M., Sonntag, C., Abdel-Hamid, M. et al. (2008). Non-verbal behavior during standardized interviews in patients with schizophrenia spectrum disorders. *Journal of Nervous and Mental Disease*, 196, 282–288.

Burns, J. K. (2004). An evolutionary theory of schizophrenia: cortical connectivity, metarepresentation, and the social brain. *Behavioral and Brain Sciences*, 27, 831–855; discussion 855–885.

Cantor-Graae, E. and Selten, J. P. (2005). Schizophrenia and migration: a meta-analysis and review. *American Journal of Psychiatry*, 162, 12–24.

Crespi, B. and Badcock, C. (2008). Psychosis and autism as

diametrical disorders of the social brain. *Behavioral and Brain Sciences*, 31, 241–320.

Crespi, B., Summers, K. and Dorus, S. (2007). Adaptive evolution of genes underlying schizophrenia. *Proceedings, Biological Sciences*, 274, 2801–2810.

Crow, T. J. (1990). The continuum of psychosis and its genetic origin. The sixty-fifth Maudsley Lecture. *British Journal of Psychiatry*, 156, 788–797.

Crow, T. J. (1995). A Darwinian approach to the origins of psychosis. *British Journal of Psychiatry*, 167, 12–25.

Crow, T. J. (1999). Commentary on Annett, Yeo et al., Klar, Saugstad and Orr: cerebral asymmetry, language and psychosis – the case for a *Homo sapiens*-specific sex-linked gene for brain growth. *Schizophrenia Research*, 39, 219–231.

Crow, T. J. (2012). Schizophrenia as variation in the *sapiens*-specific epigenetic instruction to the embryo. *Clinical Genetics*, 81, 319–324.

Crow, T. J., Done, D. J. and Sacker, A. (1995). Childhood precursors of psychosis as clues to its evolutionary origins. *European Archives of Psychiatry and Clinical Neuroscience*, 245, 61–69.

Crow, T. J., Done, D. J. and Sacker, A. (1996). Cerebral lateralization is delayed in children who later develop schizophrenia. *Schizophrenia Research*, 22, 181–185.

Davis, J., Eyre, H., Jacka, F. N. et al. (2016). A review of vulnerability and risks for schizophrenia: beyond the two hit hypothesis. *Neuroscience and Biobehavioral Reviews*, 65, 185–194.

Del Giudice, M. (2010). Reduced fertility in patients' families is consistent with the sexual selection model of schizophrenia and schizotypy. *PLoS ONE*, 5, e16040.

Del Giudice, M. (2017). Mating, sexual selection, and the evolution of schizophrenia. *World Psychiatry*, 16, 141–142.

Delgado García, G. and García Landa, J. (1979). [Reactivity of the intradermal test with toxoplasmosis in schizophrenic patients]. *Revista Cubana de Medicina Tropical*, 31, 225–231.

DeLisi, L. E. (1997). Gender and age at onset of schizophrenia. *British Journal of Psychiatry*, 171, 188.

DeLisi, L. E., Shaw, S., Sherrington, R. et al. (2000). Failure to establish linkage on the X chromosome in 301 families with schizophrenia or schizoaffective disorder. *American Journal of Medical Genetics*, 96, 333–341.

Doi, N., Hoshi, Y., Itokawa, M. et al. (2009). Persistence criteria for susceptibility genes for schizophrenia: a discussion from an evolutionary viewpoint. *PLoS ONE*, 4, e7799.

Ferdowsian, H., Durham, D. and Brüne, M. (2013). Mood and anxiety disorders in chimpanzees: a response to Rosati et al. (2012). *Journal of Comparative Psychology*, 127, 337–340.

Ferdowsian, H. R., Durham, D. L., Johnson, C. M. et al. (2012). Signs of generalized anxiety and compulsive disorders in chimpanzees. *Journal of Veterinary Behavior: Clinical Applications and Research*, 7, 353–361.

Flegr, J. (2007). Effects of toxoplasma on human behavior. *Schizophrenia Bulletin*, 33, 757–760.

Flint, J. and Munafò, M. (2014). Schizophrenia: genesis of a complex disease. *Nature*, 511, 412–413.

Goldstein, J. M., Seidman, L. J., O'Brien, L. M. et al. (2002). Impact of normal sexual dimorphisms on sex differences in structural brain abnormalities in schizophrenia assessed by magnetic resonance imaging. *Archives of General Psychiatry*, 59, 154–164.

Haselton, M. G. and Miller, G. F. (2006). Women's fertility across the cycle increases the short-term attractiveness of creative intelligence. *Human Nature*, 17, 50–73.

Hjorthøj, C., Stürup, A. E., McGrath, J. J. et al. (2017). Years of potential life lost and life expectancy in schizophrenia: a systematic review and meta-analysis. *Lancet Psychiatry*, 4, 295–301.

Howes, O., McCutcheon, R. and Stone, J. (2015). Glutamate and dopamine in schizophrenia: an update for the 21st century. *Journal of Psychopharmacology*, 29, 97–115.

Hung, C. C., Chen, Y. H., Tsai, M. T. et al. (2001). Systematic search for mutations in the human tissue inhibitor of metalloproteinase-3 (TIMP-3) gene on chromosome 22 and association study with schizophrenia. *American Journal of Medical Genetics*, 105, 275–278.

Huxley, J., Mayr, E., Osmond, H. et al. (1964). Schizophrenia as a genetic morphism. *Nature*, 204, 220–221.

Jablensky, A. (2006). Subtyping schizophrenia: implications for genetic research. *Molecular Psychiatry*, 11, 815–836.

Jarvik, L. F. and Deckard, B. S. (1977) The Odyssean personality. A survival advantage for carriers of genes predisposing to schizophrenia? *Neuropsychobiology*, 3, 179–191.

Jaynes, J. (1976). *The Origin of Consciousness in the Breakdown of the Bicameral Mind*. Boston, MA: Houghton Mifflin.

Jennen-Steinmetz, C., Löffler, W. and Häfner, H. (1997). Demography and age at onset of schizophrenia. *British Journal of Psychiatry*, 170, 485–486.

Juckel, G., Manitz, M. P., Brüne, M. et al. (2011). Microglial activation in a neuroinflammational animal model of schizophrenia – a pilot study. *Schizophrenia Research*, 131, 96–100.

Kano, S. I., Hodgkinson, C. A., Jones-Brando, L. et al. (2020). Host–parasite interaction associated with major mental illness. *Molecular Psychiatry*, 25, 194–205.

Karlsson, J. L. (1968). Genealogic studies of schizophrenia. In *The Transmission of Schizophrenia*, D. Rosenthal and S. S. Kety (eds.). London: Pergamon Press, pp. 85–94.

Keller, M. C. and Miller, G. (2006). Resolving the paradox of common, harmful, heritable mental disorders: which evolutionary genetic models work best? *Behavioral and Brain Sciences*, 29, 385–404; discussion 405–452.

Kellett, J. M. (1973). Evolutionary theory for the dichotomy of the functional psychoses. *Lancet*, 1, 860–863.

Kety, S. S., Wender, P. H., Jacobsen, B. et al. (1994). Mental illness in the biological and adoptive relatives of schizophrenic adoptees. Replication of the Copenhagen Study in the rest of Denmark. *Archives of General Psychiatry*, 51, 442–455.

Khaitovich, P., Lockstone, H. E., Wayland, M. T. et al. (2008). Metabolic changes in schizophrenia and human brain evolution. *Genome Biology*, 9, R124.

Khashan, A. S., Abel, K. M., McNamee, R. et al. (2008). Higher risk of offspring schizophrenia following antenatal maternal exposure to severe adverse life events. *Archives of General Psychiatry*, 65, 146–152.

Kim, H. S., Wadekar, R. V., Takenaka, O. et al. (1999). *SINE-R.C2* (a *Homo sapiens* specific retroposon) is homologous to CDNA from postmortem brain in schizophrenia and to two loci in the Xq21.3/Yp block linked to handedness and psychosis. *American Journal of Medical Genetics*, 88, 560–566.

Krabbendam, L. and van Os, J. (2005). Schizophrenia and urbanicity: a major environmental influence – conditional on genetic risk. *Schizophrenia Bulletin*, 31, 795–799.

Krause, R., Steimer, E., Sanger-Alt, C. and Wagner, G. (1989). Facial expression of schizophrenic patients and their interaction partners. *Psychiatry*, 52, 1–12.

Kretschmer, E. (1926/1960). *Hysteria, Reflex, and Instinct.* New York: Philosophical Library.

Laval, S. H., Dann, J. C., Butler, R. J. et al. (1998). Evidence for linkage to psychosis and cerebral asymmetry (relative hand skill) on the X chromosome. *American Journal of Medical Genetics*, 81, 420–427.

Lawn, R. B., Sallis, H. M., Taylor, A. E. et al. (2019). Schizophrenia risk and reproductive success: a Mendelian randomization study. *Royal Society Open Science*, 6, 181049.

Lee, J., Jimenez, A. M., Reavis, E. A. et al. (2018). Reduced neural sensitivity to social vs nonsocial reward in schizophrenia. *Schizophrenia Bulletin*, 45, 620–628.

Leonhard, K. (2003). *Aufteilung der endogenen Psychosen und ihre differenzierte Ätiologie*, 8th ed. Stuttgart/New York: Georg Thieme Verlag.

Liu, C., Everall, I., Pantelis, C. et al. (2019). Interrogating the evolutionary paradox of schizophrenia: a novel framework and evidence supporting recent negative selection of schizophrenia risk alleles. *Frontiers in Genetics*, 10, 389.

McGlashan, T. H. and Hoffman, R. E. (2000). Schizophrenia as a disorder of developmentally reduced synaptic connectivity. *Archives of General Psychiatry*, 57, 637–648.

McGrath, J. J. (2006). Variations in the incidence of schizophrenia: data versus dogma. *Schizophrenia Bulletin*, 32, 195–197.

McGuire, M. T. and Polsky, R. H. (1979). Behavioral changes in hospitalized acute schizophrenics. An ethological perspective. *Journal of Nervous and Mental Disorders*, 167, 651–657.

Medicus, G. (2015). *Being Human. Bridging the Gap between the Sciences of Body and Mind.* Berlin: Verlag für Wissenschaft und Bildung.

Menninger, K. A. (1926). Influenza and schizophrenia: an analysis of post-influenzal 'dementia praecox,' as of 1918, and five years later. *American Journal of Psychiatry*, 82, 469–529.

Mittal, V. A., Dhruv, S., Tessner, K. D. et al. (2007). The relations among putative biorisk markers in schizotypal adolescents: minor physical anomalies, movement abnormalities, and salivary cortisol. *Biological Psychiatry*, 61, 1179–1186.

Moritz, S. and Woodward, T. S. (2006). A generalized bias against disconfirmatory evidence in schizophrenia. *Psychiatry Research*, 142, 157–165.

Moskowitz, A. K. (2004). 'Scared stiff': catatonia as an evolutionary-based fear response. *Psychological Review*, 111, 984–1002.

Murray, R. M. (1994). Neurodevelopmental schizophrenia: the rediscovery of dementia praecox. *British Journal of Psychiatry. Supplement*, (25), 6–12.

Nesse, R. M. (2005). Maladaptation and natural selection. *Quarterly Review of Biology*, 80, 62–70.

Nesse, R. M. (2013). Tinbergen's four questions, organized: a response to Bateson and Laland. *Trends in Ecology and Evolution*, 28, 681–682.

Nilsson, E., Hultman, C. M., Cnattingius, S. et al. (2008). Schizophrenia and offspring's risk for adverse pregnancy outcomes and infant death. *British Journal of Psychiatry*, 193, 311–315.

Odegaard, O. (1932). Emigration and insanity: a study of mental disease among the Norwegian-born population of Minnesota. *Acta Psychiatrica Scandinavica*, 4, 1–206.

Ostermann, S., Herbsleb, M., Schulz, S. et al. (2013). Exercise reveals the interrelation of physical fitness, inflammatory response, psychopathology, and autonomic function in patients with schizophrenia. *Schizophrenia Bulletin*, 39, 1139–1149.

Owen, M. J., Craddock, N. and Jablensky, A. (2007). The genetic deconstruction of psychosis. *Schizophrenia Bulletin*, 33, 905–911.

Pardiñas, A. F., Holmans, P., Pocklington, A. J. et al. (2018). Common schizophrenia alleles are enriched in mutation-intolerant genes and in regions under strong background selection. *Nature Genetics*, 50, 381–389.

Parker, G. (1982). Re-searching the schizophrenogenic mother. *Journal of Nervous and Mental Disease*, 170, 452–462.

Patel, S., Khan, S., Saipavankumar, M. et al. (2020). The association between cannabis use and schizophrenia: causative or curative? A systematic review. *Cureus*, 12, e9309.

Pearlson, G. D. and Folley, B. S. (2008). Schizophrenia, psychiatric genetics, and Darwinian psychiatry: an

evolutionary framework. *Schizophrenia Bulletin*, 34, 722–733.

Pitman, R. K., Kolb, B., Orr, S. P. and Singh, M. M. (1987). Ethological study of facial behavior in nonparanoid and paranoid schizophrenic patients. *American Journal of Psychiatry*, 144, 99–102.

Poirotte, C., Kappeler, P. M., Ngoubangoye, B. et al. (2016). Morbid attraction to leopard urine in *Toxoplasma*-infected chimpanzees. *Current Biology*, 26, R98–R99.

Polimeni, J. and Reiss, J.P. (2002). How shamanism and group selection may reveal the origins of schizophrenia. *Medical Hypotheses*, 58, 244–248.

Polimeni, J. and Reiss J.P. (2003). Evolutionary perspectives on schizophrenia. *Canadian Journal of Psychiatry*, 48, 34–39.

Post, F. (1994). Creativity and psychopathology. A study of 291 world-famous men. *British Journal of Psychiatry*, 165, 22–34.

Power, R. A., Kyaga, S., Uher, R. et al. (2013). Fecundity of patients with schizophrenia, autism, bipolar disorder, depression, anorexia nervosa, or substance abuse vs their unaffected siblings. *JAMA Psychiatry*, 70, 22–30.

Preti, A. and Wilson, D. R. (2011). Schizophrenia, cancer and obstetric complications in an evolutionary perspective – an empirically based hypothesis. *Psychiatry Investigations*, 8, 77–88.

Radcliffe-Brown, A. R. (1948). *The Andaman Islanders: A Study in Social Anthropology*. Cambridge: Cambridge University Press.

Randall, P. L. (1998). Schizophrenia as a consequence of brain evolution. *Schizophrenia Research*, 30, 143–148.

Sanders, A. R., Duan, J., Levinson, D. F. et al. (2008). No significant association of 14 candidate genes with schizophrenia in a large

European ancestry sample: implications for psychiatric genetics. *American Journal of Psychiatry*, 165, 497–506.

Saugstad, L.F. (1999). A lack of cerebral lateralization in schizophrenia is within the normal variation in brain maturation but indicates late, slow maturation. *Schizophrenia Research*, 39, 183–196.

Schiefenhövel, W. (1995). Aggression und Aggressionskontrolle am Beispiel der Eipo aus dem Hochland von West-Neuguinea. In *Töten im Krieg*, H. von Stietencron and J. Rüpke (eds.). Freiburg/München: Verlag Karl Alber, pp. 339–362.

Schizophrenia Working Group of the Psychiatric Genomics Consortium (2014). Biological insights from 108 schizophrenia-associated genetic loci. *Nature*, 511, 421–427.

Sei, Y., Ren-Patterson, R., Li, Z. et al. (2007). Neuregulin1-induced cell migration is impaired in schizophrenia: association with neuregulin1 and catechol-o-methyltransferase gene polymorphisms. *Molecular Psychiatry*, 12, 946–957.

Shaner, A., Miller, G. and Mintz, J. (2004). Schizophrenia as one extreme of a sexually selected fitness indicator. *Schizophrenia Research*, 70, 101–109.

Shiloh, R., Schwartz, B., Weizman, A. and Radwan, M. (1995). Catatonia as an unusual presentation of posttraumatic stress disorder. *Psychopathology*, 28, 285–290.

Stevens, A. and Price, J. (2000). *Evolutionary Psychiatry. A New Beginning*, 2nd ed. New York: Routledge.

Susser, E. S. and Lin, S. P. (1992). Schizophrenia after prenatal exposure to the Dutch Hunger Winter of 1944–1945. *Archives of General Psychiatry*, 49, 983–988.

Svensson, A. C., Lichtenstein, P., Sandin, S. et al. (2007). Fertility of first-degree relatives of patients with schizophrenia: a three generation perspective. *Schizophrenia Research*, 91, 238–245.

Tienari, P., Wynne, L. C., Moring, J. et al. (2000). Finnish adoptive family study: sample selection and adoptee DSM-III-R diagnoses. *Acta Psychiatrica Scandinavica*, 101, 433–443.

Tienari, P., Wynne, L. C., Sorri, A. et al. (2004). Genotype–environment interaction in schizophrenia-spectrum disorder. Long-term follow-up study of Finnish adoptees. *British Journal of Psychiatry*, 184, 216–222.

Tomasello, M. (2014). The ultra-social animal. *European Journal of Social Psychology*, 44, 187–194.

Torrey, E. F., Bartko, J. J., Lun, Z. R. et al. (2007). Antibodies to *Toxoplasma gondii* in patients with schizophrenia: a meta-analysis. *Schizophrenia Bulletin*, 33, 729–736.

Torrey, E. F., Torrey, B. B. and Burton-Bradley, B. G. (1974). The epidemiology of schizophrenia in Papua New Guinea. *American Journal of Psychiatry*, 131, 567–573.

Troisi, A., Pompili, E., Binello, L. and Sterpone, A. (2007). Facial expressivity during the clinical interview as a predictor functional disability in schizophrenia. A pilot study. *Progress in Neuro-psychopharmacology and Biological Psychiatry*, 31, 475–481.

Troisi, A., Spalletta, G. and Pasini, A. (1998). Non-verbal behaviour deficits in schizophrenia: an ethological study of drug-free patients. *Acta Psychiatrica Scandinavica*, 97, 109–115.

van Os, J. and Kapur, S. (2009). Schizophrenia. *Lancet*, 374, 635–645.

van Os, J., Verdoux, H., Maurice-Tison, S. et al. (1999). Self-reported psychosis-like symptoms and the continuum of psychosis. *Social Psychiatry and Psychiatric Epidemiology*, 34, 459–463.

Wahlbeck, K., Osmond, C., Forsen, T., Barker, D. J. and Eriksson, J. G. (2001). Associations between childhood living circumstances and schizophrenia: a population-based cohort study. *Acta Psychiatrica Scandinavica*, 104, 356–360.

Webster, J. P., Kaushik, M., Bristow, G. C. et al. (2013). *Toxoplasma gondii* infection, from predation to schizophrenia: can animal behaviour help us understand human behaviour? *Journal of Experimental Biology*, 216, 99–112.

Wrangham, R. W. (1999). Evolution of coalitionary killing. *American Journal of Physical Anthropologu*, (29), 1–30.

Yao, Y., Yang, J., Xie, Y. et al. (2020). No evidence for widespread positive selection signatures in common risk alleles associated with schizophrenia. *Schizophrenia Bulletin*, 46, 603–611.

Yeo, R. A., Gangestad, S. W., Edgar, C., et al. (1999). The evolutionary genetic underpinnings of schizophrenia: the developmental instability model. *Schizophrenia Research*, 39, 197–206.

Zelt, D. (1981). First person account: the Messiah quest. *Schizophrenia Bulletin*, 7, 527–531.

Zimmer, A., Youngblood, A., Adnane, A. et al. (2021). Prenatal exposure to viral infection and neuropsychiatric disorders in offspring: a review of the literature and recommendations for the COVID-19 pandemic. *Brain Behavior, and Immunity*, 91, 756–770.

Zolotova, J. and Brüne, M. (2006). Persecutory delusions: reminiscence of ancestral hostile threats? *Evolution and Human Behavior*, 27, 185–192.

Evolutionary Perspectives on Eating Disorders

Riadh Abed and Agnes Ayton*

Abstract

The focus of this chapter is on evolutionary theories and models of anorexia nervosa (AN), bulimia nervosa (BN) and obesity. Although obesity is not considered a mental health problem, its link with binge eating disorder and its massively increased prevalence in recent decades, in association with modernisation and Westernisation together with increased morbidity and mortality, have stimulated much evolutionary theorising. Disorders of eating and weight are of particular interest to evolutionary scholars for a number of reasons. These include the claim that many of these disorders are evolutionarily novel, that they have increased in prevalence in developed countries in recent decades, that they have a large female preponderance, particularly of AN and BN, and that they have an increased risk of mortality. Our poor understanding of the aetiology of eating disorders together with poor outcomes (especially for AN) has been associated with a proliferation of proximate theories/models within mainstream psychiatry but without any one theory gaining wide acceptance. This presents an opportunity for evolutionary models to propose new ways of thinking and new avenues for research on these disorders. A review of the current evolutionary literature on AN and BN shows that despite the wide range and variety of models, the sexual competition hypothesis has, so far, had the strongest empirical support from clinical and non-clinical studies. While other evolutionary theories focus on AN, the sexual competition hypothesis provides an explanation for both AN and BN, as well as for the widespread dieting seen in the population. Furthermore, it uniquely makes sense of the specific presentations of eating disorders in males. Nevertheless, it seems increasingly clear that intrasexual competition is not the whole story. More recent work that considers other areas of mismatch in the modern environment represents a necessary extension to this theoretical perspective. It is concluded that larger-scale studies on clinical populations are required to put these theoretical formulations to the test and to explore their potential clinical utility.

Keywords

anorexia nervosa, bulimia nervosa, eating disorders, evolution, intrasexual competition, mismatch, obesity

Key Points

- The aetiology of eating disorders remains in contention despite the multitude of theories.
- The recent emergence/increase of eating disorders and obesity and their association with Westernisation and modernisation suggest an important role for mismatch in their causation. In females, the increase in intrasexual competition leads to a fear of weight gain and attempts at controlling weight to maintain a youthful appearance, whilst in males it can lead to the drive for muscularity.
- Evolutionary theories on eating disorders and obesity have attempted to identify the nature of this mismatch.
- Evolutionary theories on eating disorders and obesity demonstrate how understanding ultimate causation can guide and enhance our understanding of proximate causation.
- Future research into evolutionary theories on eating disorders and obesity could lead to novel interventions.

* We are grateful to David Geaney for reading and commenting on previous drafts of this chapter.

11.1 Introduction

The Diagnostic and Statistical Manual of Mental Disorders (DSM-5; American Psychiatric Association, 2013) classification of eating disorders (EDs) includes the following categories: anorexia nervosa (AN), bulimia nervosa (BN), binge eating disorder (BED) and avoidant and restrictive food intake disorders (ARFIDs), with partial or atypical syndromes labelled as OSFEDs (other specified feeding or eating disorders). The DSM-5 OSFEDs include atypical AN, sub-threshold BN, sub-threshold BED, purging disorder and night eating syndrome. The focus of this chapter will primarily be on AN and BN as these are the main categories of EDs that have

been discussed in the current evolutionary literature. We also briefly discuss evolutionary aspects of obesity, which is not included in DSM-5. However, obesity is linked with a number of mental disorders, including depression and EDs, particularly BED (e.g. Marcus and Wildes, 2012; Volkow and O'Brien, 2007). In this chapter, the term 'eating disorders' refers to AN and BN collectively, whereas obesity will be referred to separately.

The DSM-5 criteria for AN and BN are outlined in Boxes 11.1 and 11.2. It will be noted that AN and BN share core features of morbid fear of fatness, distorted body image and a pattern of behaviour aimed at weight reduction, including

---

Box 11.1 DSM-5 criteria for anorexia nervosa

(A) Restriction of energy intake relative to requirements, leading to a significantly low body weight in the context of age, sex, developmental trajectory and physical health. Significantly low weight is defined as a weight that is less than minimally normal or, for children and adolescents, less than that minimally expected.

(B) Intense fear of gaining weight or of becoming fat or persistent behaviour that interferes with weight gain even though at a significantly low weight.

(C) Disturbance in the way in which one's body weight or shape is experienced, undue influence of body weight or shape on self-evaluation or persistent lack of recognition of the seriousness of the current low body weight.

AN restricting type (AN-R): during the last three months, the individual has not engaged in recurrent episodes of binge eating or purging behaviour (i.e. self-induced vomiting or the misuse of laxatives, diuretics or enemas). This subtype describes presentations in which weight loss is accomplished primarily through dieting, fasting and/or excessive exercise.

AN binge eating/purging type (AN-BP): during the last three months, the individual has engaged in recurrent episodes of binge eating or purging behaviour (i.e. self-induced vomiting or the misuse of laxatives, diuretics or enemas).

Box 11.2 DSM-5 criteria for bulimia nervosa

(A) Recurrent episodes of binge eating. An episode of binge eating is characterized by both of the following:

   (1) Eating, in a discrete period of time (e.g. within any two-hour period), an amount of food that is definitely larger than what most individuals would eat in a similar period of time under similar circumstances.

   (2) A sense of lack of control over eating during the episode (e.g. a feeling that one cannot stop eating or control what or how much one is eating).

(B) Recurrent inappropriate compensatory behaviours in order to prevent weight gain, such as self-induced vomiting; misuse of laxatives, diuretics or other medications; fasting; or excessive exercise.

(C) The binge eating and inappropriate compensatory behaviours both occur, on average, at least once a week for three months.

(D) Self-evaluation is unduly influenced by body shape and weight.

(E) The disturbance does not occur exclusively during episodes of anorexia nervosa.

purging, restriction of food intake or excessive exercise – and this is also true for the International Classification of Diseases, 11th Revision (ICD-11) classification (World Health Organization, 2019). AN is characterized by malnutrition, whereas BN is associated with binge eating and various compensatory behaviours without significantly low body weight. The DSM-5 classifies AN into the restricting (AN-R) and binge eating/purging (AN-BP) subtypes (Box 11.1). AN and BN have a marked female preponderance, reported to be around 10:1 in clinical samples (Gordon, 1990), but this has been revised down to around 3:1 in population-based studies. BN is more common than AN in both females and males (Hudson et al., 2007; Qian et al., 2021). Nevertheless, those presenting for treatment are overwhelmingly female, and EDs have the highest female-to-male ratio of any psychiatric disorder.

AN is known to run a more chronic course, has a poorer prognosis compared to BN (Steinhausen, 2002) and is also associated with lower remission rates (50% for AN as opposed to 75% for BN) at 10-year follow-up (Keel and Brown, 2010). Both AN and BN can result in severe and debilitating physical consequences, such as electrolyte disturbances, infertility, worn tooth enamel, cardiac damage, brain damage or, in extreme cases, multi-organ failure (National Institute of Mental Health, 2020; Sugermeyer, 2020). However, it is important to note that these serious symptoms are the consequences of AN and BN (listed in Boxes 11.1 and 11.2) and are not the core symptoms of these disorders. It is of particular concern that AN has the highest mortality of any mental disorder of around 5.9–10.0% (Fichter and Quadflieg, 2016; Insel, 2012). In addition, the evidence suggests significant heritability of AN and BN (Bulik et al., 2019), with estimates of 33–84% for AN and of 28–83% for BN.

Besides the marked female preponderance, AN and BN show a number of distinctive epidemiological features, including the fact that they are both vastly more prevalent in Western, developed countries, particularly when considering sub-threshold phenotypes (Katzman et al., 2004), and there is evidence that there has been a significant increase in all EDs in recent decades (Russell, 2000; Wu et al., 2020). Furthermore, recent studies show that this increase is spreading

to developing countries in association with urbanisation and Westernisation (Erskine et al., 2016; Sugermeyer, 2020).

These rather puzzling features, together with the claim of their recent emergence, make EDs of particular interest to evolutionary scholars. The aim of the present chapter is to survey a range of extant evolutionary models of EDs and obesity. The models surveyed provide explanations at the ultimate or evolutionary level, which can be compatible with a range of proximate, non-evolutionary theories (Abed, 1998). Hence, the chapter will explore the evolutionary roots of EDs through an examination of both the phylogenetics and function of the presumed evolved psychological mechanisms involved in these disorders (Abed, in press; see also Chapter 1 of this volume). The large and diverse literature on proximate (non-evolutionary) models of EDs is beyond the remit of this chapter. Interested readers are advised to consult standard texts this literature.

11.2 Mismatch and Phylogenetic Roots of Female Competition

Evolutionary theories relating to AN and BN are generally distinct from those that focus on obesity. However, one common factor that connects most evolutionary explanations of disordered eating and weight regulation in the modern environment is that of evolutionary mismatch (see Chapters 1, 2 and 5; also see Table 11.1). The other evolutionary concepts relevant mostly to AN and BN are female competition, the theory of sexual selection and the evolution of the distinctive human mating system (Abed, 1998, in press).

The relevance of mismatch stems from the claim that all EDs are novel phenomena that have recently emerged specifically within modern, industrialised, Western societies (Rantala et al., 2019). Also relevant is the claim that BN is a disorder that first appeared in the second half of the twentieth century in developed, Western societies and that there had been a significant rise in the incidence of both AN and BN across the Western world over recent decades (Russell, 2000). Taken together, these observations support the view that EDs represent prime examples of 'Western diseases' or 'diseases of civilization' (Pollard, 2008) where evolutionary mismatch

Table 11.1 Summary of the main characteristics of selected evolutionary theories on eating disorders (source: Abed, in press)

	Mismatch	Female competition	Relevant to AN	Relevant to BN	Relevant to other EDs	Relevant to male syndromes	Supported by empirical evidence
Reproductive suppression hypothesis	Yes	Yes	Yes	No	No	No	Yes, non-clinical studies
Adapted to flee famine hypothesis	Yes	Possibly	Yes	No	No	No	No
Parental manipulation hypothesis	No	No	Yes	No	No	No	No
Insurance hypothesis	Yes	No	Yes	No	Yes (obesity)	No	No
Social threat hypothesis	Yes	Possibly	Yes	No	No	No	No
Sexual competition hypothesis	Yes	Yes	Yes	Yes	Possibly	Yes	Yes, clinical and non-clinical studies
Extended mismatch hypotheses	Yes	Yes	Yes	Yes	Yes	Yes	No

AN: anorexia nervosa; BN: bulimia nervosa; ED: eating disorder.

plays a significant role. Fiji provides an interesting example of this: there was a rapid increase of obesity and increasing rates of BN following the introduction of US trade agreements that introduced Westernised food and culture (Becker, 2004).

To understand mismatch, we should note that the human lineage lived for 99% of its evolutionary history in relatively small, mobile, foraging, kin-based groups (see Chapter 1). It is under these conditions that human psychological mechanisms were shaped by selection. The seeds for mismatch were sown with the advent of agriculture, which resulted in permanently settled living around 10,000–12,000 years ago, and this radically altered the human physical and social environment with major implications for EDs (Abed, 1998; Li et al., 2018).

Taking an evolutionary perspective brings into sharp relief how the modern human environment diverges from the ancestral environment in a number of important ways and that the interaction of evolved human psychological mechanisms with novel conditions can lead to maladaptive outcomes in some individuals. Examples of such novel conditions include: living in much higher population densities; living among many strangers; reduced levels of kin support; constant abundance of food; loss of seasonality due to international trade in the food industry; exposure to mass media images; and many others. For example, social and mass media in the modern environment present women with a steady stream of virtual, hyper-attractive females that can be mistaken for real competitors, and this 'super-normal stimulus' can lead to maladaptive and self-damaging competitive responses in some women (Yong et al., 2017; see Figure 1.1 for an illustration of mismatch in nutrition).

Other evolutionary processes relevant to EDs include the evolution of the distinctive human mating system, which helps us to understand the roots of female competition (Abed, in press). The universal and core feature of the human mating system is the pair-bond between a male and female. Despite the variety of social arrangements across human societies and through human history, marriage is common to all human societies and forms the public acknowledgement of who has sexual access to whom, with divorce often resulting from extramarital relationships (Marlowe, 2003).

It is important to note that the human mating system is distinctive and peculiar compared to those of all other great apes and has resulted in the evolution of a suite of psychological mechanisms to manage the challenges it presented. The distinctive feature of the human pair-bonded mating system was the evolution of paternal investment and male provisioning.

Studies of foragers provide evidence for the positive effects of paternal investment on reproductive success (fitness). For example, it has been shown that men provide 85% of the protein and 65% of the total calories (Kaplan et al., 2000; Marlowe, 2003), with positive effects on female fecundity and offspring immune function, health and survival (Gurven and Hill, 2009). It should be noted, however, that the effects of fathers on correlates of offspring fitness can vary across social and ecological contexts (e.g. Bribiescas et al., 2012).

It is these conditions in our evolutionary past that shaped female psychology to be sensitive to cues of ability and willingness to invest in offspring when assessing long-term mates, where traits such as kindness, industriousness and the ability to acquire resources became highly valued and attractive (Buss and Schmitt, 1993). These are the phylogenetic roots of the human mating system (specifically long-term mating strategies) that can help us to understand the origins of the distinctive human psychology related to mate attraction, retention and mate choice. It also demonstrates that these traits are evolutionarily novel and have emerged distinctively and uniquely within the human lineage as they are not shared by our closest primate relatives (chimpanzees and bonobos), let alone other mammals.

Importantly, the demands of the human pair-bonded mating system have impacted both male and female mate value but in different ways. In the promiscuous mating system of the chimpanzees and bonobos, where paternal investment/male provisioning is absent and all mating is short term, any ovulating female is worth copulating with from a male's perspective regardless of age and condition as the male investment in mating is trivial (Muller and Pilbeam, 2017). In contrast, in the human pair-bonded system, a male's fitness became dependent on his female mate's fertility and fidelity, and a female's fitness became related to her mate's ability and willingness to provide resources. Hence, the basis of the human mating system became an exchange of paternal investment in return for paternity assurance (Abed, in press).

Consequently, female reproductive potential (number of fertile years remaining) became a crucial indicator of female mate value as the longer a man could monopolise a given woman's reproductive years, the greater would be his fitness returns. Hence, men evolved a particular sensitivity to cues of high reproductive potential, primarily cues of youth and good health. In ancestral human environments, this constituted the nubile hourglass body shape with evidence of a thin waist and fat deposits in the breasts, thighs and buttocks, each of which is associated with increased fertility and forms the basis of the human sexual dimorphism (Jasienska et al., 2004). The epidemiological evidence for sexual dimorphism in humans is extensive. Sexual dimorphism in body composition is already evident in infancy: males tend to be heavier than females at birth and have longer bodies and larger head circumferences. By early adulthood, sexual dimorphism in fat distribution is highly evident (Pulit et al., 2017; see Section 11.3.3).

These are the evolutionary roots of male sensitivity to visual cues of female physical attractiveness and also of women's motivation to display, preserve and improve their physical attractiveness and thus increase their perceived mate value[1] (Sugiyama, 2016). The extreme end of this adaptation gives rise to the risk of EDs in the modern environment.

As a result, both females and males must compete with members of the same sex for access to high-quality and high-investing mates, as poor long-term mate choice can result in high fitness costs for both sexes. This has shaped a mating psychology of choosiness in both males and females, which is strikingly different from the relatively indiscriminate mating behaviour of chimpanzees and bonobos, where female competition for mates and male choosiness are either weak or absent (Parker, 1983).

While female competition in humans may appear less extravagant and more covert compared to males, research suggests that intrasexual competition among ancestral women was a significant determinant of reproductive success (Salmon, 2017). Therefore, men who paid close attention to the female's youth, health and other signs of fertility such as the nubile hourglass body shape and were able to monopolise the reproductive years of a female of high reproductive potential would have left more progeny than their rivals. Similarly, women who correctly evaluated men for their ability and willingness to acquire and provide resources and who successfully attracted and retained such men in long-term mateships (marriages) would have had greater reproductive success than their rivals (Abed, in press).

It should be added that while in the discussion thus far the emphasis has been on the evolution of psychological mechanisms governing the long-term human mating system, both men and women may simultaneously pursue a complementary strategy of short-term mating that can yield sex-specific fitness pay offs (Buss and Schmitt, 1993).

The remainder of the chapter will discuss specific evolutionary theories relevant to nutrition, weight and EDs.

11.3 Evolutionary Models of Obesity, Overeating and Eating Disorders

11.3.1 Evolutionary Models of Obesity

Free living animals in nature eat to nutritional requirements (de Araujo et al., 2020). Fat accumulation is seasonal in species adapted to northern latitudes and in migratory birds. Humans have a higher rate of fat mass than other primates (Swain-Lenz et al., 2019), but obesity was rare until recently.

There is an intense debate concerning the evolutionary origins of the current obesity epidemic (Castillo et al., 2017; Qasim et al., 2018; Reddon et al., 2018). Over the last 50 years, 60–80% of adults and 20–30% of children have become overweight and obese in most Western

---

[1] The ability to evaluate one's physical appearance in comparison to others around them and to embark on self-improvement assumes a certain level of cognitive capacity (Abed, 1998). Together with the particular characteristics of intrasexual competition in humans, these are of particular importance when thinking of animal models of EDs.

countries, which is unprecedented in human history (Huse et al., 2018; Peralta et al., 2018; Rodgers et al., 2018). This trend is international, with very few exceptions, such as Japan and South Korea. The rapid increase over the last few decades is clearly environmental, but there is also a genetic component (Brandkvist et al., 2020), which presents a question: how did genetic variants with a detrimental impact on human health persist through evolutionary time?

In this section we outline existing theories explaining the evolutionary origins of obesity and explore the novel environmental conditions that can help us to understand the modern-day distribution of obesity-predisposing variants.

Although obesity is not an ED, one can argue that it is ultimately the result of disordered eating: the normal satiety mechanisms are not functioning to maintain an optimal weight. Furthermore, several epidemiological studies have shown that EDs are most common among people who are obese (NHS Digital, 2020).

A recent population-based Australian study focusing on the trends between 1995 and 2015 showed significant increases in the prevalence of both obesity and binge eating. The highest increases were in the prevalence of obesity with comorbid binge eating or obesity with comorbid strict dieting/fasting (Figure 11.1) (da Luz et al., 2017).

11.3.1.1 The Thrifty Gene Hypothesis

Neel (1962, 1999) proposed the thrifty genotype hypothesis, which states that genes that maximise energy extraction and conservation would have been selected for during human evolution due to recurrent periods of food shortages. Thrifty genes would be positively selected because of the survival and reproductive fitness advantages conferred by fat deposited between famines. However, in modern society, where there is a perpetual abundance of food, these genes prepare their bearers for famines that never materialise, and the consequence is widespread obesity. He advocated a 'Palaeolithic Prescription' to reverse the obesity epidemic, recognising the need for changing the food environment and public health campaigns similar to the public health policies that curtailed smoking (Neel, 1999).

A recent study of human obesity gene risk variants in 13 populations has provided support for the thrifty gene hypothesis (Castillo et al., 2017). The results of this study were consistent with obesity genes that encode proteins possessing a fundamental role in maintaining energy metabolism and survival during the course of human evolution, and they provide evidence for the selection of ancestral risk variants both before and after the migration from Africa.

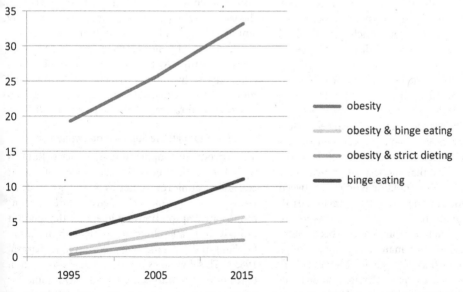

Figure 11.1 Prevalence (%) of obesity and comorbid eating disorder behaviours in South Australia from 1995 to 2015 (source: Ayton and Ibrahim, 2020)

11.3.1.2 Seasonality Hypotheses

Consistent with the thrifty gene hypothesis is the observed seasonal pattern of weight gain in many species – from birds to mammals – to survive the winter. For example, hibernating mammals become obese, insulin resistant and hyperinsulinaemic to store fat.

Seasonal fat storage is dependent on the seasonality of foods. In today's society, the intake of fructose, primarily in the form of added sugars, has skyrocketed, and this may be responsible for the obesity epidemic today. The impact of the recent loss of the seasonality of nutrients in the modern food environment is probably grossly underestimated, and this has been furtheraggravated by the introduction of ultra-processed (foods, which have been gradually replacing unprocessed and minimally processed foods over the last 40 years (Monterio et al., 2018). These products now constitute 50–60% of food consumption in Westernised countries, resulting in increased intakes of various sugars and food additives and reduced energy from protein, triggering multiple neurobiological and metabolic consequences (Ayton and Ibrahim, 2020).

11.3.1.3 The Drifty Gene Hypothesis

Speakman (2008) criticised the thrifty gene hypothesis, arguing that, given the long duration of positive selection, everyone would have inherited these thrifty genes and should be obese. He proposes that obesity must be under some counterbalancing selection, such as reduced fecundity or greater susceptibility to disease. If there was a bias in reproductive fitness towards obese individuals during famines, this would probably be offset by the detrimental effects of obesity between famines, which span much longer periods. Furthermore, he argues that if there had been selection for 'thrifty genes', then a population carrying these genes must become obese between famines, whereas data show that modern hunter-gatherer communities eating traditional diets between famines do not become obese (Speakman, 2013). However, there is abundant evidence that exposure to the modern food environment has been metabolically devastating for many indigenous groups (Wood, 2006), such as Aboriginals (Merema et al., 2019), Native Americans (Lavigne-Robichaud et al., 2018), Fijians (Taylor et al., 2018) and the Alaskan Inuits (DiNicolantonio and O'Keefe,

2017). Moreover, in many Western societies only 20–25% of the population remain of normal weight.

Speakman's 'drifty genotype' hypothesis proposes that, due to the advent of fire and the development of weapons, humans became less vulnerable to predation, thereby increasing the upper limit of body weight set points (Speakman, 2008, 2013). However, this hypothesis minimises the importance of natural and sexual selection and ignores seasonality (see the Section 11.3.2.4 for the insurance hypothesis of obesity).

11.3.2 Evolutionary Theories of AN and BN

There is a wide range of evolutionary theories and models for EDs in the literature (see Table 11.1). By their very nature, these theories deal with ultimate or evolutionary causation, attempting to answer the 'why' question. The evolutionary approach recognises that food restriction can be harmful and even deadly; nevertheless, the motivation to restrict food intake may still be adaptive under certain circumstances and for limited periods. Evolutionary formulations attempt to explore the possible evolved mechanisms underlying such motivations and the circumstances in which they can become overactivated and/or dysfunctional. Importantly, theories of ultimate causation are compatible with a range of proximate theories (i.e. both types of theories can apply simultaneously and are not mutually exclusive).

As Table 11.1 shows, most evolutionary theories focus on AN; the exceptions are the sexual competition hypothesis (Abed, 1998) and the more recent extended mismatch hypotheses (Ayton and Ibrahim, 2020; Rantala et al., 2019).

11.3.2.1 Reproductive Suppression Hypothesis

The reproductive suppression hypothesis (RSH) is one of the earliest evolutionary models of AN. It considers eating restriction as a strategy to delay reproduction in times when environmental conditions are unpropitious by lowering the amount of body fat to a level incompatible with ovulation (Voland and Voland, 1989; Wasser and Barash, 1983). This hypothesis rests on the observation that not all conditions are equally favourable for reproduction. Hence, according to the RSH, AN is not itself an adaptation, and what was selected for was the ability of females to alter the timing of reproduction, with AN being a by-product of this process that arises through mismatch due to the unnaturally prolonged engagement of the reproductive suppression mechanisms as a result of novel environmental conditions (Salmon et al., 2008). Consistent with the RSH, women who perceive low levels of support from their romantic partners and families are prone to dieting and do not feel ready for parenthood, suggesting that poor environmental conditions may be causal in the development of AN (Juda et al., 2004).

Predictions arising from the RSH were tested in a study by Salmon et al. (2008). They hypothesised that two main cues in the modern environment signalled unfavourable reproductive conditions: intense female competition and unwanted sexual attention from males. They also hypothesised that these two novel conditions, which are prevalent in modern urbanised environments, signal low levels of support and potential subversion of female choice, respectively, and lead to delaying reproduction through mismatch (Salmon et al., 2008). Their findings offered some support for their hypotheses and hence for the RSH, but the authors noted that other, more neutral kinds of stress also had the potential to increase concern and dissatisfaction over weight and body shape (Salmon et al., 2008). Hence, the RSH suggests that whereas in ancestral environments such cues would have led to a temporary postponement of reproduction, in the modern environment the intensity and duration of such experiences can escalate to anorexic-type behaviours and symptoms. The emphasis of the RSH on the pivotal role of mismatch and the abnormally intense female competition in the modern environment shows an overlap with the sexual competition hypothesis (SCH), and hence the two hypotheses are not necessarily mutually exclusive. However, unlike the SCH, the explanatory scope for the RSH is limited to AN, given that it is the only variant of EDs that involves suppression of ovulation.

Although plausible, the RSH has some limitations: aside from its exclusive focus on AN, it does not explain the basis for distorted body image or why some men are also afflicted (Li et al., 2014).

11.3.2.2 Parental Manipulation Hypothesis

The parental manipulation hypothesis is a variant of the RSH in which dominant parents, who are highly involved in controlling resources, induce reproductive suppression in their daughter(s) (Voland and Voland, 1989). Demaret (1991) suggested that AN may be an analogue to the phenomenon of 'the helper at the nest' found in a number of species. This model draws on kin selection theory (Hamilton, 1964) and asserts that AN may be adaptive insofar as it increases the helping behaviour of an individual with AN towards her own kin and thus aids their survival and reproduction while suppressing her own reproductive activity.

Studies conducted in pre-industrial societies have found that daughters who are born earlier (thus being able to make a greater contribution to the care of younger siblings) tend to increase their parents' reproductive success (Turke, 1989). However, the model does not account for the drive for thinness or AN behaviours that derive from sources external to the family. Nor does it explain the recent increase in the incidence of AN precisely in societies where overall fertility as well as parental influence have plummeted. Finally, no studies to date have demonstrated increased fertility in parents of AN patients (Abed, in press).

11.3.2.3 Adapted to Flee Famine Hypothesis

Guisinger (2003) proposed the adapted to flee famine hypothesis (AFFH), which states that the symptoms of AN evolved to cope with famine and food shortages, whereby food restriction, denial of starvation and hyperactivity represent adaptive behaviours that helped with migration to more promising surroundings. The AFFH was prompted by the curious features of AN that include self-starvation coupled with hyperactivity. Li et al. (2014) suggest that findings from a range of studies are consistent with the possibility of the existence of adaptations that deactivate desires for eating and activate desires for travelling at times of food shortages, motivating individuals to overcome the pain of hunger and energising them to migrate to more food-abundant locations.

However, the AFFH is problematic for a variety of reasons, not least the fact that prolonged food restriction is dangerous and potentially deadly, and this would have been even more hazardous in the ancestral environment (Del Giudice, 2018). Also, the AFFH fails to explain why individuals with AN resist eating when food is readily available (Del Giudice, 2018; Li et al., 2014). A further weakness is the fact that the AFFH appears to confound consequences with causation (or primary with secondary symptoms), as the features of 'fleeing famine' (e.g. restlessness and hyperactivity) may represent the consequences of starvation that arise in AN as a result of a self-imposed restriction of food intake (Nettersheim et al., 2018). Also, Guisinger's explanation for the sex difference in AN is unsatisfactory as it relies on the assumption of universal human patrilocality, which implies a greater exploration range for females, whereas studies show that marital residence patterns in foragers are quite flexible and variable (Alvarez, 2004), and, contrary to AFFH, the anthropological record shows that it is not women but men who have the larger exploration range. Finally, Guisinger's explanation for the trigger of AN appears to rely on female competition to attract mates in a modern environment, which renders the AFFH more or less indistinguishable from the SCH (Abed, in press).

11.3.2.4 Insurance Hypothesis

The insurance hypothesis (IH) is primarily an evolutionary theory of obesity, similar to the thrifty gene hypothesis. It proposes that the function of storing fat is to provide a buffer against shortfalls in the food supply (Nettle et al., 2017). Thus, individuals should store more fat when they receive cues that access to food is uncertain. Nettle et al. (2017) suggest that the IH predicts that an extremely lean body will be favoured when the individual's estimate of food security is unusually high and when there is a perception that shortfalls will never occur. The hypothesis suggests that the perception of absolute food security (arising from mismatch) leads to the 'shutting down' of food consumption mechanisms, which in turn leads to AN.

This prediction is supported by the evidence that families of relatively high socioeconomic position have the highest risk of AN, and that this risk is higher in high-income countries (Goodman et al., 2014); however, a recent study by Mitchison et al. (2020) did not confirm the relationship between AN and socioeconomic position.

Nevertheless, the model has considerable face validity, but it also suffers from limitations. Besides its exclusive relevance to AN, it offers little explanation for AN's large female preponderance or for its clinical features, such as distorted body image.

11.3.2.5 Social Threat Hypothesis

Gatward (2007) proposed the social threat hypothesis, which suggests that AN is the outcome of competition for status within the group. As a social species, human survival depended on group membership and acceptance by others, as exclusion from the group was risky, even potentially fatal in the ancestral past. Maintaining or improving status is thus of paramount importance, as status is an indicator of one's worth to the group and is strongly linked with access to reproductive resources. The argument is that, unlike in pre-industrial environments (where plumpness was a sign of status), in modern Western environments (where there is an abundance of food), status becomes linked to self-control. The hypothesis, based on mismatch, shares a number of weaknesses with the AFFH, is difficult to test and does not rule out alternatives (Li et al., 2014).

11.3.2.6 Sexual Competition Hypothesis

The SCH attempts to explain both AN and BN as well as the phenomenon of the drive for thinness that includes a spectrum of subclinical states (Abed, 1998). Intrasexual competition occurs in both males and females, but some of the behavioural manifestations are sex-specific. The importance of physical attractiveness and a youthful, nubile shape as visual cues for high female reproductive potential have already been alluded to in Section 11.2. We also noted that the importance of female reproductive potential (remaining fertile years) in determining mate value relates specifically to the human mating system characterised by pair-bonding, long-term mating strategies and high paternal investment. Uniquely, this system has given rise to the distinctive female intrasexual competition for mates. The SCH proposes that modern Western environments create a plethora of mismatches that crucially includes abnormally intense and persistent female intrasexual competition.

The SCH proposes that intense female intrasexual competition is the biological root for the drive for thinness as an adaptive response originally suited to small-scale, ancestral environments, and that the extreme version of this manifests itself in what we now recognise as EDs. Hence, the SCH proposes that a range of EDs (AN, BN, partial syndromes of both as well as the drive for thinness) are manifestations of abnormally intense female intrasexual competition whereby females of reproductive age compete with each other in the novel environment of modern (Western and Westernised) cities through a strategy of 'the pursuit of thinness' as a signal of youth. This is claimed to lead to a state of 'runaway female intrasexual competition', the extreme versions of which are EDs (Abed, 1998).

The SCH is based on the fact that throughout human evolutionary history the female shape has been a reliable indicator of the female's reproductive history and reproductive potential (Bovet and Raymond, 2015; Singh, 1994). The same is not true for men, where physical appearance, while relevant, is much less useful in assessing a man's reproductive potential. The visual signal for a female's peak reproductive potential in ancestral environments was the female's nubile shape, which was generally short-lived and declined with the repeated cycles of gestation and lactation (Symons, 1995).

The SCH proposes that a number important socioecological factors serve to upregulate the intensity of female intrasexual competition in modern societies. These include (Abed, 2012; Nettersheim et al., 2018): (1) female autonomy, which refers to the freedom of individual females to make mating decisions with relatively little interference from kin, which contrasts markedly with the situation during the majority of human evolutionary history (Apostolou, 2007); (2) living in modern cities where females coexist in close proximity to and encounter abnormally high densities of other autonomous females; (3) reduced fertility (birth rates) (Vining, 1986), which has meant that females have increasingly managed to preserve their nubile shape beyond the age of nubility, thus creating the novel phenomenon of the older but still nubile-looking woman, which further intensifies female intrasexual competition (Abed, 1998); (4) the particular Western brand of socially sanctioned monogamy, which, in contrast to polygamy, creates a shortage of eligible men in the marriage market (Henrich, 2020); and (5) the ubiquity of super-attractive youthful nubile female images in the media that are mistaken for competitors (Li et al., 2018).

Therefore, the SCH is based on the idea of a primary mismatch between the design of the female's psychological adaptations for mate attraction and retention and for competing with rival females on the one hand and the novel circumstances of the modern, Westernised urban environment on the other.

The explanatory value the SCH claims to offer extends to AN and BN and partial syndromes of both, and also provides an explanation for the drive for thinness, the female preponderance and the fact that these disorders affect primarily females of reproductive age, as well as their geographical distribution. However, the SCH does not explain why individuals present with different EDs in response to intense female intrasexual competition. Life history factors have been proposed as a promising avenue to explore (Abed et al., 2012; Nettersheim et al., 2018; see also Chapter 1 of this volume).

Life history theory (LHT) posits that organisms allocate resources to either somatic effort or reproduction (Stearns, 1992). Somatic effort includes growth and body maintenance/defence, whereas reproductive effort includes mating, parenting and nepotistic effort, each of which can be offset or delayed in favour of the other (Del Giudice, 2018). This yields what has been termed the 'fast–slow spectrum' of life history strategies.

Accordingly, individuals with BN are more likely to fall into a fast life history, whereas those with AN more likely display a slow life history strategy (Abed et al., 2012; Nettersheim et al., 2018). Support for this contention comes from BN's association with heightened impulsivity, sensation-seeking, novelty-seeking and borderline personality disorder (Cassin and von Ranson, 2005), as well as with early menarche and early sexual experiences (Kaltiala-Heino et al., 2001). Also consistent with this view is AN's association with low impulsivity, at least in AN-R (Waxman, 2009).

The predictions of the SCH and LHT have been examined in a few non-clinical studies and in one explorative clinical study. Faer et al. (2005) found that intrasexual competition for mates was the determining factor for both anorexic and bulimic tendencies in a non-clinical population of female American undergraduates, which is consistent with the SCH. A further study of female undergraduates in the UK testing the relationship between intrasexual competition, LHT and abnormal eating behaviour showed that a slow life history strategy was negatively correlated with disordered eating behaviour and that intrasexual competition was related to disordered eating behaviour, which are consistent with the SCH (Abed et al., 2012).

In another study of undergraduate students in the USA by Li et al. (2010), male and female participants were exposed to profiles of individuals of average attractiveness with either high or low intrasexual competition cues. The high intrasexual competition cues led to more restrictive eating attitudes and body image concerns in heterosexual women and homosexual men, whereas homosexual women and heterosexual men showed no differences between the two sets of conditions. These findings are consistent with the predictions of the SCH (Abed, 1998).

There has so far been only one small explorative study of a clinical population of AN and BN patients testing the predictions of the SCH and LHT (Nettersheim et al., 2018). This study found that BN was associated with several measures typical of a fast life history strategy, whereas AN did not significantly differ from controls, suggesting that AN lies on the slow end of the life history continuum. There was evidence of high intrasexual competition in BN but not in AN. The negative finding regarding intrasexual competition in AN is clearly problematic for the SCH. However, when taking the whole sample of ED patients together (AN and BN combined) there was a significant correlation between intrasexual competition for mates and higher scores of abnormal eating behaviour, thus lending partial support to the SCH in a clinical population with EDs. A major limitation of this study was that it was small and underpowered, which might explain the negative finding regarding intrasexual competition in the AN group.

11.3.2.7 Extended Mismatch Hypotheses

A number of authors have suggested that despite the explanatory power of the SCH it remains incomplete, and so they have proposed *extended mismatch hypotheses*. These evolutionists accept that intense female intrasexual competition is a necessary factor in the causation of EDs, but they argue that it is not sufficient (Ayton and Ibrahim, 2020; Rantala et al., 2019). Ayton and Ibrahim (2020) propose that intrasexual competition is driven by the effects of the modern industrialised food environment, which override normal satiety mechanisms and result in increasing risk of abdominal obesity and in widespread dieting. The conflict between maintaining sexual attractiveness and increased risk of obesity is further exploited by the diet and weight-loss industries and contributes to the causation of EDs via

multiple mechanisms. Similarly, Rantala et al. (2019) have proposed a multifaceted mismatch theory that includes modern nutrition but also incorporates the effects of stress, stress hormones, immune responses, proinflammatory cytokines and disruption in the composition of the microbiota, as well as the additional effects of a range of comorbidities. The explanatory scope of these evolutionary mismatch hypotheses goes well beyond AN and BN and includes BED, obesity and other EDs and extends to a range of medical conditions such as type 2 diabetes, coronary heart disease and many other health problems prevalent in the modern environment (Rantala et al., 2019).

Rantala et al.'s mismatch hypothesis for EDs proposes that the modern environment has led to an 'adaptive metaproblem' (Al-Shawaf, 2016) through creating a fundamental conflict between the evolved psychological mechanisms for food consumption and those for mating. They propose that the evolved psychological mechanisms responsible for food intake and those responsible for mating, which functioned harmoniously in ancestral environments, became conflicted in the conditions of the modern environment (Al-Shawaf, 2016; King, 2013; Rolls, 2017). The novel condition of the abundance of calorically dense nutrients creates a situation where the previously co-adapted mechanisms of food intake and mating become antagonistic and where individuals become torn between food rewards and mating rewards. This antagonism, Rantala et al. (2019) suggest, drives the adaptive metaproblem in contemporary humans, manifesting ultimately in various forms of EDs.

These recently proposed mismatch models build on the SCH and integrate a wide range of data that improve the original SCH's explanatory power. The models are important additions to the evolutionary literature on EDs and show considerable promise in terms of furthering our understanding of both the proximate and ultimate causation of EDs as well as for future therapeutic interventions.

11.3.3 Males and Eating Disorders

The existence of EDs in males has been a problem for a number of evolutionary formulations, especially those based on reproductive suppression and female competition. Interestingly, unlike females who present with the female-typical 'drive for thinness' disorders that include AN and BN, males present (though less frequently) with two variants of body dissatisfaction. In addition to the 'drive for thinness' variant that afflicts a proportion of males and is known to be associated with homosexuality (Abed, 1998; Calzo et al., 2018; Li et al., 2010), there is a second, newly recognised male-typical variant of body dissatisfaction where young men focus on their upper-body musculature, feeling it to be too small (Karazsia et al., 2017; Pope et al., 2002). A particular strength of the SCH is that it is the only evolutionary theory that can claim to explain both of these variants. In the case of the drive for thinness in males (in both AN and BN) the SCH's explanation is a partial one, as it can account for the existence of these disorders in homosexual men, who, like heterosexual women, aim to attract men and hence rely heavily on visual cues of attractiveness (Abed, 1998). The fear of fatness and the drive for muscularity in men fits well into the SCH framework. It is argued that this particular variant of body dissatisfaction has evolutionary roots in male intrasexual competition, where intense competition between males is influenced by some of the same socioecological factors that affect female competition in the modern environment but with a sex-specific bias.

The evolutionary roots of the drive for muscularity in males are based on the process of sexual selection that explains the origins of sexual dimorphism in humans. Humans are moderately sexually dimorphic, with men, on average, being around 20% heavier than women (Puts et al., 2016). This is below the threshold of dimorphism for polygynous species (60%) but above that for monogamous species (10%) (Marlowe and Berbesque, 2012). However, the fat-free sexual dimorphism (i.e. the dimorphism that excludes fatty tissue) in humans is significantly higher at 31–43% (Lassek and Gaulin, 2009), and men possess 61% more lean muscle mass than women, including 50% more lower-body muscle mass and 75% more arm muscle mass (Lassek and

Gaulin, 2009). It has been suggested that these sex differences in muscularity are comparable to those of gorillas, a highly sexually dimorphic, polygynous species (Puts et al., 2016). Furthermore, sex differences in aggression and violent behaviour are evident cross-culturally, and this is particularly the case when examining the data on extreme violence resulting in homicide (Daly and Wilson, 1988).

Taken together, this evidence points to the importance of physical strength and specifically upper-body strength in males over human evolutionary history for use in male intrasexual competition both for direct physical contests and for visual signalling of formidability to intimidate male rivals, as well as for attracting to females (Puts et al., 2016).

Hence, the SCH uniquely provides a parsimonious explanation for both the ultimate causation of the drive for thinness in male homosexuals and the phenomenon of the 'drive for muscularity' that can afflict some young men.

11.4 Conclusion

EDs and obesity may be considered paradigmatic examples of diseases of modernity arising from evolutionary mismatch. As such, their explanation must involve reference to ultimate causation to make sense. Without a theory that can organise the disparate and seemingly unconnected tangle of complex data, little progress can be made. Thus, EDs and obesity may be ideal grounds where the value and power of evolutionary thinking can be demonstrated in psychiatry and medicine generally. However, psychiatry and medicine do not progress by theories alone. Evolutionarily inspired theories must be rigorously tested and their possible therapeutic implications carefully evaluated and shown to be clinically effective before they can be fully incorporated into mainstream psychiatry. This is the challenge that evolutionary psychiatry must tackle head-on.

References

Abed, R. T. (1998). The sexual competition hypothesis for eating disorders. *Br J Med Psychol* 71, 525–547.

Abed, R. T. (in press). Evolutionary perspectives on eating disorders.

In: L. Al-Shawaf and T. Shackelford (eds.), *The Oxford Handbook on Evolution and Emotions*. Oxford: Oxford University Press.

Abed, R. T., Mehta, S., Figueredo, A. J., Aldridge, S., Balson, H., Meyer, C. and Palmer, R. (2012).

Eating disorders and intrasexual competition: testing an evolutionary hypothesis among young women. *Sci World J* 2012, 290813.

Al-Shawaf, L. (2016). The evolutionary psychology of hunger. *Appetite* 105, 591–595.

Alvarez, H. P. (2004). Residence groups among hunter-gatherers: a view of the claims and evidence for patrilocal bands. In: B. Chapais and C. Berman (eds.), *Kinship and Behavior in Primates*. Oxford: Oxford University Press, pp 420–442.

American Psychiatric Association (2013). *Diagnostic and Statistical Manual of Mental Disorders*, 5th ed. Arlington, VA: APA.

Apostolou, M. (2007). Sexual selection under parental choice: the role of parents in the evolution of human mating. *Evol Hum Behav* 28, 403–409.

Ayton, A. and Ibrahim, A. (2020). The Western diet: a blind spot of eating disorder research?-a narrative review and recommendations for treatment and research. *Nutr Rev* 78, 579–596.

Becker, A. E. (2004). Television, disordered eating, and young women in Fiji: negotiating body image and identity during rapid social change. *Cult Med Psychiatry* 28, 533–559.

Bielemann, R. M., Santos, L. P., Costa, C. D. S., Matijasevich, A., and Santos, I. S. (2018). Early feeding practices and consumption of ultraprocessed foods at 6 y of age: findings from the 2004 Pelotas (Brazil) Birth Cohort Study. *Nutrition* 47, 27–32.

Bovet, J. and Raymond, M. (2015). Preferred women's waist-to-hip ratio variation over the last 2,500 years. *PLoS ONE* 10, e0123284.

Brandkvist, M., Bjorngaard, J. H., Odegard, R. A., Brumpton, B., Smith, G. D., Asvold, B. O., et al. (2020). Genetic associations with temporal shifts in obesity and severe obesity during the obesity epidemic in Norway: a longitudinal population-based cohort (the HUNT study). *PLoS Med* 17, e1003452.

Bribiescas, R. G., Ellison, P. T. and Gray, P. B. (2012) Male life history, reproductive effort, and the evolution of the genus *Homo*: new directions and perspectives. *Curr Anthropol* 53, 424–435.

Bruch, H. (1988). *Conversations with Anorexics*. Northvale, NJ: Aronson.

Bulik, C. M., Blake, L. and Austin, J. (2019). Genetics of eating disorders: what the clinician needs to know. *Psychiatr Clin North Am* 42, 59–73.

Buss, D. M. and Schmitt, D. P. (1993). Sexual strategies theory: an evolutionary perspective on human mating. *Psychol Rev* 100, 204–232.

Calzo, J. P., Austin, S. B. and Micali, N. (2018). Sexual orientation disparities in eating disorder symptoms among adolescent boys and girls in the UK. *Eur Child Adolesc Psychiatry* 27, 1483–1490.

Cassin, S. E. and von Ranson, K. M. (2005). Personality and eating disorders: a decade in review. *Clin Psychol Rev* 25, 895–916.

Castillo, J. J., Hazlett, Z. S., Orlando, R. A. and Garver, W. S. (2017). A global evolutionary and metabolic analysis of human obesity gene risk variants. *Gene*, 627, 412-419.

da Luz, F. Q., Sainsbury, A., Mannan, H., Touyz, S., Mitchison, D., and Hay, P. (2017). Prevalence of obesity and comorbid eating disorder behaviors in South Australia from 1995 to 2015. *Int J Obes (Lond)* 41, 1148–1153.

Daly, M. and Wilson, M. (1988). *Homicide*. New York: Aldine de Gruyter.

de Araujo, I. E., Schatzker, M. and Small, D. M. (2020). Rethinking food reward. *Annu Rev Psychol*, 71, 139–164.

Del Giudice, M. (2018). *Evolutionary Psychopathology: A Unified Approach*. New York: Oxford University Press.

Demaret, A. (1991). De la grossesse nerveuse a l'anorexie mentale. *Acta Psychiatr Belg* 91, 11–22.

DiNicolantonio, J. J. and O'Keefe, J. (2017). Markedly increased intake of refined carbohydrates and sugar is associated with the rise of coronary heart disease and diabetes among the Alaskan Inuit. *Open Heart* 4, e000673.

Erskine, H. E., Whiteford, H. A. and Pike, K. M. (2016). The global burden of eating disorders. *Curr Opin Psychiatry* 29, 346–353.

Faer, L. M., Hendriks, A., Abed, R. T. and Figueredo, A. J. (2005). The evolutionary psychology of eating disorders: female competition for mates or for status? *Psychol Psychother* 78, 397–417.

Fichter, M. M. and Quadflieg, N. (2016). Mortality in eating disorders: results of a large prospective clinical longitudinal study. *Int J Eat Disord* 49, 391–401.

Gatward, N. (2007). Anorexia nervosa: an evolutionary puzzle. *Eur Eat Disord Rev* 15, 1–12.

Goodman, A., Heshmati, A. and Koupil, I. (2014) Family history of education predicts eating disorders across multiple generations among 2 million Swedish males and females. *PLoS ONE* 9, e106475.

Gordon, R. A. (1990). *Anorexia and Bulimia: Anatomy of a Social Epidemic*. Cambridge: Wiley-Blackwell.

Guisinger, S. (2003). Adapted to flee famine: adding an evolutionary perspective on anorexia nervosa. *Psychol Rev* 110, 745–761.

Gurven, M. and Hill, K. (2009). Why do men hunt? A reevaluation of 'Man the Hunter' and the sexual division of labor. *Curr Anthropol* 50, 51–74.

Hamilton, W. D. (1964). The genetical evolution of social behavior. II. *J Theor Biol* 7, 17–52.

Henrich, J. (2020) *The Weirdest People in the World: How the West Became Psychologically*

Peculiar and Particularly Prosperous. London: Allen Lane.

Hudson, J. I., Hiripi, E., Pope, H. G. Jr and Kessler, R. C. (2007). The prevalence and correlates of eating disorders in the national comorbidity survey replication. *Biol Psychiatry* 61, 348–358.

Huse, O., Hettiarachchi, J., Gearon, E., Nichols, M., Allender, S. and Peeters, A. (2018). Obesity in Australia. *Obes Res Clin Pract* 12, 29–39.

Insel, T. (2012). National Institute of Mental Health (NIMH). Spotlight on eating disorders. Retrieved from www.nimh.nih.gov/about/directors/thomas-insel/blog/2012/spotlight-on-eating-disorders.shtml

Jasieńska, G., Ziomkiewicz, A., Ellison, P. T., Lipson, S. F. and Thune, I. (2004). Large breasts and narrow waists indicate high reproductive potential in women. *Proc Biol Sci* 271, 1213–1217.

Juda, M. N., Campbell, L. and Crawford, C. B. (2004). Dieting symptomatology in women and perceptions of social support: an evolutionary approach. *Evol Hum Behav* 25, 200–208.

Kaltiala-Heino, R., Rimpelä, M., Rissanen, A. and Rantanen, P. (2001). Early puberty and early sexual activity are associated with bulimic-type eating pathology in middle adolescence. *J Adolesc Health* 28, 346–352.

Kaplan, H. S., Hill, K. R., Lancaster, J. B. and Hurtado, A. M. (2000). A theory of life history evolution: diet intelligence and longevity. *Evol Anthropol* 9, 156–185.

Karazsia, B. T., Murnen, S. K. and Tylka, T. L. (2017). Is body dissatisfaction changing across time? A cross-temporal meta-analysis. *Psychol Bull* 143, 293–320.

Katzman, M. A., Hermans, K. M. E., van Hoeken, D. and Hoek, H. W. (2004). Not your 'typical island woman': anorexia nervosa is reported only in subcultures in Curaçao. *Cult Med Psychiatry* 28, 463–492.

Keel, P. K. and Brown, T. A. (2010). Update on course and outcome in eating disorders. *Int J Eat Disord* 43, 195–204.

King, B. M. (2013). The modern obesity epidemic, ancestral hunter-gatherers, and the sensory/reward control of food intake. *Am Psychol* 68, 88–96.

Lassek, W. D. and Gaulin, S. J. C. (2009). Costs and benefits of fat-free muscle mass in men: relationship to mating success, dietary requirements, and natural immunity. *Evol Hum Behav* 30, 322–328

Lavigne-Robichaud, M., Moubarac, J. C., Lantagne-Lopez, S., Johnson-Down, L., Batal, M., Laouan Sidi, E. A. and Lucas, M. (2018). Diet quality indices in relation to metabolic syndrome in an Indigenous Cree (Eeyouch) population in northern Quebec, Canada. *Public Health Nutr* 21, 172–180.

Li, N. P., Smith, A. R., Griskevicius, V., Cason, M. J. and Bryan, A. (2010). Intrasexual competition and eating restriction in heterosexual and homosexual individuals. *Evol Hum Behav* 31, 365–372.

Li, N. P., Smith, A. R., Yong, J. C. and Brown, T. A. (2014) Intrasexual competition and other theories of eating restriction. In: V. Weekes-Shackelford and T. Shackelford (eds.), *Evolutionary Perspectives on Human Sexual Psychology and Behavior*. New York: Springer, pp. 323–346.

Li, N. P., van Vugt, M. and Colarelli, S. M. (2018) The evolutionary mismatch hypothesis: implications for psychological science. *Curr Dir Psychol Sci* 27, 38–44.

Marcus, M. D. and Wildes, J. E. (2009). Obesity: is it a mental disorder? *Int J Eat Disord* 42, 739–753.

Marlowe, F. W. (2003) The mating system of foragers in the cross-cultural Standard Cross-Cultural Sample. *Cross Cult Res* 37, 282–306.

Marlowe, F. W. and Berbesque, J. C. (2012). The human operational sex ratio: effects of marriage, concealed ovulation, and menopause on mate competition. *J Hum Evol* 63, 834–842.

McCuen-Wurst, C., Ruggieri, M. and Allison, K. C. (2018). Disordered eating and obesity: associations between binge-eating disorder, night-eating syndrome, and weight-related comorbidities. *Ann N Y Acad Sci* 1411, 96–105.

Merema, M., O'Connell, E., Joyce, S., Woods, J. and Sullivan, D. (2019). Trends in body mass index and obesity prevalence in Western Australian adults, 2002 to 2015. *Health Promot J Austr* 30, 60–65.

Mitchison, D., Mond, J., Bussey, K., Griffiths, S., Trompeter, N., Lonergan, A., et al. (2020). DSM-5 full syndrome, other specified, and unspecified eating disorders in Australian adolescents: prevalence and clinical significance. *Psychol Med* 50, 981–990.

Monteiro, C. A., Cannon, G., Moubarac, J. C., Levy, R. B., Louzada, M. L. C. and Jaime, P. C. (2018). The UN Decade of Nutrition, the NOVA food classification and the trouble with ultra-processing. *Public Health Nutr* 21, 5–17.

Moodie, R., Stuckler, D., Monteiro, C., Sheron, N., Neal, B., Thamarangsi, T., et al. (2013). Profits and pandemics: prevention of harmful effects of tobacco, alcohol, and ultra-processed food and drink industries. *Lancet*, 381, 670–679.

Muller, M. N. and Pilbeam, D. R. (2017). The evolution of the human mating system. In: M. N. Muller, R. W. Wrangham and

D. R. Pilbeam (eds.), *Chimpanzee and Human Evolution*. Cambridge, MA: Belknap Press of Harvard University Press, pp. 427–463.

Murdock, G. P. and White, D. R. (1969). Standard cross-cultural sample. *Ethnology* 8, 329–369.

National Institute of Mental Health (2020). Eating disorders. Retrieved from www.nimh.nih .gov/health/publications/eating-disorders/index.shtml

Neel, J. V. (1962). Diabetes mellitus: a 'thrifty' genotype rendered detrimental by 'progress'? *Am J Hum Genet* 14, 353–362.

Neel, J. V. (1999). The 'thrifty genotype' in 1998. *Nutr Rev* 57, S2–S9.

Nettersheim, J., Gerlach, G., Herpertz, S., Abed, R., Figueredo, A. and Brüne, M. (2018). Evolutionary psychology of eating disorders: an explorative study in patients with anorexia nervosa and bulimia nervosa. *Front Psychol* 9, 2122.

Nettle, D., Andrews, C. and Bateson, M. (2017). Food insecurity as a driver of obesity in humans: the insurance hypothesis. *Behav Brain Sci* 40, E105.

Nghiem, S., Vu, X. B. and Barnett, A. (2018). Trends and determinants of weight gains among OECD countries: an ecological study. *Public Health* 159, 31–39.

NHS Digital (2020). Health Survey for England 2019. Retrieved from https://digital.nhs.uk/data-and-information/publications/statistical/health-survey-for-england/2019/health-survey-for-england-2019-data-tables

Parker, G. A. (1983). Mate quality and mating decisions. In: P. Bateson (ed.), *Mate Choice*. New York: Cambridge University Press, pp. 141–164.

Peralta, M., Ramos, M., Lipert, A., Martins, J. and Marques, A. (2018). Prevalence and trends of overweight and obesity in older adults from 10 European countries from 2005 to 2013. *Scand J Public Health* 46, 522–529.

Pollard, T. (2008). *Western Diseases: An Evolutionary Perspective*. Cambridge: Cambridge University Press.

Pope, H. G., Phillips, K. A. and Olivardia, R. (2002) *The Adonis Complex: How to Identify, Treat, and Prevent Body Obsession in Men and Boys*. New York: Free Press.

Pulit, S. L., Karaderi, T. and Lindgren, C. M. (2017). Sexual dimorphisms in genetic loci linked to body fat distribution. *Biosci Rep* 37, BSR20160184.

Puts, D. A., Bailey, D. H. and Reno, P. L. (2016). Contest competition in men. In D. M. Buss (ed.), *The Handbook of Evolutionary Psychology*. Hoboken, NJ: John Wiley and Sons, pp. 385–402.

Qasim, A., Turcotte, M., de Souza, R. J., Samaan, M. C., Champredon, D., Dushoff, J., et al. (2018). On the origin of obesity: identifying the biological, environmental and cultural drivers of genetic risk among human populations. *Obes Rev* 19, 121–149.

Qian, J., Wu, Y., Liu, F., Zhu, Y., Jin, H., Zhang, H., et al. (2021). An update on the prevalence of eating disorders in the general population: a systematic review and meta-analysis. *Eat Weight Disord*. doi: 10.1007/s40519-021-01162-z.

Rantala, M. J., Luoto, S., Krama, T. and Krams, I. (2019) Eating disorders: an evolutionary psychoneuroimmunological approach. *Front Psychol* 10, 2200.

Reddon, H., Patel, Y., Turcotte, M., Pigeyre, M. and Meyre, D. (2018). Revisiting the evolutionary origins of obesity: lazy versus peppy-thrifty genotype hypothesis. *Obes Rev* 19, 1525–1543.

Rodgers, A., Woodward, A., Swinburn, B. and Dietz, W. H. (2018). Prevalence trends tell us what did not precipitate the US obesity epidemic. *Lancet Public Health* 3, e162–e163.

Rolls, B. J. (2017). Dietary energy density: applying behavioral science to weight management. *Nutr Bull* 42, 246–253.

Russell, G. (2000) Disorders of eating. In: M. G. Gelder, J. J. Lopez-Ibor Jr and N. C. Andreasen (eds.), *New Oxford Textbook of Psychiatry*, Vol. 1. Oxford: Oxford University Press, pp. 835–855.

Salmon, C. (2017). Is female competition at the heart of reproductive suppression and eating disorders? In: M. L. Fisher (ed.), *The Oxford Handbook of Women and Competition*. Oxford: Oxford University Press, pp. 764–796.

Salmon, C., Crawford, C., Dane, L., and Zuberbier, O. (2008). Ancestral mechanisms in modern environments: impact of competition and stressors on body image and dieting behavior. *Hum Nat* 19, 103–117.

Singh, D. (1994). Ideal body shape: role of body weight and waist-to-hip ratio. *Int J Eat Disord* 16, 283–288.

Speakman, J. R. (2008). Thrifty genes for obesity, an attractive but flawed idea, and an alternative perspective: the 'drifty gene' hypothesis. *Int J Obes (Lond)* 32, 1611–1617.

Speakman, J. R. (2013). Evolutionary perspectives on the obesity epidemic: adaptive, maladaptive, and neutral viewpoints. *Annu Rev Nutr* 33, 289–317.

Stearns, S. C. (1992). *The Evolution of Life Histories*. Oxford: Oxford University Press.

Steinhausen, H. C. (2002) The outcome of anorexia nervosa in the 20th century. *Am J Psychiatry* 159, 1284–1293.

Sugermeyer, J. (2020). Eating disorders (ED), a global epidemic, de-stigmatizing ED to save lives. In: S. Okpaku (ed.), *Innovations in Global Mental Health*. Cham: Springer, pp. 191–201.

Sugiyama, L. A. (2016) Physical attractiveness: an adaptational perspective. In: D. Buss (ed.), *The Handbook of Evolutionary Psychology*. Hoboken, NJ: John Wiley and Sons, pp 317–384.

Swain-Lenz, D., Berrio, A., Safi, A., Crawford, G. E. and Wray, G. A. (2019). Comparative analyses of chromatin landscape in white adipose tissue suggest humans may have less beigeing potential than other primates. *Genome Biol Evol* 11, 1997--2008.

Symons, D. (1995). Beauty is in the adaptations of the beholder. In P. R. Abramson and S. D. Pinkerson (eds.), *Sexual Nature, Sexual Culture*. Chicago, IL: University of Chicago Press, pp. 80–118.

Taylor, R., Lin, S., Linhart, C. and Morrell, S. (2018). Overview of trends in cardiovascular and diabetes risk factors in Fiji. *Ann Hum Biol* 45, 188–201.

Turke, P. (1989). Evolution and the demand for children. *Popul Dev Rev* 15, 61–90.

Vining, D. R. (1986). Social versus reproductive success: the central theoretical problem of human sociobiology. *Behav Brain Sci* 9, 167–216.

Voland, E. and Voland, R. (1989). Evolutionary biology and psychiatry: the case for anorexia nervosa. *Ethol Sociobiol* 10, 223–240.

Volkow, N. D. and O'Brien, C. P. (2007). Issues for DSM-V: should obesity be included as a brain disorder? *Am J Psychiatry* 164, 708–710.

Wasser, S. K. and Barash, D. P. (1983). Reproductive suppression among female animals: implications for biomedicine and sexual selection theory. *Q Rev Biol* 58, 513–538.

Waxman, S. E. (2009). A systematic review of impulsivity in eating disorders. *Eur Eat Disord Rev* 17, 408–425.

Wood, L. E. (2006). Obesity, waist-hip ratio and hunter-gatherers. *BJOG* 113, 1110–1116.

World Health Organization (2019). The ICD-11 Classification of Mental and Behavioral Disorders. Retrieved from https://icd.who.int/en

Wu, J., Liu, J., Li, S., Ma, H. and Wang, Y. (2020). Trends in the prevalence and disability-adjusted life years of eating disorders from 1990 to 2017: results from the Global Burden of Disease Study 2017. *Epidemiol Psychiatr Sci* 29, e191.

Yong, J. C., Li, N. P., Valentine, K. A. and Smith, A. R. (2017). Female virtual intrasexual competition and its consequences: an evolutionary mismatch perspective. In M. L. Fisher (ed.), *The Oxford Handbook of Women and Competition*. Oxford: Oxford University Press, pp. 657–680.

Chapter 12

Substance Abuse and Evolution

Paul St John-Smith and Riadh Abed

Abstract

An evolutionary perspective on drug use and addiction poses two primary questions that complement the proximate models of mainstream medicine. These are: why are humans motivated to repetitively seek out and consume non-nutritional substances, and why do plants (which are the sources of the majority of such chemicals) manufacture substances that can alter the functioning of the human nervous system? We propose that these questions can have a real bearing on our understanding of the phenomena of abuse and addiction that complements models of proximate causation. The evolutionary perspective recognises that addiction can only arise through the interaction of substances with evolutionarily ancient systems designed to promote the pursuit of rewards associated with increased fitness[1] in the ancestral environment. Thus, neglecting the phylogenetic history and function of such systems necessarily results in an incomplete understanding of this phenomenon. Evolution can also help us to understand human uniqueness and especially the role of cumulative culture and gene–culture co-evolution in shaping the human body and mind. Hence, the evolutionary perspective enables a deeper understanding of the human vulnerability to substance abuse and addiction. The chapter concludes by considering the clinical and public policy implications of the evolutionary perspective presented.

Keywords

addiction, co-evolutionary arms race, drug misuse, evolution, mismatch, pharmacophagy, plant neurotoxins

Key Points

- The evolutionary perspective explores why humans are vulnerable to drug misuse and become addicted to a range of non-nutritional substances.
- The evolutionary approach highlights the paradox as to why humans should procure and become addicted to plant toxins that are designed by selection to deter consumption by other organisms.
- Evolutionary models of addiction such as pharmacophagy, mismatch and costly signalling are theories of ultimate causation that can complement rather than replace theories of proximate causation.

- Considering evolutionary factors helps to inform future public health approaches to the problems of drug abuse and addiction.

12.1 Background

12.1.1 Introduction

The use of drugs is one of the most intriguing human behaviours. Some drugs are used positively for therapeutic purposes, others cause immense harm to individuals and societies (e.g. heroin, cocaine and methamphetamine) or inflict a terrible social burden in the form of preventable illnesses (e.g. alcohol and tobacco), while yet others appear to be mostly harmless and are widely enjoyed by people around the world (e.g. coffee and chocolate) (Sullivan et al., 2002).

Problem drug use clearly causes many harms to users with no obvious benefits. Drug abuse would therefore appear to be uniformly maladaptive.

---

[1] The term 'fitness' will be used throughout this chapter to refer to the Darwinian concept of reproductive success and not to individual good health and well-being.

However, more careful inspection shows that some drugs are beneficial in some contexts. Stimulants such as caffeine and nicotine reduce fatigue and suppress appetite, alcohol can relieve anxiety and reduce stress and opiates can alleviate pain. Furthermore, the extensive comorbidity between drug use and other mental disorders may be partly explained as an attempt at symptom alleviation or self-medication (Khantzian, 2003). In the UK, when surveying community mental health team patients, 44% (95% confidence interval (CI) 38.1–49.9%) reported past-year problem drug use and/or harmful alcohol use, and 75% (95% CI 68.2–80.2%) of drug service and 85% of alcohol service patients (95% CI 74.2–93.1%) had a past-year psychiatric disorder (Weaver et al., 2003). These characteristics of drug use have led some researchers to suggest that humans may have evolved specific adaptations that motivate individuals to consume psychoactive substances at certain times (Sullivan et al., 2002). Drug use has been found in all human societies throughout historical and prehistorical times, as well as being evident in closely related species. These observations warrant serious evolutionary exploration.

12.1.2 What Is Drug Misuse and Addiction?

A drug is any chemical substance that, after administration, causes a biological effect or change in an organism's physiology or psychology. Drugs are distinguished from food and substances that provide nutrition, but this is not an absolute distinction. For instance, alcohol may be viewed as both a food as well as a drug, and caffeine is found in a variety of foodstuffs. In this chapter, we will concentrate on those psychoactive drugs not customarily regarded as nutrition and where the use of the drug/substance is harmful to the individual or to others. Both biological criteria as well as sociocultural value judgements are required to decide whether substance use is a misuse, and the definition varies across societies and legal jurisdictions.

Drug misuse is defined by the World Health Organization as the use of a substance for a purpose not consistent with legal or medical guidelines, such as the non-medical use of prescription medications or the recreational use of illegal drugs. Inappropriate drug consumption is viewed as a major public health problem not only undermining economic and social development, but also contributing to crime, mental disorder and medical problems, including heart disease, lung cancer, hepatitis C, HIV and tuberculosis (Roberts et al., 2014).

The related phenomenon of addiction occurs secondarily to substance use initiation and is characterised by two core behavioural patterns: intensification and reinstatement (Berridge, 1997). Hence, addiction involves a pattern of behaviour aimed at inducing pleasure and/or reducing discomfort and is characterised by: (1) recurrent failure to control the behaviour (powerlessness); and (2) continuation of the behaviour despite significant negative consequences (unmanageability) (Goodman, 1990).

The choice to use a substance is initially voluntary; however, because chronic substance use can alter a user's metabolism (dependency) and also permanently affect structures in the prefrontal cortex associated with decision-making and judgement, a person becomes driven to use drugs and/or alcohol (Muñoz-Cuevas et al., 2013).

The evolutionary perspective draws attention to two interesting facts. The first is the observation that the drugs most often associated with abuse or addiction are plant derivatives. Salient examples include cocaine, opiates, caffeine, cannabis (tetrahydrocannabinol; THC) and tobacco (nicotine), all of which are plant defensive neurotoxins (Sullivan et al., 2008). The second observation is that these psychoactive drugs can induce or alter emotions that in human evolutionary history signalled increases in fitness and then potentially became substitutes for the real thing. These observations hold important insights.

There is the additional contemporary problem of synthetic chemical entities to consider (e.g. benzodiazepines, pain killers and designer drugs or novel psychoactive substances; NPSs). A designer drug is a structural or functional analogue of a controlled substance that has been designed to mimic the pharmacological effects of the original drug while avoiding classification as illegal and/or detection in standard drug tests (St John-Smith et al., 2013). Evolutionary models of drug use are unique in that they emphasise the effects drugs had on fitness over human evolution. For substance abuse – a seemingly maladaptive trait – to persist, either there must be a 'trade-off' where the harm is counterbalanced by a fitness benefit (St John-Smith et al., 2013) or substance-taking must be a by-product of other adaptive processes.

12.1.3 Causation

Following Tinbergen's causal system, a complete understanding of any biological phenomenon requires the understanding of both proximate and ultimate (evolutionary) causes (see Chapter 1). Therefore, for a given trait to evolve in a population, three conditions should be present: a genetic component, variation in the trait and effects of the trait on reproductive success. Indeed, it is a central tenet of neo-Darwinian evolutionary theory that a trait cannot evolve if it reduces the overall reproductive success of its carrier. So, the question is: how can a seemingly maladaptive trait with negative fitness costs such as drug use arise and persist in all human populations? One putative hypothesis is that there must be a 'trade-off' (i.e. some other selective advantages/benefits outweighing risk) leading to enhanced reproductive success even at the expense of long-term better health (Trevathan et al., 2008). Other explanations rely on a range of evolutionary pathways for the persistence of disease and disorder (see Chapter 1).

12.1.4 Epidemiology

Worldwide, around 230 million adults between the ages of 15 and 64 use an illegal drug at least once a year, and about 27 million of these are 'problem' drug users. The most frequently used substances are alcohol and nicotine, which are generally legal, and cannabis, amphetamines or ecstasy, followed by cocaine and opiates, which are generally illegal (European Monitoring Centre for Drugs and Drug Addiction, 2012; United Nations Office on Drugs and Crime, 2012). Universally, the use of drugs such as cannabis, cocaine, amphetamines and opiates is more prevalent among males than females. The problem affects rich and poor nations and is geographically ubiquitous, suggesting that vulnerability is species-wide and a human-universal.

The UK has relatively high levels of drug use compared to many comparable developed countries. In 2014/2015, it was estimated that more than 11 million adults aged between 16 and 59 in England and Wales had taken illegal drugs in their lifetime, including nearly 3 million who had taken an illicit drug in the past year (Gromyko, 2015). This level of drug use is associated with significant levels of mortality and morbidity and represents an escalating public health problem.

Nearly 4,400 drug poisoning deaths were registered in England and Wales in 2019, the highest number since records began in 1993 (Mahase, 2020).

Psychological and psychiatric problems such as early conduct disorder symptoms, antisocial behaviour, depression, anxiety and childhood disruptive disorders such as attention deficit hyperactivity disorder are associated with the onset of cannabis and other drug use. Furthermore, deficits in the ability to modulate emotions or behaviours when dealing with stress have been found to be related to the initiation of drug use (Huang et al., 2014).

12.1.5 Genes, Twin Studies and the Heritability of Addictions

An evolutionary explanation can be sought for any disorder that occurs universally in all human populations, but it is a mistake to assume that the disorder itself was shaped by selection. The medical model views substance abuse as a biological phenomenon, and its focus has therefore been on questions such as genetic factors, neurochemical mechanisms and other brain abnormalities. Evidence from family, adoption and twin studies converges on the relevance of genetic factors in the development of addictions. Twin studies have shown that the heritability of addictions (in ascending order: hallucinogens, stimulants, cannabis, sedatives, smoking, alcohol, caffeine, opiates and cocaine), ranges from 0.39 to 0.72 (Ducci and Goldman, 2012).

Kendler et al. (2007) have researched the concordance between twins of the use of caffeine, nicotine, cannabis and cocaine in a portion of the Virginia Twin Sample including 5,000 participants. Genetic risk could not be explained by one factor acting across all substances. Rather, two shared factors were found: an 'illicit' agent factor mainly explaining vulnerability to cannabis and cocaine dependence; and a 'licit' agent factor primarily explaining vulnerability to alcohol, caffeine and nicotine. However, genetic and environmental influences modulating risk of substance use disorders change developmentally and across the lifespan (Ducci and Goldman, 2012). Genes influencing diverse aspects of addiction neurobiology including anxiety, impulsivity and reward and including genes such as monoamine oxidase A, the serotonin transporter (*SLC6A4*) and catechol-O-methyl transferase, have been implicated in the shared genetic liability between addictions and other psychiatric disorders (Ducci and Goldman, 2012). The evolutionary questions as to why these alleles that predispose to addiction and other disorders remain within the genome have yet to be asked or researched formally.

Genome-wide association studies have shown that addiction is highly polygenic with each allelic variant contributing in a small, additive fashion to addiction vulnerability. In addition, addiction vulnerability shows substantial genetic heterogeneity (Hall et al., 2013). Studies of opioid, stimulant and co-occurring substance use disorders have identified several promising genes and pathways to guide future investigations into the biological mechanisms underlying these disorders (Jensen, 2016).

12.1.6 Phylogeny: Plant–Animal Co-evolutionary Arms Races

Organisms can be classified into those that synthesise their nutrients from primary inorganic ingredients through photosynthesis (autophytes) and those that feed on them (heterophytes) (Hagen et al., 2018). The autophytes include plants, while all animals are heterophytes. Hence, while it is in the interest of a heterophyte to consume all of the nutrients it needs from plant sources, the plant must protect itself against a myriad of predators. Thus, the relationship between plants and the animals that feed on them is understandably antagonistic, although this does not preclude the possibility of some mutually beneficial interactions (symbiosis or cultivation). Plants that evolved the capacity to synthesise compounds such as alkaloids (e.g. nicotine, morphine, cocaine) appear to have had advantages, in some environments, over more palatable variants or species because they contained poisons, including animal neurotoxins, to deter their consumption by bacteria, fungi, worms, insects and herbivores (Patel et al., 2013; Sullivan et al., 2008). Natural plant toxins are often present in unripe fruits or vegetables that are common food sources.

However, in the mammalian clade, herbivores have evolved a range of countermeasures to combat plants' chemical defences in what can be described as a co-evolutionary arms race. These measures include enzymatic deactivation, sequestration, selective eating and co-consumption of neutralising substances (St John-Smith et al., 2013). It is not surprising that a number of plant alkaloids consumed by humans, including caffeine, nicotine and arecoline/betel nut, demonstrate activity against other organisms and have insecticidal or antihelminthic properties when tested in vitro. This occurrence arises because of the deep shared or common ancestry and conservation of basic biological mechanisms that occur in all animals. It is worth noting that the targets of this arms race were primarily invertebrates (insects and worms), which represented the greatest threat to the survival of such plants. The hypothesis can be formulated that in the parasite-rich human ancestral environment, the toxicity arising from consuming small quantities of plants containing these toxins may have been outweighed by the attendant antiparasitic benefits (Sullivan et al., 2008).

However, the evolutionary adaptations proposed for animals to cope with poisonous plants only seem to occur in a limited number of situations. To spread the overall toxin load, a generalised or widely ranging diet often prevents ingestion of a significantly toxic amount of any single poisonous plant species, but this broad dietary strategy cannot always be relied upon. Natural selection has selected certain characteristics so that all large herbivores have the ability to detect and avoid poisonous plants. They also have the ability to detoxify or otherwise render ineffective a certain level of some ingested poisons. However, poisoning does occur even in native wild herbivores that evolved alongside any given local species of vegetation. Aversive conditioning appears to be one principal co-evolutionary adaptation that may protect both the plant and the animal (Laycock, 1978).

Different plant compounds interfere with nearly every step in animal neuronal signalling, including: (1) neurotransmitter synthesis, storage, release, binding and reuptake; (2) receptor activation and function; and (3) key enzymes involved in signal transduction. In many cases, plant compounds achieve these effects because they have evolved to resemble endogenous neurotransmitters (Wink, 2000).

Plant secondary metabolites have been shaped by evolution for more than 500 million years. As a result, many of them have distinctive biochemical and pharmacological properties. As already mentioned in this section, many of the plant defence compounds primarily defend against consumption by insects. However, other animals – including humans – that consume such plants may also experience negative effects. Aversive tastes such as bitterness and hotness may protect a plant from consumption and, if the plants are also poisonous, these act as warnings that protect animals too (Lewis and Elvin-Lewis, 1977).

12.1.7 Animal Defences: Cytochrome P450

Cytochromes P450 enzymes (CYPs) are a super-family of enzymes. In mammals, they oxidise steroids, fatty acids and xenobiotics. They are important for the clearance of toxic compounds and for hormone synthesis and breakdown (Danielson, 2002). CYPs have been identified in all kingdoms of life – animals, plants, fungi, protists, bacteria and archaea – as well as in viruses. More than 300,000 distinct CYP proteins are known, and the P450 group is thought to have originated from an ancestral gene that existed over 3 billion years ago. Repeated gene duplications have subsequently given rise to one of the largest of the multigene families. These enzymes are notable both for the diversity of reactions that they catalyse and for the range of chemically dissimilar substrates upon which they act. CYPs support the oxidative, peroxidative and reductive metabolism of both endogenous and xenobiotic substrates (Danielson, 2002).

The mammalian CYP phylogenetic data provide compelling evidence of a long evolutionary history of exposure to plant toxins and support the hypothesis that exposure to plant neurotoxins is not evolutionarily novel for humans. Nevertheless, one can argue that there is now a mismatch between contemporary drug-profligate and ancestral drug-limited environments. The domestication of plants in the Neolithic Revolution with the move from hunting and gathering to farming led to large-scale cultivation of various plants and hence greater potential availability of plant toxins than could have been present in the wild (Mummert et al., 2011). If plant toxins were not a recent selection pressure on humans then loss of enzyme function through genetic drift would be expected. However, for the majority of phenotypes, loss of function from drift does not appear to have occurred (Sullivan

et al., 2008); on the contrary, there is evidence of recent exposure to plant toxins and stabilising selection (Solus et al., 2004). In some cases, high-frequency polymorphisms can be plausibly associated with the local plant ecology. Ethiopia, Saudi Arabia and Turkey, for example, have very high frequencies of 2D6 ultra-metabolisers: individuals with multiple functional copies of 2D6 genes (Aynacioglu et al., 1999).

12.1.8 Palaeogenetic and Archaeological Evidence for Prehistoric Psychoactive Drug Use

Archaeology offers a deep time perspective on drug use and human–plant interactions. The first written record of opium is dated to 3400 BCE, and the early use of other psychoactive substances such as cannabis, coca, betel net and a variety of hallucinogens is well documented (Dobkin de Rios, 1990). Even earlier, the 'flower burial' at Shanidar Cave in northern Iraq, which dates to Middle Palaeolithic times (circa 60,000 BCE), is widely regarded as the earliest possible evidence of shamanistic intoxicant plant use in the world. The burial contained the skeleton of an adult male Neanderthal (*Homo neanderthalensis*) who is argued to have been a shaman because of the presence of a wide range of medicinal plant 'pollen clusters', including *Ephedra altissima* (Merlin, 2003).

Humans worldwide have also been using psychoactive substances such as opium, alcohol and 'magic mushrooms' since prehistoric times (see Chapter 13). There is much archaeological data supporting their consumption in prehistoric times (Guerra-Doce, 2015). Without written records, chemical and DNA analysis of ancient remains (such as the fossils of psychoactive plants, the residues of alcohol and other psychoactive chemicals) and prehistoric artefacts and drawings are used to investigate if and how drugs were used. Key examples of prehistoric drug use include (Guerra-Doce, 2015):

(1) Hallucinogens: hallucinogenic San Pedro cactus remains were found in a cave in Peru dating back to between 8600 and 5600 BCE. Also found were seeds of mescal beans from southern Texas and northern Mexico dating to the end of the ninth millennium BCE to 1000 CE.

(2) Opium: in Italy, fossilised remains of the opium plant have been found dating to the mid-sixth millennium BCE. Other remains of poppy seed capsules and traces of opiates have been discovered in the plaque and bones of human skeletons dating back to the fourth millennium BCE, along with prehistoric art showing parts of the poppy being used in religious ceremonies.

(3) Coca leaves: human coca use in South America dates back to around 8,000 years ago. The remains of pieces of coca leaves have been found in the floors of houses in Nanchoc Valley, Peru, and in human dental remains and mummy hair.

(4) Tobacco: smoking pipes dating back to around 2000 BCE have been found in north-western Argentina, and remnants of nicotine have been found in pipes dating back to 300 BCE.

Thus, our propensity for using addictive psychoactive substances is attested to in the genome and, more recently, in the archaeological records. In classical antiquity, psychoactive substances were used by priests in religious ceremonies (e.g. *Amanita muscaria*), by healers for medicinal purposes (e.g. opium) and by the general population in a socially approved way (e.g. alcohol, nicotine and caffeine). Our ancestors appear to have refined more potent compounds and devised faster routes of administration that today contribute to abuse. Pathological use was described by as early as classical antiquity (Hagen and Tushingham, 2019).

The cultural and learning aspects of drug misuse seem important. Humans are good at communicating with each other as to the immediate effects of plants, adverse or otherwise. Plant food choice was undoubtedly one of the selection pressures for the evolution of social learning in the human lineage through cumulative cultural evolution (see Chapter 1) influenced by local ecological and cultural factors. This would explain, for example, why addiction to nicotine and alcohol is much more prevalent in Western societies than addiction to all other drugs (Kessler et al., 2005). If there was natural selection on the human lineage to deliberately consume neurotoxic plants for medicinal or other purposes, the resulting adaptations for regulated neurotoxin intake would certainly also rely heavily on social learning

to identify substances that maximise the benefits of ingestion and minimise the costs (St John-Smith et al., 2013).

12.1.9 Darwinian Fitness and Emotions

Emotions have common substrates in humans and animals (Darwin, 1890; Panksepp, 2004). The neurobiological systems implicated in emotional states have been shaped by selection because they generate positive emotional states when stimuli in the world signal improved chances of survival and reproductive success for the organism (e.g. food, sex and positive social relations), and they generate negative states when events in the world are unpropitious. Hence, from an evolutionary perspective, it makes sense that neural circuitry has undergone strong selective pressure and extensive modification towards behaviours that promote survival and reproduction and away from fitness-reducing behaviours (St John-Smith et al., 2013). These primary emotional systems often have specific neurotransmitter signatures (Panksepp, 2004).

Interestingly, drugs of abuse act to override the adaptive functions of the primary emotional systems through diminishing negative or aversive affect (e.g. opiates) or increasing positive affect (e.g. stimulant drugs that increase dopamine). Thus, the drug-taker experiences the increase in positive affect or decrease in negative affect independently of any change in environmental success or threat, leading to the decoupling of the emotional system from environmental success or threat. In other words, these drugs bypass the evolved protective mechanisms used to signal real success or danger and lead drug-takers to continue to consume substances despite mounting harm (Nesse, 1994). This usurpation of the emotional system by drugs forms the basis of the 'hijack model' (see Section 12.2.1.1).

The pursuit of emotion-associated goals tends to move organisms up a hedonic and adaptive gradient, but neurobehavioral systems are designed to maximise fitness, not happiness, so our pleasures are often fleeting and we experience much unnecessary suffering. The neurochemical mechanisms that mediate these states confer intrinsic vulnerability to substance abuse in environments where drugs are available. Therefore, a better understanding of the mechanisms, origins and functions of the emotions will enhance our ability to cope with substance abuse and our ability to make decisions about the therapeutic use of psychoactive drugs (Nesse, 1994).

12.1.10 The Reward versus Poison Paradox

Sullivan et al. (2008) highlight the conflict between the fact that drugs of abuse are neurotoxins that have evolved in plants as defences against overgrazing by herbivores on the one hand and the neurobiological reward model of substance misuse on the other. Why should mammals be attracted to those plant alkaloids whose initial consumption is associated with clear aversive effects? For example, neophyte drug users typically report a range of unpleasant subjective effects on initial use of a psychoactive compound. Sullivan et al. (2008) argue that multiple mechanisms and levels of ecological understanding are required to distinguish neophyte use from chronic drug use and that co-evolution (e.g. pharmacophagy) may have an explanatory role. It is notable that most first-time users of cigarettes report adverse reactions, including nausea, dizziness, sickness and headache; two-thirds of subjects rate inhaling their first cigarette as bad and nearly three-quarters report that their first cigarette made them not want to smoke again.

These observations seemingly contradict the reward model of drug use and suggest that mechanisms other than a false perception of an increased fitness benefit via hijacking of the brain's mesolimbic dopamine system (MDS) lead to continued tobacco use. These factors include sociocultural aspects such as advertising, peer pressure and parental and other high-status adult role models. Greater exposure to promotion leads to higher risk. The evidence indicates that exposure to tobacco promotion causes children to initiate tobacco use, which may generalise to other substances. However, sociocultural factors can only represent a partial explanation of tobacco use given its prevalence and use across cultures and societies. Universally, dopamine plays an instrumental role in the processing of reward-related stimuli, and drug-induced dopamine stimulation explains at least some drug abuse phenomena. How the primary emotional systems are affected are discussed in Section 12.2.1.1 (DiFranza et al., 2006).

12.2 Specific Evolutionary Models of Substance Misuse (see Box 12.1)

> **Box 12.1** Evolutionary models of substance misuse and addiction[2]
>
> **Mismatch-based models**
>
> Generic mismatch
> Hijack model
> Novel psychoactive substances
>
> **Trade-off-based models**
>
> Pharmacophagy
> Neurotoxin regulation
>
> **Models based on selection for risk-taking behaviour and signalling**
>
> Sexual selection
> Costly signalling
> Life history-based models
>
> **Others**
>
> Foetal protection hypothesis
> Shamanic model of psychedelic drug use

12.2.1 Mismatch and Mismatch-Based Models

Mismatch theory is arguably the predominant evolutionary paradigm regarding drug abuse (see Chapter 1). According to this model, drug addiction is a consequence of the (novel) interaction either of NPSs or highly purified, mass-produced plant neurotoxins with (ancient) evolved reward systems, causing alteration of brain biochemical mechanisms and processes and resulting in the maladaptive outcome of dependency in a proportion of the population (St John-Smith et al., 2013). Thus, according to the mismatch model, the novelty of the compounds (in terms of structure, purity or quantity) implies the lack of evolved mechanisms for limiting reward experiences, as such scenarios did not occur over human evolutionary history.

---

[2] Some of the proposed models are conceptually similar or overlapping, are not mutually exclusive and may interact in unpredictable ways (St John-Smith et al., 2013).

12.2.1.1 The Hijack Model

The hijack model of drug abuse is based on mismatch. It proposes that drugs of abuse hijack the ancient and evolutionarily conserved neural mechanisms associated with positive emotions that evolved to mediate incentive behaviour (Nesse and Berridge, 1997). The theory focuses on the MDS, a collection of dopamine neurons in the midbrain of humans and many other animals that plays a central role in Pavlovian conditioning and similar types of reinforcement learning. Research on the molecular pathways of addiction suggests that drugs of abuse, despite their diverse chemical substrates, converge on this common circuitry in the brain's limbic system. Specifically, drugs are thought to activate the mesolimbic dopamine pathway, facilitating dopamine transmission in the nucleus accumbens via disinhibition, excitation and uptake blockade to produce a dopamine-like yet dopamine-independent effect. According to this model, the MDS evolved to reinforce behaviours that increased access to natural rewards that improved our ancestors' fitness (food, mates, allies, etc.; Sullivan et al., 2008).

Phylogenetically, reward systems are evolutionarily ancient and shared across species, which accounts for the relevance of rodent models in studying the neurobiology of substance use disorders in humans. It is notable that rodents and humans both respond to sugar with hedonia (liking) and to dopaminergic agents with salience motivation (wanting). The central role of neurotransmitters such as dopamine (which exists in most multicellular organisms) has endured over hundreds of millions of years, with pathways gradually being modified to maximise fitness in each species (Barron et al., 2010). Available evidence dates the emergence of dopamine as a neurotransmitter back to the earliest appearance of the nervous system, over 500 million years ago in the Cambrian Period (Cottrell, 1967).

The hijack model proposes that drugs of abuse utilise and usurp these evolutionarily ancient systems, creating a signal in the brain (such as euphoria or ecstasy) that indicates – falsely – the arrival of a huge fitness benefit. This changes behavioural propensities so that drug-seeking increases in frequency and displaces adaptive behaviours. In other words, psychoactive drugs can induce emotions that, in human evolutionary history, signalled increases in fitness and thereby potentially became substitutes for the real thing (Durrant et al., 2009).

Considering aversive or negative but protective emotions, Nesse's 'smoke detector principle' explains why evolved systems that regulate protective responses often give rise to false alarms and apparently excessive responses (Nesse, 2019; see also Chapter 7 of this volume), which in turn enable self-medication to reduce these responses, often without immediate penalties.

Therefore, instead of only seeking explanations for substance abuse in individual differences such as genes, temperament, early experiences, social conditions, cultural setting or exposure to drug use, an evolutionary perspective suggests that we should also consider how these factors interact with the emotional and behavioural mechanisms that make all humans vulnerable to substance abuse. This view encourages therapeutic attention to the diversity of factors that influence people's emotions, including relationships, social support, social inequity, the experience of discrimination and opportunities or blocked opportunities. Therefore, there are good evolutionary reasons why people who are not succeeding in social competition are less likely to experience positive emotions and consequently have more frequent negative emotions, and so they will take drugs more often and also be less responsive to treatment.

12.2.1.2 Novel Psychoactive Substances

The effects on humans of NPSs is another example of mismatch. Increasing levels of taking NPSs worldwide represents an evolutionary challenge to our evolved biological systems. Our ability to synthesise new mind-altering drugs proceeds at a rate far faster than natural selection operates, which requires hundreds of generations for the evolution of protective responses. There is therefore concern over the ability of our body to defend against or detoxify entirely novel compounds that have unknown harmful effects on humans (Orsolini et al., 2017).

Psychostimulant and amphetamine-like drugs (e.g. novel stimulants such as 4,4-DMAR, methiopropamine, modafinil, ethylphenydate, synthetic cathinones and synthetic cocaine substitutes and MDMA-like drugs) may simulate and provide false responses to what appear to be adaptive advantages represented by feelings of improved control over the natural environment, increased perceptual skills, improved time reactions to stimuli and resistance to stressors. They also produce decreased feelings of fatigue and improvements in competitive strategies, including perceived academic performance (Schifano et al., 2015). The sedatives, anxiolytics and hypnotics such as novel benzodiazepines, synthetic opioids and the naturally occurring gamma-hydroxybutyrate represent another group that may produce euphoria, increased sex drive and tranquillity responses and a perceived increased control of fear and enhanced control of painful stimuli (Schifano et al., 2015).

The latest hallucinogens and entheogens include the synthetic cannabinoids known as 'Spice' drugs, and they also include psychedelic phenethylamines such as 25I-NBOMe (2C-I-NBOMe or Cimbi-5, also shortened to '25I'), a synthetic hallucinogen that is used in biochemistry research for mapping type 2A serotonin receptors in the brain. Others include tryptamine derivatives and phencyclidine and ketamine-like dissociative drugs. These drugs cause not only acute responses and toxicity but also delayed responses that may be harmful or beneficial depending on the circumstances and doses used. Nevertheless, we hypothesise that using chemicals that give out false signals of fitness or attachment, confidence or well-being is a risky and potentially harmful long-term strategy (see Chapter 20).

12.2.2 Models Based on Trade-Offs

12.2.2.1 Pharmacophagy Hypothesis and Infection Control

It appears that even our earliest ancestors consumed herbs to relieve pain or used plants in a variety of ways. Fossil records reveal that the human use of plants as traditional medicines dates back to the Middle Palaeolithic, approximately 60,000 years ago (Solecki et al., 1975).

Using appropriate plants could provide fitness benefits. Nowadays, many pharmaceutical drugs are still derived from plants (Maridass and De Britto, 2008). Proponents of the pharmacophagy hypothesis/medicinal model of drug use suggest that pharmacophagy (the consumption of pharmacological substances for medicinal purposes) evolved in the context of human–plant co-evolution as a form of self-medication. Theorists propose that the reason humans learned to ignore the cues of plant toxicity (e.g. bitter

taste) and consumed bioactive and potentially lethal substances with little to no energetic content was because ingesting the bioactive compounds of plants in small amounts was therapeutic (Hagen et al., 2013).

The proponents of the self-medicating model of drug use suggest that it is possible that at some stages in our evolutionary history self-regulated consumption of plant neurotoxins may have been advantageous and selected for. It has been hypothesised that the human brain evolved to control and regulate the intake of psychoactive plant toxins in such a way as to increase fitness. This is demonstrated by parallel evidence from CYP studies and other genetic studies. They suggest that plant toxins were deliberately ingested by ancestral humans to combat parasites or disease-carrying vectors (e.g. mosquitos; Sullivan et al., 2008).

Primates, too, appear to engage in pharmacophagy. Detailed behavioural, pharmacological and parasitological investigations of two such behaviours – bitter pith chewing and leaf swallowing – have been conducted on three East African chimpanzee populations. These behaviours are now known to occur widely among chimpanzees, bonobos and lowland gorillas. For both bitter pith chewing and leaf swallowing, selection of the same plant species tends to occur among neighbouring groups of same ape species. These local cultural traditions of plant selection may be transmitted when females of the same species transfer into non-natal groups. However, selection of the same plant species or species of related plant genera by two sympatric ape species or between regional populations of great ape subspecies strongly suggests common criteria of medicinal plant selection. Along with the intriguing observation that the same medicinal plants are selected by apes and humans with similar illnesses, this provides insight into the evolution of medicinal behaviour in modern humans and the possible nature of self-medication in early hominids. The occurrence of these and other specific self-medicative behaviours, such as geophagy, in primates and other animal taxa suggests the existence of an underlying mechanism for the recognition and use of plants and soils with common medicinal or functional properties (Huffman, 1997).

Sullivan and Hagen (2002) hypothesised that hominins may have exploited plant toxins to overcome nutritional and energetic constraints on central nervous system signalling. Nicotine and other popular plant drugs are powerfully insecticidal and anti-helminthic. Furthermore, some recreational drugs remain remarkably effective treatments for mammalian pathogens. For example, nicotine, arecoline (the principal psychoactive component of betel nut, which is widely chewed in Asia and the Pacific) and THC – three of the world's most popular plant drugs – are potent anti-helminthics. Nicotine, arecoline and their close chemical relatives have been widely used to deworm livestock, and there is evidence that tobacco and cannabis use is associated with reduced helminthic infestation in studies of hunter-gatherers (Roulette et al., 2014, 2016).

Perhaps the widespread recreational use of tobacco, betel nut and cannabis could be a vestigial form of human pharmacophagy – an evolved response to chronic infections of helminths or other parasites with nicotinic or muscarinic receptors – in ancestral human populations. There is doubt, however, that there was selection for use of any one plant drug specifically; instead, there could have been selection to seek out and use plants rich in cholinergic agents. Psychoactive plant substances could be especially valued because these clearly interfere with neuronal signalling in humans and hence might be expected to also interfere with the nervous systems of pathogens such as helminths and arthropods.[3]

Finally, the pharmacophagy hypothesis proposes that the consumption of chemicals with medicinal properties is contingent on human–plant co-evolution. Self-medication advantages arose when humans learned to overcome cues of plant toxicity (e.g. bitter taste) and consumed potentially toxic substances with little energetic content because ingesting the toxins in small amounts was therapeutic. Thus, the consumption of plant alkaloids may have contributed to increased fitness and a taste for these substances could have been selected for.

12.2.2.2 The Neurotoxin Regulation Hypothesis

Psychoactive substance use has been typical of most traditional and modern societies and is maintained in the population despite the potential for abuse and related harms, raising the possibility that it confers fitness benefits that offset its costs. As described in Section 12.1.6, the efficacy of plant neurotoxins evolved over 500 million years, and therefore they are not evolutionarily novel. Consequently, human physiology can identify plant toxins and activate defences that involve genes, tissue barriers, neural circuits, organ systems and behaviours to protect against them. However, the unpleasant symptoms of drug toxicity and related immediate aversive responses (e.g. headache, sweating, nausea and vomiting) still occur in humans (despite the protective systems), and because they are not immediately pleasant or rewarding, they are not consistent with a simplistic theory of drug use, such as those postulated in immediate or simple instrumental reward models. Thus, other mechanisms, such as trade-offs, must be considered as explanations.

The neurotoxin regulation hypothesis (NRH) proposes that the parallel consumption of both the nutrients and neurotoxins in plants selected for a system capable of maximising the benefits of plant energy extraction while mitigating the costs of plant toxicity. The NRH of human drug use is similar to the pharmacophagy hypothesis with which it is linked. It also proposes that during the course of human evolution plant consumption was important for fitness. In order to achieve this, humans evolved a defence system in which plant consumption is mediated by cues of toxicity in a manner sensitive to the individual's toxicity threshold, maintaining blood toxin concentrations below a critical level (Hagen et al., 2018).

The mammalian body has also evolved to develop defences against toxicity, such as exogenous substance metabolism and vomiting reflexes (Hagan et al., 2013). The NRH of drug use is a response to advocates of the hijack model. This is largely because the neurobiological reward theory of drug use specifies actions between plant neurotoxins and human reward systems as novel and rewarding. The NRH emphasises the evolutionary biology of plant–human co-evolution and maintains that secondary plant metabolites, such as nicotine, morphine and cocaine, are potent neurotoxins that evolved to deter and punish herbivore consumption of the plant soma, not encourage or reward it. Hence, the NRH highlights that it is evolutionarily disadvantageous for

---

[3] See St John-Smith et al. (2013) for information on psychotropic drugs that affect insects, parasites and bacteria.

plants to produce toxins that plant predators (e.g. humans) are attracted to, and that it runs contrary to evolutionary logic that plant predators would evolve neurobiological systems unprotected from plant toxin consumption.

12.2.3 Models Based on Selection for Risk-Taking and Signalling

12.2.3.1 Life History Factors

Understanding individual difference factors has been an important focus in theories of addiction. Life history factors (see Chapter 1) are known to play a significant role in drug initiation. Evolution also endows organisms with the capacity to learn from the environment. Those who have experienced abusive and unpredictable care in childhood view the world as perilous and unpredictable (St John-Smith et al., 2013). Under these conditions, a strategy of immediate gratification and 'future discounting' is frequently adopted. Such risk-taking behaviour represents a 'fast life history' strategy. Life history theory can explain the male preponderance in drug use as female drug users incur much higher fitness costs through reduced parenting capacity, potential teratogenic effects and potential circumvention of female mate choice.

In addition to the male preponderance in illicit drug taking, misuse tends to be higher in adolescents and young adults than for other age groups. The prevalence of substance use disorders is also significantly higher in unmarried individuals and individuals of lower socioeconomic status (as measured according to education and income). The broad patterns of risk found for substance use problems are also largely mirrored for a range of other risky behaviours, including dangerous driving and risky sex (Reyna and Farley, 2006).

12.2.3.2 Sexual Selection and Its Consequences

Although psychoactive substances may have facilitated survival among ancestral humans, it is not clear that this has enhanced fitness through improved mating success. Sexual selection (see Chapter 1) and cultural theories concerning drug use suggest individuals might consume drugs to increase reproductive opportunities. The assumption is that some drug use can increase fitness because consumption may: (1) advertise biological/genetic quality, sexual maturity or availability; (2) decrease inhibitions in mating contexts; and/or (3) enhance associative learning behaviours that in turn increase mating opportunities (Richardson et al., 2017). Richardson et al.'s findings suggest that substance use provides little predictive value about the individual's current prospects for acquiring sexual partners or future reproductive success. Thus, if adaptations for substance use were shaped by selection, their adaptive value does not seem to be found in mating success.

It has been suggested that individuals might use drug substances to signal maturity. Sexually selected cues of quality often emerge in adolescence and reliably signal developmental maturity. Psychoactive substances are most harmful for individuals who are developmentally immature (Hagen et al., 2013). Although this hypothesis remains untested, evidence in support of it comes from age at onset of drug use. Tobacco consumption rarely occurs prior to the age of 11, and in almost all cases this aligns with age at onset of drug use, as cigarette addicts report having first smoked in adolescence. Hagen et al. (2013) suggest that this is due to the developmental maturity of the adolescent nervous system as well as increased competition for mates. Consistent with these notions, researchers have found that adolescents with alcohol use disorders were more sexually active, had more sexual partners and initiated sexual activity at slightly younger ages (Bailey et al., 1999).

12.2.3.3 Costly Signalling and the Handicap Hypothesis

Zahavi and Zahavi's (1997) handicap hypothesis is one possible explanation for the evolution of honest and costly signalling. The general idea is that individuals honestly signal their quality because signalling is costly and therefore low-quality individuals cannot afford to produce such signals. Within evolutionary biology, signalling theory represents a body of theoretical work examining communication between individuals, both within and across species.[4] Costly signalling

---

[4] Stotting in Thomson's gazelles is a classic example of an honest signal. Gazelles that stot advertise their condition both to predators and conspecifics and are less likely to be pursued by predators than those that do not stot (FitzGibbon and Fanshaw, 1988).

proposes that humans engage in substance use despite its health costs in part to advertise that they can afford to do so. This idea was tested in relation to the Darwinian fitness of those people using such drugs and whether it increased their reproductive success, with negative results being found. This suggests that drug use does not signal genetic quality and therefore does not lend support to the handicap model (Borkowska and Pawlowski, 2014).

12.2.4 Other Evolutionary Models

12.2.4.1 Foetal Protection Hypothesis

Recreational drugs are nearly all embryotoxic or teratogenic, potentially causing congenital abnormalities as well as other reproductive harms. The foetal protection hypothesis proposes that, given sex-specific vulnerabilities and fitness costs, selection for increased drug avoidance could have evolved in women to protect them from harming their developing foetuses and nursing infants (Hagen et al., 2013).

Over half of all pregnancies involve heightened food aversions and up to 80% involve nausea and vomiting. This is a conundrum given the increased requirements for nutrition in pregnancy. Nausea and vomiting in pregnancy commonly occur in the first trimester but are ironically associated with good pregnancy outcomes. Widespred aversions to toxic plant products in the diet or in plant-derived drugs, especially during organogenesis, suggest that morning sickness may be a mechanism for protecting mother and embryo that has evolved because these chemicals pose a risk to the developing foetus (Patil et al., 2012). Pregnancy-related aversions include drugs such as alcohol, coffee and tobacco, and these aversions appear to reduce drug intake. Women smokers, for example, often reduce or cease smoking during pregnancy, and one important reason for this seems to be sensory aversion to tobacco smoke (Pletsch et al., 2008).

In the environment of evolutionary adaptedness, the need for women, especially pregnant women, to avoid teratogenic substances would have been high. Evidence from evolutionary anthropology suggests that ancestral women, similar to women in extant hunter-gatherer populations, experienced high fertility and high infant mortality (Wishard, 2012). Given the high reproductive costs, the fitness cost of ingesting neurotoxins is higher for women than men. The result is increased selected defences, including aversion to toxins in women of childbearing age. An illustration of this can be found in the Aka, a hunter-gatherer population who have incredibly high smoking prevalence rates among men (95%) but very low rates among women (5%; Roulette et al., 2014). Women detect the presence of toxins at lower concentrations than men (Benowitz et al., 2006). Women also generally metabolise toxins faster than men (Dempsey et al., 2002). Research on pregnant women has documented that hormone levels in pregnancy alter the levels of CYPs, thereby increasing drug metabolism (Choi et al., 2013).

Changes in xenobiotic metabolism in women using birth control also suggest hormonally mediated influences (Hagen et al., 2013). The NRH is supported by the finding that sex differences in drug use are partly a consequence of maternal toxin defence mechanisms that function to protect the foetus and infant. Research on the treatment of substance abuse might specifically benefit from investigating the manipulation and enhancement of toxin defence mechanisms.

12.2.4.2 Psychedelic Use in Shamanic Practices

Plant-derived 'herbal highs' such as *Salvia divinorum* and *Mitragyna speciosa* (or 'Kratom') are still used and produce responses that mimic increased empathy levels. They are putatively used for the strengthening of attachment bonds and the improvement of one's own social status within specific environments (Schifano et al., 2015). Shamans are often chosen for having visions or receiving signs from the gods whilst going through trance states induced using a variety of procedures, which typically include hallucinogen or entheogen intake (Polimeni, 2012). Entheogens are drugs that are psychedelic and hallucinogenic, and they generate transcendental feelings or hallucinatory experiences. A variety of hallucinogenic mushrooms and plants, such as psilocybin mushrooms, ayahuasca, peyote, cannabis and *Salvia divinorum*, have been used in rituals by shamans throughout history. Interestingly, club drugs (e.g. ecstasy and ketamine) have been associated in 'rave' settings with a spiritual awakening of self-awareness, a sense of liberation and mystical experiences. It has been hypothesised that the use of hallucinogens in groups improves group cohesion in tribes, leading to cultural selective advantages, and this may have therapeutic implications (Polimeni, 2012).

12.3 Clinical Implications for Treatment and the Future

By examining drug misuse from an evolutionary perspective, we aim to understand its underlying significance and evaluate its threefold nature: biology, psychology and social influences. In this chapter, we have considered some aspects of the co-evolution of mammalian brains and ancient psychotropic plants as well as human characteristics that lead to abuse. Thereby, we hope to move towards more effective treatment and early prevention, perhaps through public health measures that take greater account of known human vulnerabilities.

Further research on the neurobiological mechanisms of addiction in other species from an evolutionary perspective and investigating salience and reward systems remain valuable. An evolutionarily informed view on NPSs suggests that mismatch between novel pharmacological hyper-incentives and ancient brain mechanisms is likely to worsen with the discovery of new drugs and new routes of administration.

In psychiatric settings, a range of interventions are compatible with the evolutionary perspective. Medicines that substitute for drugs of abuse or that attempt to disrupt the rewarding effects of substances highlight our growing understanding of the neurochemical and neurophysiological underpinnings of addiction. Psychological and social interventions attempt to weaken cued associations, strengthen response inhibition and consciously increase the salience of the negative consequences of use.

Broader lifestyle changes also facilitate recovery. The literature on natural recovery, for instance, highlights the importance of life experiences in treatments. A more positive approach to treatment that promotes the pursuit of 'natural' rewards may assist in relapse prevention through reducing the relative reward salience of drugs and increasing the perceived costs of use (Klingemann and Sobell, 2007).

Life history theory explains why adolescence is a period of heightened vulnerability for the development of substance use problems and may promote initiatives that enable families and communities to act as 'surrogate frontal lobes' that can temper risk-taking proclivities (Durrant et al., 2009). Furthermore, improving the prospects of disadvantaged adolescents may reduce their propensity towards risk-taking. This strategy straddles individual treatment interventions and also has wider societal and policy implications.

We suggest that it is crucial to investigate the evolutionary basis of this epidemic of substance misuse before we make the mistake of only investigating the necessary but insufficient proximate mechanistic causes and immediate environmental stimuli that may be associated with individual cases. Strategies for reducing the harm caused by addiction to drugs and other behavioural compulsions can be made more effective through a combination of targeting the mesocorticolimbic reward pathway with pharmacological agents, enhancing self-regulatory capacities and restructuring of the social environment to regulate availability and promote increased levels of social control (Durrant et al., 2009). We propose, therefore, that an evolutionary understanding is required if we are to achieve a comprehensive plan to tackle the worldwide problem of drug misuse and addiction.

12.4 Conclusions

From an evolutionary perspective, it is not surprising that plants evolved the capacity to produce chemicals that are toxic to their predators (primarily against bacteria, worms, insects and herbivores but also affecting humans). Plant predators in turn co-evolved mechanisms to take advantage of some of these deterrent plant toxins. Benefits to plant predators of limited consumption include anti-parasitic, anti-bacterial, endurance-enhancing and emotional effects. Under these circumstances, beneficial consumption of plant toxins (pharmacophagy) would be selected for by evolution, and so their use becomes adaptive if not rewarding.

Other plant toxins may be consumed because of direct hedonic effects achieved by disruption of the primary emotional systems in the brains of the plant predators. Our common ancestry and the high degree of conservation of biological operating systems between species explains why substances that affect our brains can also affect and be toxic to other animals. Counter-exploitation of plant toxins (pharmacophagy) during the course of human evolution may have been a factor in their cultivation and the extended use of toxin-producing plants. In an environment where short life expectancy was normal and parasites were common, some phytochemicals may have had adaptive advantages.

Environmental mismatch and trade-off theories explain how benefits in one environment may be outweighed by harms in another. Furthermore, pharmacological manipulation of the brain's emotional systems may create false emotional indicators of increased fitness, including feelings of positive emotions (e.g. attachment, security or achievement), or alternatively a reduction of protective negative emotions (e.g. pain, loneliness, fear and anxiety). These emotional effects may be the initial reason for these substances being used despite some initial negative or aversive responses. Thereafter, classical conditioning, receptor density changes and epigenetic modifications may lead to cycles of increasing drug use. Finally, one can imagine that ancestors who tolerated and benefitted from moderate/limited drug use may have had other selective advantages such as pain relief obtained with opiates or increased energy obtained with stimulants. Such advantages could have been useful during a hunt, during foraging or in situations requiring physical endurance or privation (St John-Smith et al., 2013).

Why humans seek out and at times develop addictions to drugs that harm them remains an open question. Evolutionary models of drug use are unique in that they emphasise the effects drugs had on fitness over human evolutionary history. The models and hypotheses discussed in this chapter need to be evaluated through empirical research to determine the relative merits and effect sizes, if any, of each of these processes (Saah, 2005). The clinical implications of these theories remain in the explanatory rather than the clinical domain. However, they are consistent with a range of current mainstream psychosocial and medical interventions and could also inform future possibilities for treatment.

References

Aynacioglu, A. S., Sachse, C., Bozkurt, A., Kortunay, S., Nacak, M., Schröder, T., Kayaalp, S. O., Roots, I. and Brockmöller, J., 1999. Low frequency of defective alleles of cytochrome P450 enzymes 2C19 and 2D6 in the Turkish population. *Clinical Pharmacology & Therapeutics*, 66, 185–192.

Bailey, S. L., Pollock, N. K., Martin, C. S. and Lynch, K. G., 1999. Risky sexual behaviors among adolescents with alcohol use disorders. *Journal of Adolescent Health*, 25, 179–181.

Barron, A. B., Søvik, E. and Cornish, J. L., 2010. The roles of dopamine and related compounds in reward-seeking behavior across animal phyla. *Frontiers in Behavioral Neuroscience*, 4, 163.

Benowitz, N. L., Lessov-Schlaggar, C. N., Swan, G. E. and Jacob, P., III, 2006. Female sex and oral contraceptive use accelerate nicotine metabolism. *Clinical Pharmacology & Therapeutics*, 79, 480–488.

Berridge, V., 1997. Addiction history. *Addiction*, 92, 253–255.

Borkowska, B. and Pawlowski, B., 2014. Recreational drug use and fluctuating asymmetry: testing the handicap principle. *Evolutionary Psychology*, 12, 769–782.

Choi, S. Y., Koh, K. H. and Jeong, H., 2013. Isoform-specific regulation of cytochromes P450 expression by estradiol and progesterone. *Drug Metabolism and Disposition*, 41, 263–269.

Cottrell, G. A., 1967. Occurrence of dopamine and noradrenaline in the nervous tissue of some invertebrate species. *British Journal of Pharmacology and Chemotherapy*, 29, 63–69.

Danielson, P. Á., 2002. The cytochrome P450 superfamily: biochemistry, evolution and drug metabolism in humans. *Current Drug Metabolism*, 3, 561–597.

Darwin, C. R., 1890. *The Expression of the Emotions in Man and Animals*. London: John Murray.

Dempsey, D., Jacob, P. and Benowitz, N. L., 2002. Accelerated metabolism of nicotine and cotinine in pregnant smokers. *Journal of Pharmacology and Experimental Therapeutics*, 301, 594–598.

DiFranza, J. R., Wellman, R. J., Sargent, J. D., Weitzman, M., Hipple, B. J. and Winickoff, J. P., 2006. Tobacco promotion and the initiation of tobacco use: assessing the evidence for causality. *Pediatrics*, 117, e1237–e1248.

Dobkin de Rios, M., 1990. *Hallucinogens: Cross-Cultural Perspectives*. Prospect Heights, IL: Waveland Press.

Ducci, F. and Goldman, D., 2012. The genetic basis of addictive disorders. *Psychiatric Clinics*, 35, 495–519.

Durrant, R., Adamson, S., Todd, F. and Sellman, D., 2009. Drug use and addiction: evolutionary perspective. *Australian & New Zealand Journal of Psychiatry*, 43, 1049–1056.

European Monitoring Centre for Drugs and Drug Addiction, 2012. *Annual Report 2012: The State of* the Drug Problem in Europe. Luxembourg: Publications Office of the European Union.

FitzGibbon, C. D. and Fanshawe, J. H., 1988. Stotting in Thomson's gazelles: an honest signal of condition. Behavioral Ecology and Sociobiology, 23, 69–74.

Goodman, A., 1990. Addiction: definition and implications. British Journal of Addiction, 85, 1403–1408.

Gromyko, D., 2015. Extent and trends in illicit drug use. In: D. Lader (ed.), Drug Misuse: Findings from the 2014/15 Crime Survey for England and Wales, 2nd ed. London: Home Office, pp. 1–7. Retrieved from https://assets.publishing.service.gov.uk/government/uploads/system/uploads/attachment_data/file/462885/drug-misuse-1415.pdf

Guerra-Doce, E., 2015. Psychoactive substances in prehistoric times: examining the archaeological evidence. Time and Mind, 8, 91–112.

Hagen, E. H. and Tushingham, S., 2019. The prehistory of psychoactive drug use. In: T. B. Henley, M. J. Rossano and E. P. Kardas (eds.), Handbook of Cognitive Archaeology: Psychology in Prehistory. New York: Routledge, pp. 471–498.

Hagen, E. H., Roulette, C. J. and Sullivan, R. J., 2013. Explaining human recreational use of 'pesticides': the neurotoxin regulation model of substance use vs. the hijack model and implications for age and sex differences in drug consumption. Frontiers in Psychiatry, 4, 142.

Hagen, E. H., Sullivan, R. J., Ahmed, S. and Pickard, H., 2018. The evolutionary significance of drug toxicity over reward. In: H. Pickard and S. H. Ahmed (eds.), The Routledge Handbook of Philosophy and Science of Addiction. New York: Routledge, pp. 102–120.

Hall, F. S., Drgonova, J., Jain, S. and Uhl, G. R., 2013. Implications of genome wide association studies for addiction: are our a priori assumptions all wrong? Pharmacology & Therapeutics, 140, 267–279.

Haug, S., Núñez, C. L., Becker, J., Gmel, G. and Schaub, M. P., 2014. Predictors of onset of cannabis and other drug use in male young adults: results from a longitudinal study. BMC Public Health, 14, 1202.

Huffman, M. A., 1997. Current evidence for self-medication in primates: a multidisciplinary perspective. American Journal of Physical Anthropology, 104, 171–200.

Jensen, K. P., 2016. A review of genome-wide association studies of stimulant and opioid use disorders. Molecular Neuropsychiatry, 2, 37–45.

Kendler, K. S., Myers, J. and Prescott, C. A., 2007. Specificity of genetic and environmental risk factors for symptoms of cannabis, cocaine, alcohol, caffeine, and nicotine dependence. Archives of General Psychiatry, 64, 1313–1320.

Kessler, R. C., Berglund, P., Demler, O., Jin, R., Merikangas, K. R. and Walters, E. E., 2005. Lifetime prevalence and age-of-onset distributions of DSM-IV disorders in the National Comorbidity Survey Replication. Archives of General Psychiatry, 62, 593–602.

Khantzian, E. J., 2003. The self-medication hypothesis revisited: the dually diagnosed patient. Primary Psychiatry, 10, 47–54.

Klingemann, H. and Sobell, L. C., 2007. Promoting Self-Change from Addictive Behaviors. Berlin: Springer Science+Business Media.

Laycock, W. A., 1978. Coevolution of poisonous plants and large herbivores on rangelands. Rangeland Ecology &

Management/Journal of Range Management Archives, 31, 335–342.

Lewis, W. H. and Elvin-Lewis, M. P. F., 1977. Medical Botany: Plants Affecting Man's Health. New York: Wiley.

Mahase, E., 2020. Drug deaths: England and Wales see highest number since records began. BMJ, 371, m3988.

Maridass, M. and De Britto, A. J., 2008. Origins of plant derived medicines. Ethnobotanical Leaflets, 2008, 44.

Merlin, M. D., 2003. Archaeological evidence for the tradition of psychoactive plant use in the old world. Economic Botany, 57, 295–323.

Mummert, A., Esche, E., Robinson, J. and Armelagos, G. J., 2011. Stature and robusticity during the agricultural transition: evidence from the bioarchaeological record. Economics & Human Biology, 9, 284–301.

Muñoz-Cuevas, F. J., Athilingam, J., Piscopo, D. and Wilbrecht, L., 2013. Cocaine-induced structural plasticity in frontal cortex correlates with conditioned place preference. Nature Neuroscience, 16, 1367–1369.

Nesse, R. M., 1994. An evolutionary perspective on substance abuse. Ethology and Sociobiology, 15, 339–348.

Nesse, R. M., 2019. The smoke detector principle: signal detection and optimal defense regulation. Evolution, Medicine, and Public Health, 2019, 1.

Nesse, R. M. and Berridge, K. C., 1997. Psychoactive drug use in evolutionary perspective. Science, 278, 63–66.

Orsolini, L., Francesconi, G., Papanti, D., Giorgetti, A. and Schifano, F., 2015. Profiling online recreational/prescription drugs' customers and overview of drug vending virtual marketplaces. Human

Psychopharmacology: Clinical and Experimental, 30, 302–318.

Orsolini, L., St John-Smith, P., McQueen, D., Papanti, D., Corkery, J. and Schifano, F., 2017. Evolutionary considerations on the emerging subculture of the e-psychonauts and the novel psychoactive substances: a comeback to the shamanism? *Current Neuropharmacology*, 15, 731–737.

Panksepp, J., 2004. *Affective Neuroscience: The Foundations of Human and Animal Emotions*. Oxford: Oxford University Press.

Patel, S., Nag, M. K., Daharwal, S. J., Singh, M. R. and Singh, D., 2013. Plant toxins: an overview. *Research Journal of Pharmacology and Pharmacodynamics*, 5, 283–288.

Patil, C. L., Abrams, E. T., Steinmetz, A. R. and Young, S. L., 2012. Appetite sensations and nausea and vomiting in pregnancy: an overview of the explanations. *Ecology of Food and Nutrition*, 51, 394–417.

Pletsch, P. K., Pollak, K. I., Peterson, B. L., Park, J., Oncken, C. A., Swamy, G. K. and Lyna, P., 2008. Olfactory and gustatory sensory changes to tobacco smoke in pregnant smokers. *Research in Nursing & Health*, 31, 31–41.

Polimeni, J., 2012. *Shamans among Us: Schizophrenia, Shamanism and the Evolutionary Origins of Religion*. Morrisville, NC: Lulu Press.

Reyna, V. F. and Farley, F., 2006. Risk and rationality in adolescent decision making: implications for theory, practice, and public policy. *Psychological Science in the Public Interest*, 7, 1–44.

Richardson, G. B., Chen, C. C., Dai, C. L., Swoboda, C. M., Nedelec, J. L. and Chen, W. W., 2017. Substance use and mating

success. *Evolution and Human Behavior*, 38, 48–57.

Roberts, C., Lepps, H., Strang, J. and Singelton, N., 2014. Drug use and dependence. NHS Digital. Retrieved from https://files .digital.nhs.uk/pdf/3/k/adult_ psychiatric_study_ch11_web.pdf

Roulette, C. J., Kazanji, M., Breurec, S. and Hagen, E. H., 2016. High prevalence of cannabis use among Aka foragers of the Congo Basin and its possible relationship to helminthiasis. *American Journal of Human Biology*, 28, 5–15.

Roulette, C. J., Mann, H., Kemp, B. M., Remiker, M., Roulette, J. W., Hewlett, B. S., Kazanji, M., Breurec, S., Monchy, D., Sullivan, R. J. and Hagen, E. H., 2014. Tobacco use vs. helminths in Congo basin hunter-gatherers: self-medication in humans? *Evolution and Human Behavior*, 35, 397–407.

Saah, T., 2005. The evolutionary origins and significance of drug addiction. *Harm Reduction Journal*, 2, 1–7.

Schifano, F., Orsolini, L., Duccio Papanti, G. and Corkery, J. M., 2015. Novel psychoactive substances of interest for psychiatry. *World Psychiatry*, 14, 15–26.

Solecki, R.S., 1975. Shanidar IV, a Neanderthal flower burial in northern Iraq. *Science*, 190, 880–881.

Solus, J. F., Arietta, B. J., Harris, J. R., Sexton, D. P., Steward, J. Q., McMunn, C., Ihrie, P., Mehall, J. M., Edwards, T. L. and Dawson, E. P., 2004. Genetic variation in eleven phase I drug metabolism genes in an ethnically diverse population. *Pharmacogenomics*, 5, 895–931.

St John-Smith, P., McQueen, D., Edwards, L. and Schifano, F., 2013. Classical and novel psychoactive substances:

rethinking drug misuse from an evolutionary psychiatric perspective. *Human Psychopharmacology: Clinical and Experimental*, 28, 394–401.

Sullivan, R. J. and Hagen, E. H., 2002. Psychotropic substance-seeking: evolutionary pathology or adaptation? *Addiction*, 97, 389–400.

Sullivan, R. J., Hagen, E. H. and Hammerstein, P., 2008. Revealing the paradox of drug reward in human evolution. *Proceedings of the Royal Society B: Biological Sciences*, 275, 1231–1241.

Trevathan, W., Smith, E. O. and McKenna, J. J. (eds.), 2008. *Evolutionary Medicine and Health: New Perspectives*. Oxford: Oxford University Press.

United Nations Office on Drugs and Crime, 2012. World Drug Report 2012. Vienna: United Nations publication. Retrieved from www .unodc.org/unodc/en/data-and-analysis/WDR-2012.html

Weaver, T., Madden, P., Charles, V., Stimson, G., Renton, A., Tyrer, P., Barnes, T., Bench, C., Middleton, H., Wright, N. and Paterson, S., 2003. Comorbidity of Substance Misuse and Mental Illness Collaborative study team. Comorbidity of substance misuse and mental illness in community mental health and substance misuse services. *The British Journal of Psychiatry*, 183, 304–313.

Wink, M., 2000. Interference of alkaloids with neuroreceptors and ion channels. In: Atta-ur-Rahman (ed.), *Studies in Natural Products Chemistry*, Vol. 21. Amsterdam: Elsevier, pp. 3–122.

Wishard, G., 2012. *The Evolution of Childhood: Relationships, Emotion and Mind*. Abingdon-on-Thames: Taylor & Francis.

Zahavi, A. and Zahavi, A., 1997. *The Handicap Principle*. New York: Oxford University Press.

Chapter 13

The Social Function of Alcohol from an Evolutionary Perspective

Robin I. M. Dunbar

Abstract

Humans and alcohol share a deep evolutionary history: our capacity to convert alcohol into useable sugars is a trait we share with the African great apes (gorillas and chimpanzees) and is unique to this taxonomic family among the primates. Although the archaeological record only allows us to date the production of alcohol back about 9,000 years (by which time it is already on an industrial scale), a cottage industry of alcohol production must date back a great deal further. With the exception of where its consumption has been prohibited on religious grounds, alcohol use occurs in every culture and society. Notwithstanding its hedonic properties, its real functional benefit is primarily social, playing an important role in rituals and group bonding. I review studies that demonstrate its functional consequences in terms of social bonding, mediated by alcohol's ability to trigger the brain's endorphin system. The endorphin system is the central basis for social bonding in primates. The health and other benefits that arise from social bonding are considerable.

Keywords

alcohol dehydrogenase (ADH), endorphins, friendship, health benefits, mental health, social bonding

Key Points

- The relationship between humans and alcohol dates much further back than recorded history.
- The African great apes (including humans) are unique among primates in possessing enzymatic systems capable of metabolising and detoxifying alcohol.
- While being fully cognisant of the undoubted harm that excessive alcohol consumption poses to health and social well-being, it is also important to recognise the role that alcohol has played (over evolutionary history) and continues to play in human social life in many societies.
- The chapter serves as a reminder that the health benefits of well-functioning social bonds are as important or more so than other known determinants of health such as healthy diet, exercise, refraining from smoking, etc. Facilitators of social bonding in human societies include such activities as social eating, religious services, music, dance and social consumption of alcohol.

- This chapter is not intended as a guide to the assessment and/or treatment of alcohol misuse.

It is no exaggeration to say that alcohol has had a less than savoury reputation down through the ages. The medical profession has decried its destructive consequences for health, judicial authorities have condemned its social consequences and the violence it sometimes gives rise to and governments and religious communities have made determined efforts to limit its consumption or even ban it altogether. In this it shares much in common with salt, sugar, fatty foods, tobacco and class A drugs as one of many villains in the self-destructive downfall of humankind – not to mention the costs paid by society to repair the damage or absorb the consequences of alcohol-fuelled aggression. While there are obviously good grounds for holding so negative a view, we should perhaps pause before we throw the baby out with the bathwater and ask why the consumption of alcohol has come to be so near-universal a feature of human societies the world over. Is it simply that the stuff is addictive? But, if so, why aren't we all completely addicted to it? Why is it that it is always so essential a feature of social occasions? This should prompt us to ask what role alcohol has played in our evolutionary history and what role it plays in our contemporary lives. In this chapter, I want to explore both the deep history of humans and their love affair with alcohol and the social role that alcohol has played in facilitating friendships and community bonding.

13.1 A Short History of Alcohol Consumption

Our species' association with alcohol consumption, as well as many other psychoactive drugs from psilocybin to opium, has a very long history. In the archaeological record, the preparation of alcoholic drinks can be dated back at least 9,000 years. At Göbekli Tepe in south-eastern Turkey, stone fermentation vessels of enormous size (160 litres in solid stone) date from 7000 to 8000 BCE (Dietrich and Dietrich, 2019). The fermentation residues recovered from inside these jars have allowed chemists to determine the original recipes. Similarly, there is evidence that fruit wines (with honey or rice components and herbal flavourings) were being produced and drunk in the early Neolithic in China's Red River Valley (McGovern, 2019).

Wines are technically easier to produce than beers, which involve a more complex processing sequence. Nonetheless, archaeologists have wondered whether the einkorn and emmer wheats and primitive barleys that were first farmed in the Levant during the early Neolithic might have been cultivated for beer-making rather than bread-making: they have a different gluten structure from their modern counterparts and, as a result, make a very poor form of unleavened bread at best. However, they make an excellent gruel that would have provided the perfect mash for brewing (Hayden et al., 2013). Though less common now, the fermentation of honey to make mead was widely known historically. Indeed, there is circumstantial evidence for its production in Border Cave, South Africa, as early as 40,000 years ago (Rusch, 2020). The main problem with the preparation of alcoholic drinks is the need for vessels. As a result, unequivocal archaeological evidence doesn't appear until the

Neolithic when settlements allowed larger, more robust vessels to be made. Prior to that, hunter-gatherers may well have used small, fragile vessels such as ostrich eggshells and gourds that do not preserve well, especially in open occupation sites. Historically, the production of mead was certainly known to the San hunter-gatherers of southern Africa (Rusch, 2020). Alternatively, they may simply have relied on collecting naturally fermenting fruits.

The consumption of naturally occurring alcohols in overripe fruit may be extremely ancient. Fruits that have fallen to the forest floor and overripe fruits on the branch ferment naturally as the spores of natural yeasts settle on them and exploit the sugars they contain. Most fermenting fruits contain around 4% alcohol – about the same strength as beers. Alcohol is a waste product of fermentation by yeasts. Although alcohol is essentially a poison and on its own is of little use, around 10 million years ago the ancestors of the African apes (the gorillas, chimpanzees and humans) evolved a pair of enzymes that allowed them to convert alcohol back into useable sugars. This involves a two-step process: first using the alcohol dehydrogenase (ADH) enzyme to convert the alcohol into an aldehyde, and then using the aldehyde dehydrogenase (ALDH) enzyme to convert the aldehyde into acetic acid for use in the Krebs cycle (Carrigan, 2019; Carrigan et al., 2015). These two processes need to be in very close lockstep. If the ADH enzymes are slow or inefficient, alcohol builds up in the system and has the well-known adverse effects on cognition; but if ALDH doesn't keep pace with ADH, then highly toxic aldehydes build up. The African great ape lineage (including humans) is unique among the primates in having evolved these two correlated enzymes. The Asian apes (orangutans and gibbons) and all the monkeys lack them.

This obviously begs the question as to why the African apes, and no one else, evolved this unique adaptation. The most plausible reason is competition from monkeys and the abundance of fermenting fruit on the forest floor dropped by other species as well as from natural falls. Until around 10 million years ago, the Old World primate fauna was dominated by the apes, with the monkeys being a small side branch. Then, around 10 million years ago, the world's climate underwent a dramatic drying and cooling (Andrews and Van Couvering, 1975). The huge tropical forests that dominated Africa and South America underwent a massive contraction, forcing primate species into competition with each other and with other frugivores (squirrels, birds). However, the Old World monkeys had evolved the capacity to detoxify the tannins and other phenolic compounds in unripe fruit, whereas apes (and, hence, humans) lack the enzymes to do this and are only able to feed on ripe fruit (Wrangham et al., 1998). This dietary handicap will be familiar as the drying sensation in the mouth and the stomach ache and diarrhoea that we experience on eating unripe fruit. Monkeys were thus at a significant advantage, since they could eat the fruits that were available long before the apes could. When fruiting trees were in short supply, monkeys were able to clean out the available supply long before apes were able to access any. The result was a major wave of ape extinctions, with only around 10% of the ape species surviving to the present time (Fleagle, 2013). Those that made it through this intense winnowing seem to have done so by being able to exploit fermenting fruits on the ground. In Africa, none of the smaller arboreal ape species survived, with all of the surviving African great apes being species that make extensive use of terrestrial forest floor habitats.

Thus, an adaptation to handle mildly alcoholic foods seems to be very ancient in the hominin lineage, and indeed seems to predate its separation from the African great ape stock some 6–8 million years ago. An ape-like ecology continued to dominate the hominin lineage from these earliest times until around 2 million years ago, when the genus *Homo* (to which modern humans belong; see Chapter 4) appeared and rapidly replaced the bipedal apes known as australopithecines that were their immediate ancestors. The exploitation of fermented fruits from the forest floor is likely to have continued to be a major source of high-energy foods for all of the australopithecines, but this would have been more challenging for the various *Homo* species who were more nomadic and spent much of their time ranging out into the woodlands and savannahs beyond the forest edge. Nonetheless, they had the genetic adaptation and are likely to have continued to make at least occasional use of fermenting fruits whenever they ventured into the forests.

The big gap, of course, is in what happened between this point and the time when the first evidence for alcohol production appears in the archaeological record, possibly as early as 40,000 years ago and certainly by 9,000 years ago (see earlier in this section). By the latter stage, however, we are already in industrial production mode, and this cannot have appeared out of the blue. It will have been preceded by a very lengthy period of family-level cottage industry production. Nonetheless, by the time the evidence for alcohol production does appear in the archaeological record, it is on a scale that reflects large-scale feasting. Its distribution is so widespread as to suggest that it had played such a role for some considerable time. This raises the question of just what role alcohol consumption played and whether it still plays that role.

13.2 The Mechanisms of Social Bonding

Conventionally, there has been a tendency to emphasise the destructive medical consequences of alcohol consumption, varying from disapproval to outright prohibition. There can be little doubt about the fact that excessive alcohol consumption is socially destructive and can have life-threatening medical consequences. These are not, of course, to be underestimated, but they raise the question of whether resort to alcohol is simply a consequence of the hedonic effects of alcohol or represents some wider benefit. I argue here that alcohol consumption evolved as part of a suite of activities used to bond large communities. To understand why this might be so, we need to briefly consider the scale of the problem faced by ancestral humans.

Primates are an intensely social group of animals whose sociality has been the key to their evolutionary success. For most animals, group living is a response to external threats, usually predation. Lone animals are highly vulnerable to predators. This can be dealt with by forming casual herds, which allow animals to dissipate the costs of group living by dispersing once the threat has past. However, such a strategy leaves animals at risk of being caught on their own. A herd left to its own devices will end up scattered over distances too great to easily reconvene when the next predator appears. Primates have adopted a more risk-averse strategy that ensures that animals will always have companions close by.

They achieve this by creating bonded social groups whereby individuals' emotional attachment to each other ensures that they will remain close rather than drifting apart during foraging (see Chapter 1).

Primates create this bonding through social grooming – an activity that can occupy as much as 20% of the entire day in some of the most social species. The light brushing of the fur that occurs during social grooming stimulates the receptors of a unique set of neurons embedded in the hairy skin: the C-tactile neural system (Olausson et al., 2010). These are unmyelinated and hence slow-firing, with no return motor loop, and they go directly to the insula in the brain (Björnsdotter et al., 2009). From there, they activate the brain's endorphin-producing centres. Being opioids, endorphins (and β endorphins in particular) create opiate-like feelings of warmth, relaxation, calmness and trust that facilitate the development of a bonded relationship. Social touch remains a crucial basis for human social bonding (Suvilehto et al., 2015, 2019) and is underpinned by the same endorphin mechanism (Nummenmaa et al., 2016), though in the absence of body fur it takes the form of stroking, hugging and caressing.

Grooming is not random in primate groups; instead, it is mainly directed to very specific individuals within the group, with these relationships remaining extremely stable over time (Dunbar and Shultz, 2010; Massen et al., 2010). This results in bonded individuals constantly monitoring each other's whereabouts (Dunbar and Shultz, 2010) and being anxious to maintain physical contact. In this respect, we are reminded of Sternberg's (1997) triangular theory of love, two key components of which are 'being close' and 'feeling close': animals that have bonded relationships want to maintain close physical proximity. They have what, in humans, we would recognise as 'friendships' (Massen et al., 2010; Silk, 2002).

Primates create bonded groups out of these dyadic friendships by creating a network of bonded relationships that function as a cascade of links to create a spider's web of interlinked individuals. There are, however, two problems with grooming in this respect. One is that, even in humans, grooming (or any kind of physical touch) has an intimate quality to it that means it is a strictly one-on-one activity: neither monkeys, apes nor humans groom (or cuddle) more than one individual at a time with any frequency. The second issue is that the strength of a relationship with a specific individual depends on the time invested in grooming that individual (Dunbar, 1980; Sutcliffe et al., 2012). The combination of these two issues limits the size of groups that can be bonded by grooming, with the upper limit in primates set at about 50 individuals.

To evolve larger social groups, our ancestors needed to find ways to break through this glass ceiling so as to allow more individuals to be bonded without the need to increase the time required for social interaction. It seems that, over time, they lit upon a suite of behaviours that all trigger the endorphin system at a distance, thereby allowing us to 'groom' with several (in some cases, many) individuals simultaneously. These include laughter, singing, dancing, feasting, the rituals of religion and emotional storytelling. These did not appear all together but over a period of several million years, beginning with laughter (probably around 2 million years ago, since we share it with the great apes; Dunbar, in press) and ending with storytelling and the rituals of religion after the evolution of fully modern language (around 200,000 years ago: Dunbar, 2009), allowing community size to increase by a series of stages.

The important feature about all of these activities in the present context is that they all trigger the endorphin system. This has been demonstrated either using changes in pain threshold after performing the activity (laughter: Dunbar et al., 2012; singing: Weinstein et al., 2016; dancing: Tarr et al., 2015, 2016; religious rituals: Charles et al., under review; storytelling: Dunbar et al., 2016), indirectly using an endorphin antagonist (naltrexone) to block endorphin uptake (dance: Tarr et al., 2017; religious rituals: Charles et al., 2020) or directly using positron emission tomography (PET) neuroimaging (with carfentanil as the radioligand) to confirm endorphin uptake (laughter: Manninen et al., 2017; eating: Tuulari et al., 2017). In addition, all of these activities have been shown to increase the perceived sense of social bonding with the individuals involved (laughter: Dunbar et al., 2021; singing: Pearce et al., 2015; Weinstein et al., 2016; dance: Tarr et al., 2015, 2016; eating:

Dunbar, 2017; religious rituals: Charles et al., under review; storytelling: Dunbar et al., 2016). It is notable that this sense of enhanced bonding applies only to those with whom the subject is doing the activity in question and not to close friends who are not actually present (Tarr et al., 2016).

One important feature of our social world is that it is tightly constrained by both our cognitive ability to manage relationships and by our ability to create social bonds with individuals by investing time and emotional capital in them (Dunbar, 2018). While the overall size of our social networks is limited to around 150 individuals, the way we distribute our time among these individuals results in a series of circles of friendship of increasing intensity but decreasing size (Dunbar, 2020b). These circles have very distinct sizes (counting cumulatively, roughly 5, 15, 50 and 150) that are very robust and do not seem to change much across the lifespan. The most important of these circles is the innermost one of 5 – the support clique or 'shoulders to cry on' friends. We devote approximately 40% of our total social time and emotional capital to these five individuals, with a further 20% devoted to the 10 additional people that make up the circle of 15 (Sutcliffe et al., 2012). Thus, just 15 people receive approximately 60% of our social effort.

Although individuals vary somewhat in the sizes of the individual circles, the average sizes are extremely consistent across samples from a variety of sources and modes of contact (including face-to-face, telephone, texting and social media; Dunbar, 2020b). Each circle is associated broadly with different social functions, identified broadly with the support clique of 5 (those who will drop everything to come to your aid when your world implodes), the sympathy group of 15 (often defined as those whose death tomorrow would be genuinely upsetting), the affinity group of 50 (who provide the pool from which regular social companions are drawn) and the full social network of 150 friends and family (those who feel sufficient obligation towards you to want to come to those once-in-a-lifetime celebrations such as weddings and funerals; Dunbar, 2018; Sutcliffe et al., 2012).

13.3 The Social Role of Alcohol

Both archaeologically and ethnographically, it is clear that alcohol has, and has had, a close association with feasting (Guerra-Doce, 2015). The presence in the earliest settlements of fermentation vats of a size and weight that would only be worthwhile if their products were being used in large feasts implies a social role for alcohol not too different from that found in contemporary societies. Much of the literature has, perhaps inevitably, focused on the socially disinhibiting effects of alcohol consumption – alcohol as a social lubricant. This, of course, is beyond question: alcohol does loosen tongues and makes people more voluble and social – and in excessive quantities excessively voluble. However, whatever its hedonic properties might be, this alone does not explain why societies should continue to use it in a social context. If it was simply a matter of pleasure, private use of alcohol would be more important than consumption in public contexts.

In fact, the issue has much more to do with the fact that researchers have, almost without exception, focused on dyadic relationships as the social norm. How we respond to another individual's social cues and how we relate to an offspring or parent, a lover or a best friend seem to define the social world. But this is to miss most of what is actually interesting about the social world, namely how the individual and their intimate relationships fit into the larger social network within which they are embedded. And part of the challenge we face is turning this extended network into a bonded social group. It seems that the consumption of alcohol became part of the toolkit that we evolved to do this.

There has been a long-standing interest dating back to the 1970s in the role that the endorphin system might play in alcoholic addiction. The plethora of studies carried out since then now suggests fairly uncontroversially that alcohol triggers the endorphin system and that endorphin uptake in the nucleus accumbens then activates the dopaminergic pathway (Gianoulakis, 2009; Gonzales and Weiss, 1998; Modest-Love and Fritz, 2005), thereby creating both the pleasure and the buzz. Most of these studies have involved demonstrating that naltrexone or other μ-opioid receptor antagonists reduce alcohol consumption in both rodents and humans, whereas δ-opioid receptor antagonists (for which β-endorphins have only a very weak affinity) have an inconsistent effect at best. These findings have largely been borne out by knockout studies using genetically engineered mutant mice: mutants lacking the genes for the μ-opioid receptors, for example, have an aversion to alcohol (Roberts et al., 2000). Other studies have shown dose–response effects of alcohol consumption on β-endorphin secretion from the pituitary and hypothalamus (its two principle sources). In contrast, studies that have assayed for plasma oxytocin found no evidence that alcohol consumption triggers the release of oxytocin (Dolder et al., 2017).

Identifying the endorphin and dopamine systems as being activated by alcohol consumption immediately raises the question as to whether the alcohol itself is instrumental in increasing social bonding. One obvious problem in this context is that it is usually difficult to dissociate effects due to alcohol consumption from those due to the other activities commonly involved in social contexts such as laughter that are also known to trigger both the endorphin and psychological bonding systems. However, some insights are provided by a large-scale national survey into the use of pubs. The survey (carried out by YouGov and commissioned by the campaigning organisation Campaign for Real Ale (CAMRA)) asked 2254 respondents to rate aspects of their drinking habits and to answer a number of standard sociological questions related to life satisfaction based on the questions used by the UK Office of National Statistics. The data indicate that regular drinkers, and especially those with a 'local' that they visit regularly, were significantly happier, more satisfied with life, felt their life was more worthwhile, felt more engaged with the wider community within which they lived, trusted the members of that community more and had more close friends than non-drinkers. Notably, those who had a regular 'local' to which they went (where they were likely to know the clientele as well as the staff) rated themselves higher on most of these measures than those who were more peripatetic in their drinking habits. Causality is difficult to establish from data of this kind, but some insights can be gained by exploratory path analysis. This suggests that those who are more satisfied with their lives are more likely to be happier and to trust their wider community, but there is also a strong independent effect of the frequency of pub visits on engagement with the local community, trust in this wider community and the number of close friends.

A parallel *in vivo* study of the clientele of a sample of pubs (87% of whom were below the UK legal drink-drive limit for blood alcohol level, as assayed on the spot by breathalyser) suggested that the environment of the pub itself has an important effect: drinkers in quieter traditional community pubs differed from drinkers in city centre bars (where the emphasis is typically on high volume throughput) in their engagement in conversations and with each other, as well as in the duration and stability of conversations (Dunbar et al., 2017). Those frequenting community pubs seemed to be social drinkers who were there to engage with each other, whereas city centre bars were more likely to attract those simply aiming to get drunk as fast as possible. Aside from the difference in the quantity of alcohol consumed (and hence the negative health effects), the distinction is likely to be important in terms of the social and health benefits derived from the consumption of alcohol.

In sum, however detrimental overconsumption might be in health terms, modest alcohol consumption in a social context has demonstrable benefits in terms of a number of standard psychological and social metrics. These benefits reflect directly the size of social circle – and especially the number of close friends ('shoulders to cry on' friends) – that anyone is likely to have. The question this raises is exactly what these benefits might be.

13.4 Some Benefits of Endorphins

In addition to facilitating the processes of social bonding and community cohesion, alcohol seems to have direct benefits at the personal level in two key respects. One is in terms of enhanced cognitive performance; the other is in respect of health benefits. This is not, of course, to say that excessive alcohol consumption does not have the adverse consequences that have so frequently been highlighted in the medical literature. There can be no doubt about these. Rather, the point I highlight here is the distinction between moderate consumption and overconsumption.

There is considerable experimental and survey evidence that modest alcohol consumption is correlated with beneficial consequences in terms of cognition. Lang et al. (2007) examined data from the English Longitudinal Study of Ageing (ELSA) and found that, for respondents in their 60s, cognitive function (memory recall, numerical reasoning) showed an inverted-U-shaped relationship with alcohol consumption, with those having moderate consumption (one to two drinks per day) performing best. They also had higher ratings of well-being and lower frequencies of symptoms associated with depression. Similar results were obtained from the UK Whitehall II Study of some 10,000 civil servants aged 46–68 when assessed: moderate drinkers (up to 30 drinks (240 g of alcohol) a week) performed better than both those who rarely drank and those who drank significantly more on a range of cognitive and verbal fluency tasks, even when adjusting for age, physical health, smoking status and employment grade (Britton et al., 2004). Similarly, a US study of ageing women found that those who had at least one drink per day had higher cognitive function on a battery of tests designed to detect mild cognitive impairment and dementia risk than those who did not drink or had lower intake levels (Espeland et al., 2005). Similarly, a large-scale longitudinal US study of retired nurses in their 70s revealed higher cognitive function among moderate drinkers (intake of less than 15 g of alcohol per day) compared to both non-drinkers and those who drank 15–30 g per day (Stampfer et al., 2005). In a naturalistic study, Carlyle et al. (2017) tested memory for previously learnt facts both after a 'normal' social drinking evening (mean consumption of ~83 g of alcohol) and the following morning. They found that performance was higher, especially on recall the following day, for those who drank socially than a matched control group who remained sober.

In addition, there is considerable survey evidence from longitudinal studies to suggest that modest alcohol consumption may protect against later dementia (Sabia et al., 2018) as well as cardiovascular disease (Haseeb et al., 2017; O'Keefe et al., 2014). In both cases, those who consumed little or no alcohol and those who overconsumed experienced adverse consequences compared to moderate drinkers.

It is notable that many of these studies report an inverted-U-shaped relationship between alcohol consumption and ill health. Such relationships are common in biology. No salt is bad for you, some salt is good for you, but too much salt is toxic. Often these kinds of relationships reflect trade-offs between two opposing forces that correlate in opposite directions with the same independent variable. In the present case, these are the benefits provided both by social bonding and by

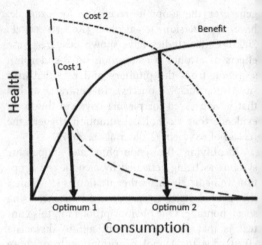

Figure 13.1 There is no perfect solution in the biological world because most things are a trade-off between the costs and benefits of consumption. Here, the benefits and costs of consuming something (e.g. alcohol) are both measured in terms of the effects that they each independently have on health (e.g. on future lifespan). The optimum level of consumption (the point at which the health benefits equal the health costs) will depend on the shapes of the two curves. Benefits (solid line) often have an asymptotic shape (they rise rapidly to a maximum and then flatten off with no further increase in the benefit). If the cost curve is steep (Cost 1, long-dashed line: even a small amount of the substance adversely affects health), the optimum level of consumption will be low (Optimum 1). If the cost curve is shallow (Cost 2, short-dashed line: adverse effects are only felt after consuming a great deal), then the optimum level of consumption will be higher (Optimum 2)

the fact that some aspect of alcohol protects against at least some diseases (health and longevity increase with alcohol consumed as a result) and the costs incurred by consuming what is essentially a poison (with the result that health and longevity decrease with alcohol consumed). The optimal balance will depend on the exact slopes of the two functions and the way they work against each other. The steeper the cost curve (or the shallower the benefit curve), the lower will be the optimal level of consumption (Figure 13.1).

In addition to these direct benefits, there are also significant benefits that arise indirectly through the creation of friendships. There is now a wealth of evidence that the best predictor of both mental health and well-being and physical health and well-being, and even longevity, is the number and quality of close friendships (Dominguez and Arford, 2010; House, 2001; Pinquart and Duberstein, 2010; Reblin and Uchino, 2008; Smith and Christakis, 2008). Holt-Lunstad et al. (2010), for example, collated data from 148 epidemiological studies of mortality and reported that the risk of mortality from cardiovascular causes in particular was most strongly influenced by the quality of close friendships, with giving up smoking being a close second, but all other factors that the medical profession conventionally worry about (obesity, diet, lack of exercise, alcohol consumption, prescribed medication, local air quality) lagged far behind. These effects extend both to physical ailments, such as cancer (Chou et al., 2012; Liu and Newschaffer, 2011), as well as to the dementias and the general mortality associated with old age (Min et al., 2007; Rodriguez-Laso et al., 2007; Tilvis et al., 2012). Many of these studies are based on longitudinal studies of large national samples. It is important to appreciate that these effects derive not from the total number of friends one has but specifically the number of close (or 'shoulders to cry on') friends.

The significance of these social effects on health are given added significance by the fact that the protective effects of close social relationships are not confined to humans. Similar effects have been reported from wild primates: females who have more grooming partners (i.e. friends) have better health, lower stress levels and quicker recovery times from injuries, are more fertile, have better offspring survival rates and themselves live longer (Crockford et al., 2008; Silk et al., 2003, 2009, 2010; Wittig et al., 2008). Similar findings have been reported for wild horse (Cameron et al., 2009; Nuñez et al., 2015) and dolphin populations (Frère et al., 2010).

To the extent that alcohol is used as part of the bonding process, these benefits will derive from this source. This does not, of course, imply that the consumption of alcohol is essential (i.e. both necessary and sufficient) to obtain these benefits. Humans bond their friendships through a suite of social behaviours and activities. In large-scale survey studies, we have shown that both eating socially (especially in the evening) and being religiously active (as indexed by the frequency of attending religious services) lead to higher self-ratings of happiness and satisfaction with life as well as less frequent reports of feeling depressed (Dunbar, 2017, 2020a). The point here is simply that all of these activities involve engaging socially with other people.

In a very large-scale multinational survey across 13 European countries, Santini et al. (2021) reported that, among people aged 50 years and older, future symptoms of depression were minimised for those who had around five close friends or were involved in about three voluntary community activities (e.g. helping with Scouts, being involved in hobby clubs, religious centres or political organisations). These two factors could be offset against each other (the effect of having fewer friends could be offset by being involved in more organisations), but they were not additive: having five friends *and* being involved in three organisations resulted in *higher* levels of depression. Being involved in voluntary and other communal organisations most likely works because these are social rather than strictly functional environments, such that people meet and engage socially with each other and hence create friendships of some kind. Having more than five friends or being involved in more than three activities results in one's social capital being spread too thinly, such that the benefits of social engagement are not fully realised.

While these obviously need not involve the consumption of alcohol, it is clear nonetheless that the consumption of alcohol often does play a role in these social processes. Dunbar (2017) found that evening meals were considered to be especially productive for bonding old friendships. When asked what activities were most important in these contexts, respondents identified three in particular: laughter, reminiscences and the consumption of alcohol.

The mechanism(s) involved in these buffering effects remains unclear, however, mainly because the benefits of the endorphin system outside of pain modulation and hedonic pleasure have not featured prominently enough to warrant detailed exploration of the biochemical mechanisms that underpin them. Nonetheless, there is some evidence to suggest that endorphins promote the production of 'natural killer' (NK) cells by the immune system (Mandler et al., 1986), although this process can be impeded by excessive consumption of alcohol (Boyadjieva et al., 2001; Sarkar et al., 2012). Functionally, NK cells target and destroy viruses and cancer cells, which might explain in part the beneficial effects that friendship and modest alcohol consumption have on both general morbidity levels and mortality risk.

13.5 Conclusion

Alcohol has been a part of the human social world for a great deal longer than those beverages such as tea and coffee that we associate both with refreshment and entertainment. It has formed one of the suite of activities that we use for building and maintaining friendships. The social role of alcohol, however, is not simply that it makes us more social and voluble. While that is certainly true, it misses the far more important point that, directly and indirectly (through the creation of friendships), alcohol can influence our health and well-being. The large cultural component of *how* we use alcohol does, however, mean that it can be used to excess by a minority of the population (McShane, 2019), and this can have significant consequences both for the costs of treating the conditions that result from this and for the costs borne by the wider society from drink-fuelled violence.

Of course, it is by no means the case that social life would end without alcohol. None of the behaviours that form the core of our social world (laughter, singing, dancing, feasting, emotional storytelling, the rituals of religion) are sacrosanct in these terms, and at one time or another different societies have tried to suppress most of them – albeit largely without success. The production of alcohol does, of course, involve more technical skill than most of these other behaviours, and cultures do sometimes lose these skills. That said, alcohol is only one of a very large number of psychotropic drugs (opium, cannabis, psilocybin, mescaline, morning glories, henbane, belladonna, mandrake) that humans have discovered and used in social contexts (Dunbar, 2022; Dunbar and Hockings, 2019), all of which share with alcohol both beneficial properties (many were originally discovered for their medicinal properties) and destructive consequences when overused. As with most things biological, the use of alcohol has always been a trade-off between these social benefits and personal costs.

References

Andrews, P. and Van Couvering, J. A. (1975). Palaeoenvironments in the East African Miocene. In: F. S. Szalay (ed.), *Approaches to Primate Paleobiology*, Vol. 5. Basel: Karger, pp. 62–103.

Björnsdotter, M., Löken, L., Olausson, H., Vallbo, Å. and Wessberg, J. (2009). Somatotopic organization of gentle touch processing in the posterior insular cortex. *Journal of Neuroscience* 29: 9314–9320.

Boyadjieva, N., Dokur, M., Advis, J. P., Meadows, G. G. and Sarkar, D. K. (2001). Chronic ethanol inhibits NK cell cytolytic activity. Role of opioid peptide-endorphin. *Journal of Immunology* 167: 5645–5652.

Britton, A., Singh-Manoux, A. and Marmot, M. (2004). Alcohol consumption and cognitive function in the Whitehall II Study. *American Journal of Epidemiology* 160: 240–247.

Cameron, E. Z., Setsaas, T. H. and Linklater, W. L. (2009). Social bonds between unrelated females increase reproductive success in feral horses. *Proceedings of the National Academy of Sciences of the United States of America* 106: 13850–13853.

Carlyle, M., Dumay, N., Roberts, K., McAndrew, A., Stevens, T., Lawn, W. and Morgan, C.J. (2017). Improved memory for information learnt before alcohol use in social drinkers tested in a naturalistic setting. *Scientific Reports* 7: 6213.

Carrigan, M. (2019). Hominoid adaptation to dietary ethanol. In: K. Hockings and R. I. M. Dunbar (eds.), *Alcohol and Humans: A Long and Social Affair*. Oxford: Oxford University Press, pp. 24–44.

Carrigan, M. A., Uryasev, O., Frye, C. B., Eckman, B. L., Myers, C. R., Hurley, T. D. and Benner, S. A. (2015). Hominids adapted to metabolize ethanol long before human-directed fermentation. *Proceedings of the National Academy of Sciences of the United States of America* 112: 458–463.

Charles, S. J., Farias, M., van Mulukom, V., Saraswati, A., Dein, S., Watts, F. and Dunbar, R. I. M. (2020). Blocking mu-opioid receptors inhibits social bonding in rituals. *Biology Letters* 16: 20200485.

Charles, S. J., van Mulukom, V., Farias, M., Brown, J. E., Delmonte, R., Maraldi, E., et al. (under review). Religious rituals increase social bonding and pain threshold.

Chou, A., Stewart, S., Wild, R. and Bloom, J. (2012). Social support and survival in young women with breast carcinoma. *Psycho-Oncology* 21: 125–133.

Crockford, C., Wittig, R. M., Whitten, P. L., Seyfarth, R. M. and Cheney, D. L. (2008). Social stressors and coping mechanisms in wild female baboons (*Papio hamadryas ursinus*). *Hormones and Behavior* 53: 254–265.

Dietrich, O. and Dietrich, L. (2019). Rituals and feasting as incentives for cooperative action at early Neolithic Göbekli Tepe. In: K. Hockings and R. I. M. Dunbar (eds.), *Alcohol and Humans: A Long and Social Affair*. Oxford: Oxford University Press, pp. 93–114.

Dolder, P. C., Holze, F., Liakoni, E., Harder, S., Schmid, Y. and Liechti, M. E. (2017). Alcohol acutely enhances decoding of positive emotions and emotional concern for positive stimuli and facilitates the viewing of sexual images. *Psychopharmacology* 234: 41–51.

Dominguez, S. and Arford, T. (2010). It is all about who you know: social capital and health in low-income communities. *Health Sociology Review* 19: 114–129.

Dunbar, R. I. M. (1980). Determinants and evolutionary consequences of dominance among female gelada baboons. *Behavioral Ecology and Sociobiology* 7: 253–265.

Dunbar, R. I. M. (2009). Why only humans have language. In: R. Botha and C. Knight (eds.), *The Prehistory of Language*. Oxford: Oxford University Press, pp. 12–35.

Dunbar, R. I. M. (2017). Breaking bread: the functions of social eating. *Adaptive Human Behavior and Physiology* 3: 198–211.

Dunbar, R. I. M. (2018). The anatomy of friendship. *Trends in Cognitive Sciences* 22: 32–51.

Dunbar, R. I. M. (2020a). Religiosity and religious attendance as factors in wellbeing and social engagement. *Religion Brain and Behavior* 11: 17–26.

Dunbar, R. I. M. (2020b). Structure and function in human and primate social networks: Implications for diffusion, network stability and health. *Proceedings of the Royal Society A: Mathematical, Physical and Engineering Sciences* 476: 20200446.

Dunbar, R. I. M. (2022). *The Evolution of Religion*. London: Pelican.

Dunbar, R. I. M. (in press). Laughter and its role in the evolution of human social bonding. *Philosophical Transactions of the Royal Society B: Biological Sciences*.

Dunbar, R. I. M. and Hockings, K. (eds.) (2019). Introduction. In: K. Hockings and R. I. M. Dunbar (eds.), *Alcohol and Humans: A Long and Social Affair*. Oxford: Oxford University Press, pp. 1–8.

Dunbar, R. I. M. and Shultz, S. (2010). Bondedness and sociality. *Behaviour* 147: 775–803.

Dunbar, R. I. M., Baron, R., Frangou, A., Pearce, E., van Leeuwen, E.J.C., Stow, J., et al. (2012). Social laughter is correlated with an elevated pain threshold. *Proceedings of the Royal Society B: Biological Sciences* 27: 1161–1167.

Dunbar, R. I. M., Frangou, A., Grainger, F. and Pearce, E. (2021). Laughter influences social bonding but not prosocial generosity to friends and strangers. *PLoS ONE* 16: e0256229.

Dunbar, R. I. M., Launay, J., Wlodarski, R., Robertson, C., Pearce, E., Carney, J. and MacCarron, P. (2017). Functional benefits of (modest) alcohol consumption. *Adaptive Human Behavior and Physiology* 3: 118–133.

Dunbar, R. I. M., Teasdale, B., Thompson, J., Budelmann, F., Duncan, S., van Emde Boas, E. and Maguire, L. (2016). Emotional arousal when watching drama increases pain threshold and social bonding. *Royal Society Open Science* 3: 160288.

Espeland, M. A., Gu, L., Masaki, K. H., Langer, R. D., Coker, L. H., Stefanick, M. L., et al. (2005). Association between reported alcohol intake and cognition: results from the Women's Health Initiative Memory Study. *American Journal of Epidemiology* 161: 228–238.

Fleagle, J. G. (2013). *Primate Adaptation and Evolution*, 3rd ed. New York: Academic Press.

Frère, C. H., Krützen, M., Mann, J., Connor, R. C., Bejder, L. and Sherwin, W. B. (2010). Social and genetic interactions drive fitness variation in a free-living dolphin population. *Proceedings of the National Academy of Sciences of the United States of America* 107: 19949–19954.

Gianoulakis, C. (2009). Endogenous opioids and addiction to alcohol and other drugs of abuse. *Current Topics in Medicinal Chemistry* 9: 999–1015.

Gonzales, R. A. and Weiss, F. (1998). Suppression of ethanol-reinforced behavior by naltrexone is associated with attenuation of the ethanol-induced increase in dialysate dopamine levels in the nucleus accumbens. *Journal of Neuroscience* 18: 10663–10671.

Guerra-Doce, E. (2015). The origins of inebriation: archaeological evidence of the consumption of fermented beverages and drugs in prehistoric Eurasia. *Journal of Archaeological Method and Theory* 22: 751–782.

Haseeb, S., Alexander, B. and Baranchuk, A. (2017). Wine and cardiovascular health: a comprehensive review. *Circulation* 136: 1434–1448.

Hayden, B., Canuel, N. and Shanse, J. (2013). What was brewing in the Natufian? An archaeological assessment of brewing technology in the Epipaleolithic. *Journal of Archaeological Method and Theory* 20: 102–150.

Holt-Lunstad, J., Smith, T. and Bradley Layton, J. (2010). Social relationships and mortality risk: a meta-analytic review. *PLoS Medicine* 7: e1000316.

House, J. (2001). Social isolation kills, but how and why? *Psychosomatic Medicine* 63: 273–274.

Inagaki, T. K., Ray, L. A., Irwin, M. R., Way, B. M. and Eisenberger, N. I. (2016). Opioids and social bonding: naltrexone reduces feelings of social connection. *Social Cognitive and*

Affective Neuroscience 11: 728–735.

Lang, I., Wallace, R. B., Huppert, F. A. and Melzer, D. (2007). Moderate alcohol consumption in older adults is associated with better cognition and well-being than abstinence. *Age and Ageing* 36: 256–261.

Liu, L. and Newschaffer, C. J. (2011). Impact of social connections on risk of heart disease, cancer and all-cause mortality among elderly Americans: findings from the Second Longitudinal Study of Aging (LSOA II). *Archives of Gerontology and Geriatrics* 53: 168–173.

Mandler, R. N., Biddison, W. E., Mandler, R. and Serrate, S. A. (1986). Endorphin augments the cytolytic activity and interferon production of natural killer cells. *Journal of Immunology* 136: 934–939.

Manninen, S., Tuominen, L., Dunbar, R. I. M., Karjalainen, T., Hirvonen, J., Arponen, E., et al. (2017). Social laughter triggers endogenous opioid release in humans. *Journal of Neuroscience* 37: 6125–6131.

Massen, J., Sterck, E. and de Vos, H. (2010). Close social associations in animals and humans: functions and mechanisms of friendship. *Behaviour* 147: 1379–1412.

McGovern, P. E. (2019). Uncorking the past: alcoholic fermentation as humankind's first biotechnology. In: K. Hockings and R. I. M. Dunbar (eds.), *Alcohol and Humans: A Long and Social Affair*. Oxford: Oxford University Press, pp. 81–92.

McShane, A. (2019). Through the drinking glass: a long history of pints and performative materialities in England. In: K. Hockings and R. I. M. Dunbar (eds.) *Alcohol and Humans: A Long and Social Affair*. Oxford: Oxford University Press, pp. 178–195.

Min, S.-Y., Whitecraft, E., Rothbard, A. B. and Salzer, M. S. (2007). Peer support for persons with co-occurring disorders and community tenure: a survival analysis. *Psychiatric Rehabilitation Journal* 30: 207–213.

Modesto-Lowe, V. and Fritz, E. M. (2005). The opioidergic–alcohol link. *CNS Drugs* 19: 693–707.

Nummenmaa, L., Tuominen, L., Dunbar, R. I. M., Hirvonen, J., Manninen, S., Arponen, E., et al. (2016). Reinforcing social bonds by touching modulates endogenous μ-opioid system activity in humans. *NeuroImage* 138: 242–247.

Nuñez, C. M. V., Adelman, J. S. and Rubenstein, D. I. (2015). Sociality increases juvenile survival after a catastrophic event in the feral horse (*Equus caballus*). *Behavioral Ecology* 26: 138–147.

O'Keefe, J. H., Bhatti, S. K., Bajwa, A., DiNicolantonio, J. J. and Lavie, C. J. (2014). Alcohol and cardiovascular health: the dose makes the poison… or the remedy. *Mayo Clinic Proceedings* 89: 382–393.

Olausson, H., Wessberg, J., Morrison, I., McGlone, F. and Vallbo, A. (2010). The neurophysiology of unmyelinated tactile afferents. *Neuroscience and Biobehavioral Reviews* 34: 185–191.

Pearce, E., Launay, J. and Dunbar, R. I. M. (2015). The ice-breaker effect: singing mediates fast social bonding. *Royal Society Open Science* 2: 150221.

Pinquart, M. and Duberstein, P. R. (2010). Association of social networks with cancer mortality: a meta-analysis. *Critical Review of Oncology and Haematology* 75: 122–137.

Reblin, M. and Uchino, B. N. (2008). Social and emotional support and its implication for health. *Current Opinion in Psychiatry* 21: 201–205.

Roberts, A. J., McDonald, J. S., Heyser, C. J., Kieffer, B. L., Matthes, H. W., Koob, G. F. and Gold, L. H. (2000). μ-Opioid receptor knockout mice do not self-administer alcohol. *Journal of Pharmacology and Experimental Therapeutics* 293: 1002–1008.

Rodriguez-Laso, A., Zunzunegui, M. V. and Otero, A. (2007). The effect of social relationships on survival in elderly residents of a Southern European community: a cohort study. *BMC Geriatrics* 7: 19.

Rusch, N. (2020). Controlled fermentation, honey, bees and alcohol: archaeological and ethnohistorical evidence from southern Africa. *South African Humanities* 33: 1–31.

Sabia, S., Fayosse, A., Dumurgier, J., Dugravot, A., Akbaraly, T., Britton, A., et al. (2018). Alcohol consumption and risk of dementia: 23 year follow-up of Whitehall II cohort study. *BMJ* 362: k2927.

Santini, Z., Jose, P., Koyanagi, A., Meilstrup, C., Nielsen, L., Madsen, K., et al. (2021). The moderating role of social network size in the temporal association between formal social participation and mental health: a longitudinal analysis using two consecutive waves of the Survey of Health, Ageing and Retirement in Europe (SHARE). *Social Psychiatry and Psychological Epidemiology* 56: 417–428.

Sarkar, D. K., Sengupta, A., Zhang, C., Boyadjieva, N. and Murugan, S. (2012). Opiate antagonist prevents μ- and δ-opiate receptor dimerization to facilitate ability of agonist to control ethanol-altered natural killer cell functions and mammary tumor growth. *Journal of Biological Chemistry* 287: 16734–16747.

Silk, J. (2002). Using the 'F'-word in primatology. *Behaviour* 139: 421–446.

Silk, J. B., Alberts, S. C. and Altmann, J. (2003). Social bonds of female baboons enhance infant survival. *Science* 302: 1232–1234.

Silk, J. B., Beehner, J. C., Bergman, T. J., Crockford, C., Engh, A. L., Moscovice, L. R., et al. (2009). The benefits of social capital: close social bonds among female baboons enhance offspring survival. *Proceedings of the Royal Society B: Biological Sciences* 276: 3099–3104.

Silk, J. B., Beehner, J. C., Bergman, T. J., Crockford, C., Engh, A. L., Moscovice, L. R., et al. (2010). Strong and consistent social bonds enhance the longevity of female baboons. *Current Biology* 20: 1359–1361.

Smith, K. P. and Christakis, N. A. (2008). Social networks and health. *American Journal of Sociology* 34: 405–429.

Stampfer, M. J., Kang, J. H., Chen, J., Cherry, R. and Grodstein, F. (2005). Effects of moderate alcohol consumption on cognitive function in women. *New England Journal of Medicine* 352: 245–253.

Sternberg, R. J. (1997). Construct validation of a triangular love scale. *European Journal of Social Psychology* 27: 313–335.

Sutcliffe, A., Dunbar, R. I. M., Binder, J. and Arrow, H. (2012). Relationships and the social brain: integrating psychological and evolutionary perspectives. *British Journal of Psychology* 103: 149–168.

Suvilehto, J., Glerean, E., Dunbar, R. I. M., Hari, R. and Nummenmaa, L. (2015). Topography of social touching depends on emotional bonds between humans. *Proceedings of the National Academy of Sciences of the United States of America* 112: 13811–13816.

Suvilehto, J., Nummenmaa, L., Harada, T., Dunbar, R. I. M., Hari, R., Turner, R., et al. (2019). Cross-cultural similarity in relationship-specific social touching. *Proceedings of the Royal Society B: Biological Sciences* 286: 20190467.

Tarr, B., Launay, J., Cohen, E. and Dunbar, R. I. M. (2015). Synchrony and exertion during dance independently raise pain threshold and encourage social bonding. *Biology Letters* 11: 20150767.

Tarr, B., Launay, J. and Dunbar, R. I. M. (2016). Silent disco: dancing in synchrony leads to elevated pain thresholds and social closeness. *Evolution and Human Behavior* 37: 343–349.

Tarr, B., Launay, J. and Dunbar, R. I. M. (2017). Naltrexone blocks endorphins released when dancing in synchrony. *Adaptive Human Behavior and Physiology* 3: 241–254.

Tilvis, R., Routasalo, P., Karppinen, H., Strandberg, T., Kautiainen, H., and Pitkala, K. (2012). Social isolation, social activity and loneliness as survival indicators in old age: a nationwide survey with a 7-year follow up. *European Geriatric Medicine* 3: 18–22.

Tuulari, J. J., Tuominen, L., de Boer, F. E., Hirvonen, J., Helin, S., Nuutila, P. and Nummenmaa, L. (2017). Feeding releases endogenous opioids in humans. *Journal of Neuroscience* 37: 8284–8291.

Weinstein, D., Launay, J., Pearce, E., Dunbar, R. I. M. and Stewart, L. (2016). Singing and social bonding: changes in connectivity and pain threshold as a function of group size. *Evolution and Human Behavior* 37: 152–158.

Wittig, R. M., Crockford, C., Lehmann, J., Whitten, P. L., Seyfarth, R. M. and Cheney, D. L. (2008). Focused grooming networks and stress alleviation in wild female baboons. *Hormones and Behavior* 54: 170–177.

Wrangham, R. W., Conklin-Brittain, N. L. and Hunt, K. D. (1998). Dietary response of chimpanzees and cercopithecines to seasonal variation in fruit abundance. I. Antifeedants. *International Journal of Primatology* 19: 949–970.

Chapter 14

Evolutionary Perspectives on Childhood Trauma

Annie Swanepoel, Michael J. Reiss, John Launer, Graham Music and Bernadette Wren

Abstract

Throughout human evolutionary history, infants and children have been dependent on adult caregivers for survival. The care that adults give is greatly influenced by prevailing conditions, including the availability of food and their social contacts, and also by their own experience of care. We use an evolutionary perspective to discuss possible reasons why children may suffer trauma at the hands of their parents and consider how children have adapted in response to such trauma to maximise their chances of survival in order to reach reproductive age and produce their own offspring. We examine how child maltreatment might differ at the hands of mothers, fathers and step-parents and discuss parent–offspring conflict, life history theory, attachment theory and differential susceptibility to help explain the complexity of childhood trauma. We end with recommendations for clinical practice.

Keywords

abuse, attachment theory, childhood trauma, evolutionary perspectives, life history theory, parent–offspring conflict

Key Points

- Adverse childhood experiences lead to trauma in sensitive individuals. Adverse contexts lead to parental stress, which in turn can give rise to abuse and neglect.
- While harmful to the children who are its victims, such behaviour may be adaptive for adults in some contexts and advantageous to siblings.
- Infants have evolved to survive so far as is possible, whatever their environments. It is adaptive to be securely attached and trusting in a benign environment. In contrast, it is adaptive to avoid annoying a rejecting mother and to plead with an ambivalent one. Infants can become attached to abusive caregivers and use a variety of strategies, even if disorganised, to try to find an approach that works.
- Individuals have differing levels of sensitivity to the environment. Some are like dandelions and will manage regardless. Others are more like orchids and will struggle very much in a non-ideal environment, but if

given a benign environment will do exceptionally well – outperforming the more resilient types.

- An evolutionary perspective does not consider one single developmental pathway or attachment pattern as normal and the others as abnormal – nor one as functional and the others as dysfunctional. Nature requires different strategies to cope with different circumstances.
- A more nuanced understanding of adult behaviours and their determinants may enable clinicians, patients and clients alike to take a less idealistic but more realistic and more compassionate view.

14.1 An Evolutionary Perspective on Why Parents May Maltreat Their Children

As therapists and scholars interested in how evolutionary thinking might inform clinical work in psychiatry, we have been meeting regularly at the Tavistock Clinic for a number of years to look at ways that evolutionary thinking might inform theory and practice in the field of mental health (Swanepoel et al., 2016, 2017; Wren et al., 2019, 2021). We are interested in how such thinking might enhance other ways of understanding these issues and contribute to reducing stigma by making sense of feelings and behaviours that might otherwise merely seem aberrant. We believe that this approach also has something of value to add to our understanding of childhood trauma.

A growing body of research has identified the harmful effects that adverse childhood experiences (ACEs) have on physical and mental health throughout life (Danese and McEwen, 2012). Such forms of trauma are wide-ranging and encompass parental separation, household mental illness or domestic violence and alcohol or drug abuse, as well as verbal, physical and sexual abuse and physical or emotional neglect. These all have complex causes. In this chapter, we specifically address physical abuse and neglect of children, where we believe evolutionary influences play a part and where evolutionary thinking may be helpful to clinicians (see also Chapter 16). Our focus is mainly on: (1) how abusive or neglectful behaviour may have been adaptive (over evolutionary history) for adults under stress and/or advantageous to siblings; and (2) how children respond to abuse and neglect in a variety of ways that make sense in evolutionary terms and may lead to intergenerational patterns of trauma. We do not address sexual abuse since its causes are likely to be more multifactorial (Mathews, 2019) and it is as yet unclear how or whether an evolutionary perspective adds to our understanding of it.

Child abuse is a common and serious problem. The majority of published contributions on the issue focus on describing what happens and how that influences the child as well as the risks of intergenerational transmission (WHO, 2020). Few thinkers in child psychiatry or psychology have focused on how evolutionary science may provide a wider perspective (e.g. van IJzendoorn et al., 2020). Tinbergen described four aspects that need to be considered in order to understand a behaviour from an evolutionary perspective (Tinbergen, 1963): causation (mechanism), survival value (function), ontogeny (development) and its evolutionary history (see Chapter 1). Most of the thinking about child abuse (as is the case for the whole of mainstream mental health) currently focuses on mechanism and development alone. Thus, while we now have a better understanding of how exposure to trauma affects stress systems and can lead to long-term physical and emotional ill health (Heim et al., 2019) and know that stressed and unsupported mothers are at higher risk of abusing their children (St-Laurent et al., 2019), little attention has been paid to the underlying factors as to why this might be so – what Tinbergen referred to as the 'survival value' of a behaviour, both for mothers and for children.

While concentrating on 'survival value', we emphasise that it is *not* our contention that pursuing an evolutionary understanding of maltreatment means that we deem it to be acceptable; nor do we advocate doing nothing to help change the situation. Rather, what we are proposing is that the issue of abuse and neglect be considered not just through a safeguarding lens (if focusing on the child(ren)) or legal lens (if focusing on the abuser), but also by trying to make sense of these behaviours. Our approach, in line with all evolutionary psychiatry scholarship, is therefore not normative but explanatory. We should also stress that abuse and neglect are deeply harmful for children, and we would therefore argue that a deeper understanding of this phenomenon can improve the efficacy of prevention and management. However, we will argue that there are specific circumstances under which we might expect abuse of children to occur for reasons that, from an evolutionary perspective, may be adaptive for the abuser.

In order to explain our evolutionarily informed thinking, we will refer to: (1) parent–offspring conflict; (2) life history theory; (3) conditional adaptation as described by attachment theory; and (4) differential susceptibility (see also Chapter 1). Our aim is to show that children are shaped by the environments they are born into and that the parental care they receive transmits information about the environment prenatally and for many years after. If, as professionals, we want to improve children's lives, far from working only with children, we need also to improve their physical and emotional environments.

14.2 Parent–Offspring Conflict: Can Child Maltreatment Be Adaptive for the Parent?

14.2.1 Introduction

Parents' and children's interests are not always fully aligned (see Chapter 1). Even the most committed mother will find that her baby wants more from her than she is able to give. Mothers have other commitments too, which may include a relationship with the father, other children, wider caring responsibilities in the family, friendships and paid employment. Babies want their mothers to be available at their beck and call. This is not and has never been possible all of the time. Parent–offspring conflict refers to the difference in the level of optimal parental investment from the viewpoint of the parent and that of the offspring. In general terms, the greater the biological relationship, the greater the investment. Having surviving children allows parental genes to remain in the gene pool and not die out. From an evolutionary perspective, those parents who invested optimally in their children's survival are the ones whose genes survived and whose descendants we are.

14.2.2 Step-Parents

This raises the question of childcare by non-related step-parents. In the 1970s, data gradually accumulated that appeared to show that stepchildren were far more at risk of harm from a step-parent than from a biological parent. The phenomenon became known as the 'Cinderella effect' after the tale recounted by Perrault in the seventeenth century and Jacob and Wilhelm Grimm in the nineteenth century. In Cinderella, it is a stepmother who makes life a misery for her stepchild. Interestingly, there is more of a stigma attached to stepmothers than to stepfathers, which may make it more difficult for stepmothers to engage with their stepchildren for fear of being seen as trying to push the biological mother from her pedestal (van Houdt et al., 2020).

In a series of publications produced in the 1980s and 1990s, the evolutionary psychologists Martin Daly and Margo Wilson presented data to substantiate the idea that step-parents are about one order of magnitude more likely to harm stepchildren than they are likely to harm their own children or other parents are to harm their biological children (e.g. Daly and Wilson, 1996). The reason, they argued, followed directly from evolutionary biology. Parental investment is very costly for humans. To be blunt, it therefore makes less sense to invest in children to whom one is not genetically related than in one's own children. Daly and Wilson also drew direct comparisons with non-humans. For example, when, as happens quite often, a pride of female lions is taken over by a new group of male lions, the new males often kill all of the lion cubs in the pride. The result is that the lionesses come back into oestrus and mate with the new adult males, producing offspring that now have these new adult males as their fathers.

Daly and Wilson's ideas, though highly controversial at the time, have been broadly accepted by many. Nevertheless, and as is so often the case when we come to considering humans rather than lions or other members of the non-human animal kingdom, things are not as straightforward as might initially be supposed (Nobes et al., 2019). For a start, we can't do controlled experiments in this area, so we are reduced to making inferences from correlations. We may not, though, be comparing like with like. For example, step-parents are generally younger than biological parents, and younger parents are more likely to harm their children (Ganong et al., 2019). Then there is the fact that the overwhelming majority of step-parents do not harm their stepchildren – quite the opposite. Many children do extremely well in stepfamilies (Ganong and Coleman, 2003), especially when the new relationship is close and stable.

Nevertheless, it does seem that from a child's point of view it is, on average, safer to be brought up by both of one's biological parents than by one biological parent and one step-parent. Children living with a stepfather and their mother, compared to those living with a biological father, on average have worse outcomes, including lower academic achievement, more criminal behaviour, substance misuse and teenage pregnancy (Hofferth and Anderson, 2003).

This might partly be explained by the likelihood of children in 'reconstituted' families having already often lived in less harmonious circumstances and having suffered dislocations. But step-parents have also been consistently shown in the research to be on average less warm and nurturing and less likely to become attached to their stepchildren (Pryor and Rodgers, 2001).

14.2.3 Fathers

Moving from step-parents to biological fathers, it might be supposed that, from an evolutionary perspective, fathers should be no more likely to harm their biological children than mothers are to harm their biological children. However, things aren't necessarily quite so simple. For a start, in common with many other 'monogamous' animals, in humans the offspring that result from a heterosexual partnership are not necessarily the putative father's. Rigorous determinations in humans of the incidence of what is termed 'paternal discrepancy' come up with figures that are generally smaller than the oft-quoted 10%; figures in the 2–4% range seem more likely (Bellis et al., 2005; Larmuseau et al., 2013). Nevertheless, 2–4% in evolutionary terms is a very large driving force for natural selection (see Chapter 11 for further discussion on the role of paternal investment in human evolutionary history).

What this means is that we would expect, consciously or otherwise, an evolutionary pressure for fathers, unlike mothers, to be open to the possibility that one or more of their children are not their biological children. We would therefore expect fathers to be less likely than mothers, on average, to continue to invest in 'their' offspring, and we would predict that they would be more likely, on average, to harm them. Somewhat more mundanely, there is also the point that there is greater 'distance' between a father and his children compared to between a mother and her children. Fathers don't get pregnant, they don't breastfeed and, even in the most sex-equal of societies, they, on average, spend less time with their children than do mothers. All of this means that the bonds between fathers and their children are, on average, weaker than those between mothers and their children.

14.2.4 Mothers

In our evolutionary past, environments were often uncertain, unstable and stress-inducing. At times, maternal responses of ambivalence or abandonment towards their infants might have increased the likelihood of survival for the mother as well as for her other, stronger children (whether born or yet to be born). By contrast, the contemporary contexts in many countries where mothers and their children live involve dramatic differences from these earlier circumstances (see Chapter 1 for a discussion of the concept of the environment of evolutionary adaptedness (EEA)). In our view, it is likely that current environmental demands may often not fit well with what evolution has prepared mothers to cope with. For example, a woman today may be the sole carer for her children, with little community support available, perhaps being employed outside the home on a wage that cannot adequately support a family and requiring her to call on professional childcare. Such a mother may experience particular kinds of stress and may, in consequence, behave towards her children in withdrawn, rejecting or punitive ways. While it is hard to think of this as 'adaptive' in an evolutionary sense, we have argued elsewhere (Swanepoel et al., 2017) that adaptation always depends on trade-offs, and in some circumstances the 'least worst' trade-off may be the best available.

A particular obstacle when considering such a view of abuse is that many associate maternal attachment with the idea that mothers and infants have evolved a need to remain closely bonded in order to protect offspring during the vulnerable early stages of life (Bowlby, 1969/1997). The modern evolutionary approach is considerably more nuanced than this. Perhaps the most influential research in this respect has been that of the primatologist Sarah Blaffer Hrdy (1999, 2009). Hrdy has argued on empirical grounds that maternal responses to their infants may lie anywhere on a spectrum from close bonding to ambivalence or abandonment, largely according to circumstances, including the degree of safety or danger. In considering the different factors that determine maternal responses to their infants, including abuse, the anthropologist Daniela Sieff (2019; see also Chapter 16 of this volume) addresses these in terms of maternal factors and those relating to the children.

An analogy in modern Western societies might be the favouring of one child over another in terms of either material or social investment. Typically, but not necessarily, we would expect that the younger of a pair of siblings is more likely to be the weaker of the two, meaning that, from an evolutionary perspective, we would predict that younger siblings are more likely to be the focus of maternal abuse unless there are other factors involved (e.g. the older sibling is less healthy or the present sexual partner of the mother is the parent of the younger sibling but not the older).

14.3 A Life History Take on Child Maltreatment

A further evolutionary perspective is relevant. There are a series of non-conscious 'choices' that an individual (in any species) has to make – when to start reproducing, how far apart to space off-spring, how many offspring to nurture and so on – that are also part of navigating life. Will an individual leave more surviving offspring if it waits before starting to reproduce until it has grown to a larger size and has a more extensive social network? Or if it waits, does it face too great a risk of being killed by a predator (or dying from other hazards) before it has a chance to have any progeny? The body of research that addresses these kinds of questions is called life history theory (Reiss, 1990; Stearns, 1992; see Box 14.1).

Humans, like all animals, constantly adapt to their environments. Such very early adaptations trigger neurobiological patterns that have a profound effect throughout the lifespan at the levels of the psychological and biological systems. Those born into highly stressed environments, especially when there is a high level of unpredictability (McCullough, 2013), tend later in life to have a speeded-up metabolism, faster resting heart rate and more activated stress response system and to develop what some call a fast as opposed to a slow life course strategy, being more susceptible to physical and mental disease and typically dying at an younger age. Contrary to what some might presume, this is a survival strategy, and it is seen in a range of mammals, not just humans (Ellis et al., 2017). Any too trusting and complacent individual might well have met a violent end before they could reproduce (strictly speaking, reproduce as much as would otherwise have been the case). In some situations, wariness, vigilance and lack of trust enhance immediate survival, but at psychological and health costs.

Girls raised in dangerous, stressed or abusive environments are more likely to have a range of mental health issues, are typically more avoidant or reactive and are less able subsequently to parent as successfully as might otherwise have been the case. In the West, girls with insecure attachments often reach puberty earlier (Ellis and Del Giudice, 2019), as do those born into highly stressed families or adopted from poor-quality orphanages, and they are more likely to be sexually active younger and to reproduce earlier and more often. One evolutionary explanation for early reproduction is that, in a dangerous and unpredictable world, those who leave it too long before they reproduce might well die before they have the chance to do so. Similarly, an evolutionary explanation for why women in such situations have more children is because it is likely that each individual child has a lower chance of surviving to reproduce than it would have had had it been born in a better environment. All of this links to why animals, including humans, tend to take more risks when their environments are unstable and stress-inducing or why they become more involved in violence or sexually promiscuous behaviour. Such behaviour may be considered adaptive, and girls who grow up in harsh, unstable environments can be seen as being more successful at getting pregnant early (Ellis et al., 2017).

Children living in safe, relatively stable and therefore predictable environments non-consciously pick up very different messages, such as that it is better to wait until later to reproduce, that it is fine to have fewer children but to invest more in each one and that one can rely on long-term, stable relationships (Music, 2016). When given cues that suggest a dangerous or uncertain situation, those brought up in poorer and less predictable socioeconomic circumstances tend to take more risks, while those brought up in economically advantaged and more predictable circumstances tend to take the slower, more risk-averse strategy (Griskevicius et al., 2011). A faster

---

Box 14.1 'Fast' and 'slow' life histories

- 'Fast life history' individuals begin reproducing at a young age and tend to have more offspring, each of whom is nurtured less. They can be described as following a biologically embodied unconscious strategy that prioritises 'quantity' over 'quality'.
- 'Slow life history' individuals defer reproduction and tend to have fewer offspring, in whom they invest considerable resources. They can be described as following a biologically embodied, unconscious strategy that prioritises the 'quality' of offspring over their 'quantity'.

life course can therefore be an adaptive response, enhancing the chances of surviving in threatening environments, but it comes with substantial costs. Childhood adversity has profound long-term effects on both physical and mental health, including future parenting capacities, the number of children conceived and the investment in each.

It is in early childhood that the seeds of huge differences in health outcomes and emotional well-being are sown. Studies of ACEs provide perhaps the most marked evidence of the costs of damaging childhoods (Danese and McEwen, 2012). Thus, from an evolutionary perspective, we see a trade-off. Immediate survival trumps people's long-term physiological and mental health, undermining empathic parenting. The good news is that these cycles, when recognised, can be broken. For example, the stress systems of adolescents adopted from orphanages into caring homes can be recalibrated in puberty (Gunnar et al., 2019), and while early stress predisposes girls (at least in the West) to early menarche, this effect is buffered by secure early attachment relationships (Sung et al., 2016). Early menarche linked to adversity and stress is seen as a transdiagnostic indicator of likely mental health problems, which can interfere with the ability to parent successfully (Colich et al., 2020).

The evidence is clear that the more adverse the early experiences a child has, the greater the likelihood of a faster life course, which entails a greater likelihood of physical and mental illness, less stable relationships and work lives and, on average, dying younger (Dube et al., 2003). There are severe costs to following the 'fast' pathway, many of which have been quantified for humans (Chisholm and Sieff, 2015). These costs are known to Western governments that try to minimise teenage pregnancy rates. But bearing these costs would have made adaptive sense for those of our ancestors who were living in a dangerous world where adult life was precarious and child mortality was 40% or more.

14.4 How Children Have Adapted, with Reference to Attachment Theory

There is substantial evidence that environmental sensitivity in infants and children helps them to develop in the ways that will be most adaptive given the circumstances into which they have been born. In this section, we explore these dynamics. In particular, we focus on how the physical and social environment of parents affects their parenting styles and how an infant's environment (which consists mainly of the parent(s)) affects development and attachment patterns. We also outline the evolutionary logic underlying these dynamics, arguing that although it is ideal to be loved by one's immediate family and reared in circumstances where there are no material shortages, evolution does not only prepare us for the optimum. We suggest that an evolutionary understanding might be helpful in discriminating between adaptive responses and pathological ones.

Humans can survive in a wide range of physical environments, from the Arctic to rainforests to the Sahara. They can also survive in a wide range of emotional environments, from loving to neglectful to violent ones. In adapting to specific environments, certain characteristics and genetic potentials will be activated through epigenetic mechanisms, whereas others will be suppressed.

From birth onwards – indeed, even prenatally (Glover, 2015; Music, 2013) – the human organism is continually deciphering signals about their emotional environment, and their bodies and minds are then adapting to them. Living in a nurturing environment will activate particular genetic pathways and psychological states, whereas living in a violent or unloving environment will activate different ones. The pathways activated in hostile environments are typically regarded as pathological. Although they do indeed have profoundly negative effects on longer-term physical and psychological health (Weder et al., 2014), when we look at them through an evolutionary lens we can begin to understand why these pathways exist and how they can be adaptive in some circumstances. Ellis et al. (2017) make the point that the prevailing deficit model of childhood adversity misses the unique strengths and abilities that develop in high-stress environments. We illustrate this point in relation to attachment theory.

Attachment theory was formulated by the child psychiatrist John Bowlby (1969/1997). At its core was the observation that infants are born with a need to form a strong bond to their main caregiver (usually the mother). If they are to become psychologically healthy, their caregiver has to respond to this need by providing dependable, sensitive and loving nurturance. Bowlby showed that when such care is available children grow up to become what we regard as psychologically healthy. He called such children 'securely attached'. In contrast, Bowlby felt that when such care is not available children are pushed towards psychopathology. He called children who grew up without sensitive care 'insecurely attached'.

Bowlby was influenced both by the study of other animals and by evolutionary theory. In formulating attachment theory, he was adamant that we need to take account of the environment in which *Homo sapiens* evolved. He called that environment the EEA, and he primarily envisioned it as the 2 million years when humanity's ancestors lived as hunter-gatherers. Bowlby argued that in the EEA attachment evolved to keep infants close to mothers who would not only feed them but also protect them from predators (see Chapter 1).

Bowlby's work was further developed by his colleague Ainsworth (1978), who identified two different kinds of insecure attachment in children: 'insecure-avoidant' and 'insecure-ambivalent'. Main and Solomon (1986) described a further category that they termed 'disorganised' and found to be prevalent in children who suffered abuse or neglect. This classification of attachment patterns has been validated around the world in many studies, although interesting cultural variations exist (Cassidy and Shaver, 2010). See Box 14.2 for the different attachment styles in children.

Bowlby and Ainsworth believed that secure attachment was 'normal' and evolutionarily adaptive, whereas insecure attachment was abnormal and maladaptive. Mary Main was the first to propose that the attachment system would need to be capable of calibration to a variety of environments, both favourable and adverse. Sensitive caregiving is optimal, and the provision of a secure base would help a child to explore and learn. However, less sensitive caregiving could be expected to elicit responses that would support survival even in adverse conditions (Duschinsky, 2020).

The vigilance of infants in ambivalent/resistant dyads was readily explicable in this account, as such vigilance helped retain proximity to a caregiver in potentially dangerous environments. It is also conceivable that evolutionary processes would have selected for avoidance as one part of

---

Box 14.2 Secure and insecure attachment (percentages reflective of UK and US populations)

- Children with secure attachments (approximately 50%) have caregivers who are generally sensitive and attuned to their needs. Such children see themselves as worthy of being loved. They generally develop good social skills and high levels of empathy. They form unconscious internal models that see their parents (and other people) as trustworthy.
- Children with insecure-avoidant attachments (approximately 25%) tend to have neglectful, distant and unresponsive caregivers. Such children learn to block the need for human connection and grow up determinedly self-sufficient. Typically, such children struggle to feel empathetic.
- Children with insecure-ambivalent attachments (approximately 15%) tend to have inconsistent caregivers who swing between being intrusive and being dismissive. These children generally become hyper-tuned to their attachment figures. They can be extremely sensitive to any hint of withdrawal or intrusion. They consequently tend to struggle to relate empathically.
- Children with disorganised attachments (approximately 10%) typically experience abuse and/or neglect or caregiving by a parent with mental illness. Such children experience 'fear without solution', as their caregiver – to whom they are primed to turn when they are scared – is also the source of their fear. They often spend long periods of time being emotionally dysregulated and have a high chance of psychiatric and physical disorders later in life (Danese et al., 2009).

---

the infant repertoire for responding to caregivers, since infants who are able to avoid antagonising their caregivers or making demands that their caregiver will rebuff are more likely to have survived. Infants successfully utilising an avoidant strategy maintain an indirect but real proximity to their caregiver as well as the regulatory control to continue to be responsive to the environment (Duschinsky, 2020). These lines of enquiry were taken further in the early 1990s when evolutionarily minded researchers, in particular James Chisholm (1999) and Jay Belsky (1997), began to ask whether the trajectory embodied in insecure attachment is really an abnormal and maladaptive artefact of 'inadequate' parenting or has rather been shaped by natural selection because it has evolutionary value.

One reason for asking this question was that it had become well established in the field of animal behaviour that a developmental trajectory that was adaptive in one environment would not necessarily be adaptive in a different environment. Moreover, studies had shown that development was plastic enough for individuals to follow the pathways that would most likely be adaptive given the environment into which they had been born. Zoologists called the different forms of morphology, physiology and behaviour that result from such plasticity 'conditional adaptations'.

An environmental feature discovered to be commonly associated with conditional adaptations is the relative benevolence or harshness of that environment. In a diverse array of species, the developmental trajectories that give individuals the best chance of surviving and reproducing in harsh, unpredictable or dangerous environments are different from the ones that are successful in mild, stable and benign environments. This discovery is relevant to humans because we now know that the environment in which we evolved was not always benevolent. In fact, during the long period when our ancestors lived as hunter-gatherers the climate was particularly unstable (Potts and Sloan, 2010). As a result, life was often very precarious indeed. It was not only the physical environment that brought uncertainty and danger to ancestral infants and children; the family environment was just as crucial (Chisholm, 1999; Hrdy, 1999). Some children were born to mothers who were healthy and adept at gathering food and who had a network of relations who could help with childcare and provisioning. Others were born to mothers who struggled with their health, were less adept at gathering food or had little social support (Chisholm, 1999; Hrdy, 1999, 2009). In fact, life could be particularly precarious for human children (compared to other great apes) because they remain dependent on parents long after weaning. During times of dire shortage, ancestral mothers would have needed to favour one child over another if such mothers were to have at least some surviving children (Hrdy, 1999, 2015). A child living in the EEA who was less favoured than their

siblings would have been in a life-threatening situation (Sieff, 2015).

We now turn to some of the key features of attachment patterns – the fear system and internal models – and examine how the characteristics of insecure attachment might actually be adaptive in certain circumstances.

14.4.1 Fear System

Early attachment stress contributes to shaping an individual's fear reactivity through calibrating the hypothalamic–pituitary–adrenal (HPA) axis (Rincón-Cortés and Sullivan, 2014). Attachment security during early life is associated with creating a resilient fear system that responds less reactively to threats and returns quickly to a calm state when the threat has passed. In contrast, early emotional insecurity is generally associated with having a sensitised HPA axis that leaves the individual forever on the lookout for danger, meaning that even after a perceived threat has passed it takes a long time for fear levels to return to base levels (Oosterman et al., 2010).

This pattern is not unique to humans. In harsh conditions, individuals of many species develop a fear system that is particularly sensitised to danger (LeDoux, 2014). For example, rat mothers who are stressed spend less time licking and grooming their pups than do unstressed mothers. In response to this relative lack of maternal nurturance, epigenetic mechanisms are activated that calibrate the pups' HPA axes in ways that build a reactive fear system (Diorio and Meaney, 2007; Francis et al., 1999). Behaviourally, the HPA-sensitised pups grow into adults who are reticent about exploring new ground, reluctant to go out into open spaces and more fearful generally.

Although the costs associated with this fearful behaviour are significant, wild rats become stressed when living in an environment that contains large numbers of predators, and under such conditions a sensitised fear system enhances the chances of surviving. Evolutionary thinking suggests that this heightened sensitivity to fear is adaptive. The same adaptive logic is relevant to our own species (Evans and Kim, 2013; Flinn et al., 2011).

Among humans, a highly reactive HPA axis has costs in terms of physical health and mental well-being (Lanius et al., 2010). It increases the risk of suffering from cardiovascular and other diseases and from anxiety disorders and it causes the loss of neurons in the hippocampus, which plays a central role in memory. Additionally, people with a reactive fear system spend more energy anxiously scanning their world for possible threats. They are at risk of seeing danger where none exists and then behaving in ways that create self-fulfilling prophecies. They also have less time and energy to invest in more fulfilling and creative pursuits (Sieff, 2015). However, for individuals born into dangerous environments, these disadvantages are insignificant compared to dying young and childless (Chisholm, 1999).

14.4.2 Internal Models

As a result of attachment relationships, humans acquire 'internal models' of the relational world. Sarah Hrdy (1999, 2009) argues that the different forms that these models can take are best understood as part of a conditional adaptation to the social environment into which an individual has been born. She calls humans 'cooperative breeders', meaning that ancestral mothers depended on help to raise offspring. This help was necessary because of the long period of post-weaning dependency, which in turn meant that human mothers (unlike other primates) had to provision several children simultaneously. Thus, Hrdy argues, a mother's social network was a hugely important environmental factor; although ancestral children born to mothers with limited social support could have survived, their chances of surviving would have been better if they used different ways of relating compared to children who benefitted from being born into a large social network (see Box 14.3).

In summary, in a benign environment where parents are well and have adequate support, they will likely be capable of providing sensitive and responsive care to their children, which allows them to follow a slow life history. These children will as a result be more likely to become trusting, open and loving (i.e. securely attached). However, if parents are stressed, whether due to ill health, poverty or having less social support, they are typically less able to provide consistent and high levels of care to their offspring. Such children will then adapt to their harsh environment by becoming either compulsively self-reliant (avoidant attachment) or clingy and compulsively care-

> **Box 14.3 The effects of social support on internal models**
>
> - A child who is born to a mother with considerable social support will generally grow up believing other people are trustworthy. Such a child will feel that it is fine to ask for help and that they are worthy of being helped.
> - A child born to a mother with a limited social network is more likely to have an unconscious internal model of being unwilling to go to others for help. This is adaptive in situations where help is not available. However, it can hinder children from seeking and accepting support that becomes available later in life, including through therapy. This has been termed 'double deprivation' (Williams, 1974).

seeking (ambivalent attachment). In these cases, children will also develop highly activated stress systems – mirroring their parents' stress and hence adapting to the more stressful circumstances they are exposed to.

We know that chronic high stress levels contribute to mental and physical disorders in later life (Danese et al., 2009); however, this process does not necessarily inhibit reproduction, and thus the cycle is perpetuated unless the environment changes as natural selection does not select for happiness, but only for survival and reproduction.

It is more difficult to see the adaptive value of disorganised attachment. This is the predominant pattern in children who have been abused, neglected or raised by caregivers who were traumatised themselves. Hrdy (2009) has argued that, in previous times, children would not have survived such adversity. As such, she suggests, the pathology seen is not adaptive, since it would not have resulted in the ability to reproduce and raise offspring who survived. However, other thinkers have argued that freezing (or 'attentive immobility') is a functional response that could play a protective role in high-risk contexts in which caregiver behaviour may be potentially harmful (Haltigan et al., 2021). Furthermore, it is conceivable that in high-stress situations, risky, last-resort strategies may be adaptive in exploring alternative coping mechanisms in order to – hopefully – arrive upon behaviours that reduce the risk to the child (Haltigan et al., 2021).

However, it is important to note that a disorganised attachment is not proof of maltreatment (van IJzendoorn et al., 2020). A parent who has unresolved trauma may have flashbacks and periods of dissociation. A child observing a frightened caregiver can be traumatised and develop a disorganised attachment even where no maltreatment occurs. Furthermore, Crittenden and Landini (2011) have argued that the disorganised category does not exist as a separate entity and can be understood as an extreme variation of the avoidant and ambivalent styles that can allow individuals to survive and adapt to highly traumatising environments. At its extreme it includes psychopathy, in which individuals survive and even thrive by caring only about themselves and exploiting others. As with any adaptation to the environment, these strategies are then continued and learnt by the offspring, resulting in the intergenerational transmission of trauma.

It is also important to note that not all pathological presentations are caused by the environment. A child may have underlying difficulties such as intellectual disabilities or other neurodevelopmental disorders (see Chapter 15). On the other hand, just because a child has survived unscathed does not mean that the environment was benign. We know that some children are naturally less sensitive to environmental influences and as such are more resilient to harsh environments.

14.5 How Does an Evolutionary Perspective View Epigenetics, Differential Susceptibility and Resilience?

According to Barker's hypothesis (Hales and Barker, 1992), the metabolism of an unborn foetus is programmed by the mother's diet. Hence, mothers who were pregnant during a famine will tend to have babies who have a 'thrifty phenotype'. These babies would be adapted to survive on less food than average. If food were to become abundant, they would be more likely than other babies to develop metabolic complications. Through signals picked up during intrauterine life, foetal programming prepares the infant to adapt to the environment it is likely to be born into (Glover, 2011, 2015) – a

phenomenon also referred to as 'developmental mismatch' (Gluckman and Hanson, 2006). The same principles function after birth. Such a perspective views maternal behaviour as a crucial (albeit unwitting) part of conditional adaptation, arguing that the bodies and minds of infants have evolved to use the quality of their early experiences as information about the environment they expect to find themselves in later in life. This information indicates to the developing brain and body something about the benevolence or harshness of the social and physical world that each infant has been born into and might therefore expect to encounter in future (Belsky, 1997; Chisholm, 1999; Chisholm and Sieff, 2015; Simpson and Belsky, 2008).

However, this is not about blaming mothers. Such a view of foetal programming simply argues that in harsh environments, either socially or physically, mothers are preoccupied and as a result are not able to nurture their infants as responsively and patiently as they would if they were less stressed. We discussed this in Section 14.3 in terms of a stressful environment leading to a fast life history, in which the investment in a particular child is reduced. This view also suggests that over many millennia (perhaps going all the way back to the origin of mammals) infants evolved embodied systems that responded in ways that would enhance their survival given that they had been born into a challenging world.

Another twist to the evolutionary story is that, although all infants show a degree of adaptability, some infants and children are more 'plastic' than others (Bakermans-Kranenburg and van IJzendoorn, 2011; Belsky and Hartman, 2014). Previously, it was thought that adverse experiences predisposed some children and adults to stressful responses more than others – that some children were simply born more 'vulnerable'. In fact, we have learnt that some children are not just more vulnerable but are more 'plastic', and so they are more influenced by their environments generally. These individuals might show higher than average stress responses when receiving insensitive parenting but lower than average responses given good parenting (Beaver and Belsky, 2012). Such children have been likened to 'orchids' – compared to 'dandelion' children who are robust, resilient and survive even in harsh environments (Kennedy, 2013). Parents will raise their children to survive in the current

Box 14.4 Vignette

Marsha was 18. She had just given birth to her third child, Jo, her first son. The first two had been taken into care within six months of their births on the grounds of neglect. Marsha had an edgy feel, a tough exterior belying a fragile emotional state hidden beneath reactive emotional dysregulation. She had been in and out of care herself, her mother being a drug-using sex worker and her father being violent and probably a pimp. In an assessment centre, Marsha was self-conscious and trying hard to impress but struggled to spend time with Jo, and when she did, her seemingly loving gestures had, on close inspection, a tough harshness about them. When feeding, she held Jo too tightly and thrust him away afterwards. When he cried, Marsha seemed to flinch and then flashed bared teeth and looked as if she might hit him before trying to soothe him in a way she seemed to think that others expected of her. Her ability to think about Jo was limited, showing little capacity for mind-mindedness and manifesting low empathy and little love. She was controlling, trying to force her expectations and pace on her son and unable to pick up on his discomfort or tension. Jo seemed to have given up, not expecting softness or loving responses, and his eyes already had a glazed look. While it was the bruises and soiled nappies that evoked social services action, it was the emotional mis-attunement that was most painful and worrying.

Witnessing violence has a profound effect on a child's brain and nervous system. Marsha's stress system would have been affected even prenatally due to the violence and fear in her environment, leading stress hormones to cross the placenta and resulting in her being born with a highly activated HPA axis. Marsha's early life was lived in an atmosphere of fear, indeed terror, oscillating with profound neglect when she was left alone for hours, patterns she was repeating with Jo.

It is easy to condemn mothers such as Marsha, but Marsha was in fact the victim of her own history and that of previous generations. She had been exposed to violence and inappropriate sexuality from early in her life, and she too became, as is common, a classic victim turned perpetrator. But there is another way of looking at Marsha's development: in evolutionary terms she had developed an effective way to survive in her early environment.

She would have developed a personality rooted in the expectation of danger, giving rise to a constant state of high alert, a hyper-aroused sympathetic nervous system and a reactive 'fight' system. Marsha exhibited massive wariness and distrust and had had little familiarity with giving or receiving love and understanding. People like Marsha experience life as one lived-in, constant life threat and neither trust in nor recognise the presence of benign figures. For understandable reasons they do not trust softness, kindness or vulnerability and often glorify strength, power and aggression. This makes sense of how Marsha struggled to be with Jo in a kindly way; the harsh and frankly abusive set of exchanges, which looked like callousness, can be seen as explicable adaptations to a terrifying early life.

Marsha and Jo were referred to an intensive parenting programme and Marsha learnt to be curious about Jo and to think about how he might be feeling. Staff treated Marsha with kindness and understanding and helped her to do the same with Jo. Marsha was able to become more attuned and reflective, which had a positive impact on her relationship with Jo.

environment, but there is no guarantee that the world might not change dramatically. If the world is benign, then the 'sensitive orchid' children may do better, but if it becomes hostile, fitness is enhanced for the 'resilient dandelion' type.

New research also suggests that this has implications for treatment (see Box 14.4). Some children will be more influenced than others by certain treatments (Kennedy, 2013), such as some parenting interventions and drug treatments. Research strongly suggests that this variation is due to underlying genetic differences and that individuals with more plastic genetic variants are much more affected by some treatments than are those with alternative alleles (Bakermans-Kranenburg and van IJzendoorn, 2015). Candidate genes in this process are the serotonin receptor gene *5HT* (Lesch, 2011) and the dopamine receptor gene (Bakermans-Kranenburg, 2011).

14.6 Conclusion

'It takes a village to raise a child.' Even if the relationship with the mother is difficult, children can benefit greatly from good relationships with fathers, grandparents or other caring people. Children also differ greatly, with some who are easy-going and resilient and others who are very difficult to care for due to a challenging temperament or underlying neurodevelopmental disorders (see Chapter 15). We hope that the chapters in this volume and our other writing show that, far from blaming mothers, an evolutionary view reveals how mothers generally do the best they can in difficult circumstances. If we want to help children, we also need to address the emotional, social and physical environments they find themselves in.

References

Ainsworth, M. D. (1978). *Patterns of Attachment: A Psychological Study of the Strange Situations.* Mahwah, NJ: Lawrence Erlbaum Associates.

Bakermans-Kranenburg, M. J. and van IJzendoorn, M. H. (2011). Differential susceptibility to rearing environment depending on dopamine-related genes: new evidence and a meta-analysis. *Development and Psychopathology,* 23, 39–52.

Bakermans-Kranenburg, M. J. and van IJzendoorn, M. H. (2015). The hidden efficacy of interventions: gene × environment experiments from a differential susceptibility perspective. *Annual Review of Psychology,* 66, 381–409.

Beaver, K. M. and Belsky, J. (2012). Gene–environment interaction and the intergenerational transmission of parenting: testing the differential-susceptibility hypothesis. *Psychiatric Quarterly,* 83, 29–40.

Bellis, M. A., Hughes, K., Hughes, S. and Ashton, J. R. (2005). Measuring paternal discrepancy and its public health consequences. *Journal of Epidemiology and Community Health,* 59, 749–754.

Belsky, J. (1997). Attachment, mating, and parenting: an evolutionary interpretation. *Human Nature,* 8, 361–381.

Belsky, J. and Hartman, S. (2014). Gene–environment interaction in evolutionary perspective: differential susceptibility to environmental influences. *World Psychiatry,* 13, 87–89.

Bowlby, E. J. M. (1969/1997). *Attachment and Loss: Attachment.* London: Pimlico.

Cassidy, J. and Shaver, P. R. (2010). *Handbook of Attachment: Theory, Research and Clinical Applications,* 2nd ed. New York: Guilford Press.

Chisholm, J. S. (1999). *Death, Hope and Sex: Steps to an Evolutionary Ecology of Mind and Morality.* Cambridge: Cambridge University Press.

Chisholm, J. S. and Sieff, D. F. (2015). Live fast, die young; an evolved response to hostile environments? In: D. F. Sieff (ed.), *Understanding and Healing Emotional Trauma: Conversations with Pioneering Clinicians and Researchers.* London: Routledge, pp. 163–181.

Colich, N. L., Platt, J. M., Keyes, K. M., Sumner, J. A., Allen, N. B. and McLaughlin, K. A. (2020). Earlier age at menarche as a transdiagnostic mechanism linking childhood trauma with multiple forms of psychopathology in adolescent girls. *Psychological Medicine,* 50, 1090–1098.

Crittenden, P. M. and Landini, A. (2011). *Assessing Adult Attachment: A Dynamic Maturational Approach to Discourse Analysis.* New York: Norton.

Daly, M. and Wilson, M. (1996). Evolutionary psychology and marital conflict: the relevance of stepchildren. In: D. M. Buss and N. Malamuth (eds.), *Sex, Power, Conflict: Feminist and Evolutionary Perspectives.* Oxford: Oxford University Press, pp. 9–28.

Danese, A. and McEwen, B. S. (2012). Adverse childhood experiences, allostasis, allostatic load, and age-related disease. *Physiology & Behavior,* 106, 29–39.

Danese, A., Moffitt, T. E., Harrington, H., Milne, B. J., Polanczyk, G., Pariante, C. M., Poulton, R. and Caspi, A. (2009). Adverse childhood experiences and adult risk factors for age-related disease. *Archives of Pediatrics & Adolescent Medicine,* 163, 1135–1143.

Diorio, J. and Meaney, M. J. (2007). Maternal programming of defensive responses through sustained effects on gene expression. *Journal of Psychiatry and Neuroscience,* 32, 275–284.

Dube, S. R., Felitti, V. J., Dong, M., Giles, W. H. and Anda, R. F. (2003). The impact of adverse childhood experiences on health problems: evidence from four birth cohorts dating back to 1900. *Preventive Medicine,* 37, 268–277.

Duschinsky, R. (2020). *Cornerstones of Attachment Research.* Oxford: Oxford University Press.

Ellis, B. J. and Del Giudice, M. (2019). Developmental adaptation to stress: an evolutionary perspective. *Annual Review of Psychology,* 70, 111–139.

Ellis, B. J., Bianchi, J., Griskevicius, V. and Frankenhuis, W. E. (2017). Beyond risk and protective factors: an adaptation-based approach to resilience. *Perspectives on Psychological Science,* 12, 561–587.

Evans, G. W. and Kim, P. (2013). Childhood poverty, chronic stress, self-regulation, and coping. *Child Development Perspectives,* 7, 43–48.

Flinn, M. V., Nepomnaschy, P. A., Muehlenbein, M. P. and Ponzi, D. (2011) Evolutionary functions of early social modulation of hypothalamic–pituitary–adrenal axis development in humans. *Neuroscience and Biobehavioral Reviews*, **35**, 1611–1629.

Francis, D. D., Champagne, F. A., Liu, D. and Meaney, M. J. (1999). Maternal care, gene expression, and the development of individual differences in stress reactivity. *Annals of the New York Academy of Sciences*, **896**, 66–84.

Ganong, L. H. and Coleman, M. (2003) *Stepfamily Relationships*. New York: Springer.

Ganong, L., Jensen, T., Sanner, C., Russell, L. and Coleman, M. (2019). Stepfathers' affinity-seeking with stepchildren, stepfather–stepchild relationship quality, marital quality, and stepfamily cohesion among stepfathers and mothers. *Journal of Family Psychology*, **33**, 521–531.

Glover, V. (2011). Annual research review: prenatal stress and the origins of psychopathology: an evolutionary perspective. *Journal of Child Psychology and Psychiatry*, **52**, 356–367.

Glover, V. (2015). Prenatal stress and its effects on the fetus and the child: possible underlying biological mechanisms. In: V. Glover and M. C. Antonelli (eds.), *Perinatal Programming of Neurodevelopment*. Dordrecht: Springer, pp. 269–283.

Gluckman, P. and Hanson, M. (2006). *Mismatch: Why Our World No Longer Fits Our Bodies*. Oxford: Oxford University Press.

Griskevicius, V., Tybur, J. M., Delton, A. W. and Robertson, T. E. (2011). The influence of mortality and socioeconomic status on risk and delayed rewards: a life history theory approach. *Journal of Personality and Social Psychology*, **100**, 1015–1026.

Gunnar, M. R., DePasquale, C. E., Reid, B. M., Donzella, B. and Miller, B. S. (2019). Pubertal stress recalibration reverses the effects of early life stress in postinstitutionalized children. *Proceedings of the National Academy of Sciences of the United States of America*, **116**, 23984–23988.

Hales, C. N. and Barker, D. J. (1992). Type 2 (non-insulin-dependent) diabetes mellitus: the thrifty phenotype hypothesis. *Diabetologia*, **35**, 595–601.

Haltigan, J. D., Del Giudice, M. and Khorsand, S. (2021). Growing points in attachment disorganization: looking back to advance forward. *Attachment & Human Development*, **23**, 438–454.

Heim, C. M., Entringer, S. and Buss, C. (2019). Translating basic research knowledge on the biological embedding of early-life stress into novel approaches for the developmental programming of lifelong health. *Psychoneuroendocrinology*, **105**, 123–137.

Hofferth, S. L. and Anderson, K. G. (2003) Are all dads equal? Biology versus marriage as a basis for paternal investment, *Journal of Marriage and the Family*, **65**, 213–232.

Hrdy, S. B. (1999). *Mother Nature: Natural Selection and the Female of the Species*. London: Chatto & Windus.

Hrdy, S. B. (2009). *Mothers and Others: The Evolutionary Origins of Mutual Understanding*. Cambridge, MA: Belknap Press of Harvard University Press.

Hrdy, S. B. (2015). Variable postpartum responsiveness among humans and other primates with 'cooperative breeding': a comparative and evolutionary perspective. *Hormones and Behavior*, **77**, 272–283.

Kennedy, E. (2013). Orchids and dandelions: how some children are more susceptible to environmental influences for better or worse, and the implications for child development. *Clinical Child Psychology and Psychiatry*, **18**, 319–321.

Lanius, R. A., Vermetten, E. and Pain, C. (2010). *The Impact of Early Life Trauma on Health and Disease: The Hidden Epidemic*. Cambridge: Cambridge University Press.

Larmuseau, M. H., Vanoverbeke, J., Van Geystelen, A., Defraene, G., Vanderheyden, N., Matthys, K., Wenseleers, T. and Decorte, R. (2013) Low historical rates of cuckoldry in a Western European human population traced by Y-chromosome and genealogical data. *Proceedings of the Royal Society B: Biological Sciences*, **280**, 20132400.

LeDoux, J. E. (2014). Coming to terms with fear. *Proceedings of the National Academy of Sciences of the United States of America*, **111**, 2871–2878.

Lesch, K. P. (2011). When the serotonin transporter gene meets adversity: the contribution of animal models to understanding epigenetic mechanisms in affective disorders and resilience. *Current Topics in Behavioral Neuroscience*, 7, 251–280.

Main, M. and Solomon, J. (1986). Discovery of an insecure disoriented attachment pattern: procedures, findings and implications for the classification of behaviour. In: T. B. Brazelton and M. Youngman (eds.), *Affective Development in Infancy*. Norwood, NJ: Ablex, pp. 95–124.

Mathews, B. (2019). *New International Frontiers in Child Sexual Abuse*. Cham: Springer.

McCullough, M. E., Pedersen, E. J., Schroder, J. M., Tabak, B. A., and Carver, C. S. (2013). Harsh childhood environmental characteristics predict exploitation and retaliation in humans. *Proceedings of the Royal Society B: Biological Sciences*, **280**, 20122104.

Music, G. (2013). Stress pre-birth: how the fetus is affected by a mother's state of mind.

International Journal of Birth and Parent Education, **1**, 12–15.

Music, G. (2016). *Nurturing Natures: Attachment and Children's Emotional, Social and Brain Development*, 2nd ed. London: Psychology Press.

Nobes, G., Panagiotaki, G. and Russell Jonsson, K. (2019). Child homicides by stepfathers: a replication and reassessment of the British evidence. *Journal of Experimental Psychology: General*, **148**, 1091–1102.

Oosterman, M., de Schipper, J. C., Fisher, P., Dozier, M. and Schuengel, C. (2010). Autonomic reactivity in relation to attachment and early adversity among foster children. *Development and Psychopathology*, **22**, 109–118.

Potts, R. and Sloan, C. (2010). *What Does It Mean to Be Human?* Washington, DC: National Geographic Society.

Pryor, J. and Rodgers, B. (2001) *Children in Changing Families: Life after Parental Separation*. Oxford: Blackwell Publishers.

Reiss, M. J. (1990). Size, growth and reproduction: the logic of allometry. *Evolutionary Theory*, **9**, 279–297.

Rincón-Cortés, M. and Sullivan, R. M. (2014). Early life trauma and attachment: immediate and enduring effects on neurobehavioral and stress axis development. *Frontiers in Endocrinology*, **5**, 33.

Sieff, D. F. (2015) Connecting conversations: expanding our understanding to transform our trauma-worlds. In: D. F. Sieff (ed.), *Understanding and Healing Emotional Trauma: Conversations with Pioneering Clinicians and Researchers*. London: Routledge, pp. 221–236.

Sieff, D. F. (2019). The death mother as nature's shadow: infanticide, abandonment, and the collective unconscious. *Psychological Perspectives*, **62**, 15–34.

Simpson, J. A. and Belsky, J. (2008). Attachment theory within a modern evolutionary framework. In: P. R. Shaver and J. Cassidy (eds.), *Handbook of Attachment: Theory, Research and Clinical Applications*, 2nd ed. New York: Guilford Press, pp. 131–157.

St-Laurent, D., Dubois-Comtois, K., Milot, T. and Cantinotti, M. (2019). Intergenerational continuity/discontinuity of child maltreatment among low-income mother–child dyads: the roles of childhood maltreatment characteristics, maternal psychological functioning, and family ecology. *Developmental Psychopathology*, **31**, 189–202.

Stearns, S. (1992). *The Evolution of Life Histories*. Oxford: Oxford University Press.

Sung, S., Simpson, J. A., Griskevicius, V., Kuo, S. I.-C., Schlomer, G. L. and Belsky, J. (2016). Secure infant-mother attachment buffers the effect of early-life stress on age of menarche. *Psychological Science*, **27**, 667–674.

Swanepoel, A., Music, G., Launer, J. and Reiss, M. (2017). How evolutionary thinking can help us understand ADHD. *BJPsych Advances*, **23**, 410–418.

Swanepoel, A., Sieff, D. F., Music, G., Launer, J., Reiss, M. and Wren B. (2016). How evolution can help us understand child development and behaviour. *BJPsych Advances*, **22**, 36–43.

Tinbergen, N. (1963). On aims and methods of ethology. *Zeitschrift für Tierpsychologie*, **20**, 410–433.

van Houdt, K., Kalmijn, M. and Ivanova, K. (2020). Stepparental support to adult children: the diverging roles of stepmothers and stepfathers. *Journal of Marriage and the Family*, **82**, 639–656.

van IJzendoorn, M. H., Bakermans-Kranenburg, M. J., Coughlan, B. and Reijman, S. (2020). Annual research review: umbrella synthesis of meta-analyses on child maltreatment antecedents and interventions: differential susceptibility perspective on risk and resilience. *Journal of Child Psychology and Psychiatry*, **61**, 272–290.

Weder, N., Zhang, H., Jensen, K., Yang, B. Z., Simen, A., Jackowski, A., Lipschitz, D., Douglas-Palumberi, H., Ge, M., Perepletchikova, F., O'Loughlin, K., Hudziak, J. J., Gelernter, J. and Kaufman, J. (2014). Child abuse, depression, and methylation in genes involved with stress, neural plasticity and brain circuitry. *Journal of the American Academy of Child and Adolescent Psychiatry*, **53**, 417–424.

WHO (2020). Child Maltreatment. Retrieved from: www.who.int/en/news-room/fact-sheets/detail/child-maltreatment (accessed: 2 April 2021).

Williams, G. (previously Henry, G.) (1974). Doubly deprived. *Journal of Child Psychotherapy*, **3**, 15–28.

Wren, B., Launer, J., Music, G., Reiss, M. J. and Swanepoel, A. (2021). Can an evolutionary perspective shed light on maternal abuse of children? *Clinical Child Psychology and Psychiatry*, **26**, 283–294.

Wren, B., Launer, J., Reiss, M. J., Swanepoel, A. and Music, G. (2019). Can evolutionary thinking shed light on gender diversity? *BJPsych Advances*, **25**, 351–362.

Evolutionary Perspectives on Neurodevelopmental Disorders

Annie Swanepoel, Michael J. Reiss, John Launer, Graham Music and Bernadette Wren

Abstract

We discuss evolutionary perspectives on two neurodevelopmental disorders: attention deficit hyperactivity disorder (ADHD) and autism spectrum disorder (ASD). Both have a genetic background, and we explore why these genes may have survived the process of natural selection. We draw on the concept of evolutionary mismatch, in which a trait that may have conferred advantages in the past can become disadvantageous when the environment changes. We also describe the non-genetic influences on these conditions. We point out that children with neurodevelopmental conditions are more likely to suffer maltreatment, so it is important to consider both the genes and the environment in which children have grown up. In hunter-gatherer societies, ADHD may have favoured risk-taking, which may explain why it has survived. The contemporary model of schooling, in which children are expected to sit still for many hours a day, does not favour this. Understanding ADHD in terms of an evolutionary mismatch therefore raises ethical issues regarding both medication and the school environment. ASDs are far more heterogeneous and are characterised by high heritability and low reproductive success. At the severe end of the spectrum, ASD is highly disadvantageous and often co-occurs with intellectual disability. On the other hand, high-functioning ASD may have been adaptive in our evolutionary past in terms of the potential for the development of specialist skills and can still be so today in the right environment.

Keywords

ADHD, autism spectrum disorders, evolutionary mismatch, evolutionary perspectives, neurodevelopmental disorders

Key Points

- Evolutionary thinking can deepen our understanding and aid our clinical treatment of childhood developmental disorders.
- The concept of evolutionary mismatch can be particularly helpful in understanding the relatively high prevalence of certain neurodevelopmental disorders. The concept refers to traits that may have conferred advantages in the past but now, given changes in the environment, may be disadvantageous.
- In our evolutionary past, children were not expected to sit still and concentrate on academic tasks for many hours a day. Attention deficit hyperactivity disorder (ADHD) may have favoured adaptive novelty-seeking and risk-taking. Understanding

ADHD in terms of an evolutionary mismatch raises significant issues regarding the management of childhood ADHD, including ethical ones.

- Autism spectrum disorders (ASDs) are highly heterogeneous but are characterised by high heritability and low reproductive success. At the more severe end of the spectrum, if accompanied by intellectual disability, ASDs can be highly disadvantageous. On the other hand, high-functioning autism may have been adaptive in our evolutionary past and can be so today in the right environments.

15.1 Introduction

As clinicians and scholars, we believe that the traditional disease model – still dominant in psychiatry – is less than ideal for making sense of a range of psychological issues, including developmental problems in childhood (Swanepoel et al., 2016). We also believe that a model based on evolutionary thinking can deepen understanding and aid clinical practice by showing how behaviours, bodily responses and psychological beliefs tend to occur for reasons that are evolutionarily adaptive, even when these might on first appearance seem pathological. Our wish is to demonstrate the way that evolutionary arguments can make a contribution to helping young people who present with patterns of behaviour that indicate neurodevelopmental diversity or atypicality.

We draw particularly on the concept of 'evolutionary mismatch'. This is said to occur when the environment in which an organism lives is significantly different from that in which it evolved, so that traits that were once adaptive may become, in effect, pathological. One widely accepted example of this is that humans evolved to survive periods of food scarcity by craving and eating high-calorie foods when these were available. In the current environment of plentiful food for many of us, this leads to widespread obesity. Thus, a trait that conferred survival advantage in the past can lead to vulnerability to disorder if the environment changes (Cofnas, 2016). Here, we apply this reasoning to the two most commonly diagnosed neurodevelopmental disorders: attention deficit hyperactivity disorder (ADHD) and autism spectrum disorder (ASD).

We do not argue for a single explanation for these conditions. Indeed, we caution against too simplistic an understanding of them, including the belief that all such diagnoses are faulty or that the conditions can always be objectively identified and straightforwardly treated. Instead, our hope is that an evolutionary perspective will prove useful to clinicians and others working with children (or adults) presenting with these problems.

15.2 Attention Deficit Hyperactivity Disorder

15.2.1 Identification and Classification

ADHD is characterised by hyperactivity, impulsivity and inattention, and it appears not infrequently to be linked with serious consequences, including educational failure, substance abuse and criminal involvement. Few childhood conditions designated as psychiatric disorders are as controversial (Timimi and Taylor, 2004). While diagnosis is generally made on the basis of behavioural checklists, there are ongoing debates about the status of such diagnoses. The prevalence of diagnosis seems to be increasing, but the reasons for this are hotly disputed (Thapar and Cooper, 2016). Some mental health professionals see ADHD as a developmental disorder, some as being genetically driven, while others see it as a set of symptoms that are indistinguishable from the effects of trauma on children.

In the fourth edition of the Diagnostic and Statistical Manual of Mental Disorders (DSM-IV), ADHD fell under 'disruptive behaviour disorders'. In DSM-5, ADHD was moved into the category of neurodevelopmental disorders, alongside ASD and intellectual disabilities. A neurodevelopmental disorder is one in which the development of the central nervous system is disturbed. Common characteristics of ADHD are onset in early childhood, cognitive as well as behavioural deficits and symptomatic and functional impairments that tend to persist. There is typically a male preponderance, and these disorders tend to have a degree of heritability. There is a large overlap with different neurodevelopmental disorders – co-occurrence is the rule rather than the exception (Dyck et al., 2011; Posner et al., 2014).

In support of a neurodevelopmental view, the Ben-Gurion Infant Development Study showed that sons of fathers with ADHD are more irritable and responses to their needs are less adequate than in sons of fathers without ADHD (Auerbach et al., 2004). At-risk infants were both more irritable and indicated less clearly what was bothering them, making parenting more difficult. This was confirmed by Elberling et al. (2014), who found that mother–infant interaction problems were more likely. Interestingly, expressed emotion (parental hostility) is child-specific not parent-specific (Cartwright et al., 2011).

Only 10% of clinic samples of preschoolers diagnosed with ADHD are back in the normal range at 15–18 years (Lahey et al., 2016). In England, ADHD in preschool boys is associated with a 10-point reduction in General Certificate of Secondary Education (age 16) scores (Washbrook et al., 2013) and there is a 7–12-point average IQ deficit in individuals with ADHD

(Simonoff et al., 2007). It has also been shown that preschool ADHD incurs a 17-fold lifetime economic burden to the state due to increased needs in health, education and social care, and preschool ADHD makes it more likely that children will be bullies or the victims of bullying (Verlinden et al., 2015).

15.2.2 Epidemiological Issues

One notable fact about ADHD is that rates of recognition, diagnosis and treatment vary widely between and within countries. In 2012, at least 9% of school-aged children in the USA were diagnosed with ADHD; the corresponding figure for France was less than 0.5% (Wedge, 2012). The rate of ADHD diagnosis in preschoolers varies too, even between quite similar countries: in Denmark it is 1% (Elberling et al., 2016), while it is 3.8% in Iceland (Gudmundsson et al., 2013). The rates even differ substantially across states in the USA (Fulton et al., 2015). They have also increased considerably in many countries, including the USA and UK. Such variations may be due to differences in how the condition is defined and the ways data are gathered (Polanczyk et al., 2014).

Another significant finding is that in many countries there is a substantially increased likelihood of ADHD diagnosis if a child is in the youngest group in a school-year cohort. For example, children in Denmark born just before the cut-off for the next year were about 2.5 times more likely to have an ADHD diagnosis (Krabbe et al., 2014). Similar results have been seen in other countries, including Germany (Schwandt and Wuppermann, 2016), Canada (Chen et al., 2015), Taiwan (Chen et al., 2016) and Israel (Hoshen et al., 2016). This suggests an increase in diagnoses in children who are less emotionally mature and less able to be still.

There are also cultural differences in diagnosis rates (Ghosh et al., 2015), which might be explained by some cultures placing higher value on emotional regulation as a value and/or other factors. Problems with self-regulation are identified as being more common in US than Asian males, for example (Wanless et al., 2013). Cultures that value close bodily contact and a quick response to signals of distress and where there are clear imperatives for children to abide by rules are ones where self-regulation develops earlier and more fully. Children in more interdependent cultures are also quicker to develop skills in compliance and emotional regulation (Wanless et al., 2013), especially boys. It is nevertheless clear that there are children, principally boys, who show symptoms identified as ADHD that cause concern everywhere and whose longer-term trajectories are often not good (Thapar and Cooper, 2016).

15.2.3 Genes, Adaptation and Epigenetics

According to evolutionary thought, behaviour traits that have survived and been passed down the generations must have had adaptive value in the past and possibly have such value today. It is certainly conceivable that more adventurous individuals in hunter-gatherer society sometimes did better in terms of leaving viable offspring, perhaps because they were more willing to explore (see Box 15.1).

It is worth asking why it might be adaptive for a child to have a version of a gene or set of genes that appears to give rise to such a poor prognosis as ADHD. The likely answer is that such a temperament might be advantageous in some environments. For example, when we examine the genes of people involved in major migrations, such as refugees, we see that a higher proportion than average have the same 'novelty-seeking' genetic variant associated with ADHD in children (Matthews and Butler, 2011). Being a carrier of that novelty-seeking variant might have increased the likelihood of survival by making such individuals more predisposed to seek out a new place to make a home when danger loomed, and hence survive to pass on this variant.

> **Box 15.1 Example of how a gene associated with ADHD may have been adaptive**
>
> About one-seventh of a Kenyan tribe, the Ariaal, have the long version of the *DRD4* gene, which is associated with novelty-seeking. The Ariaal have either a nomadic life, moving from place to place, or a more settled, pastoral life. Those with the novelty-seeking allele and who lived a nomadic life were well nourished and healthy. In contrast, those with the novelty-seeking allele but living a settled, pastoral life were on average less well nourished (Eisenberg et al., 2008).

Genes alone do not cause ADHD symptoms, and gene–environment interactions look increasingly likely to play a central role. It seems, for example, that carriers of the long allele of the *DRD4* gene (the 7-repeat allele) are more likely to show ADHD symptoms (Faraone et al., 2014), and this genetic variant also increases the likelihood that children will be novelty-seeking. For these children, insensitive parenting in the early years predicts more externalising behaviours, although this is not the case for carriers of the short variant (Windhorst et al., 2015). Inheriting the long allele also predicts worse emotional regulation and a greater likelihood of disorganised attachment presentations (Pappa et al., 2015). Hence, this and other genes may predispose for ADHD, but this can only ever be a partial explanation.

Another study looked at hyperactive children who were adopted (Harold et al., 2013). Where these children received sensitive and attuned parenting, the symptoms of hyperactivity were not subsequently seen. Again, we find that nature and nurture interact to produce their effects (van IJzendoorn and Bakermans-Kranenburg, 2015). Thus, what we are seeing is that some children are born with more genetic susceptibility for ADHD-type symptoms, but also that certain kinds of environmental influences can greatly reduce the potential effects of genes.

Epigenetic research shows that some children are more susceptible to the influence of their environment than others – what Belsky and others have called 'differential susceptibility to rearing' (Belsky, 2005). Belsky has also argued that successful reproduction of one's genes is more likely if some of one's offspring are more influenced by the current environment than others. In such scenarios, at least some offspring will survive to pass on their genes. Thus, we now think not in terms of vulnerability genes but relative plasticity (Belsky and Hartman, 2014).

15.2.4 Environmental Influences

There have been a number of studies linking quality of parenting to ADHD diagnosis, suggesting that ADHD is related to insecure attachment relationships (e.g. Roskam et al., 2014). What the research makes clear is that children with a relaxed disposition are less likely to be vigilant in an environment that is stressful or dangerous. Research has

also shown how even young infants, when feeling less emotionally held, move around more and are less able to concentrate (Miller, 1989; Tronick, 2007). Infants and children feel calm and are stiller when their emotional and physiological states are regulated by an adult attuned to them. Studies show that having a stressful or traumatic childhood is highly predictive of being impulsive and dysregulated and having poor executive functioning (Ersche et al., 2012). In families displaying high levels of negativity, anger or aggression, children tend to struggle much more with emotional regulation (Morris et al., 2007). Indeed, where there is violence and aggression we see extreme sympathetic nervous system arousal alongside externalising behaviours (El-Sheikh et al., 2009; Panzer and Viljoen, 2005).

From the perspective of life history theory (Belsky et al., 2012), a speeded-up metabolism, less trust, less relaxation and more suspicion and risk-taking might be adaptive for abusive homes or violent neighbourhoods. In such environments there is little emotional security or expectation that things will work out well. This is a strategy that ensures short-term survival, though at the cost of long-term physical and mental health. Our responses can therefore be seen as adaptive to our environments, triggering neurobiological patterns that have a profound effect on the rest of our lives (Belsky et al., 2012). Those born into highly stressed worlds tend to have not just a speeded-up metabolism and more activated stress response systems; they may also develop what some call a 'fast' as opposed to a 'slow' life history strategy. This also happens in a range of other mammals as a strategy that aids survival. Without it, any too trusting and complacent ancestors might have met a violent end before they had time to reproduce.

Evidence shows that ADHD symptoms can increase due to social and economic influences. For example, Mischel (2014) found that children from low-income families in violent parts of the Bronx tended to have a below average ability to self-regulate compared to more privileged children. Early severe institutional deprivation is associated with adult ADHD (Kennedy et al., 2016). Other studies have found a link between low socioeconomic status and the growth of executive parts of the brain (Noble et al., 2005), linking poverty with chronic stress and neurocognitive outcomes into adulthood (Evans and Schamberg, 2009). At six months, infants from socioeconomically deprived environments are less able to pay attention (Clearfield and Jedd, 2013). Childhood poverty and its associated stress levels have a big effect on capacities for emotional regulation, the development of inhibitory brain networks (Kim et al., 2013) and the likelihood of increased risk-taking (Griskevicius et al., 2011). Being able to defer gratification depends on feeling sufficiently relaxed (high vagal tone) and being helped to bear and regulate one's emotions (Moore and Macgillivray, 2004).

ADHD can be thought of in part as a deficit of executive functions (Barkley, 2006). Those diagnosed with ADHD struggle, for example, with planning, emotional regulation, focusing, concentrating and putting plans into action (Brown, 2013). Those able to delay gratification have more activity in prefrontal brain regions, which are central to abstract thinking, planning, working memory and emotional regulation (Barkley, 2012). Those with more impulsive character traits tend to lack these prefrontal 'brakes' on their impulsivity (McClure et al., 2004). Instead, more primitive subcortical brain areas are active. This also is seen in trauma and in stressful situations generally, which is partly why many children who display symptoms that fit with ADHD checklists for other reasons are misdiagnosed as having ADHD (DeJong, 2010).

15.2.5 Social Changes

The social environment for children has altered dramatically over the past two centuries. Whereas boys would typically have learnt a trade from their father or other relative, this changed with universal schooling. One result is that there is a mismatch between the strengths of children with ADHD (i.e. their tendency to explore, to challenge and to try out new ways of doing things) and their environment.

Why are male rates for ADHD typically higher than those for females? One common evolutionary explanation is that, as in many species, males have had to be more risk-taking to compete for mates, since a higher proportion of males than females fail to have children and pass on their genes (Bateman, 1948). Thus, sexual competition between adult males is high. This can be compounded when males have to leave their families to seek out mates. Boys are also more sensitive

than girls to the consequences of suboptimal parental care. From birth onwards girls, on average, are better equipped to regulate their emotions and better able to cope with disruptions in parenting. Parents may need to work harder to imitate and respond to their sons than their daughters, and boys need more input in order to feel emotionally regulated (Tronick and Weinberg, 2000). Following postnatal depression, it seems boys fare worse, having less capacity for object constancy at 18 months and showing more behavioural problems at school age (Murray et al., 1993). Sander (2007) looked at newborns separated from their parents and placed with new carers. After a few days the girls had all entrained to their new carers' day–night rhythms, but the boys took several days longer to adjust, suggesting that they were more vulnerable following disruptions of care.

Tronick (2007) found that depressed mothers were consistently angrier with sons than daughters. By six months sons were gesturing more anxiously and were three times more likely than daughters to resort to self-comforting strategies such as sucking their thumbs. A study in France showed that mothers with a propensity for depression were more likely to become depressed if they had male babies (de Tychey et al., 2008). Such research might suggest a trade-off in evolutionary history between the need to be risk-taking and to explore and the capacity to concentrate and be still. Some ADHD symptoms might still make adaptive sense today, such as being vigilant and wary in the face of violence, thus prioritising survival and safety over capacities such as empathy, self-reflection and emotional regulation (Music, 2016). However, it is also possible that these adaptations could backfire in contemporary society where schooling and academic pressure are so important. A diagnosis of ADHD is most often made in the context of schooling, with most cases being diagnosed in children between the ages of 6 and 12 (NHS, 2018). In a typical school classroom with 25 or more young people, ADHD symptoms will affect other children in the classroom and a teacher's capacity to teach.

The standard model of schooling in which 20 or more young people of the same age are taught in classrooms for about 5 hours a day on most days of the year for 10 years certainly runs counter some of our evolved behavioural strategies. Schooling therefore favours some young people at the expense of others, including those with ADHD (Swanepoel et al., 2017). To add to this issue, schools – especially primary ones – can be seen as feminised institutions, with the large majority of teachers being women. In England in 2019, 76% of the total teaching workforce in state-funded schools was female (DfE, 2020). As has been noted, ADHD predominantly affects males, with childhood and adolescent ADHD male: female identification ratios varying from 3 in Norway to 16 in Austria (ADHD Institute, 2019). This gender imbalance decreases with age. It is likely that schools typically favour the sorts of passive, acquiescent behaviours that society often deems particularly appropriate for females. A 'good student' is essentially defined as a slow life history strategist with traits such as self-management, relationship skills, responsible decision-making and setting and achieving positive goals (Ellis et al., 2017). This leads to a mismatch between what schools want and what children with ADHD are adapted for.

15.2.6 Treatment

The main treatment approaches for ADHD are medication and psychological interventions. Methylphenidate improves irritability in ADHD (de la Cruz, 2015). A Cochrane meta-analysis showed that methylphenidate improves teacher ratings of ADHD and does not cause serious adverse effects; however, the data quality is poor (Storebø et al., 2016). Psychological interventions for ADHD show small effects on un-blinded outcomes but no effects on blinded outcomes (Abikoff et al., 2015).

There is a lot of controversy about the treatment of ADHD, with two main opposing camps. On the one hand, there is some evidence to show that ADHD has a biological component and responds to stimulant treatment (at least in the short term) and that children who are treated with medication have generally better educational outcomes and are less likely to abuse drugs or get in trouble with the law (Thapar and Cooper, 2016). On the other hand, many clinicians argue that normal children are being medicated to make them compliant and that medication is being used as a form of social control. We ourselves are not of one mind on these questions.

We would all argue, however, that a 'one-size-fits-all' approach to school instruction is not appropriate and that the standard practice of teaching and evaluating children under quiet, controlled environmental conditions can disadvantage children with ADHD. Indeed, some studies have shown that children with ADHD may show improved performance if they are allowed to learn while moving around (Ellis et al., 2017). It has been reported that people in the military who do well in the classroom often perform poorly in the field, where they need quickly to switch from task to task in a stressful environment (Ellis et al., 2017). People with ADHD can outperform others in stressful, changing conditions that require a lot of physical activity.

There is differential susceptibility regarding the development of oppositional defiant disorder and conduct disorder in children genetically more susceptible to developing ADHD (Bakermans-Kranenburg and van IJzendoorn, 2015). These children are more likely to develop ADHD with its serious behavioural complications if they experience low warmth in their relationships with their caregivers. They will be less likely than average children to develop these difficulties if they experience warm parenting. It is therefore too simplistic just to link genetic traits to outcomes: once again, there are significant gene–environmental interactions at play.

A serious ethical question to be asked is: should psychiatrists prescribe medication to help a child fit into an environment that is not ideal? Many ADHD services do not have behavioural support services to which they can refer. This puts pressure on psychiatrists to prescribe, even if social measures might have been more appropriate. It is also questionable whether prescribing is ethically justifiable when it is undertaken because of the shortcomings of the school environment. Furthermore, there can be a conflict of interest between what is best for the child and what is easiest for teachers. In a rare study that examined the views of children with ADHD, Singh (2012) found that in both the UK and the USA, children wanted more treatment options apart from medication, but these were not available. The question of informed consent becomes difficult with younger children. Some of the complexities involved in assessment and treatment are illustrated by the case vignette in Box 15.2 (Swanepoel, 2021). (Both vignettes in this chapter are composite and fictionalised.)

Box 15.2 Case vignette 1

Ethan (10) is placed with his grandparents under a special guardianship order as his mother is unable to look after him due to her dependence on drugs. Ethan was previously under a child protection plan due to neglect from his mother and physical abuse from her partner. His grandparents struggle to manage him and often think he is naughty and should be punished by not being allowed to go to football, which he loves. His school has referred him to Child and Adolescent Mental Health Services (CAMHS) as he is on the verge of exclusion: he is unable to sit still and concentrate and is constantly active. He also gets into fights with other children and is rude to teachers. One of his maternal cousins has recently been diagnosed with ADHD.

Ethan presents with clear symptoms of ADHD. He is constantly on edge and jumps at the slightest noise. When he explains his interactions with other children and teachers it is clear that he feels that he is defending himself and gives as good as he gets. He admits to having nightmares of the domestic abuse he witnessed and of the physical abuse he experienced. His greatest wish is to be returned to his mother's care to protect her. He believes this will happen if he is excluded from school, as he knows his grandparents won't be able to cope with him at home all of the time.

Care plan:

(1) Ethan is given a diagnosis of ADHD due to his long-standing symptoms of hyperactivity, impulsivity and inattention. He is started on the non-stimulant medication atomoxetine as he needs cover 24 hours a day and is unlikely to cope with the rebound effects of stimulants.
(2) Ethan is given a diagnosis of post-traumatic stress disorder due to his symptoms of hypervigilance and re-experiencing of the trauma (nightmares), and he is put forward for therapy with the aim of him feeling less threatened and less likely to respond to fear by fighting.
(3) His grandparents are referred to a parenting course for children with ADHD to help them understand him better. They are advised not to stop him from playing football as exercise is likely to help him be calmer at home.
(4) The social worker is informed. She arranges to meet Ethan to explain that if the placement with his grandparents fails he will go into foster care, as going back to his mum is not an option.
(5) A letter is written to the community mental health team looking after his mother to inform them of Ethan's diagnosis of ADHD, suggesting that she is screened as well, since untreated ADHD can be a factor in unmanageable substance abuse.

Follow-up at three months:

Ethan is much more settled at school and with his grandparents. Exclusion from school and placement breakdown have been avoided. He is happy to continue taking his medication.

In sum, we believe that an evolutionary view can help both professionals and patients understand ADHD in a broader sense, where it can be thought about as both a liability and a strength and where the environment should be adapted as much as possible before using medication to adapt the individual.

15.3 Autism Spectrum Disorder

15.3.1 Introduction

ASDs are a heterogeneous group of neurodevelopmental conditions. Those affected can range from profoundly intellectually disabled individuals who are non-verbal to high-functioning individuals who excel in their chosen profession. ASD is characterised by difficulties in social and emotional communication and restrictive and repetitive interests. The ability to maintain focus on a specific interest can be a real strength and can lead to high-functioning people with ASD outperforming neurologically typical ones.

However, it is important to note that most people with any one neurodevelopmental condition will also meet criteria for other neurodevelopmental conditions and that comorbidity is the norm rather than the exception.

The resemblance between some aspects of infant attachment disorganisation and behaviours typically found in neurodevelopmental disorders (such as freezing, atypical postures and behavioural stereotypies) was recognised by Main in her analysis of attachment styles in children diagnosed with autism (as discussed by Haltigan et al., 2021). There are now codified procedures to address this overlap, which are used when examining individuals with established neurodevelopmental disorders or who are at a high risk of these (Haltigan et al., 2021).

Autism exists on a spectrum – hence the increasing use of the term ASD. Unfortunately, early descriptions of these conditions suggested that they were the result of childhood psychoses or psychodynamic disturbances of parent–child relationships. This led to unhelpful and erroneous blaming of mothers. Advances in medical science helped to establish ASD as a neurobiological disorder of early brain development, the precise causes of which are still unclear. There are many genetic, epigenetic, metabolic, hormonal, immunological, neuroanatomical and neurophysiological aetiologies of ASD, as well as an array of gastrointestinal and other systemic comorbid disorders.

In line with the current understanding of gene–environment interactions, there is emerging evidence that maternal psychological distress may potentiate the effects of genes carrying a neurodevelopment risk via altered expression of regulatory genes in these networks prenatally (Breen et al., 2018). Thus, people with ASD form a heterogeneous population with extensive neurodiversity (Modabbernia et al., 2017).

15.3.2 Aetiology

We know that autism is a heritable neurodevelopmental disorder with deleterious effects on reproductive success. The combination of high heritability and low reproductive success raises the question: why was autism not eliminated by natural selection (Ploeger and Galis, 2011)? Autism risk genes do not seem to have evolved recently; they exhibit physical features related to their age, including large gene and protein sizes and regulatory sequences that help to control gene expression (Casanova et al., 2019).

It could be that autism is a 'disorder' or 'disease', and so is not adaptive, or that autism is an adaptation conferring some sort of selective advantage. The National Autistic Society (2021) gives a figure of 1% for the prevalence of ASD in the UK. In evolutionary terms, this is high for a condition that is reproductively disadvantageous. The prevalence of autism suggests that the second reason (that autism is an adaptation) plays a part, but this does not rule out the first (that autism is a disorder or disease).

It seems highly likely that autism is a disorder for those with single-mutation genetic changes and genetic syndromes. These individuals often have significant intellectual disabilities. Studies have found that at least 3–10% of cases of autism are related to *de novo* and rare genetic variants (De la Torre-Ubieta et al., 2016). Equally, environmental factors such as prenatal teratogens (e.g. valproate or alcohol) can cause syndromes that often classify as autism. Thurm et al. (2019) point out that autism accompanied by intellectual disability points towards the presence of a specific aetiological factor and cannot be classed as evolved or adaptive.

So-called high-functioning autism may, from an evolutionary perspective, be adaptive. We know that high-functioning autism is highly heritable and due to multiple genes that each have a small effect. A suite of studies has reported positive genetic correlations between the likelihood of developing autism and measures of enhanced mental ability (Crespi, 2016). These findings indicate that alleles for autism overlap broadly with alleles for high intelligence. Polimanti and Gelernter (2017: 4) state that 'using genome-wide data, we observed that common alleles associated with increased risk for ASD present a signature of positive selection in European populations. This strongly suggests that these variants have undergone positive selection during the course of human evolutionary history.'

ASD is sufficiently common that there may often have been one or two autistic individuals in each of our ancestral hunter-gatherer groups (which probably numbered 100–150 individuals). We know that ASD appears young, is lifelong and is more likely to appear in children born to older parents. High-functioning people with autism often show outstanding abilities in memory and spatial skills and develop expertise in their area of special interest. This may have been of survival value in traditional societies if food was sparse and solitary foraging increased the chances of survival (Reser, 2011). Ploeger and Galis (2011) hypothesise that, from an evolutionary point of view, men with well-developed systemising skills may have had an advantage. Systemising may have been important for developing tools and weapons and in hunting, tracking and trading. It is indeed the case that ASD seems to be more common in men than in women, though this may be at least partly due to misdiagnosis.

The suggestion that ASD has persisted because it was advantageous for ancestral hunter-gatherer tribes despite being deleterious for the individuals concerned is based on the theory of group selection. This proposes that traits may exist even if they are disadvantageous to the individuals themselves because they benefit the group in which the individual lives. This theory dates back to Darwin, but it fell into disfavour in the 1970s when it was widely presumed that the forces of natural selection operated much more strongly on individuals. More recently, however, there has been a resurgence in group selection theory (Wilson and Sober, 1994). Nowadays, the benefits of having people with high-functioning autism in quite a wide range of jobs are increasingly being appreciated.

Other evolutionary arguments for ASD have also been proposed. One such argument is connected with the fact that the genetic component of autism is polygenic, with at least 30 genes being involved. In most people, the interactions between these genes result in individuals with who are neurotypical or who have high-functioning ASD. Inevitably, however, in some individuals the result is 'the development of autism, low intelligence, or other pathologies' (Ploeger and Galis, 2011: 41). This argument sees autism as an unintended consequence of evolution – a bit like being substantially shorter or taller than is optimal as a result of the random assortment of chromosomes during gamete formation.

There is little doubt that over the course of our species' evolutionary history there has been selection for increased intelligence. Humans do not have the physical prowess of many other large mammals; we rely on our wits, including our social skills. However, it is worth pointing out that what is meant by 'intelligence' may not have been the same throughout our evolutionary history. Today's intelligence tests, for example, do not measure such important skills as persistence, truthfulness or reliability – all traits that may have been even more valuable when we lived in groups where everyone knew each other.

The case vignette in Box 15.3 illustrates what might be the consequences of a mismatch between a child with high-functioning ASD and their environment.

15.3.3 Development and Life History Theory

We know that mothering infants with autism (who are less likely to make eye contact and

---

Box 15.3 Case vignette 2

Erin (12) presented to accident and emergency after a serious suicide attempt. She had a diagnosis of high-functioning ASD and attempted to end her life by hanging herself in her cupboard in the middle of the night in her room at her boarding school. Thankfully, the rail did not hold her weight, and the crash woke her roommate, who told the teachers.

Erin was highly gifted in music and was placed in a specialist residential school for this. However, she was uninterested in the social chit-chat of the other girls. She was seen as aloof and arrogant and was bullied. Erin did not have a close relationship with her high-performing parents and had no friends. When she became suicidal she did not tell anyone.

The outcome was that Erin was admitted to a psychiatric hospital and eventually placed in a specialist school for autistic children closer to home, which she attended daily. Care was taken to adapt the environment so as not to overwhelm her and to support her social skills as well as her musical gifts.

---

reciprocate a social smile) is more difficult (Shepherd et al., 2018). This results in a greater chance of psychiatric disorder in the mother (Fairthorne et al., 2016). In our recent evolutionary past, mothers needed to make difficult choices in order to raise at least some surviving offspring. We also know that infant characteristics play a role in maternal decisions in this respect. Hrdy and Burkart (2020) explain how, across traditional societies, mothers adjust parental investment in line with social and ecological circumstances. Those infants who are most skilled at appealing to their mothers and attracting other carers are most likely to survive. This must have led to selection pressure to smile, babble, develop theory of mind and engage in social interactions with others. Children with autism would have been at a disadvantage if they were born to mothers who did not have adequate social support. The pressures of natural selection may therefore have led to the consistent finding that most children with high-functioning autism are born to older fathers (Kong et al., 2012). An autistic child being born to older parents may well have been at an advantage because they were likely to be born with older siblings who would help them to get through their early years until their specific abilities were fully developed (Meilleur et al., 2015).

15.3.4 Complex Nature–Nurture Interactions

Many traumatised and neglected children show a range of developmental difficulties that can be confused with those of neurodevelopmental disorders such as ASD (DeJong, 2010; Oswald et al., 2010). This has led researchers such as Tarren-Sweeney (2010) to argue that these children do not access the correct services sufficiently because they are not well enough understood and to develop alternative ways of conceptualising the range of issues that such children have.

McCullough et al. (2014, 2016) researched looked-after children with a diagnosis of ASD. They were given a battery of tests including the Autistic Spectrum Quotient and tests of theory of mind abilities. On such measures there was no diagnosis of ASD. These children had all been maltreated and were typical in displaying 'sub-threshold' levels of behavioural difficulties, inattention, poor symbolic and imaginary capacities and basic levels of language skills, and they also struggled with peer relationships. Similarly, a large proportion of children adopted from Eastern European orphanages showed symptoms that were strikingly like autism (Rutter et al., 2007), including self-stimulating behaviours, rocking and an inability to manage change, as well as having limited verbal ability and little desire to be close to others, to seek comfort or to understand their own and others' emotions. Unlike ASD, these 'quasi'-autistic symptoms often improved when children were adopted into caring families, particularly if this happened when they were under two years of age.

We know that trauma and abuse can give rise to hypervigilance with accompanying strong amygdala activation, high cortisol levels and difficulties in concentrating that can seem rather like ADHD (Perry et al., 1995). Trauma often leads to high stress levels, a difficulty in focusing and concentrating, problems with executive functions and regulating emotions as well as interpersonal difficulties. Such children are easily over-aroused and can seem particularly ill-suited to the structured and ordered learning environment of the classroom or to chaotic playgrounds. Stimuli such as the loud voice of a teacher, the stare of a peer or

the humiliation of not understanding something can quickly trigger disturbed behaviour. Such traumatised children can easily see threat where there is none, leading to an escalation of challenging behaviour. As a result, many maltreated children often are misdiagnosed as having ADHD or ASD (DeJong, 2010; Music, 2011). Evolved adaptive responses, such as being hyperactive in the face of danger or self-soothing by rocking in extreme neglect, can easily be misconstrued as an organic psychiatric disorder. On the other hand, it is important to acknowledge that children with neurodevelopmental conditions can also suffer trauma and that the presence of trauma does not invalidate the presence of a neurodevelopmental disorder or vice versa.

To complicate matters, some neurodevelopmental issues have their origins in prenatal life. For example, a high level of prenatal stress has a powerful effect on the developing foetus, at least partly due to cortisol crossing the placenta and affecting the hypothalamic–pituitary–adrenal axis of the unborn baby, programming it for stress postnatally and altering brain structure and functioning. Stressful adverse experiences such as maternal trauma are predictive of premature birth (Christiaens et al., 2015), which in turn is linked to many neurodevelopmental issues. Low-birthweight babies born to very anxious mothers are likely to have higher cortisol levels throughout their lifespan and a permanently altered stress response system. Severe antenatal stress affects levels of hormones such as dopamine and serotonin that regulate mood, and such stress has been increasingly linked to a range of childhood emotional and behavioural problems (Beijers et al., 2014) into adolescence and adulthood (Bosch et al., 2012). Such influences are independent of variables such as gender, parental educational level, smoking in pregnancy, birthweight and postnatal maternal anxiety. Such effects might themselves be seen as evolutionary adaptations. Sapolsky (2017), for example, suggests that the foetus primed for stress is more likely to survive in a stressful postnatal environment. It is as if the foetus is preparing for the life it is likely to live.

Prenatal factors that might not be evolutionarily adaptive include the effects of maternal use of alcohol and both legal drugs, such as antidepressants (Huybrechts et al., 2014) and antipsychotics (Kulkarni et al., 2014), and illegal drugs (Ross et al., 2015). Particularly pernicious is foetal alcohol syndrome (Mohammadzadeh and Farhat, 2014), with its devastating effects on many brain areas, including those central to memory and impulse control (Rangmar et al., 2015). Finally, nothing in our evolutionary history prepared us for the likelihood of premature foetuses surviving after being born as early as they sometimes are nowadays, and many premature babies show serious neurodevelopmental issues (Jarjour, 2015).

15.4 Conclusion

We maintain that an evolutionary perspective has much to contribute to debates about ADHD and ASD. Understanding these as biological variants that can have adaptive value for living in certain situations may help to shift perceptions of children from being 'naughty' or 'abnormal' to being seen as caught in an evolutionary mismatch. Behavioural strategies in school, for example, could then focus on allowing plenty of physical activity for children with ADHD and providing for the special skills of those with ASD. Longer term, we may need to rethink how schools are conceptualised and run. For people with ADHD and ASD, an evolutionary perspective might also help them to understand their strengths and to seek occupations where these are valued. There will inevitably be downsides to these conditions, as there probably are for all human temperaments. However, reframing such conditions in evolutionary terms paves the way for a more informed discussion of the complexities of their aetiology, diagnosis and treatment and of our ethical and social responsibilities towards the people in these groups.

References

Abikoff, H. B., Abikoff, H. B., Thompson, M., Laver-Bradbury, C., Long, N., Forehand, R. L., Miller Brotman, L., Klein, R. G., Reiss, P., Huo, L. and Sonuga-Barke, E. (2015). Parent training for preschool ADHD: a randomized controlled trial of specialized and generic programs. *Journal of Child Psychology and Psychiatry*, **56**, 618–631.

ADHD Institute (2019). Epidemiology. Retrieved from www.adhd-institute.com/burden-of-adhd/epidemiology/ (accessed 12 March 2021).

Auerbach, J. G., Atzaba-Poria, N., Berger, A. and Landau, R. (2004). Emerging developmental pathways to ADHD: possible path markers in early infancy. *Neural Plasticity*, **11**, 29–43.

Bakermans-Kranenburg, M. J. and van IJzendoorn, M. H. (2015). The hidden efficacy of interventions: gene × environment experiments from a differential susceptibility perspective. *Annual Review of Psychology*, **66**, 381–409.

Barkley, R. A. (2006). *Attention-Deficit Hyperactivity Disorder: A Handbook for Diagnosis and Treatment.* New York: Guilford Press.

Barkley, R. A. (2012). *Executive Functions: What They Are, How They Work, and Why They Evolved.* New York: Guilford Press.

Bateman, A. J. (1948). Intrasexual selection in Drosophila. *Heredity*, **2**, 349–368.

Beijers, R., Buitelaar, J. K. and de Weerth, C. (2014). Mechanisms underlying the effects of prenatal psychosocial stress on child outcomes: beyond the HPA axis. *European Child & Adolescent Psychiatry*, **23**, 943–956.

Belsky, J. (2005). Differential susceptibility to rearing influence. In: B. Ellis and D. Bjorklund (eds.), *Origins of the Social Mind: Evolutionary Psychology and Child Development.* New York: Guilford Press, pp. 139–163.

Belsky, J. and Hartman, S. (2014). Gene–environment interaction in evolutionary perspective: differential susceptibility to environmental influences. *World Psychiatry*, **13**, 87–89.

Belsky, J., Schlomer, G. L. and Ellis, B. J. (2012). Beyond cumulative risk: distinguishing harshness and unpredictability as determinants of parenting and early life history strategy. *Developmental Psychology*, **48**, 662–673.

Bosch, N. M., Riese, H., Reijneveld, S. A., Bakker, M. P., Verhulst, F. C., Ormel, J. and Oldehinkel, A. J. (2012). Timing matters: long term effects of adversities from prenatal period up to adolescence on adolescents' cortisol stress response. The TRAILS study. *Psychoneuroendocrinology*, **37**, 1439–1447.

Breen, M. S., Wingo, A. P., Koen, N., Donald, K. A., Nicol, M., Zar, H. J., Ressler, K. J., Buxbaum, J. D. and Stein, D. J. (2018). Gene expression in cord blood links genetic risk for neurodevelopmental disorders with maternal psychological distress and adverse childhood outcomes. *Brain, Behavior, and Immunity*, **73**, 320–330.

Brown, T. E. (2013). *A New Understanding of ADHD in*

Children and Adults: Executive Function impairments. Abingdon-on-Thames: Routledge.

Cartwright, K. L., Bitsakou, P., Daley, D., Gramzow, R. H., Psychogiou, L., Simonoff, E., Thompson, M. J. and Sonuga-Barke, E. J. (2011). Disentangling child and family influences on maternal expressed emotion toward children with attention-deficit/hyperactivity disorder. *Journal of the American Academy of Child and Adolescent Psychiatry*, 50, 1042–1053.

Casanova, E. L., Switala, A. E., Dandamudi, S., Hickman, A. R., Vandenbrink, J., Sharp, J. L., Feltus, F. A. and Casanova, M. F. (2019). Autism risk genes are evolutionarily ancient and maintain a unique feature landscape that echoes their function. *Autism Research*, 12, 860–869.

Chen, K., Fortin, N. and Phipps, S. (2015). Young in class: implications for inattentive/hyperactive behaviour of Canadian boys and girls. *Canadian Journal of Economics*, 48, 1601–1634.

Chen, M.-H., Lan, W.-H., Bai, Y.-M., Huang, K.-L., Su, T.-P., Tsai, S.-J., Li, C.-T., Lin, W.-G., Chang, W.-H., Pan, T.-L., Chen, T.-J. and Hsu, J.-W. (2016). Influence of relative age on diagnosis and treatment of attention-deficit hyperactivity disorder in Taiwanese children. *Journal of Pediatrics*, 172, 162–167.e1.

Christiaens, I., Hegadoren, K. and Olson, D. M. (2015). Adverse childhood experiences are associated with spontaneous preterm birth: a case–control study. *BMC Medicine*, 13, 124.

Clearfield, M. W. and Jedd, K. E. (2013). The effects of socio-economic status on infant attention. *Infant and Child Development*, 22, 53–67.

Cofnas, N. (2016). A teleofunctional account of evolutionary mismatch. *Biological Philosophy*, 31, 507–525.

Crespi, B. J. (2016). Autism as a disorder of high intelligence. *Frontiers in Neuroscience*, 10, 300.

de la Cruz, L. F., Simonoff, E., McGough, J. J., Halperin, J. M., Arnold, L. E. and Stringaris, A. (2015). Treatment of children with attention-deficit/hyperactivity disorder (ADHD) and irritability: results from the Multimodal Treatment Study of Children with ADHD (MTA). *Journal of the American Academy of Child and Adolescent Psychiatry*, 54, 62–70.e3.

De La Torre-Ubieta, L., Won, H., Stein, J. L. and Geschwind, D. H. (2016). Advancing the understanding of autism disease mechanisms through genetics. *Nature Medicine*, 22, 345–361.

de Tychey, C., Briançon, S., Lighezzolo, J., Spitz, E., Kabuth, B., de Luigi, V., Messembourg, C., Girvan, F., Rosati, A., Thockler, A. and Vincent, S. (2008). Quality of life, postnatal depression and baby gender. *Journal of Clinical Nursing*, 17, 312–322.

DfE (2020). School workforce in England: November 2019. Retrieved from https://explore-education-statistics.service.gov.uk/find-statistics/school-workforce-in-england (accessed 12 March 2021).

DeJong, M. (2010). Some reflections on the use of psychiatric diagnosis in the looked after or 'in care' child population. *Clinical Child Psychology and Psychiatry*, 15, 589–599.

Dyck, M. J., Piek, J. P. and Patrick, J. (2011). The validity of psychiatric diagnoses: the case of 'specific' developmental disorders. *Research in Developmental Disabilities*, 32, 2704–2713.

Eisenberg, D. T. A., Campbell, B., Gray, P. B. and Sorenson, M. D. (2008). Dopamine receptor genetic polymorphisms and body composition in undernourished pastoralists: an exploration of nutrition indices among nomadic and recently settled Ariaal men of northern Kenya. *BMC Evolutionary Biology*, 8, 173.

El-Sheikh, M. El-Sheikh, M., Kouros, C. D., Erath, S., Cummings, E. M., Keller, P. and Staton, L. (2009). Marital conflict and children's externalizing behavior: pathways involving interactions between parasympathetic and sympathetic nervous system activity. *Monographs of the Society for Research in Child Development*, 74, vii–79.

Elberling, H., Linneberg, A., Olsen, E. M., Houmann, T., Rask, C. U., Goodman, R. and Skovgaard, A. M. (2014). Infancy predictors of hyperkinetic and pervasive developmental disorders at ages 5–7 years: results from the Copenhagen Child Cohort CCC2000. *Journal of Child Psychology and Psychiatry*, 55, 1328–1335.

Elberling, H., Linneberg, A., Rask, C. U., Houman, T., Goodman, R. and Skovgaard, A. M. (2016). Psychiatric disorders in Danish children aged 5–7 years: a general population study of prevalence and risk factors from the Copenhagen Child Cohort (CCC 2000). *Nordic Journal of Psychiatry*, 70, 146–155.

Ellis, B. J., Bianchi, J., Griskevicius, V. and Frankenhuis, W. E. (2017). Beyond risk and protective factors: an adaptation-based approach to resilience. *Perspectives on Psychological Science*, 12, 561–587.

Ersche, K. D., Turton, A. J., Chamberlain, S. R., Müller, U., Bullmore, E. T. and Robbins T. W. (2012). Cognitive dysfunction and anxious-impulsive personality traits are endophenotypes for drug dependence. *American Journal of Psychiatry*, **169**, 926–936.

Evans, G. W. and Schamberg, M. A. (2009). Childhood poverty, chronic stress, and adult working memory. *Proceedings of the National Academy of Sciences of the United States of America*, **106**, 6545–6549.

Fairthorne, J., Jacoby, P., Bourke, J., de Klerk, N. and Leonard, H. (2016). Onset of maternal psychiatric disorders after the birth of a child with autism spectrum disorder: a retrospective cohort study. *Autism*, **20**, 37–44.

Faraone, S. V., Doyle, A. E., Mick, E. and Biederman, J. (2014). Meta-analysis of the association between the 7-repeat allele of the dopamine D4 receptor gene and attention deficit hyperactivity disorder. *American Journal of Psychiatry*, **158**, 1052–1057.

Fulton, B. D., Scheffler, R. M., Hinshaw, S. P., Levine, P., Stone, S., Brown, T. T. and Modrek, S. (2015). National variation of ADHD diagnostic prevalence and medication use: health care providers and education policies. *Psychiatric Services*, **60**, 1075–1083.

Ghosh, M., Holman, C. D. and Preen, D. B. (2015). Exploring parental country of birth differences in the use of psychostimulant medications for ADHD: a whole-population linked data study. *Australian and New Zealand Journal of Public Health*, **39**, 88–92.

Griskevicius, V., Tybur, J. M., Delton, A. W. and Robertson, T. E. (2011). The influence of mortality and socioeconomic status on risk and delayed rewards: a life history theory approach. *Journal of Personality and Social Psychology*, **100**, 1015–1026.

Gudmundsson, O. O., Magnusson, P., Saemundsen, E., Lauth, B., Baldursson, G., Skarphedinsson, G. and Fombonne E. (2013). Psychiatric disorders in an urban sample of preschool children. *Child and Adolescent Mental Health*, **18**, 210–217.

Haltigan, J. D., Del Giudice, M. and Khorsand, S. (2021). Growing points in attachment disorganization: looking back to advance forward. *Attachment & Human Development*, **23**, 438–454.

Harold, G. T., Leve, L. D., Barrett, D., Elam, K., Neiderhiser, J. M., Natsuaki, M. N., Shaw, D. S., Reiss, D. and Thapar, A. (2013). Biological and rearing mother influences on child ADHD symptoms: revisiting the developmental interface between nature and nurture. *Journal of Child Psychology and Psychiatry*, **54**, 1038–1046.

Hoshen, M. B., Benis, A., Keyes, K. M. and Zoëga, H. (2016). Stimulant use for ADHD and relative age in class among children in Israel. *Pharmacoepidemiology and Drug Safety*, **25**, 652–660.

Hrdy, S. B. and Burkart, J. M. (2020). The emergence of emotionally modern humans: implications for language and learning. *Philosophical Transactions of the Royal Society B: Biological Sciences*, **375**, 20190499.

Huybrechts, K. F., Sanghani, R. S., Avorn, J. and Urato, A. C. (2014). Preterm birth and antidepressant medication use during pregnancy: a systematic review and meta-analysis. *PLoS ONE*, **9**, e92778.

Jarjour, I. T. (2015). Neurodevelopmental outcome after extreme prematurity: a review of the literature. *Pediatric Neurology*, **52**, 143–152.

Kennedy, M., Kreppner, J., Knights, N., Kumsta, R., Maughan, B., Golm, D., Rutter, M., Schlotz, W. and Sonuga-Barke, E. J. (2016). Early severe institutional deprivation is associated with a persistent variant of adult attention-deficit/hyperactivity disorder: clinical presentation, developmental continuities and life circumstances in the English and Romanian Adoptees study. *Journal of Child Psychology and Psychiatry*, **57**, 1113–1125.

Kim, P., Evans, G. W., Angstadt, M., Ho, S. H., Sripada, C. S., Swain, J. E., Liberzon, I. and Phan, K. L. (2013). Effects of childhood poverty and chronic stress on emotion regulatory brain function in adulthood. *Proceedings of the National Academy of Sciences of the United States of America*, **110**, 18442–18447.

Kong, A., Frigge, M. L., Masson, G., Besenbacher, S., Sulem, P., Magnusson, G., Gudjonsson, S. A., Sigurdsson, A., Jonasdottir, A., Jonasdottir, A., Wong, W. S. W., Sigurdsson, G., Walters, G. B., Steinberg, S., Helgason, H., Thorleifsson, G., Gudbjartsson, D. F., Helgason, A., Magnusson, O. T., Thorsteinsdottir, U. and Stefansson, K. (2012). Rate of *de novo* mutations and the importance of father's age to disease risk. *Nature*, **488**, 471–475.

Krabbe, E. E., Thoutenhoofd, E.D., Conradi, M., Pijl, S. J. and Batstra, L. (2014). Birth month as predictor of ADHD medication use in Dutch school classes. *European Journal of Special Needs Education*, **29**, 571–578.

Kulkarni, J., Worsley, R., Gilbert, H., Gavrilidis, E., Van Rheenen, T. E., Wang, W., McCauley, K. and Fitzgerald, P. (2014). A prospective cohort study of antipsychotic medications in pregnancy: the first 147 pregnancies and 100 one year old babies. *PLoS ONE*, **9**, e94788.

Lahey, B. B., Lee, S. S., Sibley, M. H., Applegate, B., Molina, B. and Pelham, W. E. (2016). Predictors of adolescent outcomes among 4–6-year-old children with attention-deficit/hyperactivity disorder. *Journal of Abnormal Psychology*, 125, 168–181.

Matthews, L. J. and Butler, P. M. (2011). Novelty-seeking *DRD4* polymorphisms are associated with human migration distance out-of-Africa after controlling for neutral population gene structure. *American Journal of Physical Anthropology*, 145, 382–389.

McClure, S. M., Laibson, D. I., Loewenstein, G. and Cohen, J. D. (2004). Separate neural systems value immediate and delayed monetary rewards. *Science*, 306, 503–507.

McCullough, E., Gordon-Jones, S., Last, A., Vaughan, J. and Burnell, A. (2016). An evaluation of neuro-physiological psychotherapy: an integrative therapeutic approach to working with adopted children who have experienced early life trauma. *Clinical Child Psychology and Psychiatry*, 21, 582–602.

McCullough, E., Stedmon, J. and Dallos, R. (2014). Narrative responses as an aid to understanding the presentation of maltreated children who meet criteria for autistic spectrum disorder and reactive attachment disorder: a case series study. *Clinical Child Psychology and Psychiatry*, 19, 392–411.

Meilleur, A. A., Jelenic, P. and Mottron, L. (2015) Prevalence of clinically and empirically defined talents and strengths in autism. *Journal of Autism and Developmental Disorders*, 45, 1354–1367.

Miller, L. (1989). *Closely Observed Infants*. London: Duckworth.

Mischel, W. (2014). *Marshmallow Test*. New York: Little, Brown and Company.

Modabbernia, A., Velthorst, E. and Reichenberg, A. (2017). Environmental risk factors for autism: an evidence-based review of systematic reviews and meta-analyses. *Molecular Autism*, 8, 13.

Mohammadzadeh, A. and Farhat, A. (2014). Fetal alcohol syndrome. *Asia Pacific Journal of Medical Toxicology*, 3, 10.

Moore, C. and Macgillivray, S. (2004). Altruism, prudence, and theory of mind in preschoolers. *New Directions for Child and Adolescent Development*, 103, 51–62.

Morris, A. S., Silk, J. S., Steinberg, L., Myers, S. S. and Robinson, L. R. (2007). The role of the family context in the development of emotion regulation. *Social Development*, 16, 361–388.

Murray, L., Kempton, C., Woolgar, M. and Hooper, R. (1993). Depressed mothers' speech to their infants and its relation to infant gender and cognitive development. *Journal of Child Psychology and Psychiatry*, 34, 1083–1101.

Music, G. (2011). Misdiagnosed and misunderstood. *Counselling Children and Young People*, 2, 2–6.

Music, G. (2016). *Nurturing Natures: Attachment and Children's Emotional, Social and Brain Development*. London: Psychology Press.

National Autistic Society (2021). What is autism? Retrieved from www.autism.org.uk/advice-and-guidance/what-is-autism (accessed 12 March 2021).

NHS (2018). Attention deficit hyperactivity disorder (ADHD). Retrieved from www.nhs.uk/conditions/Attention-deficit-hyperactivity-disorder/Pages/Introduction.aspx (accessed 12 March 2021).

Noble, K. G., Norman, M. F. and Farah, M. J. (2005). Neurocognitive correlates of socioeconomic status in kindergarten children. *Developmental Science*, 8, 74–87.

Oswald, S. H., Heil, K. and Goldbeck, L. (2010). History of maltreatment and mental health problems in foster children: a review of the literature. *Journal of Pediatric Psychology*, 35, 462–472.

Panzer, A. and Viljoen, M. (2005). Supportive evidence for ADHD as a neurodevelopmental disorder. *Medical Hypotheses*, 64, 755–758.

Pappa, I., Mileva-Seitz, V. R., Bakermans-Kranenburg, M. J., Tiemeier, H. and van IJzendoorn, M. H. (2015). The magnificent seven: a quantitative review of dopamine receptor D4 and its association with child behavior. *Neuroscience & Biobehavioral Reviews*, 57, 175–186.

Perry, B. D., Pollard, R. A., Blakley, T. L., Baker, W. L. and Vigilante, D. (1995). Childhood trauma, the neurobiology of adaptation, and 'use-dependent' development of the brain: how 'states' become 'traits'. *Infant Mental Health Journal*, 16, 271–291.

Ploeger, A. and Galis, F. (2011). Evolutionary approaches to autism – an overview and integration. *McGill Journal of Medicine*, 13, 38–43.

Polanczyk, G. V., Willcutt, E. G., Salum, G. A., Kieling, C. and Rohde, L. A. (2014). ADHD prevalence estimates across three decades: an updated systematic review and meta-regression analysis. *International Journal of Epidemiology*, 43, 434–442.

Polimanti, R. and Gelernter, J. (2017). Widespread signatures of positive selection in common risk alleles associated to autism spectrum disorder. *PLoS Genetics*, 13, e1006618.

Posner, M. I., Rothbart, M. K., Sheese, B. E. and Voelker, P. (2014). Developing attention: behavioral and brain mechanisms. *Advances in Neuroscience*, 2014, 405094.

Rangmar, J., Hjern, A., Vinnerljung, B., Strömland, K., Aronson, M. and Fahlke, C. (2015). Psychosocial outcomes of fetal alcohol syndrome in adulthood. *Pediatrics*, 135, e52–e58.

Reser, J. E. (2011). Conceptualizing the autism spectrum in terms of natural selection and behavioral ecology: the solitary forager hypothesis. *Evolutionary Psychology*, **9**, 207–238.

Roskam, I., Stievenart, M., Tessier, R., Muntean, A., Escobar, M. J., Santelices, M. P., Juffer, F., Van IJzendoorn, M. H. and Pierrehumbert, B. (2014). Another way of thinking about ADHD: the predictive role of early attachment deprivation in adolescents' level of symptoms. *Social Psychiatry and Psychiatric Epidemiology*, **49**, 133–144.

Ross, E. J., Graham, D. L., Money, K. M. and Stanwood, G. D. (2015). Developmental consequences of fetal exposure to drugs: what we know and what we still must learn. *Neuropsychopharmacology*, **40**, 61–87.

Rutter, M., Beckett, C., Castle, J., Colvert, E., Kreppner, J., Mehta, M., Stevens, S. and Sonuga-Barke, E. (2007). Effects of profound early institutional deprivation: an overview of findings from a UK longitudinal study of Romanian adoptees. *European Journal of Developmental Psychology*, **4**, 332–350.

Sander, L. (2007). *Living Systems, Evolving Consciousness, and the Emerging Person: A Selection of Papers from the Life Work of Louis Sander*. London: Routledge.

Sapolsky, R. M. (2017). *Behave: The Biology of Humans at our Best and Worst*. London: Penguin.

Schwandt, H. and Wuppermann, A. (2016). The youngest get the pill: ADHD misdiagnosis in Germany, its regional correlates and international comparison. *Labour Economics*, **43**, 72–86.

Shepherd, D., Landon, J., Taylor, S. and Goedeke, S. (2018). Coping and care-related stress in parents of a child with autism spectrum

disorder. *Anxiety, Stress, and Coping*, **31**, 277–290.

Simonoff, E. Pickles, A., Wood, N., Gringras, P. and Chadwick, O. (2007). ADHD symptoms in children with mild intellectual disability. *Journal of the American Academy of Child & Adolescent Psychiatry*, **46**, 591–600.

Singh, I. (2012). VOICES: Voices on Identity, Childhood, Ethics and Stimulants – Children Join the Debate. Retrieved from www.basw.co.uk/system/files/resources/basw_114402-2_0.pdf (accessed 12 March 2021).

Storebø, O. J., Simonsen, E. and Gluud, C. (2016). Methylphenidate for attention-deficit/hyperactivity disorder in children and adolescents. *Journal of the American Medical Association*, **315**, 2009–2010.

Swanepoel, A. (2021). Fifteen-minute consultation: to prescribe or not to prescribe in ADHD, that is the question. *Archives of Disease in Childhood – Education and Practice Edition*, **106**, 322–325.

Swanepoel, A., Music, G., Launer, J. and Reiss, M. (2017). How evolutionary thinking can help us understand ADHD. *BJPsych Advances*, **23**, 410–418.

Swanepoel, A. Sieff, D. F., Music, G., Launer, J., Reiss, M. and Wren, B. (2016). How evolution can help us understand child development and behaviour. *BJPsych Advances* **22**, 36–43.

Tarren-Sweeney, M. (2010). It's time to re-think mental health services for children in care, and those adopted from care. *Clinical Child Psychology and Psychiatry*, **15**, 613–626.

Thapar, A. and Cooper, M. (2016). Attention deficit hyperactivity disorder. *Lancet* **387**, 1240–1250.

Thurm, A., Farmer, C., Salzman, E., Lord, C. and Bishop, S. (2019). State of the field: differentiating intellectual disability from

autism spectrum disorder. *Frontiers in Psychiatry*, **10**, 526.

Timimi, S. and Taylor, E. (2004) ADHD is best understood as a cultural construct, *British Journal of Psychiatry*, **184**, 8–9.

Tronick, E. (2007). *The Neurobehavioral and Social Emotional Development of Infants and Children*. New York: Norton.

Tronick, E. Z. and Weinberg, M. K. (2000). Gender differences and their relation to maternal depression. In: S. L. Johnson, A. M. Hayes, T. Field, M. N. Schneiderman and P. M. McCabe (eds.), *Stress, Coping, and Depression*. Mahwah, NJ: Lawrence Erlbaum, pp. 23–34.

van IJzendoorn, M. H. and Bakermans-Kranenburg, M. J. (2015). Genetic differential susceptibility on trial: meta-analytic support from randomized controlled experiments. *Development and Psychopathology*, **27**, 151–162.

Verlinden, M., Jansen, P. W., Veenstra, R., Jaddoe, V. W., Hofman, A., Verhulst, F. C., Shaw, P. and Tiemeier, H. (2015). Preschool attention-deficit/hyperactivity and oppositional defiant problems as antecedents of school bullying. *Journal of the American Academy of Child & Adolescent Psychiatry*, **54**, 571–579.

Wanless, S. B., McClelland, M., Lan, X., Son, S., Cameron, C., Morrison, F., Chen, F., Chen, J., Li, S., Lee, K. and Sung, M. (2013). Gender differences in behavioral regulation in four societies: the United States, Taiwan, South Korea, and China. *Early Childhood Research Quarterly*, **28**, 621–633.

Washbrook, E., Propper, C. and Sayal, K. (2013). Pre-school hyperactivity/attention problems and educational outcomes in adolescence: prospective longitudinal study. *British Journal of Psychiatry*, **203**, 265–271.

Wedge, M. (2012). Why French kids don't have ADHD. Psychology Today, 8 March. Retrieved from www.sakkyndig.com/psykologi/artvit/wedge2012.pdf (accessed 12 March 2021).

Wilson, D. S. and Sober, E. (1994) Reintroducing group selection to the human behavioral sciences. *Behavioral and Brain Sciences*, **17**, 585–654.

Windhorst, D. A., Mileva-Seitz, V. R., Linting, M., Hofman, A., Jaddoe, V. W., Verhulst, F. C., Tiemeier, H., van IJzendoorn, M. H. and Bakermans-Kranenburg, M. J. (2015). Differential susceptibility in a developmental perspective: DRD4 and maternal sensitivity predicting externalizing behavior. *Developmental Psychobiology*, **57**, 35–49.

Chapter 16

Maternal Negativity and Child Maltreatment

How Evolutionary Perspectives Contribute to a Layered and Compassionate Understanding

Daniela F. Sieff*

Abstract

In Western culture, both the lay public and mental health professionals tend to believe that mothers evolved to love all of their children instinctually and unconditionally. In contrast, any mother who feels ambivalence or hostility towards her child is typically seen as unnatural, and a mother who maltreats her child is seen as behaving pathologically. This chapter draws on evolutionary research to challenge this widespread view of motherhood. In particular, it describes how raising children has required mothers to negotiate a series of complex, precarious and layered trade-offs, and it argues that maternal negativity and child maltreatment can arise from this. The goal of this chapter is to foster a more evolutionarily valid, nuanced and compassionate understanding of motherhood. Such an understanding has the potential to contribute to clinical work with faltering mothers as well as to programmes focused on preventing maternal maltreatment of children.

Keywords

child abuse, child maltreatment, child neglect, evolutionary psychiatry, evolutionary trade-offs, infanticide, maternal hostility, maternal maltreatment, maternal negativity

Key Points

- Human mothers have not evolved to feel automatic and unconditional love for each and every one of their children. Instead, evolution has granted mothers with a continuum of maternal feelings, ranging from full commitment to negativity. Where a woman falls on this continuum is influenced by her circumstances. Particularly important are the resources she can garner to support her child-rearing and the characteristics of her child.

- Maternal treatment can result from the need to make a much-loved child conform to group norms. Throughout human evolutionary history being part of a group was crucial to survival.

- Maternal behaviour has evolved to be shaped by social learning. Without conscious effort or intent, girls learn about mothering through what they experience and observe during their own childhoods. The transmission of maltreatment across generations is often a maladaptive consequence of this.

- The fact that some maternal negativity and child maltreatment results from evolved influences does not make it any less harmful. Maternal negativity and child maltreatment are tremendously damaging, whatever their origins. They instigate emotional trauma (also known as complex post-traumatic stress

* I am grateful to Sarah Blaffer Hrdy, Dan Delli, Aaron Denham, Louise Holland, Bruce Lloyd and Pablo Nepomnaschy for thoughtful comments on earlier drafts. I am also grateful to those who contributed to the discussions that have followed my talks on this topic. This chapter is better for these contributions, though the final responsibility remains my own.

disorder) and pave the way for long-term psychological and physical suffering.

- An understanding of how evolved dynamics influence maternal feelings and behaviour has the potential to contribute to clinical work with faltering mothers and also to programmes focused on preventing the maltreatment of children by their mothers.

16.1 Introduction

The World Health Organization (WHO) defines child maltreatment as 'all types of physical and/or emotional ill-treatment ... which results in actual or potential harm to the child's health, survival, development or dignity in the context of a relationship of responsibility, trust or power' (WHO, 2020). In some cases, maltreatment stems from the child's own mother. This chapter explores the maternal maltreatment of children from evolutionary and anthropological perspectives.

In Western culture, both the lay public and mental health professionals tend to believe that mothers evolved to love all of their children instinctually and unconditionally and that a psychologically normal mother will do everything in her power to protect her child from maltreatment. In contrast, a mother who feels ambivalence or hostility towards her child is typically seen as unnatural, and a mother who actually maltreats her child is seen as behaving pathologically.

John Bowlby, a psychiatrist, psychologist and psychoanalyst, was the first clinician to address the mother–child relationship through an evolutionary perspective, and he supported this view:

> ... for babies to love mothers and mothers to love babies is taken for granted as intrinsic to human nature. As a result, whenever ... these standards become markedly different from the norm ... all are disposed to judge the condition as pathological. (Bowlby, 1969/1997: 242)

Bowlby was a pioneer in recognising that evolutionary thinking could make a significant contribution to the understanding of psychological well-being, but he formulated his ideas in the 1950s, and evolutionary thinking has moved on since then. Two advances are particularly important to this chapter.

First, when Bowlby was formulating his ideas, the study of animal behaviour was in its infancy and was concerned with documenting the behavioural patterns that typified an entire species. By the late 1960s, however, biologists had embarked on long-term studies in which they followed individual animals through their lives. This revealed that there is rarely a one-size-fits-all, normal way to behave; rather, evolution produces a *range* of possible behaviours, thereby allowing individuals to respond flexibly to the particular challenges and opportunities presented by their changing physical and social environments.

The second advance came from recognising that trade-offs are central to evolution. Living creatures are complex systems in which one need is traded off against another making compromises ubiquitous. At the level of physiology, for example, animals living in disease-ridden environments need to commit energy to their immune system, but that leaves less energy for growth, bodily maintenance and reproduction. A parallel example from the realm of behaviour is that animals living in predator-dense environments must be hypervigilant, but that leaves less time for feeding, maintaining social relationships and caring for offspring.

The importance of these two advances to understanding mothering became clear through the scholarship of primatologist, anthropologist and feminist Sarah Blaffer Hrdy (Hrdy, 1999, 2009). Hrdy showed that there is not just one way to be a human mother and that 'natural mothering' is not synonymous with unconditional love. Rather, depending on the environment in which a mother finds herself and the compromises she needs to make, she may feel fully committed to her child, somewhat committed, ambivalent or hostile. In the worst case, a mother might be responsible for her child's death.

It is easy to understand why evolutionary processes would have forged an emotional system in which mothers are fully committed to their infants. But why would evolution have forged an emotional system in which women sometimes feel ambivalent or hostile towards their offspring? The answer resides in the fact that most human mothers have had to manage the trade-offs between competing needs in environments very different from our own.

Anthropologists describe our society as 'WEIRD': Western, educated, industrialised, rich and democratic (Henrich et al., 2010). WEIRD societies encompass considerable diversity, but they all share characteristics that make them different from the societies in which our ancestors lived. They are also different from the societies of contemporary hunter-gatherers and subsistence horticulturalists. With respect to mothering, one such difference is the rate of child mortality. In WEIRD societies, child mortality is extremely low thanks to clean drinking water, sanitation systems, vaccinations and antibiotics. In the USA, for example, less than 1% of those born die before their 15th birthday, but in modern small-scale subsistence societies between 30% and 60% of those born do not survive to 15 years of age (Gurven and Kaplan, 2007). In pre-industrialised Western societies child mortality was just as high, and it was likely as high if not higher during our evolutionary history (Volk and Atkinson, 2013).

High child mortality rates have a profound impact on the evolutionary trade-offs involved in mothering, and negotiating these trade-offs can require mothers to withdraw commitment and care from a particular child. Thus, although some instances of maternal negativity and child maltreatment result from psychopathology, there are situations in which maternal negativity and child maltreatment are neither unnatural nor pathological. Instead, they represent an attempt to manage competing needs in a challenging environment.

The fact that some child maltreatment results from evolutionary processes does not make it any less harmful. Maternal maltreatment of children is tremendously damaging, whatever its origins. It instigates emotional trauma (also known as complex post-traumatic stress disorder) and paves the way for long-term psychological and physical suffering (Lanius et al., 2010; Sieff, 2015). However, evolution is blind to suffering (Nesse, 2019), and to judge all maternal maltreatment of children as unnatural or pathological is not only evolutionarily incorrect but clinically unhelpful. Such judgement means that mothers who feel negatively about their children believe themselves to be abnormal and sub-human, whereupon they get stuck in escalating cycles of toxic shame that make being honest about their feelings and facilitating change particularly difficult (Sieff, 2019). Equally, judging all maternal maltreatment as pathological means that programmes aimed at prevention fail to recognise the importance of environmental

factors as contributors to maternal negativity and child maltreatment. In contrast, the layered and compassionate understanding of mothering fostered by evolutionary perspectives helps address child maltreatment on both an individual and a societal level.

This chapter draws on evolutionary research to expand the understanding of four factors which have been shown to contribute to maternal negativity and child maltreatment: (1) maternal resources, (2) children's characteristics, (3) child socialisation and (4) social learning of mothering.

16.2 Maternal Resources

To raise human children requires a lengthy commitment of energy, time and attention. Resources are required to support this commitment. The resources available to ancestral mothers would have fluctuated, cycling between times of plenty and times of scarcity (Potts, 2013). The availability of resources fluctuates in many small-scale subsistence societies today as well as in sectors of WEIRD societies. A mother's judicious allocation of resources during times of scarcity has been crucial to ensuring that as many of her children survive as possible.

Two kinds of resources have been particularly important to mothers: nutritional (Section 16.2.1) and social (Section 16.2.2).

16.2.1 Nutritional Resources

It takes calories to raise a human child. Not only must mothers secure enough calories for pregnancy and breastfeeding, but also human children rarely procure all of their own food until they are in the middle of their teenage years. Therefore, adults must continue to provision children long after they have been weaned. Securing sufficient calories can be extremely challenging when food is scarce, and during such times a mother may be forced to make difficult decisions. How much food should she keep for herself and how much should she give to her children? Of the food that she gives to her children, should she divide it equitably between all of her children or should she favour certain children?

Sometimes a mother's decisions are conscious, often they are unconscious. Either way, when there is not enough food a mother's challenge is to find the most evolutionarily pragmatic response – the compromise that represents the best of a bad job.

16.2.1.1 Trade-Off between a Mother and Her Children at Times of Food Shortages

WEIRD cultures view mothers as instinctively self-sacrificing and willing to forfeit their lives to save their children. This makes evolutionary sense because in these environments child mortality is low and motherless children generally survive. In contrast, mothers who make this ultimate sacrifice in environments where child mortality is high are likely to be evolutionarily penalised in two ways: first, motherless children are at risk of dying, so a self-sacrificing mother will not necessarily save her child (e.g. Hill and Hurtado, 1996; Willführ and Gagnon, 2013); and second, a mother who gives her life for her child forgoes the opportunity to beget children in the future when food might be more plentiful and children more likely to survive.

In some situations the trade-off between a mother and her children is mediated through behavioural 'decisions' to alter the allocation of food. At other times, such as during pregnancy and breastfeeding, this trade-off is negotiated physiologically.

Human pregnancy requires around 300 extra calories per day, which is not particularly energetically expensive (Brown, 2011). However, if mothers are in very poor nutritional health then less food is passed to the foetus. As a result, these newborns will be low in weight, which leads to an increased risk of death during infancy. Furthermore, without compensatory growth during the first two years, low-birthweight infants suffer impaired physical and cognitive development as well as higher rates of adult mortality (Black et al., 2008; Crookston et al., 2011).

A similar dynamic occurs with breastfeeding. The production of breast milk requires an average of 550 extra calories per day (Sellen, 2006). This is easily managed when food is readily available, but when food shortages lead to maternal undernourishment less breast milk is produced, whereupon infants become malnourished and risk ill health and poor development. During a famine, a mother's milk may dry up altogether, condemning the infant to death.

The relationships between maternal nutritional stress, pregnancy and breastfeeding are considerably more nuanced and complex than the previous paragraphs suggest (Abu-Saad and Fraser, 2010); however, they illustrate two principles. First, negotiating trade-offs is intrinsic to mothering and starts in the womb. Second, decisions that fit the WHO's definition of maltreatment do not need to be made consciously and can be mediated entirely through physiology.

16.2.1.2 Sibling Trade-Offs

The fact that human children depend on parental provisioning long after the end of breastfeeding means that mothers must provide for several dependent siblings simultaneously. This is not true of other primates, where weaned youngsters secure the food they need through their own efforts. The unusual situation in humans can require mothers to choose between children when allocating food.

A consideration of women who live in small-scale subsistence societies helps to illustrate this. Frequent breastfeeding inhibits ovulation, and most women in such societies conceive their 'next child' only when their currently nursing child approaches weaning. Sometimes, however, the contraceptive effects of breastfeeding fail and a mother finds herself with two children who require nursing simultaneously. Any woman in this situation faces a tough decision. Should she try to breastfeed both children and take the risk that neither receives enough milk to survive or should she abandon one of her nursing children to save the life of the other? Examples of mothers who face these kinds of decisions come from across the world.

The !Kung are a modern southern African people who, until recently, secured much of their food by hunting and gathering. Data collected in the 1960s recorded that around 1 in 100 !Kung babies had been abandoned at birth and left to die (Howell, 1979). Often this was because an infant was born before the existing toddler was ready to be weaned. Among the Ache hunter-gatherers of Paraguay, newborns were also left to die if caring for them risked the life of a still-nursing child. This is poignantly described by an Ache man:

> The one who followed me [in birth order] was killed. It was a short birth spacing. My mother killed him because I was [still] small. 'You won't have enough milk for the older one,' she was told. 'You must feed the older one!' (Hill and Hurtado, 1996: 375)

Over a century earlier, an anthropologist working with a group of indigenous Australian hunter-gatherers wrote, 'Every child which was born before the one which preceded it could walk was destroyed because the mother was incapable of carrying two' (Taplin, 1874, cited in Yengoyan, 1981: 13–14).

In nineteenth-century Belgium, infants who were less than one month old and had two or more siblings under the age of five were significantly more likely to die than infants with no siblings in this age group (Helfrecht and Meehan, 2016). The cause of death was not recorded; all the same, this illustrates the reduced survival of children when birth spacing is close.

The challenge of caring for two nursing children simultaneously contributes to the fact that in some subsistence societies twins are seen as a bad omen. Typically, either one or both infants are abandoned (Barrett et al., 2002; Gabler and Voland, 1994).

In pre-modern Europe, it was not just the challenge of breastfeeding that prompted infanticide but the challenge of feeding children more generally. Kilday (2013: 163) writes that in England poverty was rife during the seventeenth to nineteenth centuries, and killing a baby (or allowing it to die of neglect) was a way to protect older children from the likelihood of starvation and death 'when the burden of an extra mouth to feed would stretch the family purse too far'. Infanticide was also common in eastern Japan during the eighteenth and nineteenth centuries, where it was popularly referred to as *mabiki* – an agricultural term that means to thin out densely planted seedlings so that remaining plants have enough light and space to thrive (Drixler, 2013).

16.2.1.3 Weaned Children

It is not only infants who are at risk from being abandoned; older children can also be vulnerable. Imagine a woman in a non-WEIRD society who has four children and is trying to navigate a severe food shortage. Does she divide her limited food equally between all of her children or does she favour a couple of them? If she allocates food fairly between all of her children none are likely to survive. But if she favours a couple of children she increases the odds that at least some of her children remain well-enough nourished to endure this difficult time. In this instance, the mother has no intention to kill any of her children, but nevertheless the children to whom she gives less food have an increased risk of death.

A different manifestation of this dynamic is abandoning daughters to an early marriage. In several sub-Saharan African countries, food shortages have resulted in young girls being taken out of school to marry: 'For the good of the rest of the family, a daughter had to be sacrificed . . . one less mouth to feed' (Chamberlain, 2017).

A mother's decisions are rarely the products of rational calculations, nor are they necessarily conscious. More often than not they are influenced by stress-related hormonal changes (Reijman et al., 2016) and cultural beliefs. For example, in many cultures infants are not seen as being fully human at the time of their birth; rather, they are believed to grow into their status as a human being. Depending on the culture, becoming fully human may take days, weeks, months or even years (Denham, 2017; Hrdy, 1999; Lancy, 2015). In such cultures, abandoning an infant to die is not considered to be murder.

Regardless of the mechanisms that mediate these harrowing maternal decisions, the fact remains that we are the descendants of mothers who did whatever was necessary to keep at least some children alive. Mothers who shunned favouritism and lost all of their children as a consequence did not leave descendants.

16.2.1.4 How Do These Evolutionary Trade-Offs Relate to Life in Industrialised, Wealthy Nation States?

Most middle-class Westerners have access to plentiful calories and struggle to envision how food shortages might hold sway in the psyche. However, food shortages have been a constant challenge in human evolution, and many families still struggle with insufficient food today (Pereira et al., 2017). Some of these families live in low- and middle-income countries, while others live in wealthier nations.

US figures from 2016 showed around 13 million children living in households suffering from food insecurity (Coleman-Jensen et al., 2018). Although there is no single measure of child malnourishment in the UK (House of Commons, 2019), UNICEF reported that around 19% of British children live with an adult who is moderately or severely food insecure (Pereira et al., 2017). Being a less-favoured child in these food-impoverished households is unlikely to result in death; however, it will compromise long-term growth and health, school performance and well-being.

Even in households where food is not scarce children are likely to be sensitive to how their parents think about them. This is because throughout humanity's existence, being a disfavoured child has been life-threatening during tough times. Perhaps this helps to explain why sibling rivalry is so common: some researchers state that violence between siblings occurs more frequently than any other form of child abuse, and also that it is the most common type of intra-familial violence (Tucker and Finkelhor, 2017).

Viewing economic resources as analogous to food offers another way to show how evolutionary dynamics might influence maternal behaviour in wealthy, industrialised societies. A meta-analysis of child maltreatment concluded that in WEIRD nations, low socioeconomic status is correlated with a significant increase in the risk of maltreatment (van IJzendoorn et al., 2020). More subtly, American mothers who live in poverty are less sensitive to their infants' needs than those who are better off (Bakermans-Kranenburg et al., 2004). The authors of the meta-analysis write, 'The burden of stresses accompanying poverty may increase the risk for child abuse and neglect' (van IJzendoorn et al., 2020: 275). This observation aligns with evolutionary predictions.

A study in South Korea reported that although the overall infant death rate declined between 2003 and 2017, the infanticide rate did not follow suit (Baek et al., 2019). Instead, it tracked the economic situation, rising when both unemployment and inequality rose. The total number of recorded infanticides were small and more research is needed; all the same, this longitudinal study also aligns with evolutionary predictions.

16.2.2 Social Resources

Humans are a profoundly social species. For most of our species' existence, isolated individuals have not been able to survive. This means that our social network and social status can be seen as valuable resources.

16.2.2.1 Social Network

The long period of dependence of human children and the fact that mothers must provide for several children simultaneously mean that human mothers have needed help raising their children. Sarah Hrdy (2009) sees this need for help as so important that she calls us 'communal breeders'. Assistance has typically come from a shifting combination of the child's father, older siblings, grandparents, cousins and aunts (Sear and Mace, 2008). Hrdy argues that because help has been vital, a woman with meagre social support is evolutionarily inclined to be reticent about committing to her child because throughout most of humanity's existence such a child would have been unlikely to survive.

A great deal of evidence supports Hrdy's hypothesis that mothering has evolved to be sensitive to the richness or paucity of a woman's support network. In some of today's small-scale subsistence societies, if a woman loses her husband whilst pregnant or shortly after giving birth the infant has a greatly increased risk of being abandoned to die (Hill and Hurtado, 1996; Schiefenhövel, 1989). A similar dynamic operated in Britain during the seventeenth to nineteenth centuries, where it was impoverished single women without family support who were most likely to commit infanticide (Kilday, 2013). In today's WEIRD societies, on the rare occasions when mothers kill their babies, the women are typically young, unemployed, lacking support and no longer involved with the father of the child (Porter and Gavin, 2010).

Other studies show that enjoying a strong support network makes a positive difference to both mothers and their children. In many of today's subsistence societies, a child whose maternal grandmother is alive is significantly more likely to survive than a child who does not have a living grandmother (Hawkes et al., 1989; Sear and Mace, 2008). In WEIRD societies, mothers who have emotional support (either from their own mothers and family or from social workers and nurses) are more nurturing and attentive to their children than mothers lacking such help (Olds et al., 2007; Spieker and Bensley, 1994; Tracy et al., 2018). Similarly, women with emotional support develop significantly stronger bonds with their infants than women without such support (Myers and Johns, 2017).

That said, one potential hurdle for programmes aiming to support struggling mothers is that if a woman grows up unable to trust her family, then her internal models and unconscious fears may prevent her from trusting the support on offer. Thus, to ensure success, a programme may need to address that lack of trust.

16.2.2.2 Social Status

In evolutionary circles, it has long been recognised that a man's status can affect the number of children he may father, but only recently have researchers begun to look at how a woman's social status affects her children. Initial research in a small-scale subsistence society found that women with greater political influence have better-nourished and healthier children than mothers with less influence (Alami et al., 2020). If this observation is replicated in other societies, then one might predict that women with political status will be less prone to maternal negativity and maltreatment than women who are less respected.

16.3 Children's Characteristics

Having explored maternal resources, this section considers how a child's characteristics can influence maternal feelings and behaviour. Three particularly influential characteristics are health and robustness, disposition and sex.

16.3.1 Health and Robustness

In non-WEIRD societies, where child mortality is typically between 30% and 60%, it is hard for even a relatively well-resourced mother to keep her children alive. It is particularly difficult when a child is small, premature or sickly. A mother of such a vulnerable child might be more evolutionarily successful – that is, leave more descendants – if she allows the child to die and directs her emotional, nutritional and economic resources towards healthier and more robust offspring (Hrdy, 1999, 2009). Disturbing though this is, examples of mothers biasing their care in this way come from diverse sources.

The social anthropologist Nancy Scheper-Hughes worked in a Brazilian shanty town with people who suffered from high levels of malnutrition, illness and death as a result of historically entrenched racism, trauma, inequality and poverty. In her classic ethnography *Death without Weeping*, Scheper-Hughes (1992) describes how mothers in this community nurtured active babies who were thought to be fighters and survivors while detaching from quiet babies who were passive, sickly, disabled or developmentally delayed. Whilst outright infanticide was met with horror, women believed it was best if quiet and poorly infants died quickly. To facilitate this process, mothers engaged in what researchers call 'delayed' or 'passive infanticide'; that is, denying an infant sufficient food, water and care. These mothers were not conscious of their actions but viewed their underweight and ailing infants as wanting to die. As one mother explained,

> Julieta ... *herself* never took hold [of life]. If she died it was because she herself, on seeing what was ahead, what was in store for her, *she* decided to die. (Scheper-Hughes, 1992: 369, original emphasis)

Scheper-Hughes' research led her to conclude that emotional scarcity can follow from material scarcity, and she warns against sentimentalising 'Mother'. She writes that the image of an all-nurturing, selfless mother is a modern artefact that has emerged only because we live in a sufficiently benevolent environment for a mother to trust that every child will probably survive. Women living in environments where mortality is high cannot afford this emotional luxury.

Aaron Denham, a medical anthropologist, worked with the Nankani subsistence farmers of northern Ghana. In this community, diseases and poverty are responsible for the majority of child deaths. However, some disabled or ailing infants and children are deemed to be 'spirit children', and some of these are given fatal poison. Spirit children are seen not as human children who have been possessed by spirits but as malevolent spirits who masquerade as humans in order to infiltrate a family and cause harm, disease and death (Denham, 2017). Although parents express pain when their child turns out to be a spirit child, in most cases the child's death is not grieved; rather, there is relief that a source of misfortune has been removed. Denham argues that one way to understand this cultural system is to realise that a child with chronic illness or special needs will place terrible pressure on a struggling family:

> When families say that a spirit child is destined to kill family members or destroy the house, this reality is not so farfetched. For a vulnerable family, a child with excessive needs can deplete limited resources, prevent the mother from working, [and] render the family more vulnerable to collapse ... (Denham, 2017: 184)

Nutritional anthropologist Katherine Dettwyler recorded a similar practice in Mali. Talking about developmentally delayed children, a village chief explained to Dettwyler:

> Well, if they don't get better after a couple of years, then you know that they are evil spirits, and you give up ... you take them out into the bush and you just leave them ... they turn into snakes and slither away ... You go back the next day and they aren't there. Then you know for sure that they weren't really children at all, but evil spirits. When you see a snake, you wonder if this used to be your child. (Dettwyler, 1994: 85–86)

European beliefs and practices concerning changelings bear a strikingly similarity to those described by Dettwyler (Hrdy, 1999; Lancy, 2015). Beginning in the Middle Ages and continuing for several centuries, sickly, disabled or otherwise challenging children risked being seen as the offspring of fairies, elves or goblins who had infiltrated human families to steal resources from human children. Infants deemed to be changelings were left in a forest so that they could return to their magical realm. The reality was that the abandoned child was likely to succumb to hypothermia or to be eaten by a wild animal.

It was not only visibly disabled or sick children who were at risk in Europe and other parts of the world; rather, several cultures developed viability tests to determine whether a newborn infant was worth nurturing. Hrdy (1999: 464) quotes Soranus (second century CE), who describes how infants in ancient Europe were subjected to ice-cold baths 'in order to let die, as not worth rearing, one that cannot bear the chilling'. Some believe that this practice was the source for the ritual of baptism. Similar practices of exposing infants to the elements arose in many other parts of the world (Hrdy, 1999).

A study by psychologist Janet Mann suggests that a mother's preference for strong children remains subtly present in contemporary Western society. Mann (1992) observed mothers of preterm twins to determine whether they treated their fragile babies equally. Her sample was small but her findings were telling: every mother gave more attention to the healthier twin but was unaware of doing so. In tougher times, the less healthy twin would likely have died from neglect.

There is evidence that in WEIRD nations children with congenital challenges, autism spectrum disorders and learning difficulties are at an increased risk of being maltreated (Dion et al., 2018; McDonnell et al., 2019; Murphy, 2011)

It is difficult for many of us to take these insights on board, in part because it is frightening to do so and in part because many of us live in WEIRD nations during unprecedented times. We have access to plentiful food and clean water, vaccinations and antibiotics, as well as birth control and safe abortions. Mercifully few of us have experienced the death of a child. Historically, this was not the case, and it is still not the case for many women living in non-WEIRD communities today; nearly every parent will have lost children, and practically every child will have experienced the deaths of siblings, cousins and friends while growing up. For most of humanity's existence, the death of children (due to one cause or another) has been part of life.

16.3.2 Disposition

Children are not the passive recipients of maternal care; rather, a child's disposition plays a significant role in determining a mother's attitudes and behaviour. A child's disposition emerges from the interweaving of genetic influence, *in utero* conditions, early experiences and cultural norms (Stevenson-Hinde, 2011).

Bowlby (1969/1997) was one of the first to highlight this. He observed that when infants of the same age and sex were placed in the same foster home together an active infant typically received more attention than a passive one. He suggested that the more active infant demanded more from the adults and in turn offered the adults more rewards when those demands were met.

A study of Kenyan Maasai by medic and anthropologist Marten De Vries (1987) showed that an infant's disposition can sometimes make the difference between life and death. During the 1973–1974 drought, Maasai infants who were classified as having a difficult temperament were more likely to survive than those with an easy temperament. De Vries suggests several reasons for this, and the one of particular interest here is that almost all crying and fussing were met with an offer of the breast. Thus, 'difficult infants' were fed more often and were better nourished. Nutritional status has a significant impact on child survival in subsistence societies at the best of times, and this is intensified in times of famine.

In contrast, in WEIRD societies today, where mothers typically have little support and help with childcare, children with 'difficult' temperaments may be more at risk of maltreatment.

16.3.3 Sex

There is much evolutionary theory about when it is adaptive for parents to favour children of one sex and disfavour children of the other (Sieff, 1990). In this chapter there is space to mention only some of the pertinent questions that evolutionary thinking brings to our attention: do daughters or sons have a greater chance of having children of their own? Do children of daughters or sons provide mothers with greater help and so result in the mother having more surviving children? Do the benefits of a daughter or son differ depending on birth order? Might a mother favour a first-born daughter because she would help with rearing other children but not a later-born daughter? Do children of the same sex compete with one another in ways that are harmful to their long-term chances of having children? Do children of the same sex support each other and increase the chances of the siblings having children?

In addition to evolutionary considerations, maternal negativity arising from a child's sex can be due to personal preference, psychodynamic influences, societal organisation, cultural values and government policies.

16.4 Child Socialisation

Having looked at how maternal resources and children's characteristics influence maltreatment, I now explore how the need to socialise a child into cultural norms and values can sometimes lead to mothers (inadvertently) maltreating children who they cherish and love.

Humans are a profoundly social species. Throughout our evolutionary history we have depended on being a member of a mutually supportive community to survive and raise children. However, there is always a risk that an individual will try to exploit their community, and to prevent this from occurring group members need to be bound together for the common good. This binding is achieved partly through collective norms and shared moral values and partly by punishing individuals who flout the norms and values (Apicella and Silk, 2019; Boyd and Richerson, 2009). Those who repeatedly flout group standards risk being thrown out of their community (Boehm, 2012). In WEIRD societies

being expelled from your community is not life-threatening, but it has been life-threatening for much of humanity's existence. Thus, a child's survival has depended on being socialised into community norms and values.

Often the socialisation of children occurs without any maltreatment, but from time to time parents turn to forms of emotional or physical punishment that constitute maltreatment (Lancy, 2015). Maltreatment may be especially likely if the child actively rebels. In some communities, when a child refuses to conform to group norms the entire family is expelled, risking the well-being not only of the dissenting child, but also of their siblings and parents (Atari, 2020). In this situation, the incentive for parents to force a child to conform is even stronger.

Additional challenges emerge when parents need to prepare a child for life in a violent or dangerous environment, and under these circumstances child socialisation can routinely include verbal or physical abuse (Lancy, 2015). One such example occurs in some 'honour cultures'. These cultures take different forms, but in many of them men respond to insults with violent aggression (Atari, 2020). This is potentially costly, because aggression can escalate; however, in certain environments, it is protective to have a reputation for being easily offended and violent. For instance, when wealth is held in livestock or some other easily stolen commodity and law enforcement has little power, a reputation for being irascible and violent can deter thieves (Nisbett and Cohen, 1996; Nowak et al., 2016). Boys are not born with an 'honour' instinct; rather, they are socialised into this ethos. Typically, both mothers and fathers play an important role in the socialisation process. For example, in the American South during the nineteenth century, parents shamed and beat their sons if they shrunk from fights. They also encouraged them to play violent physical games (Nisbett and Cohen, 1996). Given that spanking has the same impact as severe abuse (Cuartas et al., 2021) and being shamed is traumatising (Sieff, 2015), such parental behaviour fits the WHO definition of 'maltreatment'.

Alternative instances of child maltreatment can occur when parents have been impacted by personal or historic trauma. These parents often have an (unconscious) sense of what their child needs to become if they are going to be protected from suffering the same trauma. To ensure their much-loved child gains this supposed protection, a parent may cajole, shame and punish the child in a misguided expression of love.

16.5 Social Learning of Mothering

The fourth and final factor to be explored is 'social learning', which biologists formally define as any learning that is facilitated by observing or interacting with another individual (Hoppitt and Laland, 2013). In humans, social learning includes acquiring skills, behaviour, knowledge, attitudes or beliefs from others. Social learning can happen both through conscious and explicit attempts to become proficient in some area of life and through unconscious and implicit mechanisms. Either way, social learning has been crucial to human evolution: it enabled our ancestors to inhabit an extraordinarily wide range of physical, social and cultural environments and provided the building blocks for complex culture (Henrich, 2015; Laland, 2017; Terahima and Hewlett, 2016; also see Chapter 1 of this volume).

So important is social learning to our species that most aspects of human life depend on some degree of social learning, and motherhood is no exception. Women learn about mothering from what they experience and observe during their own childhoods (Lancy, 2015; LeVine et al., 1996; McKerracher et al., 2020). An advantage of this is that girls acquire the forms of maternal behaviour which fit their environments; a disadvantage is that girls who experience or observe maltreatment when growing up are at risk of maltreating their own children once they become mothers.

A considerable amount of research supports the idea that social learning contributes to the maltreatment of children by their mothers. In WEIRD societies, although the recurrence of maltreatment across generations is not inevitable, parents are significantly more likely to maltreat their children if they themselves were severely maltreated as children (Assink et al., 2018; Madigan et al., 2019; van IJzendoorn et al., 2020). Multiple factors will be contributing to the repetition of maltreatment across generations, but it is safe to assume that social learning plays an important role.

That said, it may be that the transgenerational recurrence of child maltreatment is more common in WEIRD societies than in non-WEIRD societies. There are two reasons for my speculative suggestion.

First, the high rates of child mortality that are typical of non-WEIRD societies mean that severely maltreated girls are unlikely to survive to become mothers themselves. The girls who live to become the next generation of mothers will generally be those who have been mothered with care and commitment (Hrdy, 1999).

Second, in most non-WEIRD societies, children's experiences of mothering are broad. Not only are children typically looked after by multiple carers, but because much of daily life is lived in the community, children observe a multiplicity of mothers and others caring (or not) for a variety of different children (Lancy, 1996). This diversity of caregiving will be internalised, and by the time girls become mothers they will have a range of options available to them.

In short, it is possible that the continuity of child maltreatment across generations is primarily a WEIRD phenomenon that has emerged because (1) child death rates are low and (2) children neither experience being cared for by a wide variety of people nor do they observe much maternal behaviour outside of their own homes. Research from both Western and small-scale subsistence societies would be required to assess the merit of this hypothesis.

16.6 Summary and Application of Evolutionary Insights

This chapter has explored four different factors that contribute to the maltreatment of children by their mothers: maternal resources, children's characteristics, child socialisation and social learning. The focus has been on how evolutionary perspectives can contribute new layers of understanding. The insights that have emerged will now be summarised alongside brief thoughts about how these insights might contribute to addressing the maternal maltreatment of children at both individual and societal levels.

16.6.1 Maternal Feelings and Behaviours Have Evolved to Be Sensitive to Circumstances

Western culture imagines that women have evolved to love all of their children unconditionally and to treat them accordingly. Such love is believed to arise instinctually. A woman's hormonal profile changes during pregnancy, and these changes do predispose her to bond with her infant (Bridges, 2008; Numan and Insel, 2006). However, this is not the whole story. Human mothers raise children across a range of circumstances, and as a result, a range of feelings and behaviours evolved to be part of the maternal repertoire. At one end of this range is full commitment, in the middle is ambivalence and at the other end is negativity.

Maternal negativity is best thought of as a medley of conscious and unconscious feelings and behaviours that wax and wane depending on both the resources available to a mother and the characteristics of a child.

A mother can lovingly nurture a child who appears strong and healthy but fatally neglect one who is weak and ill. She can be fiercely committed to an infant born after an older sibling is weaned but kill one whose birth would risk the life of a still-nursing toddler. In good times, when material resources are abundant and women have plentiful social support, maternal negativity has little place in the lives of women. However, in times of scarcity and/or when women are unsupported, negative feelings can emerge to colour the emotional palette and behaviour of mothers.

Another way in which circumstances can affect mothering is though the demands of socialisation. A mother may maltreat a much-loved child to prepare that child for adulthood in a particular physical and/or cultural environment. The fact that this form of maltreatment is rooted in love rather than negativity does not prevent it from causing significant harm.

Although the above insights will not, by themselves, prevent maltreatment, they can inform both clinical work with faltering mothers and preventative programmes.

Beginning with clinical work, the belief that normal mothers are naturally loving means that women who experience negativity or who harm their children typically feel that they are defective and not quite human (Parker, 2012). Such a feeling constitutes 'toxic shame': a deep, visceral and insidious conviction in being fundamentally inadequate as a human being (Kaufman, 1992).

Living with toxic shame is intolerable and, in an attempt to escape from these feelings, people risk being drawn into harmful behaviour such as addictions, grandiosity or rage (Bradshaw, 1988; Lloyd and Sieff, 2015). Shame-laden people also feel compelled to try to rid themselves of whatever

is activating their shame; in the case of mothering, this can mean wanting to rid themselves of the child. In the following account, an American woman describes how her need to escape shame led her to act out infanticidal impulses:

> I can remember hurling the baby down on the pillows once, and just screaming and not caring. I wanted to kill him really. I think it was to do with being so tormented, worried and guilty. You know, the anxiety and guilt at feeling I was getting it all wrong, and that *I was bad and useless*. I just wanted to get away from the situation. I felt unable to tolerate it. (Parker, 1995: 19, emphasis added)

An evolutionary understanding, as part of a psychoeducation process, can help to combat toxic shame, enabling a faltering mother to see herself in a larger and more self-compassionate context. Maybe she is struggling with closely spaced children; maybe her child is weak or disabled; maybe an economic downturn means that resources are scarce; maybe she is without support. Whatever the issue, although in today's WEIRD culture her child will probably survive, the child would not have done so for much of humanity's existence, and her feelings may be reflecting this. Once a woman starts to view her predicament in this evolutionary context she can begin to build the self-compassion that will allow her to face her feelings about herself and her child. This sets the stage for genuine change (Sieff, 2020).

Moving on to prevention, an evolutionary understanding of mothering highlights the role of poverty and a lack of support in predisposing mothers to maltreat their children. Although these environmental factors are well recognised in some circles, in others it remains common to view maltreating mothers through the lens of individual 'psychopathology'. This focus on mental ill health diverts attention away from societal failings, and an evolutionary perspective can redress the imbalance. Indeed, an evolutionary perspective proposes that it will be very hard to prevent maternal negativity and the maltreatment of children unless social and environmental factors are addressed.

16.6.2 Maternal Feelings and Behaviours Have Evolved to Be Sensitive to Social Learning

Human mothering has evolved to be shaped by social learning. Without conscious effort or intent, girls learn about mothering through what they experience and observe during their own childhood. Understanding this can help both individual women who are maltreating their children and programmes aimed at preventing the maltreatment of children.

Many women who were maltreated as children have no wish for their own children to suffer what they endured, and they feel particularly shameful when they find themselves behaving as their mothers did. An awareness of social learning offers such women a larger and more self-compassionate context in which to understand their own behaviour and so creates the conditions in which it can be addressed.

An awareness of our species' reliance on social learning might also contribute to the design of programmes aimed at preventing or stopping maternal maltreatment of children. A recent meta-analysis of child maltreatment concluded that when maltreatment is occurring the only programmes that reliably prevented it from continuing are those that involve parental education and training (van IJzendoorn et al., 2020). Parental education and training can be seen as compensatory social learning that redresses the learning that was not available during childhood.

16.6.3 Maternal Feelings and Behaviours Arise As a Result of Many Intersecting Factors

The four factors discussed in this chapter all contribute to the maltreatment of children by their mothers, but they do so in very different ways. The first two – maternal resources and children's characteristics – describe circumstances in which a mother's maltreatment of an unfavoured child is likely to be evolutionarily adaptive (that is, it results in a woman leaving more descendants). The third – child socialisation – is different in that maltreatment arises as a response to our evolved need to belong to a group. The fourth is different again in that child maltreatment occurs as an unintended consequence of our species' evolved dependence on social learning coupled with the limited experience of mothering that girls have in WEIRD societies.

Bringing together different evolved dynamics helps us to understand that there is no single or neat story to explain maternal maltreatment of

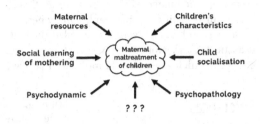

Maternal maltreatment of children: Possible contributing factors

© Daniela F. Sieff, 2021   www.danielasieff.com

Figure 16.1 Maternal maltreatment of children: possible contributing factors

children. Rather, multiple factors intersect in complicated and layered ways to either increase or decrease the risk.

In truth, the picture is even more complex than that presented in this chapter. Some factors that contribute to child maltreatment are better viewed though a psychodynamic lens than through an evolutionary one (Woodman and Sieff, 2009), whereas others are best viewed through the lens of psychopathology. This chapter has restricted itself to those factors that are amenable to evolutionary perspectives because of the nature of this edited volume. However, when working with real people, all potential contributing factors must be explored. We humans are complex creatures and we live multifaceted lives; there is rarely a single reason for any aspect of what we feel or for how we behave (Figure 16.1).

16.7 Conclusion

Viewing human mothering through an evolutionary lens highlights the fallacy of believing that biology has programmed mothers to unconditionally love each and every child to whom they give birth. It reveals the problem of seeing committed and self-sacrificing mothering as natural and ambivalent and hostile mothering as unnatural. It illuminates how raising children requires mothers to negotiate a series of complex, precarious and layered trade-offs, and it shows how maternal negativity and child maltreatment can arise from this.

The fact that evolved dynamics contribute to some instances of harmful maternal behaviour does not mean that such behaviour is either acceptable or unavoidable. To assume that a behaviour is justified or inevitable simply because it has been subject to evolution is called the 'naturalistic fallacy'. Nobody argues that we should endure the high rates of child mortality that have characterised most of humanity's existence, nor that we are destined to do so. However, just as we needed to understand disease vectors, nutrition and sanitation to reduce child mortality, we need also to understand the factors that arouse maternal negativity and child maltreatment to better address it. Evolutionary perspectives can offer an important contribution to this understanding.

References

Abu-Saad, K. and Fraser, D. 2010. Maternal nutrition and birth outcomes. *Epidemiologic Reviews*, 32, 5–25.

Alami, S., Von Rueden, C., Seabright, E., Kraft, T. S., Blackwell, A. D., Stieglitz, J., Kaplan, H. and Gurven, M. 2020. Mother's social status is associated with child health in a horticulturalist population. *Proceedings of the Royal Society B: Biological Sciences*, 287, 20192783.

Apicella, C. L. and Silk, J. B. 2019. The evolution of human cooperation. *Current Biology*, 29, R447–R450.

Assink, M., Spruit, A., Schuts, M., Lindauer, R., Van Der Put, C. E. and Stams, G. J. M. 2018. The intergenerational transmission of child maltreatment: a three-level meta-analysis. *Child Abuse and Neglect*, 84, 131–145.

Atari, M. 2020. Culture of honor. In: V. Zeigler-Hill and T. K. Shackelford, (eds.), *Encyclopedia of Personality and Individual Differences*. Cham: Springer International Publishing, pp. 977–981.

Baek, S. U., Lim, S. S., Kim, J. and Yoon, J. H. 2019. How does economic inequality affect infanticide rates? An analysis of 15 years of death records and representative economic data. *International Journal of Environmental Research and Public Health*, 16, 3679.

Bakermans-Kranenburg, M. J., Van Ijzendoorn, M. H. and Kroonenberg, P. M. 2004. Differences in attachment security between African-American and white children: ethnicity or socio-economic status? *Infant Behavior and Development*, 27, 417–433.

Barrett, L., Dunbar, R. and Lycett, J. 2002. *Human Evolutionary Psychology*. Basingstoke and New York: Palgrave Macmillan.

Black, R. E., Allen, L. H., Bhutta, Z. A., Caulfield, L. E., De Onis, M., Ezzati, M., Mathers, C. and Rivera, J. 2008. Maternal and child undernutrition: global and regional exposures and health consequences. *Lancet*, 371, 243–260.

Boehm, C. 2012. *Moral Origins: The Evolution of Virtue, Altruism and Shame*. New York: Basic Books.

Bowlby, E. J. M. 1969/1997. *Attachment and Loss: Attachment*. London: Pimlico.

Boyd, R. and Richerson, P. J. 2009. Culture and the evolution of human cooperation. *Philosophical Transactions of the Royal Society B: Biological Sciences*, 364, 3281–3288.

Bradshaw, J. 1988. *Healing the Shame That Binds You*. Deerfield Beach, FL: Health Communications, Inc.

Bridges, R. S. (ed.) 2008. *Neurobiology of the Parental Brain*. Amsterdam: Elsevier.

Brown, L. S. 2011. Nutritional requirements during pregnancy. In: J. Sharlin, and S. Edelstein (eds.), *Essentials of Life Cycle Nutrition*. Ontario: Jones and Bartlett Publishers, pp. 1–24.

Chamberlain, G. 2017. Why climate change is creating a new generation of child brides. *The Observer*, 26 November.

Coleman-Jensen, A., Rabbitt, M. P., Gregory, C. A. and Anita Singh, A. 2018. *Household Food Security in the United States in 2017*. Washington, DC: United States Department of Agriculture, Economic Research Service.

Crookston, B. T., Dearden, K. A., Alder, S. C., Porucznik, C. A., Stanford, J. B., Merrill, R. M., Dickerson, T. T. and Penny, M. E. 2011. Impact of early and concurrent stunting on cognition. *Maternal & Child Nutrition*, 7, 397–409.

Cuartas, J., Weissman, D. G., Sheridan, M. A., Lengua, L. and Mclaughlin, K. A. 2021. Corporal punishment and elevated neural response to threat in children. *Child Development*, 92, 821–832.

De Vries, M. W. 1987. Cry babies, culture and catastrophe: infant temperament among the Masai. In: N. Scheper-Hughes (ed.), *Child Survival: Anthropological Perspectives on the Treatment and Maltreatment of Children*. Dordrecht: D. Reidel Publishing Company, pp. 165–185.

Denham, A. R. 2017. *Spirit Children: Illness, Poverty, and Infanticide in Northern Ghana*. Madison: University of Wisconsin Press.

Dettwyler, K. A. 1994. *Dancing Skeletons: Life and Death in West Africa*. Long Grove, IL: Waveland Press.

Dion, J., Paquette, G., Tremblay, K.-N., Collin-VÉZina, D. and Chabot, M. 2018. Child maltreatment among children with intellectual disability in the Canadian Incidence Study. *American Journal on Intellectual and Developmental Disabilities*, 123, 176–188.

Drixler, F. 2013. *Mabiki: Infanticide and Population Growth in Eastern Japan, 1660–1950*. Berkley: University of California Press.

Gabler, S. and Voland, E. 1994. Fitness of twinning. *Human Biology*, 66, 699–713.

Gurven, M. and Kaplan, H. 2007. Longevity among hunter-gatherers: a cross-cultural examination. *Population and Development Review*, 33, 321–365.

Hawkes, K., O'Connell, J. F. and Blurton Jones, N. 1989. Hardworking Hadza grandmothers. In: V. Standen and R. A. Foley (eds.), *Comparative Socioecology: The Behavioural Ecology of Humans and Other Mammals*. London: Blackwell Scientific Publications, pp. 361–366.

Helfrecht, C. and Meehan, C. L. 2016. Sibling effects on nutritional status: Intersections of cooperation and competition across development. *American Journal of Human Biology*, 28, 159–170.

Henrich, J. 2015. *The Secret of Our Success: How Culture Is Driving Human Evolution, Domesticating Our Species, and Making Us Smarter*. Princeton, NJ: Princeton University Press.

Henrich, J., Heine, S. J. and Norenzayan, A. 2010. The weirdest people in the world? *Behavioral and Brain Sciences*, 33, 61–83.

Hill, K. and Hurtado, A. M. 1996. *Ache Life History: The Ecology and Demography of a Foraging People*. New York: Aldine de Gruyter.

Hoppitt, W. and Laland, K. N. 2013. *Social Learning: An Introduction to Mechanisms, Methods, and Models*. Princeton, NJ: Princeton University Press.

House of Commons 2019. *Hunger, Food Insecurity and Malnutrition in the UK*. Florence: UNICEF Office of Research.

Howell, N. 1979. *Demography of the Dobe !Kung*. New York: Academic Press.

Hrdy, S. B. 1999. *Mother Nature: Natural Selection and the Female of the Species*. London: Chatto & Windus.

Hrdy, S. B. 2009. *Mothers and Others: The Evolutionary Origins of Mutual Understanding*. Cambridge, MA: Belknap Press of Harvard University Press.

Kaufman, G. 1992. *Shame: The Power of Caring*. Rochester, VA: Schenkman Books, Inc.

Kilday, A.-M. 2013. *A History of Infanticide in Britain c 1600 to the Present*. Basingstoke and New York: Palgrave Macmillan.

Laland, K. N. 2017. *Darwin's Unfinished Symphony: How Culture Made the Human Mind*. Princeton, NJ: Princeton University Press.

Lancy, D. F. 1996. *Playing on Mother-Ground: Cultural Routines for Children's Development*. New York: Guilford Press.

Lancy, D. F. 2015. *The Anthropology of Childhood: Cherubs, Chattel, Changelings*. Cambridge: Cambridge University Press.

Lanius, R. A., Vermetten, E. and Pain, C. 2010. *The Impact of Early Life Trauma on Health and Disease: The Hidden Epidemic*. Cambridge: Cambridge University Press.

Levine, R., Dixon, S., Levine, S., Richman, A., Liederman, P. H., Keefer, C. H. and Brazelton, T. B. 1996. *Child Care and Culture: Lessons from Africa*. Cambridge: Cambridge University Press.

Lloyd, J. B. and Sieff, D. F. 2015. Return from exile: beyond self-alienation, shame and addiction to reconnect with ourselves. In: D. F. Sieff (ed.), *Understanding and Healing Emotional Trauma: Conversations with Pioneering Clinicians and Researchers*. London: Routledge, pp. 25–45.

Madigan, S., Cyr, C., Eirich, R., Fearon, R. M. P., Ly, A., Rash, C., Poole, J. C. and Alink, L. R. A. 2019. Testing the cycle of maltreatment hypothesis: meta-analytic evidence of the intergenerational transmission of child maltreatment. *Developmental Psychopathology*, 31, 23–51.

Mann, J. 1992. Nurturance or negligence: maternal psychology and behavioral preference among preterm twins In: J. H. Barkow, L. Cosmides and J. Tooby (eds.), *The Adapted Mind: Evolutionary Psychology and the Generation of Culture*. Oxford: Oxford University Press, pp. 367–390.

Mcdonnell, C. G., Boan, A. D., Bradley, C. C., Seay, K. D., Charles, J. M. and Carpenter, L. A. 2019. Child maltreatment in autism spectrum disorder and intellectual disability: results from a population-based sample. *Journal of Child Psychology and Psychiatry*, 60, 576–584.

Mckerracher, L. J., Nepomnaschy, P., Altman, R. M., Sellen, D. and Collard, M. 2020. Breastfeeding duration and the social learning of infant feeding knowledge in two Maya communities. *Human Nature*, 31, 43–67.

Murphy, N. 2011. Maltreatment of children with disabilities: the breaking point. *Journal of Child Neurology*, 26, 1054–1056.

Myers, S. and Johns, S. E. 2017. Trade-offs in mother–infant bonding: a life history perspective on maternal emotional investments during infancy (poster). Presented at: 5th Annual Toulouse Economics and Biology Workshop: The Evolution and Economics of the Family. Toulouse: Institute of Advanced Studies, 1–2 June.

Nesse, R. M. 2019. *Good Reasons for Bad Feelings: Insights from the Frontier of Evolutionary Psychiatry*. London: Penguin.

Nisbett, R. E. and Cohen, D. 1996. *Culture of Honor: The Psychology of Violence in the South*. Boulder, CO: Westview Press.

Nowak, A., Gelfand, M. J., Borkowski, W., Cohen, D. and Hernandez, I. 2016. The evolutionary basis of honor cultures. *Psychological Science*, 27, 12–24.

Numan, M. and Insel, T. R. 2006. *The Neurobiology of Parental Behavior*. Berlin: Springer Science+Business Media.

Olds, D. L., Sadler, L. and Kitzman, H. 2007. Programs for parents of infants and toddlers: recent evidence from randomized trials. *Journal of Child Psychology and Psychiatry*, 48, 355–391.

Parker, R. 1995. *Mother Love/ Mother Hate: The Power of Maternal Ambivalence*. New York: Basic Books.

Parker, R. 2012. Shame and maternal ambivalence. In: P. Mariotti (ed.), *The Maternal Lineage: Identification, Desire and Transgenerational Issues*. London: Routledge, pp. 85–112.

Pereira, A., Handa, S. and Holmqvist, G. 2017. *Prevalence and Correlates of Food Insecurity among Children across the Globe. Innocenti Working Papers*. Florence: UNICEF Office of Research.

Porter, T. and Gavin, H. 2010. Infanticide and neonaticide: a review of 40 years of research literature on incidence and causes. *Trauma, Violence, & Abuse*, 11, 99–112.

Potts, R. 2013. Hominin evolution in settings of strong environmental variability. *Quaternary Science Reviews*, 73, 1–13.

Reijman, S., Bakermans-Kranenburg, M. J., Hiraoka, R., Crouch, J. L., Milner, J. S., Alink,

L. R. A. and Van Ijzendoorn, M. H. 2016. Baseline functioning and stress reactivity in maltreating parents and at-risk adults: review and meta-analyses of autonomic nervous system studies. *Child Maltreatment*, 21, 327–342.

Scheper-Hughes, N. 1992. *Death without Weeping: The Violence of Everyday Life in Brazil*. Berkley: University of California Press.

SchiefenhÖVel, W. 1989. Reproduction and sex-ratio manipulation through preferential female infanticide among the Eipo, in the highlands of west New Guinea. In: A. E. Rasa, C. Vogel and E. Voland (eds.), *Sociobiology of Sexual and Reproductive Strategies*. London: Chapman and Hall, pp. 170–193.

Sear, R. and Mace, R. 2008. Who keeps children alive? A review of the effects of kin on child survival. *Evolution and Human Behavior*, 29, 1–18.

Sellen, D. W. 2006. Lactation, complementary feeding, and human life history. In: K. Hawkes and R. R. Paine (eds.), *The Evolution of Human Life History*. Santa Fe, NM: School of American Research Press, pp. 155–196.

Sieff, D. F. 1990. Explaining biased sex ratios in human populations: a critique of recent studies. *Current Anthropology*, 31, 25–48.

Sieff, D. F. 2015. *Understanding and Healing Emotional Trauma: Conversations with Pioneering Clinicians and Researchers*. London: Routledge.

Sieff, D. F. 2019. The Death Mother as nature's shadow: infanticide, abandonment and the collective unconscious. *Psychological Perspectives*, 62, 15–34.

Sieff, D. F. 2020. Trauma-worlds and their transformation: moving beyond a life built around fear, dissociation and shame [video]. YouTube. Retrieved from www.youtube.com/watch?v=QE48YTU9Ss8

Spieker, S. J. and Bensley, L. 1994. Roles of living arrangements and grandmother social support in adolescent mothering and infant attachment. *Developmental Psychology*, 30, 102–111.

Stevenson-Hinde, J. 2011. Culture and socioemotional development, with a focus on fearfulness and attachment. In: X. Chen and K. H. Rubin (eds.), *Socioemotional Development in Cultural Context*. New York: Guilford Press, pp. 11–28.

Terahima, H. and Hewlett, B. S. (eds.) 2016. *Social Learning and Innovation in Contemporary Hunter-Gatherers: Evolutionary and Ethnographic Perspectives*. Berlin: Springer.

Tracy, M., Salo, M. and Appleton, A. A. 2018. The mitigating effects of maternal social support and paternal involvement on the intergenerational transmission of violence. *Child Abuse and Neglect*, 78, 46–59.

Tucker, C. J. and Finkelhor, D. 2017. The state of interventions for sibling conflict and aggression: a systematic review. *Trauma, Violence, & Abuse*, 18, 396–406.

Van Ijzendoorn, M. H., Bakermans-Kranenburg, M. J., Coughlan, B. and Reijman, S. 2020. Annual research review: umbrella synthesis of meta-analyses on child maltreatment antecedents and interventions: differential susceptibility perspective on risk and resilience. *Journal of Child Psychology and Psychiatry*, 61, 272–290.

Volk, A. A. and Atkinson, J. A. 2013. Infant and child death in the human environment of evolutionary adaptation. *Evolution and Human Behavior*, 34, 182–192.

WHO. 2020. Child maltreatment. World Health Organization. Retrieved from www.who.int/news-room/fact-sheets/detail/child-maltreatment

Willführ, K. P. and Gagnon, A. 2013. Are stepparents always evil? Parental death, remarriage, and child survival in demographically saturated Krummhörn (1720–1859) and expanding Québec (1670–1750). *Biodemography and Social Biology*, 59, 191–211.

Woodman, M. and Sieff, D. F. 2009. Confronting Death Mother – an interview with Marion Woodman. *Spring*, 81, 177–199.

Yengoyan, A. A. 1981. Infanticide and birth order: an empirical analysis of preferential female infanticide among Australian Aboriginal populations. *Anthropology UCLA*, 7, 255–273.

Alzheimer's Disease as a Disease of Evolutionary Mismatch, with a Focus on Reproductive Life History

Molly Fox

Abstract

Risk factors for Alzheimer's disease, such as cardiovascular, metabolic and inflammatory problems, were probably less prevalent throughout much of human history compared to today in post-industrial societies. Therefore, I explore the possibility that individuals today have greater Alzheimer's disease risk compared to our age-matched, pre-modern counterparts. Additionally, a critical way in which human physiology has changed across history relates to dramatic changes in female reproductive life history norms. Reproductive life history may exert cumulative effects across an individual's lifespan, bestowing considerable influence on geriatric disease risk. A growing body of research links women's reproductive life histories with Alzheimer's disease risk. Here, I briefly discuss ways in which aspects of female reproductive life history (e.g. reproductive span, pregnancy and breastfeeding) might alter physiological pathways implicated in Alzheimer's disease aetiology, as well as how each of these aspects of female reproductive life history have shifted across our species' evolutionary past. I also explore the connections between the apolipo-protein E gene, its context-dependent role in Alzheimer's disease risk and its emerging role in women's reproductive function. In summary, some aspects of pre-modern female reproductive life history patterns could indicate lower age-matched risk in the past, but further research is needed to establish the relevant biological pathways and epidemiological patterns.

Keywords

Alzheimer's disease, dementia, female reproductive life history, longevity, mismatch

Key Points

- Diseases that manifest in the later stages of life may still be subject to selection via inclusive fitness effects because of the interconnected nature of human families and communities.
- Several Alzheimer's disease risk factors were probably less common in the pre-modern past than today in post-industrial societies, such as cardiovascular and metabolic dysfunction.
- Female reproductive life history norms have changed dramatically across human history, with implications for geriatric health via cumulative biological effects across the lifespan.
- Female reproductive life history may influence Alzheimer's disease risk through various physiological pathways, such as hormone

exposure, immune function or oxidative stress.
- The *APOE-ε4* allele may have context-dependent effects on both fertility and Alzheimer's disease risk, with risks that are unique to post-industrialised environments.

17.1 Introduction

Alzheimer's disease (AD) is a devastating neurodegenerative disorder. Here, I consider the possibility that AD may be a case of evolutionary mismatch (see Chapters 1 and 5). Although human lives are, broadly speaking, more comfortable and healthy as we have eliminated threats that afflicted us throughout much of our evolutionary history, many of the conditions that plague us today may have been rarer for most of our species' collective history (Nesse and

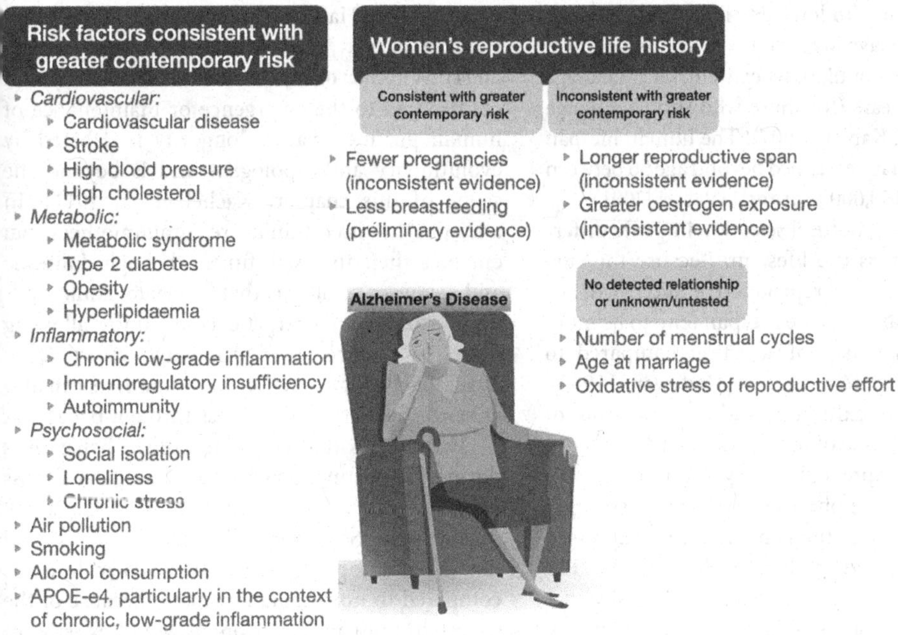

Risk factors consistent with greater contemporary risk	Women's reproductive life history	
	Consistent with greater contemporary risk	Inconsistent with greater contemporary risk

Risk factors consistent with greater contemporary risk

- *Cardiovascular:*
  - Cardiovascular disease
  - Stroke
  - High blood pressure
  - High cholesterol
- *Metabolic:*
  - Metabolic syndrome
  - Type 2 diabetes
  - Obesity
  - Hyperlipidaemia
- *Inflammatory:*
  - Chronic low-grade inflammation
  - Immunoregulatory insufficiency
  - Autoimmunity
- *Psychosocial:*
  - Social isolation
  - Loneliness
  - Chronic stress
- Air pollution
- Smoking
- Alcohol consumption
- APOE-e4, particularly in the context of chronic, low-grade inflammation

Women's reproductive life history

Consistent with greater contemporary risk
- Fewer pregnancies (inconsistent evidence)
- Less breastfeeding (preliminary evidence)

Inconsistent with greater contemporary risk
- Longer reproductive span (inconsistent evidence)
- Greater oestrogen exposure (inconsistent evidence)

Alzheimer's Disease

No detected relationship or unknown/untested
- Number of menstrual cycles
- Age at marriage
- Oxidative stress of reproductive effort

Figure 17.1 Alzheimer's disease risk factors evaluated for their consistency with an evolutionary mismatch hypothesis

Williams, 1996). While this concept has been invoked often to explain the high rates of conditions like obesity and type 2 diabetes (Stearns and Koella, 2008), there is justification to consider whether contemporary age-matched rates of AD may also be a more recent phenomenon (Figure 17.1). Firstly, AD has biological similarities with other 'diseases of civilisation'. Secondly, AD's high incidence and heavy burden on kin are inconsistent with the prevailing framework for human life history evolution, which assumes inclusive fitness benefits of longevity (Fox, 2018).

While AD is primarily problematic and feared because of its characteristic deterioration of memory and thinking ability (Gunten et al., 2018), the late stages of disease progression involve the deterioration of other somatic functions that are centrally controlled, such as the ability to swallow, walk and, eventually, breathe (Holtzman et al., 2011). Additionally, AD risk factors are not exclusively psychosocial or neurobiological but also involve peripheral biology. While early-onset AD, also known as autosomal dominant familial AD, is caused by mutations usually in one of three genes, this only accounts for <1% of AD cases (Karran et al., 2011). More than 99% of AD cases are considered sporadic and late onset. Here, I focus on late-onset AD and utilise the shorthand 'AD' to

refer to this condition. AD accounts for 60–80% of dementias, which are estimated in the USA/Europe to afflict 0.8%/0.9% of people aged 60–64, 1.7%/1.5% of people aged 65–69 and 3.3%/3.6% of people aged 70–74, and these rates exponentially increase thereafter (Ferri et al., 2005). I focus on prevalence rates among the younger age categories for AD because of their relevance for human life history evolution.

The cause(s) of AD remains mysterious. Various risk factors have been identified, but none establish precisely whether an individual will develop the disease. Well-established risk factors include cardiovascular, metabolic and inflammatory problems (Chakrabarti et al., 2015; De Bruijn and Ikram, 2014; Kinney et al., 2018; Tao et al., 2018). Other risk factors with preliminary or variable evidence include air pollution, smoking, alcohol consumption, traumatic brain injury and lower oestrogen exposure (Durazzo et al., 2014; Piazza-Gardner et al., 2013; Van Den Heuvel et al., 2007; Wu et al., 2015).

17.2 Selection Pressure and Diseases of Ageing

Humans are unique compared to other extant primates in our species' remarkable longevity. While the maximum human longevity is around 122 years (Gavrilov and Gavrilova, 2000), a composite of 8 hunter-gatherer populations exhibited a modal age at death of 72 years (for those who survived to age 14; Gurven and Kaplan, 2007). The human lifespan is estimated to have extended beyond age 50 between 1,600,000 and 150,000 years ago (Peccei, 2001).

In any species, natural selection imposes differential force across the lifespan. Because the currency of selection is reproductive success, traits that manifest earlier in the lifespan tend to be more sensitive to the force of selection compared to traits that manifest later (Medawar, 1952). Human females exhibit a sudden cessation of fecundity at the time of menopause, and so phenotypes that are expressed during pre-reproductive or reproductive life phases are subject to stronger selection pressures than phenotypes expressed during the post-reproductive life phase. For human males, the force of selection also declines with age, but not as suddenly, due to males' ongoing reproductive potential throughout adult life. Hence, diseases that emerge during later stages of the lifespan are subject to less selective pressure than those that manifest earlier, when there is greater opportunity for pathology to reduce reproductive output, and this discrepancy is starker among women. Medawar's mutation accumulation theory suggests that the genes responsible for pathology and senescence in old age may accumulate in the genome because of the weakness of selection against them (Medawar, 1952). Williams' (1957) antagonistic pleiotropy theory suggests that age-related selection bias favours genes with age-dependent effects whose benefits occur earlier and whose detriments occur later. This theory has been invoked to theorise that AD susceptibility genes may have age-dependent pleiotropic effects (Twamley et al., 2006).

However, phenotypes during women's postmenopausal life phase may be more visible to selection than the mutation accumulation and antagonistic pleiotropy theories would suggest (Fox, 2018). During the postmenopausal life phase, women are able to invest in their inclusive fitness by assisting their adult daughters and daughters-in-law with childcare towards dependent young children, allowing daughters and daughters-in-law to invest their own efforts in neonates, thereby allowing for shorter inter-birth intervals. This pattern rewards women who experience postmenopausal longevity with fitness benefits (i.e. Hawkes' grandmother hypothesis; Hawkes et al., 1997, 2000; Lahdenperä et al., 2004). Whether or how much this allocare system contributed to the emergence or maintenance of human postmenopausal longevity is debated by evolutionary anthropologists and is beyond the scope of this chapter (Kachel et al., 2011). In addition to direct childcare, grandmothers can enhance their inclusive fitness through domestic and economic labour that alleviate adult children's time and energetic constraints, allowing them to engage in reproductive effort (Fox, 2012; Reiches et al., 2009). Grandmothers can also enhance their inclusive fitness through pedagogy.

Pathologies that undermine these behaviours during the postmenopausal life phase have fitness costs, despite women's infecundity (Fox, 2018). Accordingly, Sapolsky and Finch (2000) argued that AD neuropathy may be delayed in humans compared to non-human primates because of the fitness detriments that women would experience by losing the opportunity to engage in grandmothering behaviours. Additionally, a long period of adult dependence would be burdensome for kin on whom an AD patient relies, undermining inclusive fitness beyond just lost opportunity (Fox, 2018). Typical life expectancy after AD diagnosis is 7–10 years (Zanetti et al., 2009), instigating a period of progressive loss of autonomy that imposes a costly burden to kin in addition to the loss of opportunity to benefit kin.

The prospect that AD may impose fitness consequences invites exploration of the evolutionary dynamics to explain the persistence of this trait. Furthermore, AD is more prevalent in women than men even after adjusting for survivorship bias (Andrew and Tierney, 2018). This sex bias, in the context of the adaptiveness of postmenopausal grandmothering, justifies a focus on the evolutionary dynamics of AD in women specifically.

17.3 Mismatch Hypothesis for Alzheimer's Disease

In evolutionary medicine, 'mismatch' describes the concept that human bodies are adapted to better suit a different environment from the one in which we currently reside. Biological change via natural selection is a slower process on a multigenerational timescale compared with the relatively rapid pace of human cultural modifications to lifestyles and environments (Stearns and

Koella, 2008). Depending on the trait of interest, the timescale and geographies of what is considered to be the environment of evolutionary adaptedness (EEA) (Bowlby, 1969) and of what is to be considered to be the contemporary environment may vary. Often, the Industrial Revolution is regarded as instigating the emergence of contemporary lifestyles due to its transformative global effects on aspects ranging from built environments to population density to physical activity (Rook, 2012; Stearns and Koella, 2008). Sometimes, the Agricultural Revolution is regarded as the turning point between the EEA and contemporary environments if the trait of interest is most affected by, for instance, diet or residence patterns (Rook, 2012; Stearns and Koella, 2008). Disease risk factors or causes associated with modernity may be entirely novel or at greater frequency today than in the past. In many cases, a risk factor that began to increase in frequency with the advent of agriculture or industrialisation may be accelerating in frequency or degree with the more recent globalisation trends of the twenty-first century (Fox et al., 2019).

It is difficult or impossible to determine soft-tissue disorders and women's reproductive life history (RLH) traits in the archaeological record. However, certain features may be surmised by examining these conditions among contemporary people with environments and lifestyles that more closely resemble those of our pre-industrial and pre-agricultural ancestors. However, these methods only help us surmise traits broadly because, firstly, contemporary people's environments and lifestyles inherently vary from those of the past and, secondly, peoples in the past surely exhibited variability in many domains.

There are well-established risk factors for AD that we can suppose with some confidence are either novel to post-industrial environments or are at much greater frequency (Figure 17.1). The sedentism and processed food consumption of the post-industrial era are likely to be associated with the far greater frequency of cardiovascular risk factors for AD, such as cardiovascular disease, stroke, high blood pressure and high cholesterol (De Bruijn and Ikram, 2014), and the metabolic risk factors for AD, such as metabolic syndrome, type 2 diabetes, obesity and hyperlipidaemia (Chakrabarti et al., 2015). While cardiovascular and metabolic dysfunction are not entirely novel to the post-industrial era, evidence that the

physical activity and diets of contemporary foragers and subsistence farmers are linked with dramatically superior cardiovascular and metabolic health in those populations underscores the likelihood that these AD risk factors would have been less prevalent in the past (Pontzer et al., 2012).

The typical urban lifestyles of the post-industrial era are characterised by a lack of exposure to a variety of benign microbes at young ages, which would have been more common in previous environments, due to urban living being separated from other animals and soil and the widespread sanitisation infrastructure (e.g. chemical decontamination of water; Rook, 2007). This lack of diverse, benign microbial exposure, alongside high population densities, is associated with inadequate education of the immune system, leading to lifelong, chronic, low-grade inflammation. Various inflammatory conditions – allergies, atopies and autoimmunities – have been linked to this aspect of urban dwelling. Chronic, low-grade inflammation – an established risk factor for AD (Kinney et al., 2018) – is widespread in contemporary urban populations but not among contemporary subsistence populations, such as the Tsimane forager-horticulturalists (Gurven et al., 2008). Therefore, it seems likely that this AD risk factor was less prevalent in the past (Fox et al., 2019).

Social isolation, measured by small social networks, living alone, lacking social ties or a composite of these, has been associated with increased risk of dementia and AD (Fratiglioni et al., 2000; Wilson et al., 2007). Loneliness, an emotional state related to social isolation, was associated with more than double the risk of AD in a prospective study independent of the effect of social isolation (Wilson et al., 2007). Generally, people in pre-modern human societies were less socially isolated than post-industrial norms due to their closer relationships with extended family and multigenerational family compared to the post-industrial nuclear family-based social structure, as well as their greater number of children. In contemporary developed countries, loneliness has been described as an epidemic caused by the loss of traditional social connectivity and a reliance on technology (Jeste et al., 2020). Therefore, it seems likely that the AD risk factors of social isolation and loneliness were less prevalent in the past.

Air pollution, smoking and alcohol consumption have been associated with AD risk, although the mechanisms by which these risks influence AD aetiology remain questions of debate (Durazzo et al., 2014; Piazza-Gardner et al., 2013; Wu et al., 2015). Widespread air pollution is a product of industrial manufacturing and transportation, although non-human-made forms of air pollution (e.g. dust storms) exist, and their relationships with AD merit investigation (reviewed in Fox et al., 2019). Smoking and alcohol consumption have accelerated in the post-industrial era, although exposure to smoke and alcohol is also present among contemporary foragers and subsistence farmers, such as from campfire smoke and fermented beverages (Dana Lynn, 2014; Hornsey, 2012). Thus, air pollution, smoking and alcohol consumption are less clear-cut in their history as AD risk factors.

Moderate or severe and repeated mild traumatic brain injuries have been associated with AD risk (Van Den Heuvel et al., 2007); however, there is no reason to suspect that risk of impact injuries to the head would have been systematically at greater or lower frequency across different eras of human history. Therefore, this risk factor does not support a mismatch hypothesis.

17.4 Reproductive Life History

One of the most profound ways that women's physiologies have changed across human history is the shift in female RLH norms, which can be estimated by comparing people who live today as industrialised urban dwellers with foragers and subsistence farmers. These differences in RLH have profound effects on women's lifelong biology and therefore could affect AD risk. RLH might modify later-life risk of AD through the alteration of biological pathways known to be involved in the disease's aetiology. Female RLH is linked to cardiovascular, metabolic, inflammatory and endocrine alterations to physiology in ways that have not only short-term but also long-term and, in some cases, permanent effects.

The vast majority of relevant studies have focused on the oestrogen hypothesis (Colucci et al., 2006; Fox et al., 2013a; Geerlings et al., 2001; Hong et al., 2001; Prince et al., 2018). In animal and *in vitro* studies, oestrogen has been observed to be broadly protective against a variety of pathogenic pathways implicated in AD

aetiology (Carroll et al., 2007; Greenfield et al., 2002). As a result, the medical research community has pursued clinical trials involving oestrogen administration and observational cohort studies assessing the relationship between oestrogen exposure and AD risk (Imtiaz et al., 2017; Shao et al., 2012).

The oestrogen hypothesis raises a few mostly overlooked issues. It is unclear whether the duration or quantity of oestrogen – or both – would drive a relationship between oestrogen exposure and AD risk; for example, should we expect the oestrogen exposure of pregnancy to be hundreds of times more potent in protecting against AD than the oestrogen exposure of hormone-replacement therapy due to pregnancy's oestrogen levels being hundreds of times higher (Tulchinsky and Little, 1994)? Also, there is no clear hypothesis for the timing of oestrogen's influence; for example, should we expect exposure to oestrogen at age 70 to have a greater impact compared to at age 40 or age 20? Finally, the oestrogen hypothesis implicitly suggests that women's RLH should be associated with AD risk solely because of the ways in which RLH events alter oestrogen levels; however, RLH events alter many aspects of physiology beyond oestrogen levels, some of which are also implicated in AD risk (Fox et al., 2018). Therefore, any correlations observed between RLH traits and AD risk should be considered in light of several possible physiological pathways.

There is no singular time or location at which women's RLH patterns shifted, but rather there are many transitions, with different RLH traits changing at different times. Furthermore, RLH traits are facultative, with reaction norms that reflect variability between individuals and socio-environmental contexts depending on adaptive strategies and constraints. Investigation of the individual transitions in traits in different contexts is beyond the scope of this chapter. Rather, we compare large-scale population normative ranges in 'pre-modern' contexts to reflect the vast majority of human history before the advent of agriculture with 'post-industrial' contexts to reflect the more recent, more urbanised, more industrialised context of human lives. I make no claim of uniformity in any trait (besides breast-feeding as a pre-modern universal method of early infant feeding) in any era, culture or geography.

17.4.1 Reproductive Span

Reproductive span describes the length of time between menarche and menopause. This construct offers weak or inconsistent evidence in opposition to a mismatch hypothesis. Reproductive span is likely longer in post-industrial societies than what would have been the norm for most of human evolutionary history due to younger ages at menarche and potentially older ages at menopause, although the latter is controversial (Flint, 1978; Papadimitriou, 2016). Some studies have found that earlier menarche, later menopause and/or longer reproductive span were associated with lower risk of dementia or AD (Geerlings et al., 2001; Hong et al., 2001), although several others found no such effects (Colucci et al., 2006; Prince et al., 2018), including our study of British women (Fox et al., 2013a).

Although the evidence is weak, longer reproductive span associated with reduced AD risk is consistent with what should be expected based on biomechanisms. Reproductive span has been interesting to AD researchers primarily because of the oestrogen hypothesis (i.e. long reproductive span should be protective; Colucci et al., 2006; Fox et al., 2013a; Geerlings et al., 2001; Hong et al., 2001; Prince et al., 2018). Also, longer reproductive span has been associated with lower risks of cardiovascular disease (Ley et al., 2017) and type 2 diabetes (Brand et al., 2013) and lower C-reactive protein levels (Huang et al., 2019), so this construct should be considered as a potential AD protective factor through various pathways in addition to oestrogenic neuroprotection.

17.4.2 Pregnancy

Pregnancy has been interesting to AD researchers primarily because of the oestrogen hypothesis (i.e. if quantity of oestrogen is protective, then more pregnancies – which are characterised by high oestrogen levels – should be protective). We previously suggested an alternative pathway by which expansion of immunosuppressive regulatory T-cell populations during pregnancy could explain the observed correlations between more pregnancies and lower AD risk (Fox et al., 2018). Pregnancy involves the reorganisation of several physiological systems, sometimes with long-term or even permanent effects. In addition to endocrine and immune system changes, pregnancy is also characterised by cardiovascular and metabolic alterations that should be further investigated in relation to AD risk. For instance, pregnancy induces a state of peripheral insulin resistance, and higher parity has been associated with greater risk of type 2 diabetes in postmenopausal life (Dahlgren, 2006), which could potentially increase AD risk. However, breastfeeding counteracts pregnancy-induced insulin resistance (see Section 17.4.3) (Bell and Bauman, 1997).

The practice of contraception (besides lactational amenorrhea) is a relatively recent phenomenon in human history. There is evidence of contraceptive and abortifacient practices – of varying levels of assumed efficacy – dating back to ancient Egyptian, Greek and Jewish sources, but there is no evidence of widespread contraceptive practices until nineteenth-century barrier methods and later twentieth-century hormonal methods (Himes, 1970). A composite of hunter-gatherer groups exhibited completed lifetime fertility of 5.9 compared to contemporaneous Americans' completed lifetime fertility of 1.8 (Eaton et al., 1994). The comparatively low completed fertility typical of contraceptive, post-industrial societies suggests differential health effects.

The differences in typical completed fertility have implications for geriatric women's health in two ways. Women in non-contraceptive populations exhibit greater cumulative effects of many pregnancies, whereas women in contraceptive populations would experience comparatively diminished effects. Conversely, women in contraceptive populations would exhibit greater cumulative effects of the physiological state that replaces the missing pregnancies. In post-industrial populations with sufficient or excess nutritional availability, fewer pregnancies would be associated with more ovulatory menstrual cycles, although the cumulative effects of ovulation and menstrual cycles could be altered by hormonal contraceptives. Thus, it is difficult to attribute the effects of parity on AD risk to gestational biology itself versus the deprivation of the alternative.

Several studies have investigated the relationship between parity and AD risk. While two studies found greater parity to be associated with AD or dementia risk (Prince et al., 2018; Ptok et al., 2002), several studies found no such effect (Kim et al., 2003; Waring et al., 1999). Most study designs are inadequate because it could be possible that number of pregnancies is simply a proxy for duration of oestrogen exposure, marriage or breastfeeding – constructs that are highly correlated with parity. Thus, any observed effects could be misattributed. Moreover, other ways of operationalising pregnancy history encompass more information than parity (number of completed pregnancies), especially gravidity (number of initiated pregnancies). Depending on the mechanism by which pregnancy may affect AD aetiology, it may be more meaningful to measure how many pregnancies are initiated (i.e. when major immune reorganisation occurs) instead of how many pregnancies are completed (i.e. when major sex steroid exposure occurs).

My team endeavoured to improve upon past study designs by controlling for age at first birth, reproductive span and history of breastfeeding and marriages (Fox et al., 2018). In order to clarify the oestrogen hypothesis, we deemed it crucial to distinguish between the effects of duration and quantity of oestrogen exposure by adjusting the analyses for reproductive span. Furthermore, we operationalised pregnancy history in two unique ways. Firstly, we measured cumulative number of months pregnant, combining incomplete (e.g. miscarriages) and complete (e.g. childbearing) pregnancies. Our results suggested that cumulative number of months pregnant was associated with a dose-dependent reduction in AD risk, suggesting that quantity of oestrogen exposure was a more plausible mechanism than duration of oestrogen exposure. Secondly, we compared the oestrogenic explanation with an immunoregulatory explanation. In this pursuit, we found that AD risk was significantly associated with a woman's cumulative number of first trimesters and not with third trimesters. Therefore, our results were more consistent with an immunoregulatory rather than an oestrogenic mechanism.

17.4.3 Breastfeeding

Breastfeeding has not been widely investigated in the context of AD. Nonetheless, there are a variety of physiological pathways that would potentially connect breastfeeding with AD aetiology. Breastfeeding involves alterations to the mother's peripheral glucose metabolism and lipid metabolism, beta-cell efficiency and fat mobilisation (reviewed in Fox et al., 2021). Perturbations in

each of these physiological functions have been implicated in AD pathogenesis. Furthermore, a woman's history of breastfeeding has already been connected to long-term effects on the risk of other conditions that are themselves risk factors for AD, including type 2 diabetes, cardiovascular disease, hypertension and hyperlipidaemia (Fox et al., 2021).

Of all aspects of RLH that have changed across human history, breastfeeding is arguably the domain with the largest change. Because of the combination of greater parity and longer duration of breastfeeding per child compared to post-industrial populations, pre-modern women likely spent vastly more total time breastfeeding. Women in post-industrial societies practice less breastfeeding than their pre-modern counterparts (Stuart-Macadam, 1995). In the USA, 45.9% of infants born in 2017 were exclusively breastfed through 3 months of age and 25.6% were exclusively breastfed through 6 months of age; 35.3% were still being breastfed at all by 12 months of age (Centers for Disease Control and Prevention, 2021). While 74.4% of US infants are ever breastfed, the everbreastfed rate varies across high-income countries (e.g. Ireland, 55%; France, 63%; Uruguay, 99%; UNICEF, 2018). Previous to the midnineteenth century, when infant formula was first produced, virtually all surviving infants would have been breastfed.

Breastfeeding norms across human history can be estimated based on evidence from skeletal remains and patterns among contemporary subsistence populations, although we only have limited ability to reconstruct the past from these methods. Skeletal isotope analyses of foraging populations from 12,000 to 2,500 years ago found that total breastfeeding per child was 22–68 months (Tsutaya et al., 2016). A meta-analysis of 113 contemporary non-industrialised populations found that mean length of total breastfeeding per child was 29 months (Sellen, 2001).

For example, Hadza hunter-gatherers in Tanzania exhibited a mean age at cessation of breastfeeding of 30 months and a total fertility rate of 6.3 (Jones, 2016; Sellen, 2001). Therefore, the cumulative duration of breastfeeding across a typical Hadza woman's life would be several years, possibly around a decade (not a simple matter of multiplying breastfeeding per child by number of children due to infant mortality and the potential for breastfeeding throughout a subsequent pregnancy and alongside a new sibling).

My team has conducted two relevant studies in this area. We found in a cohort of British women that longer duration of breastfeeding was associated with lower AD risk (Fox et al., 2013b). We found in a cohort of south Californian women that ever-breastfeeding was associated with superior cognitive performance after age 50 (Fox et al., 2021). Two other studies found negative relationships between breastfeeding and cognitive performance in older women (Hesson, 2012; Heys et al., 2011). While these opposite effects are perplexing, cognitive performance in non-AD cohorts is not a sufficient indicator of AD risk. Because only one study directly investigated AD risk with relation to breastfeeding, more work is needed in this area.

17.4.4 Menstrual Cycles

Menstrual cycles could plausibly be connected to AD risk because ovulation is associated with a surge in oestrogen. Menstrual cycle oestrogen exposure is small compared to pregnancy but larger than lactational amenorrhea, premenarche or postmenopause (Tulchinsky and Little, 1994). There is already evidence that cumulative number of menstrual cycles is positively associated with postmenopausal breast cancer risk, underscoring the possibility of its long-term effects on health (Clavel-Chapelon, 2002). My team conducted the only analysis (known to me) of the cumulative number of menstrual cycles and AD risk and found no relationship (Fox et al., 2013a).

Women in post-industrial contexts today typically exhibit more cumulative menstrual cycles than their hunter-gatherer peers: the mean for individuals not using hormonal contraceptives, from composites of post-industrial and hunter-gatherer groups, was found to be 450 versus 160 (Eaton et al., 1994). Therefore, I extrapolate that women in post-industrial contexts who do not use hormonal contraceptives likely experience more menstrual cycles than women in pre-modern contexts would have. This difference can be attributed to post-industrial women having younger typical age at menarche, more pregnancies, less lactational amenorrhea and older age at menopause. However, without evidence for a relationship between number of menstrual cycles and AD risk, this difference may lack relevance here.

17.4.5 Exogenous Hormone Therapies

While hormone therapies are a twentieth-century invention absent for most of our species' history, understanding their relationships with AD risk can help us to discern certain aspects of the relationship between RLH and AD. Comparing use of hormonal contraception with the equivalent duration of non-pregnant menstrual cycles could help identify the relationship between ovulation and AD risk; future studies should explore this question. While hormone therapies are administered continuously, in the human ovarian cycle hormones are naturally cyclic. Carroll et al. (2010) investigated the effects of progesterone administration in 3xTg-AD mice, distinguishing between continuous versus cyclic administration. They replicated the results of their previous study (Carroll et al., 2007) that, when both hormones are administered continuously, oestradiol lowers beta-amyloid (Aβ) accumulation and progesterone blocks this effect. However, cyclic progesterone administered alone inhibited Aβ accumulation, and when cyclic progesterone was administered with continuous oestradiol, oestradiol's reduction of Aβ accumulation was actually enhanced. Similar effects were found for working memory and visual attention. These observations suggest that menstrual cycles could potentially be neuroprotective, but human studies are needed.

An enormous body of research has explored the relationship between hormone-replacement therapy administered around the time of menopause or thereafter as a potential intervention to prevent AD-related pathogenesis. These studies are justified by the oestrogen hypothesis. While several studies that looked at exclusive oestrogen-replacement therapy found protective effects (Imtiaz et al., 2017; Shao et al., 2012), those that looked at combined oestrogen plus progestin therapy often reported either no effect (Imtiaz et al., 2017) or the opposite effect: greater risk (Shao et al., 2012). These patterns could be attributed to the phenomenon described earlier in this section: that unopposed oestrogen is neuroprotective, but when administered in conjunction with continuous progesterone the protection is attenuated.

These observations have relevance for elucidating how women's RLH may influence AD risk. For instance, it is possible that the neuroprotective oestrogenic benefits of a menstrual cycle (cyclic progesterone) may be more pronounced than the oestrogen exposure of a pregnancy (continuous progesterone).

17.4.6 Psychosocial Aspects of Reproductive Life History

Previous studies on the links between women's RLH and AD risk have neglected the potential psychosocial mechanisms. In particular, women's history of pregnancy and breastfeeding are intertwined with her relationships with romantic partners and children. Relationships with romantic partners and children are relevant for AD aetiology because a lack of social support and psychological distress have been implicated as AD risk factors (Holmen et al., 2000; Wilson et al., 2007). More pregnancies should be correlated with younger age at marriage or more years married (or in non-married romantic partnerships), which plausibly could be associated with the kind of emotional and instrumental social support that is protective against AD. Number of pregnancies should be strongly correlated with number of children. Especially at older ages, adult children are an important source of social support and have been associated with lower AD risk. A more tenuous argument could be made for breastfeeding, such that it is associated with mother–child bonding and lower maternal risk of postpartum depression (Hahn-Holbrook et al., 2013), both of which could arguably be hypothesised to lead to lower AD risk. While postpartum depression is a risk factor for major depressive disorder and history of major depressive disorder is a risk factor for AD (Green et al., 2003), the direct link between postpartum depression and AD risk remains untested. Similarly, mother–child bonding in the postpartum period could plausibly lead to better mother–child relationships in adulthood, which would plausibly be protective against AD, but these links are also untested. Future research into the connections between women's RLH and AD risk should explore psychosocial mechanisms.

Previous studies found that marriage/romantic partnerships were protective against AD risk. In a large study of over 3,000 participants, those who had been married or cohabitated with a partner exhibited significantly lower AD risk compared to those who had never done so (Helmer et al., 1999).

Relationship quality with their primary caregiver was associated with quality of life among a cohort of 50 AD patients (Mortazavizadeh et al., 2020). No association was found between age when first married or cumulative duration of all marriages with AD risk in our cohort of British women after adjusting for the effects of several RLH variables (Fox et al., 2018).

Less is known about relationships with adult children and risk of AD. One study found that strained relationships with adult children were correlated with cognitive limitations among older adults (Thomas and Umberson, 2017).

17.5 Oxidative Stress

The oxidative stress generated by greater reproductive effort among women with typical pre-modern RLH patterns compared to post-industrial counterparts is, theoretically, inconsistent with a mismatch hypothesis. Reproductive effort is metabolically costly, increasing the by-product of reactive oxygen species and thereby self-tissue damage (i.e. oxidative stress). Oxidative stress is implicated in AD pathogenesis (Huang et al., 2016). Therefore, we should examine RLH traits' long-term effects on oxidative stress to appreciate the possibility of links with AD aetiology. Ovulation produces oxidative stress, but little is known about cumulative or long-term effects in humans (Agarwal et al., 2012). Animal studies have observed oxidative stress associated with lactation, but this topic has not been adequately studied in humans (Berchieri-Ronchi et al., 2011; Ziomkiewicz et al., 2016). More is known about oxidative stress associated with pregnancy in humans. Multiparous women exhibit higher levels of bio-markers of oxidative stress during their reproductive life phase, and there is also a cumulative effect that is evident in the postmenopausal life phase (Mutlu et al., 2012; Ziomkiewicz et al., 2016). If human gestation and lactation both produce more oxidative stress than is produced during a menstrual cycle – an idea that is plausible but not yet endorsed by evidence – then women who spend more of their reproductive life phases in gestation and lactation should suffer the cumulative consequences of self-tissue damage more so than women who spend more of their reproductive life phases in menstrual cycles. Thus, differences between post-industrial and pre-modern

RLH norms would suggest that post-industrial women suffer less from the oxidative stress of reproductive effort. This is not to imply that post-industrial women would be expected to exhibit less overall lifelong oxidative stress; rather, the opposite is likely to be true due to other factors such as pollution, toxic exposures and chronic psychosocial stress, rendering post-industrial women at overall greater AD risk than their pre-modern counterparts. Nonetheless, RLH patterns may not contribute to (or may even counteract) this mismatch.

17.6 *APOE*

The apolipoprotein E (*APOE*) gene, which encodes the ApoE protein, is implicated in both AD risk and female RLH. *APOE* encodes three variants: *APOE-ε4* (the ancestral allele) and *APOE-ε3* and *APOE-ε2* (both human-specific, more recently derived alleles). Each encodes a unique isoform of the ApoE protein. In non- or semi-industrialised populations, *APOE-ε4* may give a reproductive success advantage despite its association with AD (Corbo et al., 2004b; Jasienska et al., 2015). Furthermore, there is a lack of evidence for *APOE-ε4* as an AD risk factor in non-industrialised populations, which supports the possibility of a mismatch hypothesis (Chen et al., 2010; Farrer et al., 2003; Gureje et al., 2005; Sayi et al., 1997).

Growing evidence supports a key role for *APOE* in women's differential reproductive success, although the results are often conflicting. *APOE* genotypes have been associated with earlier (Koochmeshgi et al., 2004), later (Meng et al., 2012) and no association with age at menopause (He et al., 2009) and with risk, protection and neutral effects regarding pre-eclampsia (Abyadeh et al., 2020). A meta-analysis found that the *ε4* allele was associated with recurrent pregnancy loss (Li et al., 2014).

ApoE is the primary supplier of cholesterol precursors for steroid hormone production, such as progesterone and oestrogen (Mahley and Rall Jr, 2000). The *ε4* variant is associated with the highest cholesterol levels, *ε3* with intermediate levels and *ε2* with the lowest levels (Corbo et al., 2004a). Jasienska et al. (2015) found among a natural-fertility population in rural Poland that women who carried at least one *APOE-ε4* allele exhibited 20% higher luteal progesterone, which is associated with likelihood of conception. They found no

association with oestradiol levels, possibly due to the regulatory effects of several other enzymes in the conversion pathway from cholesterol.

Consistent with the observation of the potential for greater fecundability among *APOE-ε4* carriers, in a non-industrialised natural-fertility population in Ecuador, Corbo et al. (2004b) observed the highest fertility among women with the *ε4/ε3* genotype. Contrastingly, among contraceptive populations in rural Italy and urban Denmark, women with the *ε3/ε3* genotype exhibited the highest fertility (Corbo et al., 2004a; Gerdes et al., 1996). It is possible that in more nutritionally limited natural-fertility contexts cholesterol availability has a greater impact on fertility (Jasienska et al., 2015).

ApoE and oestrogen may interact to influence AD aetiology. Oestrogen has neurotrophic effects that rely on the presence of either ApoE-ε3 or ApoE-ε2, but with only ApoE-ε4 oestrogen does not promote neuronal growth (Depypere et al., 2016). Oestrogen has neuroprotective effects via downregulation of microglial proinflammatory activity, but this protection is weaker in the presence of ApoE-ε4 compared to ApoE-ε3 and ApoE-ε2 (Brown et al., 2008). Also, oestrogen promotes ApoE production in microglia, which, in turn, participates in myelination and axon regeneration after neuronal insult (Mor et al., 1999), but ApoE-ε4 has a weaker effect in this neuronal healing cascade (Depypere et al., 2016).

ApoE is involved in various physiological functions, so the particular pathway by which it moderates AD risk must be established. Evidence against cholesterol metabolism being the primary pathway comes from studies finding that, after controlling for cholesterol level and blood pressure, the *ε4* allele remained an AD risk factor with no alteration to effect size (Kivipelto et al., 2002; Minihane et al., 2007). The evidence is stronger for the *ε4* allele exerting its impact on AD risk through its role in inflammation. Consistent with this possibility, chronic, low-grade inflammation was a risk factor for AD only among *ε4* carriers (Tao et al., 2018). Also, *ε4* was associated with risk and poor outcomes in other conditions involving neuroinflammation, such as HIV-associated dementia (Corder et al., 1998; reviewed in Fox, 2018).

The evolutionary dynamics that account for the emergence and spread of the *ε3* and *ε2* alleles and the persistence of the ancestral *ε4* allele are debated. *APOE-ε3* emerged approximately

300,000 years ago and *APOE-ε2* emerged approximately 200,000 years ago (Glass and Arnold, 2012). The ancestral *ε4* allele has been associated with a variety of pathological phenotypes, including AD (Farrer et al., 1997), coronary heart disease (Song et al., 2004) and HIV disease progression and mortality (Burt et al., 2008). On the other hand, the *ε4* allele has been associated with protection against hepatitis C-associated liver damage (Wozniak et al., 2002), cardiovascular stress (Ravaja et al., 1997), macular degeneration (Klaver et al., 1998), childhood diarrhoea (Oria et al., 2005) and malaria (Wozniak et al., 2004). Thus, while it is possible that the *ε3* and *ε2* alleles were under positive selection in certain contexts, the *ε4* allele offers other benefits that may explain its persistence, potentially dependent on regional variations in infection risks (Singh et al., 2006).

Focusing on the relationship between *ε4* and AD risk, Sapolsky and Finch (2000) proposed that the *ε3* and *ε2* alleles would have been under positive selection in humans to delay AD neuropathogenesis because of the importance of grandmothering to women's adaptive fitness. A critical question is whether the *ε4* allele promotes AD pathogenesis in pre-modern human contexts. If not, then theories that rely on its relationship with AD across human history should be rethought, although its relationship with other pathologies would remain valid.

Several non- or semi-industrialised populations demonstrate a lack of association between *APOE* genotypes and AD risk, even among some for whom the *ε4* allele is at a relatively high frequency (Fox, 2018). No correlation between *APOE* genotypes and AD risk was observed among Ibadan Yoruba Nigerians, Nyeri Kenyans, Tanzanians, Wadi Ara Arab Israelis and Bantu and Nilotic African cohorts (Chen et al., 2010; Farrer et al., 2003; Gureje et al., 2005; Sayi et al., 1997). Contrastingly, the *ε4* allele is associated with AD risk among all Western industrialised populations studied, including Americans of various ethnicities, Europeans and

Australians (Farrer et al., 1997; Martins et al., 1995; Sando et al., 2008).

17.7 Conclusion

Although there may be lower selection pressure on later parts of the lifespan, phenotypes expressed in post-reproductive human life stages can still have meaningful consequences for inclusive fitness. AD afflicts a large portion of individuals during the post-reproductive life phase and involves symptoms that render them incapable of participating in the activities that would benefit inclusive fitness. However, it is possible that AD risk may be greater today in post-industrial contexts than it would have been for age-matched individuals in pre-modern contexts. Evidence supporting this possibility comes from the observation that many established AD risk factors were most likely at lower frequencies or absent for the majority of human history. Here, I pay special attention to female RLH patterns both because of epidemiological observations of their links with AD risk and because these patterns represent a major alteration to human physiology across evolutionary history. Pregnancy and breastfeeding could plausibly exert lifelong physiological effects that are protective against AD risk, but more research is needed to establish these patterns in ways that adjust for each other as well as the psychosocial correlates of pregnancy and breastfeeding. Other underexplored areas are the ways in which menstrual cycles and the oxidative stress caused by reproductive effort may or may not contribute to AD risk. The *APOE-ε4* allele may only function as an AD risk factor in the context of chronic, low-grade inflammation, and in the absence of such inflammation, this allele may have no relationship with AD risk. The persistence of this ancestral allele may, therefore, be explained by its benefits for fecundability and protection against other diseases, thereby not requiring us to devise evolutionary theories to justify its promotion of AD.

References

Abyadeh, M., Heydarinejad, F., Khakpash, M., Asefi, Y. and Shab-Bidar, S. 2020. Association of apolipoprotein E gene polymorphism with preeclampsia: a meta-analysis. *Hypertension in Pregnancy*, 39, 196–202.

Agarwal, A., Aponte-Mellado, A., Premkumar, B. J., Shaman, A. and Gupta, S. 2012. The effects of oxidative stress on female reproduction: a review. *Reproductive Biology and Endocrinology*, 10, 49.

Andrew, M. K. and Tierney, M. C. 2018. The puzzle of sex, gender and Alzheimer's disease: why are women more often affected than men? *Women's Health*, 14, 1745506518817995.

Bell, A. W. and Bauman, D. E. 1997. Adaptations of glucose metabolism during pregnancy and lactation. *Journal of Mammary Gland Biology and Neoplasia*, 2, 265–278.

Berchieri-Ronchi, C., Kim, S., Zhao, Y., Correa, C., Yeum, K.-J. and Ferreira, A. 2011. Oxidative stress status of highly prolific sows during gestation and lactation. *Animal*, 5, 1774–1779.

Bowlby, J. 1969. *Attachment and Loss*. New York: Basic Books.

Brand, J. S., Van Der Schouw, Y. T., Onland-Moret, N. C., Sharp, S. J., Ong, K. K., Khaw, K.-T., Ardanaz, E., Amiano, P., Boeing, H., Chirlaque, M.-D., Clavel-Chapelon, F., Crowe, F. L., De Lauzon-Guillain, B., Duell, E. J., Fagherazzi, G., Franks, P. W., Grioni, S., Groop, L. C., Kaaks, R., Key, T. J., Nilsson, P. M., Overvad, K., Palli, D., Panico, S., Quirós, J. R., Rolandsson, O., Sacerdote, C., Sánchez, M.-J., Slimani, N., Teucher, B., Tjonneland, A., Tumino, R., Van Der A. D. L., Feskens, E. J. M., Langenberg, C., Forouhi, N. G., Riboli, E. and Wareham, N. J. 2013. Age at menopause, reproductive life span, and type 2 diabetes risk: results from the EPIC-InterAct study. *Diabetes Care*, 36, 1012–1019.

Brown, C. M., Choi, E., Xu, Q., Vitek, M. P. and Colton, C. A. 2008. The *APOE4* genotype alters the response of microglia and macrophages to 17β-estradiol. *Neurobiology of Aging*, 29, 1783–1794.

Burt, T. D., Agan, B. K., Marconi, V. C., He, W., Kulkarni, H., Mold, J. E., Cavrois, M., Huang, Y., Mahley, R. W. and Dolan, M. J. 2008. Apolipoprotein (apo) E4 enhances HIV-1 cell entry *in vitro*, and the *APOE ε4/ε4* genotype accelerates HIV disease progression. *Proceedings of the*

National Academy of Sciences of the United States of America, 105, 8718–8723.

Carroll, J. C., Rosario, E. R., Chang, L., Stanczyk, F. Z., Oddo, S., Laferla, F. M. and Pike, C. J. 2007. Progesterone and estrogen regulate Alzheimer-like neuropathology in female 3xTg-AD mice. *Journal of Neuroscience*, 27, 13357–13365.

Carroll, J. C., Rosario, E. R., Villamagna, A. and Pike, C. J. 2010. Continuous and cyclic progesterone differentially interact with estradiol in the regulation of Alzheimer-like pathology in female 3x transgenic-Alzheimer's disease mice. *Endocrinology*, 151, 2713–2722.

Centers for Disease Control and Prevention 2021. Data, Trend and Maps. National Center for Chronic Disease Prevention and Health Promotion, Division of Nutrition, Physical Activity, and Obesity. Retrieved from www .cdc.gov/nccdphp/dnpao/data-trends-maps/index.html

Chakrabarti, S., Khemka, V. K., Banerjee, A., Chatterjee, G., Ganguly, A. and Biswas, A. 2015. Metabolic risk factors of sporadic Alzheimer's disease: implications in the pathology, pathogenesis and treatment. *Aging and Disease*, 6, 282–299.

Chen, C. H., Mizuno, T., Elston, R., Kariuki, M. M., Hall, K., Unverzagt, F., Hendrie, H., Gatere, S., Kioy, P. and Patel, N. B. 2010. A comparative study to screen dementia and *APOE* genotypes in an ageing East African population. *Neurobiology of Aging*, 31, 732–740.

Clavel-Chapelon, F. 2002. Cumulative number of menstrual cycles and breast cancer risk: results from the E3N cohort study of French women. *Cancer Causes & Control*, 13, 831–838.

Colucci, M., Cammarata, S., Assini, A., Croce, R., Clerici, F., Novello,

C., Mazzella, L., Dagnino, N., Mariani, C. and Tanganelli, P. 2006. The number of pregnancies is a risk factor for Alzheimer's disease. *European Journal of Neurology*, 13, 1374–1377.

Corbo, R. M., Scacchi, R. and Cresta, M. 2004a. Differential reproductive efficiency associated with common apolipoprotein E alleles in postreproductive-aged subjects. *Fertility and Sterility*, 81, 104–107.

Corbo, R. M., Ulizzi, L., Scacchi, R., Martinez-Labarga, C. and De Stefano, G. 2004b. Apolipoprotein E polymorphism and fertility: a study in pre-industrial populations. *Molecular Human Reproduction*, 10, 617–620.

Corder, E. H., Robertson, K., Lannfelt, L., Bogdanovic, N., Eggertsen, G., Wilkins, J. and Hall, C. 1998. HIV-infected subjects with the *E4* allele for *APOE* have excess dementia and peripheral neuropathy. *Nature Medicine*, 4, 1182–1184.

Dahlgren, J. 2006. Pregnancy and insulin resistance. *Metabolic Syndrome and Related Disorders*, 4, 149–152.

Dana Lynn, C. 2014. Hearth and campfire influences on arterial blood pressure: defraying the costs of the social brain through fireside relaxation. *Evolutionary Psychology*, 12, 983–1003.

De Bruijn, R. F. A. G. and Ikram, M. A. 2014. Cardiovascular risk factors and future risk of Alzheimer's disease. *BMC Medicine*, 12, 130.

Depypere, H., Vierin, A., Weyers, S. and Sieben, A. 2016. Alzheimer's disease, apolipoprotein E and hormone replacement therapy. *Maturitas*, 94, 98–105.

Durazzo, T. C., Mattsson, N., Weiner, M. W. and Alzheimer's Disease Neuroimaging Initiative 2014. Smoking and increased Alzheimer's disease risk: a review of potential mechanisms.

Alzheimer's & Dementia, 10, S122–S145.

Eaton, S. B., Pike, M. C., Short, R. V., Lee, N. C., Trussell, J., Hatcher, R. A., Wood, J. W., Worthman, C. M., Jones, N. G. B. and Konner, M. J. 1994. Women's reproductive cancers in evolutionary context. *Quarterly Review of Biology*, 69, 353–367.

Farrer, L. A., Cupples, L. A., Haines, J. L., Hyman, B., Kukull, W. A., Mayeux, R., Myers, R. H., Pericak-Vance, M. A., Risch, N. and Van Duijn, C. M. 1997. Effects of age, sex, and ethnicity on the association between apolipoprotein E genotype and Alzheimer disease. *JAMA*, 278, 1349–1356.

Farrer, L. A., Friedland, R. P., Bowirrat, A., Waraska, K., Korczyn, A. and Baldwin, C. T. 2003. Genetic and environmental epidemiology of Alzheimer's disease in Arabs residing in Israel. *Journal of Molecular Neuroscience*, 20, 207–212.

Ferri, C. P., Prince, M., Brayne, C., Brodaty, H., Fratiglioni, L., Ganguli, M., Hall, K., Hasegawa, K., Hendrie, H., Huang, Y., Jorm, A., Mathers, C., Menezes, P. R., Rimmer, E. and Scazufca, M. 2005. Global prevalence of dementia: a Delphi consensus study. *Lancet*, 366, 2112–2117.

Flint, M. 1978. Is there a secular trend in age of menopause? *Maturitas*, 1, 133–139.

Fox, M. 2012. *Grandma Knows Best: The Evolution of Post-menopausal Longevity and the Preservation of Cognitive Function*. PhD thesis. Cambridge: University of Cambridge.

Fox, M. 2018. 'Evolutionary medicine' perspectives on Alzheimer's disease: review and new directions. *Ageing Research Reviews*, 47, 140–148.

Fox, M., Berzuini, C. and Knapp, L. A. 2013a. Cumulative estrogen exposure, number of menstrual cycles, and Alzheimer's risk in a cohort of British women. *Psychoneuroendocrinology*, 38, 2973–2982.

Fox, M., Berzuini, C. and Knapp, L. A. 2013b. Maternal breastfeeding history and Alzheimer's disease risk. *Journal of Alzheimer's Disease*, 37, 809–821.

Fox, M., Berzuini, C., Knapp, L. A. and Glynn, L. M. 2018. Women's pregnancy life history and Alzheimer's risk: can immunoregulation explain the link? *American Journal of Alzheimer's Disease & Other Dementias*, 33, 516–526.

Fox, M., Knorr, D. A. and Haptonstall, K. M. 2019. Alzheimer's disease and symbiotic microbiota: an evolutionary medicine perspective. *Annals of the New York Academy of Sciences*, 1449, 3–24.

Fox, M., Siddarth, P., Oughli, H., Nguyen, S., Milillo, M., Aguilar, Y., Ercoli, L. and Lavretsky, H. 2021. Women who breastfeed exhibit cognitive benefits after age 50. *Evolution, Medicine, and Public Health*, 9, 322–331.

Fratiglioni, L., Wang, H.-X., Ericsson, K., Maytan, M. and Winblad, B. 2000. Influence of social network on occurrence of dementia: a community-based longitudinal study. *Lancet*, 355, 1315–1319.

Gavrilov, L. A. and Gavrilova, N. S. 2000. Validation of exceptional longevity. *Population and Development Review*, 26, 403.

Geerlings, M. I., Ruitenberg, A., Witteman, J. C. M., Van Swieten, J. C., Hofman, A., Van Duijn, C. M., Breteler, M. M. B. and Launer, L. J. 2001. Reproductive period and risk of dementia in postmenopausal women. *JAMA*, 285, 1475–1481.

Gerdes, L. U., Gerdes, C., Hansen, P. S., Klausen, I. C. and Færgeman, O. 1996. Are men carrying the apolipoprotein ε4- or ε2 allele less fertile than ε3ε3 genotypes? *Human Genetics*, 98, 239–242.

Glass, D. J. and Arnold, S. E. 2012. Some evolutionary perspectives on Alzheimer's disease pathogenesis and pathology. *Alzheimer's and Dementia*, 8, 343–351.

Green, R. C., Cupples, L. A., Kurz, A., Auerbach, S., Go, R., Sadovnick, D., Duara, R., Kukull, W. A., Chui, H., Edeki, T., Griffith, P. A., Friedland, R. P., Bachman, D. and Farrer, L. 2003. Depression as a risk factor for Alzheimer disease: the MIRAGE study. *Archives of Neurology*, 60, 753–759.

Greenfield, J. P., Leung, L. W., Cai, D., Kaasik, K., Gross, R. S., Rodriguez-Boulan, E., Greengard, P. and Xu, H. 2002. Estrogen lowers Alzheimer β-amyloid generation by stimulating trans-Golgi network vesicle biogenesis. *Journal of Biological Chemistry*, 277, 12128–12136.

Gunten, A., Clerc, M., Tomar, R. and John-Smith, P. 2018. Evolutionary considerations on aging and Alzheimer's disease. *Journal of Alzheimer's Disease and Parkinsonism*, 8, 423.

Gureje, O., Ogunniyi, A., Baiyewu, O., Price, B., Unverzagt, F. W., Evans, R. M., Smith-Gamble, V., Lane, K. A., Gao, S. and Hall, K. S. 2005. APOE ε4 is not associated with Alzheimer's disease in elderly Nigerians. *Annals of Neurology*, 59, 182–185.

Gurven, M. and Kaplan, H. 2007. Longevity among hunter-gatherers: a cross-cultural examination. *Population and Development Review*, 33, 321–365.

Gurven, M., Kaplan, H., Winking, J., Finch, C. and Crimmins, E. M. 2008. Aging and inflammation in two epidemiological worlds. *Journals of Gerontology: Series A*, 63, 196–199.

Hahn-Holbrook, J., Dunkel Schetter, C. and Haselton, M. 2013. The advantages and disadvantages of breastfeeding for maternal mental and physical health. In: M. Spiers, P. Geller and J. Kloss (eds.), *Women's Health Psychology*. Hoboken, NJ: Wiley, pp. 414–439.

Hawkes, K., O'Connell, J. F. and Blurton Jones, N. G. 1997. Hadza women's time allocation, offspring provisioning, and the evolution of long postmenopausal life spans. *Current Anthropology*, 38, 551–577.

Hawkes, K., O'Connell, J. F., Blurton Jones, N. G., Alvarez, H. and Charnov, E. L. 2000. The grandmother hypothesis and human evolution. In: L. Cronk, N. Chagnon and W. Irons (eds.), *Adaptation and Human Behavior: An Anthropological Perspective*. Piscataway, NJ: Aldine Transaction, pp. 231–252.

He, L.-N., Recker, R. R., Deng, H.-W. and Dvornyk, V. 2009. A polymorphism of apolipoprotein E (*APOE*) gene is associated with age at natural menopause in Caucasian females. *Maturitas*, 62, 37–41.

Helmer, C., Damon, D., Letenneur, L., Fabrigoule, C., Barberger-Gateau, P., Lafont, S., Fuhrer, R., Antonucci, T., Commenges, D. and Orgogozo, J. 1999. Marital status and risk of Alzheimer's disease: a French population-based cohort study. *Neurology*, 53, 1953–1953.

Hesson, J. 2012. Cumulative estrogen exposure and prospective memory in older women. *Brain and Cognition*, 80, 89–95.

Heys, M., Jiang, C., Cheng, K. K., Zhang, W., Yeung, S. L. A., Lam, T. H., Leung, G. M. and Schooling, C. M. 2011. Life long endogenous estrogen exposure and later adulthood cognitive function in a population of naturally postmenopausal women from Southern China: the Guangzhou Biobank Cohort Study.

Psychoneuroendocrinology, 36, 864–873.

Himes, N. E. 1970. *Medical History of Contraception*. New York: Schocken Books.

Holmen, K., Ericsson, K. and Winblad, B. 2000. Social and emotional loneliness among non-demented and demented elderly people. *Archives of Gerontology and Geriatrics*, 31, 177–192.

Holtzman, D. M., Morris, J. C. and Goate, A. M. 2011. Alzheimer's disease: the challenge of the second century. *Science Translational Medicine*, 3, 77sr1.

Hong, X., Zhang, X. and Li, H. 2001. A case-control study of endogenous estrogen and risk of Alzheimer's disease. *Zhonghua liu xing bing xue za zhi = Zhonghua liuxingbingxue zazhi*, 22, 379–382.

Hornsey, I. S. 2012. *Alcohol and Its Role in the Evolution of Human Society*. Cambridge: Royal Society of Chemistry.

Huang, T., Shafrir, A. L., Eliassen, A. H., Rexrode, K. M. and Tworoger, S. S. 2019. Estimated number of lifetime ovulatory years and its determinants in relation to levels of circulating inflammatory biomarkers. *American Journal of Epidemiology*, 189, 660–670.

Huang, W. J., Zhang, X. and Chen, W. W. 2016. Role of oxidative stress in Alzheimer's disease (review). *Biomedical Reports*, 4, 519–522.

Imtiaz, B., Tuppurainen, M., Rikkonen, T., Kivipelto, M., Soininen, H., Kröger, H. and Tolppanen, A.-M. 2017. Postmenopausal hormone therapy and Alzheimer disease: a prospective cohort study. *Neurology*, 88, 1062–1068.

Jasienska, G., Ellison, P. T., Galbarczyk, A., Jasienski, M., Kalemba-Drozdz, M., Kapiszewska, M., Nenko, I., Thune, I. and Ziomkiewicz, A.

2015. Apolipoprotein E (ApoE) polymorphism is related to differences in potential fertility in women: a case of antagonistic pleiotropy? *Proceedings of the Royal Society B: Biological Sciences*, 282, 20142395.

Jeste, D. V., Lee, E. E. and Cacioppo, S. 2020. Battling the modern behavioral epidemic of loneliness: suggestions for research and interventions. *JAMA Psychiatry*, 77, 553–554.

Jones, N. B. 2016. *Demography and Evolutionary Ecology of Hadza Hunter-Gatherers*. Cambridge: Cambridge University Press.

Kachel, A. F., Premo, L. S. and Hublin, J.-J. 2011. Grandmothering and natural selection. *Proceedings of the Royal Society B: Biological Sciences*, 278, 384–391.

Karran, E., Mercken, M. and Destrooper, B. 2011. The amyloid cascade hypothesis for Alzheimer's disease: an appraisal for the development of therapeutics. *Nature Reviews Drug Discovery*, 10, 698–712.

Kim, J., Stewart, R., Shin, I. and Yoon, J. 2003. Limb length and dementia in an older Korean population. *Journal of Neurology, Neurosurgery & Psychiatry*, 74, 427–432.

Kinney, J. W., Bemiller, S. M., Murtishaw, A. S., Leisgang, A. M., Salazar, A. M. and Lamb, B. T. 2018. Inflammation as a central mechanism in Alzheimer's disease. *Alzheimer's & Dementia: Translational Research & Clinical Interventions*, 4, 575–590.

Kivipelto, M., Helkala, E. L., Laakso, M. P., Hanninen, T., Hallikainen, M., Alhainen, K., Iivonen, S., Mannermaa, A., Tuomilehto, J. and Nissinen, A. 2002. Apolipoprotein E epsilon4 allele, elevated midlife total cholesterol level, and high midlife systolic blood pressure are independent risk factors for late-life Alzheimer disease. *Annals of Internal Medicine*, 137, 149–155.

Klaver, C., Kliffen, M., Van Duijn, C. M., Hofman, A., Cruts, M., Grobbee, D. E., Van Broeckhoven, C. and De Jong, P. 1998. Genetic association of apolipoprotein E with age-related macular degeneration. *American Journal of Human Genetics*, 63, 200–206.

Koochmeshgi, J., Hosseini-Mazinani, S. M., Seifati, S. M., Hosein-Pur-Nobari, N. and Teimoori-Toolabi, L. 2004. Apolipoprotein E genotype and age at menopause. *Annals of the New York Academy of Sciences*, 1019, 564–567.

Lahdenperä, M., Lummaa, V., Helle, S., Tremblay, M. and Russell, A. F. 2004. Fitness benefits of prolonged post-reproductive lifespan in women. *Nature*, 428, 178–181.

Ley, S. H., Li, Y., Tobias, D. K., Manson, J. E., Rosner, B., Hu, F. B. and Rexrode, K. M. 2017. Duration of reproductive life span, age at menarche, and age at menopause are associated with risk of cardiovascular disease in women. *Journal of the American Heart Association*, 6, e006713.

Li, J., Chen, Y., Wu, H. and Li, L. 2014. Apolipoprotein E (Apo E) gene polymorphisms and recurrent pregnancy loss: a meta-analysis. *Journal of Assisted Reproduction and Genetics*, 31, 139–148.

Mahley, R. W. and Rall Jr, S. C. 2000. Apolipoprotein E: far more than a lipid transport protein. *Annual Review of Genomics and Human Genetics*, 1, 507–537.

Martins, R. N., Clarnette, R., Fisher, C., Broe, G. A., Brooks, W. S., Montgomery, P. and Gandy, S. E. 1995. ApoE genotypes in Australia: roles in early and late onset Alzheimer's disease and Down's syndrome. *Neuroreport*, 6, 1513–1516.

Medawar, P. B. 1952. *An Unsolved Problem of Biology*. London: HK Lewis.

Meng, F.-T., Wang, Y.-L., Liu, J., Zhao, J., Liu, R.-Y. and Zhou, J.-N. 2012. ApoE genotypes are associated with age at natural menopause in Chinese females. *AGE*, 34, 1023–1032.

Minihane, A., Jofre-Monseny, L., Olano-Martin, E. and Rimbach, G. 2007. ApoE genotype, cardiovascular risk and responsiveness to dietary fat manipulation. *Proceedings of the Nutrition Society*, 66, 183–197.

Mor, G., Nilsen, J., Horvath, T., Bechmann, I., Brown, S., Garcia-Segura, L. M. and Naftolin, F. 1999. Estrogen and microglia: a regulatory system that affects the brain. *Journal of Neurobiology*, 40, 484–496.

Mortazavizadeh, Z., Maercker, A., Roth, T., Savaskan, E. and Forstmeier, S. 2020. Quality of the caregiving relationship and quality of life in mild Alzheimer's dementia. *Psychogeriatrics*, 20, 568–577.

Mutlu, B., Bas, A. Y., Aksoy, N. and Taskin, A. 2012. The effect of maternal number of births on oxidative and antioxidative systems in cord blood. *Journal of Maternal–Fetal & Neonatal Medicine*, 25, 802–805.

Nesse, R. M. and Williams, G. C. 1996. *Why We Get Sick: The New Science of Darwinian Medicine*. New York: Random House.

Oria, R. B., Patrick, P. D., Zhang, H., Lorntz, B., De Castro Costa, C. M., Brito, G. A. C., Barrett, L. J., Lima, A. A. M. and Guerrant, R. L. 2005. APOE4 protects the cognitive development in children with heavy diarrhea burdens in Northeast Brazil. *Pediatric Research*, 57, 310–316.

Papadimitriou, A. 2016. The evolution of the age at menarche from prehistorical to modern times. *Journal of Pediatric and Adolescent Gynecology*, 29, 527–530.

Peccei, J. S. 2001. Menopause: adaptation or epiphenomenon? *Evolutionary Anthropology*, 10, 43–57.

Piazza-Gardner, A. K., Gaffud, T. J. and Barry, A. E. 2013. The impact of alcohol on Alzheimer's disease: a systematic review. *Aging & Mental Health*, 17, 133–146.

Pontzer, H., Raichlen, D. A., Wood, B. M., Mabulla, A. Z., Racette, S. B. and Marlowe, F. W. 2012. Hunter-gatherer energetics and human obesity. *PLoS ONE*, 7, e40503.

Prince, M. J., Acosta, D., Guerra, M., Huang, Y., Jimenez-Velazquez, I. Z., Rodriguez, J. J. L., Salas, A., Sosa, A. L., Chua, K.-C. and Dewey, M. E. 2018. Reproductive period, endogenous estrogen exposure and dementia incidence among women in Latin America and China; a 10/66 population-based cohort study. *PLoS ONE*, 13, e0192889.

Ptok, U., Barkow, K. and Heun, R. 2002. Fertility and number of children in patients with Alzheimer's disease. *Archives of Women's Mental Health*, 5, 83–86.

Ravaja, N., Raikkonen, K., Lyytinen, H., Lehtimaki, T. and Keltikangas-Jarvinen, L. 1997. Apolipoprotein E phenotypes and cardiovascular responses to experimentally induced mental stress in adolescent boys. *Journal of Behavioral Medicine*, 20, 571–587.

Reiches, M. W., Ellison, P. T., Lipson, S. F., Sharrock, K. C., Gardiner, E. and Duncan, L. G. 2009. Pooled energy budget and human life history. *American Journal of Human Biology*, 21, 421–429.

Rook, G. A. W. 2007. The hygiene hypothesis and the increasing prevalence of chronic inflammatory disorders. *Transactions of the Royal Society of Tropical Medicine and Hygiene*, 101, 1072–1074.

Rook, G. A. W. 2012. Hygiene hypothesis and autoimmune

diseases. *Clinical Reviews in Allergy and Immunology*, 42, 5–15.

Sando, S. B., Melquist, S., Cannon, A., Hutton, M. L., Sletvold, O., Saltvedt, I., White, L. R., Lydersen, S. and Aasly, J. O. 2008. APOE *ε*4 lowers age at onset and is a high risk factor for Alzheimer's disease; a case control study from central Norway. *BMC Neurology*, 8, 9.

Sapolsky, R. M. and Finch, C. E. 2000. Alzheimer's disease and some speculations about the evolution of its modifiers. *Annals of the New York Academy of Sciences*, 924, 99–103.

Sayi, J., Patel, N., Premukumar, D., Adem, A., Windblad, B., Matuja, W., Mitui, E., Gatere, S., Friedand, R. and Koss, E. 1997. Apolipoprotein E polymorphism in elderly east Africans. *East African Medical Journal*, 74, 668–670.

Sellen, D. W. 2001. Comparison of infant feeding patterns reported for nonindustrial populations with current recommendations. *Journal of Nutrition*, 131, 2707–2715.

Shao, H., Breitner, J. C., Whitmer, R. A., Wang, J., Hayden, K., Wengreen, H., Corcoran, C., Tschanz, J., Norton, M. and Munger, R. 2012. Hormone therapy and Alzheimer disease dementia: new findings from the Cache County Study. *Neurology*, 79, 1846–1852.

Singh, P., Singh, M. and Mastana, S. 2006. APOE distribution in world populations with new data from India and the UK. *Annals of Human Biology*, 33, 279–308.

Song, Y., Stampfer, M. J. and Liu, S. 2004. Meta-analysis: apolipoprotein E genotypes and risk for coronary heart disease. *Annals of Internal Medicine*, 141, 137–147.

Stearns, S. C. and Koella, J. C. 2008. *Evolution in Health and*

Disease. Oxford: Oxford University Press.

Stuart-Macadam, P. 1995. Biocultural perspectives on breastfeeding. In: P. Stuart-Macadam and K. A. Dettwyler (eds.), *Breastfeeding: Biocultural Perspectives*. Berlin: Walter de Gruyter & Co., pp. 1–38.

Tao, Q., Ang, T. F. A., Decarli, C., Auerbach, S. H., Devine, S., Stein, T. D., Zhang, X., Massaro, J., Au, R. and Qiu, W. Q. 2018. Association of chronic low-grade inflammation with risk of Alzheimer disease in ApoE4 carriers. *JAMA Network Open*, 1, e183597.

Thomas, P. A. and Umberson, D. 2017. Do older parents' relationships with their adult children affect cognitive limitations, and does this differ for mothers and fathers? *Journals of Gerontology: Series B*, 73, 1133–1142.

Tsutaya, T., Shimomi, A., Fujisawa, S., Katayama, K. and Yoneda, M. 2016. Isotopic evidence of breastfeeding and weaning practices in a hunter-gatherer population during the Late/Final Jomon period in eastern Japan. *Journal of Archaeological Science*, 76, 70–78.

Tulchinsky, D. and Little, A. B. 1994. *Maternal–Fetal Endocrinology*. Philadelphia, PA: W.B. Saunders.

Twamley, E. W., Ropacki, S. A. L. and Bondi, M. W. 2006. Neuropsychological and neuroimaging changes in preclinical Alzheimer's disease. *Journal of the International Neuropsychological Society*, 12, 707–735.

UNICEF 2018. *Breastfeeding: A Mother's Gift, for Every Child*. New York: United Nations Children's Fund.

Van Den Heuvel, C., Thornton, E. and Vink, R. 2007. Traumatic brain injury and Alzheimer's disease: a review. *Progress in Brain Research*, 161, 303–316.

Waring, S., Rocca, W., Petersen, R., O'Brien, P., Tangalos, E. and Kokmen, E. 1999. Postmenopausal estrogen replacement therapy and risk of AD: a population-based study. *Neurology*, 52, 965–970.

Williams, G. 1957. Pleiotropy, natural selection, and the evolution of senescence. *Evolution*, 11, 398–411.

Wilson, R. S., Krueger, K. R., Arnold, S. E., Schneider, J. A., Kelly, J. F., Barnes, L. L., Tang, Y. and Bennett, D. A. 2007. Loneliness and risk of Alzheimer disease. *Archives of General Psychiatry*, 64, 234–240.

Wozniak, M. A., Itzhaki, R. F., Faragher, E. B., James, M. W., Ryder, S. D. and Irving, W. L. 2002. Apolipoprotein E-e4 protects against severe liver disease caused by hepatitis C virus. *Hepatology*, 36, 456–463.

Wozniak, M. A., Riley, E. and Itzhaki, R. 2004. Apolipoprotein E polymorphisms and risk of malaria. *Journal of Medical Genetics*, 41, 145–146.

Wu, Y. C., Lin, Y. C., Yu, H. L., Chen, J. H., Chen, T. F., Sun, Y., Wen, L. L., Yip, P. K., Chu, Y. M. and Chen, Y. C. 2015. Association between air pollutants and dementia risk in the elderly. *Alzheimer's & Dementia: Diagnosis, Assessment & Disease Monitoring*, 1, 220–228.

Zanetti, O., Solerte, S. and Cantoni, F. 2009. Life expectancy in Alzheimer's disease (AD). *Archives of Gerontology and Geriatrics*, 49, 237–243.

Ziomkiewicz, A., Sancilio, A., Galbarczyk, A., Klimek, M., Jasienska, G. and Bribiescas, R. G. 2016. Evidence for the cost of reproduction in humans: high lifetime reproductive effort is associated with greater oxidative stress in post-menopausal women. *PLoS ONE*, 11, e0145753.

Psychopharmacology and Evolution

Paul St John-Smith, Riadh Abed and Martin Brüne

Abstract

Psychopharmacology is the scientific study of the effects of drugs on thoughts, emotions and behaviour as well as the therapeutic implications of their role in treating mental disorders. Psychopharmacology focuses on understanding relevant mental processes as the key to finding new medications and improving clinical outcomes in mental disorder. Interconnected with this, neuropsychopharmacology is the complementary discipline of the study of the basic neural mechanisms that drugs act upon to influence behaviour.[1] Progress has been slow in recent decades with no major new classes of medication being added to the psychiatric formulary. We suggest that evolutionary thinking brings novel additional scientific perspectives to psychiatry and its basic sciences that highlight the evolutionary history of cell communication, neurotransmission and substances that can alter the brain in various ways. Evolutionary perspectives of function and phylogeny also provide a deeper understanding of how natural as well as artificial chemicals (i.e. psychotropic medications) utilise evolved neuronal pathways for their actions. Evolutionary theory can thereby help us to understand the psychological effects and side effects of psychotropic medications as well as assist in the discovery and testing of new drugs.

Keywords

evolution, evolutionary psychiatry, natural selection, neuromodulators, neurotransmitters, psychopharmacology

Key Points

- Understanding the evolutionary history of neurotransmitters, receptors and the chemical agents acting on these receptors is fundamental for the understanding of the action, side effects and placebo responses of psychopharmacological drugs.
- Substances known as 'neurotransmitters' are evolutionarily ancient chemicals that originally served a range of biological functions, including defence against pathogens and hormonal activity; this multiplicity of functions complicates their therapeutic management.

- The evolutionary approach recognises that, because psychiatric disorders are grounded in complex evolved biological processes, psychopharmacological drugs do not act only on specific psychiatric syndromes or symptoms but also impact multiple neuronal processes and cell communication systems.
- An evolutionary framework can suggest practical strategies for optimising functioning and can assist in the search for and testing of new drugs.

18.1 Introduction

The prevailing biomedical approach considers psychiatric disorders as primarily brain disorders (i.e. dysfunctions that are internal to the central nervous system (CNS) and are due to diseased brain circuits). By contrast, the evolutionary psychiatrist views the brain as the organ of the mind that facilitates access to external reality and is in constant interaction with it (see Chapter 2).

---

[1] The word 'drug' is ambiguous, including both medical/therapeutic substances as well as substances for recreational purposes and substances of abuse (see Chapter 12). For the purposes of this chapter, we use the term 'drugs' to refer to chemicals developed and used for therapeutic purposes.

This allows individuals to navigate the physical and social worlds to enhance their survival and reproductive success. Thereby, mental disorders involve the relational world, not just brain chemicals and circuits. This approach mandates that the environment outside the brain can be considered as part of any pathogenesis (see Chapters 1 and 2). This difference in perspective has profound consequences not only as to what should be considered a disorder, but also as to how and when particular symptoms and syndromes can be treated and by what type of therapy. Evolutionary psychopharmacology is based on comparative pharmacology, ontogenetic pharmacology and pharmacology using (phylogenetic) animal models of function and disease. The relevant processes investigated therefore include emotions, cognition and behaviour, which are executed by the action of a highly complex, evolved CNS.

The human brain is considered to be the most complex organ that has evolved in the known universe. In order to fully understand the action of psychotropic medication it is necessary to explore not only the current structure and functions of CNSs, but also their relevant evolution and the differential activities of the drugs acting on them (Stahl, 2000). Neuropsychopharmacology is the interdisciplinary science related to psychopharmacology and fundamental neuroscience that studies the neural mechanisms upon which drugs act to influence behaviour. These studies involve consideration of neurotransmission/receptor activity, biochemical processes and neural processes and circuitry.

While CNSs integrate exteroceptive and interoceptive information (without necessarily being absolutely accurate in this regard), they do so by crosstalk between neurons and perineuronal glia utilising a broad array of substances called 'neurotransmitters', 'neuropeptides' and 'secondary messengers' (also called bio-mediators; Roshchina, 2010). These chemical activities allow organisms to navigate their physical and social worlds to enhance their survival and reproductive success. Allman (1999) stated that CNSs evolved to maintain homoeostasis as a prerequisite to help the organism fulfil its biological function (i.e. survival and reproduction). More recently, Solms (2021) proposed that homeostasis was also the primary function of consciousness.

An evolutionary approach to psychopharmacology also adds supplementary insights into the evolution of CNSs over and above conventional medical approaches. These include insights into synaptic transmission, the evolution of psychoactive substances other than the classic neurotransmitters, how and when animals (including our ancestors) intentionally began using psychoactive substances for specific purposes and what we can learn from this.

We briefly describe aspects of the evolution of CNSs and their main components that execute neuronal transmission. We also cover some of the evolutionary background knowledge of psychoactive substances and their utilisation as 'medicines'. Finally, we summarise issues around the evolutionary constraints affecting the action of psychotropic substances and examine some of the predictable and inevitable undesirable effects in psychopharmacological interventions. With regards to evolution and neuropsychopharmacology, we can now examine what is the proximate mechanism of action of a given neurotransmitter or psychoactive compound and how synaptic transmission develops in a growing organism from early developmental stages to adulthood (ontogeny). Furthermore, we can examine where that neurotransmitter or psychoactive substance comes from evolutionarily (phylogeny) and also what are its adaptive properties. It is, however, important to organise this information by employing the theoretical framework – first proposed by Nicolaas Tinbergen in 1963 – explaining why evolution is crucial for the comprehensive understanding of biological processes (see Chapter 1).

18.1.1 Tinbergen's Evolutionary Framework and Its Importance

The evolutionary theoretical framework for understanding causality proposed by Tinbergen is highly relevant to evolutionary considerations of psychopharmacology because human cognition, emotions and behaviour can only be properly understood if both proximate and evolutionary contributors are addressed (see Table 1.1 in Chapter 1).

However, we recognise that it can be difficult for clinicians to apply evolutionary models when only the perspective of dysfunction and disorder is considered because there is no obvious, immediate adaptive value of any disease or 'disorder'. Nevertheless, it becomes easier to comprehend some of these enigmatic issues when it is recognised that some conditions considered 'disorders' are not always fundamental disease processes nor necessarily categorically distinct from 'normalcy'; they may just be the unpleasant by-products of mechanisms that are adaptive (see Chapter 1). For instance, some major conditions of psychiatric concern such as anxiety develop because they represent defences, akin to cough and fever, even if the defence comes in exaggerated or dysregulated forms (Brüne, 2014; Nesse, 2011; Stearns et al., 2010; see also Chapters 1 and 2 of this volume).

18.2 Evolutionary Aspects of Neuropsychopharmacology and CNSs

18.2.1 Brain Size and Cell Communication

CNSs evolved in animals as organised collectives of specialised, excitable cells. Complex nervous systems probably evolved several times independently (Moroz, 2009). Allometric analyses suggest that there is a direct relationship between brain and body size because larger bodies require more neurons (Jerison, 1973) or because larger bodies can metabolically maintain a larger number of neurons (Watson et al., 2012). The African elephant brain contains 257 billion neurons, which is about three times the number in human brains at around 86 billion neurons (Herculano-Houzel et al., 2014). The evolution of brains is constrained by energy consumption because neurons are metabolically expensive (Fehm et al., 2006).

Cellular communication is crucial for supporting vital biological processes like homoeostasis in multicellular organisms. Excitatory cells are endowed with molecular signalling pathways for synaptic communication that probably evolved from vesicular systems and membrane ionic channels at least a billion years ago (Ryan and Grant, 2009). Cellular communication appears to have occurred early in the evolution of life, being apparent even in the most primitive organisms such as the extant prokaryotes, bacteria and archaea (Le Duc and Schöneberg, 2019). In contrast to prokaryotes, eukaryote cells possess internal organisation, which makes them more complex, structured and efficient in particular niches. Cellular communication comprises multiple routes of sending and receiving information, whereby input can come from the cell's environment (endocrine, paracrine) or from the cell itself (autocrine). Cellular

communication is energetically costly and therefore must have resulted in a substantial selective advantage (pay-off). In other words, natural selection must have acted on the chemical and physical signals in terms of energetic features (e.g. amplitude or concentration), duration and speed, as these processes are found universally throughout life and are considered to be the blueprint of all organismic communication systems (Le Duc and Schöneberg, 2019).

18.2.2 Evolutionary Origins of Receptors and Toxins

Phylogenetically, prior to the cellular utilisation of neurotransmitters, the very existence of life entailed the exchange of ions between the environment and the cell. Transmembrane-spanning peptides evolved to form ion channels and transporters. During the evolution of prokaryotes, transmembrane ion exchange became regulated by molecules that bind to the ion channel and modulate its permeability (Le Duc and Schöneberg, 2019). This prototypical receptor came in multiple forms of ligand-gated ion channels and ion pumps (Chen et al., 1999; Jaiteh et al., 2016; Tasneem et al., 2005). For example, nicotinic acetylcholine receptors are involved not only in neuron to neuron but also neuromuscular signal transduction. Given these systems' universality in nature (particularly in organisms that consume other species), it is unsurprising that their ligand-gated ion channels can be hijacked or usurped by many toxic substances that evolved in plants and other organisms as a defence against consumption by herbivores or parasites (e.g. curare). They also occur in prey species such as snails (e.g. alpha-conotoxins) and in small vertebrates such as frogs (e.g. epibatidine) and snakes (e.g. viper peptides), acting on nicotinic acetylcholine receptors and causing paralysis of the victim (Kudryavtsev et al., 2015).

18.2.3 Receptor Mechanisms

Energy-rich nucleotides and their phosphates (e.g. ATP and GTP) are also among the oldest biomolecules. They not only form the structural basis of RNA and DNA, but also serve as metabotropic molecules in signalling pathways. Nucleotide triphosphate cyclases are membrane-anchored and soluble molecules producing cAMP and cGMP, which are intracellular signalling molecules. Cyclases are regulated by a variety of molecules, including calmodulin, G proteins, nitric oxide, calcium and bicarbonate (Steegborn, 2014). These universal intracellular secondary messengers can also be targeted by drugs and toxins, including methylxanthines (e.g. caffeine), which increase the availability of cAMP and cGMP by inhibiting the phosphodiesterase. Importantly, many medical drugs act indirectly via receptors and enzymes that modulate cAMP or cGMP, including epinephrine, beta-adrenoceptor agonists and blockers, dopamine receptor agonists and antagonists and nitroglycerine (Le Duc and Schöneberg, 2019).

Over evolutionary timescales, signalling cascades have become increasingly complex and specific. Signal specificity is mainly achieved at the receptor level, where transducers decode and integrate signals into metabotropic or ionotropic information. It has been suggested that the number of components involved in cellular communication in prokaryotes and eukaryotes increased relatively to genome size (Konstantinidis and Tiedje, 2004; Tamames et al., 1996).

18.2.4 Neurones and Synaptic Transmission

Several cell types are specialised in the transmission of information over long distances, and this especially applies to neurons, whose axons may send electrical impulses at a speed of 100 metres per second. The evolution of myelin sheaths surrounding axons greatly accelerated the information transfer from one neuron to the other (Hofman, 2014). As a rule of thumb, most axosomatic synapses are inhibitory, whereas the majority of axodendritic synapses are excitatory, and axo-axonal synapses are double inhibitory, thus being disinhibitory (Zilles, 2005). Excitatory synaptic transmission is particularly expensive in terms of energetic demands, and even though it can be partly controlled by lowering the firing rate of neurons, the maintenance of membrane polarisation is costly and increases with the surface area of the membrane (Attwell and Laughlin, 2001).

Comparative analyses of the proteomic composition of synapses suggests that proto-synapses evolved earlier than the first primitive nervous systems (Ryan and Grant, 2009). Some protein families found in synapses such as calcium transporters and protein kinases also exist in unicellular organisms. Synaptic protein families are present in unicellular eukaryotes such as the yeast *Saccharomyces cerevisiae* and the amoeba *Dictyostelium discoideum* (Ryan and Grant, 2009). In chordates, several genome duplications permitted an increase in the number of synaptic gene families, including ones coding for glutamate and GABA receptors and postsynaptic membrane proteins (Emes and Grant, 2012; Ryan and Grant, 2009).

In primates, the number of synapses linked per neuron increased from 2,000 to 5,600 in non-human primates, then to 6,800–10,000 synapses per neuron in humans (Changeux, 2005).

Recent research has shown that synaptic functioning critically depends on the action of non-neuronal cells called neuroglia. Neuroglia comprise both oligodendrocytes and astrocytes. A single astrocyte cell can interact with up to 2 million synapses (Fields et al., 2014). Oligodendrocytes not only produce the myelin sheaths for up to 60 axons; they are also involved in the repair of damaged myelin sheaths after stroke (Edgar and Sibille, 2012). Moreover, oligodendrocytes maintain neuronal plasticity. Because they are rich in iron, oligodendrocytes are particularly vulnerable to oxidative stress and to glutamatergic toxicity (Haroon et al., 2017).

Astrocytes are involved in maintaining local ion concentrations and pH homoeostasis. They also support neuronal functioning by providing metabolites such as glucose and cholesterol. In addition, astroglia produce the extracellular matrix, mainly proteoglycans (Maeda, 2015), and they remove potentially toxic metabolic products, including excess glutamate (Faissner et al., 2010; Nedergaard et al., 2003). Furthermore, astroglia actively release neurotransmitters such as glutamate, steroids, lipids, neuropeptides and growth factors, which they also partly synthesise, and astroglia appear to help maintain the blood–brain barrier, rendering them 'multifunctional housekeeping cells'. In light of these complex interactions between neurons and neuroglia, Faissner et al. (2010) have suggested the term 'tripartite synapse', thus acknowledging the role of neuroglia in cell communication. This notion seems warranted from an evolutionary point of view, as the number of astroglia has significantly increased over evolutionary time. Specifically, whereas the ratio of the number of neurons to astroglia is about 6:1 in nematodes and about 3:1 in small rodents, this ratio in humans is about 1:1.4, suggesting that there are more astroglia than neurons in the human CNS. This evolutionary development cannot be explained by the metabolic demands of neurons alone (which are relatively similar among higher vertebrates). Instead, it more likely reflects the regulatory function of astroglia with regards to synaptic transmission, synaptogenesis and neurogenesis (Nedergaard et al., 2003).

18.2.5 Evolution of Neurotransmitters and Other Signalling Molecules

In multicellular organisms, chemical communication among cells is maintained by a multitude of molecules (see Table 18.1). The evolution and

Table 18.1. Some representative functions of neurotransmitters in different organisms (adapted from Roshchina, 2010)

Neurotransmitter	Microorganisms	Plants	Animals
Acetylcholine	Regulation of motility	Regulation of membrane permeability Growth and development	Carriage of nerve impulses between neurons and neuromuscular junctions Parasympathetic nervous system Arousal, attention memory and motivation
Dopamine	Bacterial growth stimulation Defensive reactions	Response to stressors Defensive reactions Growth and development	Basal ganglia movement control (humans) Prolactin inhibition (hypothalamo-pituitary) (humans) Limbic (emotional regulation) (humans) Reward mechanisms Cardiovascular effects on pulse and heart rate Embryological development
Noradrenaline	Bacterial growth stimulation	Growth and development processes Defence reactions	Sympathetic nervous system
Adrenaline	Bacterial growth stimulation	Growth and development processes Defence reactions	Vasodilatation Sympathetic nervous system
Serotonin	Cellular aggregation and regulation of membrane potentials Bacterial virulence	Growth and development processes Toxins Defence against fungi	Control of gastrointestinal function, appetite, sleep, aggression, memory, mood and temperature regulation Embryonic regulation
GABA	Cell regulation of pH	Cellular signalling	Inhibitory actions in vertebrate central nervous system
Glutamate	Stress responses Cell regulation of pH Metabolic processes	Stress responses to temperature shock, hypoxia and increased levels of calcium	Excitatory function in vertebrate central nervous system
Histamine	Stimulation of growth and cellular aggregation	Stings/defence	Bee stings and venoms Vertebrate sleep–wake cycles Bronchoconstriction Gastric acid secretion Urticaria and itch

development of sophisticated nervous systems appears not only to have been limited by or dependent upon the formation of new or better transmitter substances, receptor proteins, transducers and effector proteins, but also to have involved improved reorganisation and utilisation of these highly developed elements, producing more advanced and refined circuitry through the processes of natural and sexual selection (Roshchina, 2010; also see Chapters 3 and 4 of this volume).

Neurotransmitters are stored in vesicles located in the presynaptic neuron, and they are released into the synaptic cleft upon receiving an incoming electrical signal. The neurotransmitters subsequently diffuse across the synaptic cleft and bind to specific receptors on the surface of the postsynaptic neuron, including ion channels or G protein-coupled receptors (GPCRs). Many neurotransmitters reach high concentrations in the synaptic cleft, while their affinity for corresponding postsynaptic receptors is relatively low, such that neurotransmitters often rapidly dissolve from the receptor, which terminates signalling. In addition, several neurotransmitters are inactivated by enzymatic degradation or reuptake in the presynaptic neuron, a process that has been fine-tuned over hundreds of millions of years of evolution (Ryan and Grant, 2009).

On the postsynaptic membrane to which the neurotransmitters bind, receptor proteins excite, inhibit or otherwise modify the excitability of the postsynaptic neuron (Guyton and Hall, 2006; Raven et al., 2017). Excitation occurs directly via cation channels, whereas anion channels are opened by inhibitory neurotransmitters. Thus, while some neurotransmitters produce rather short, sharply peaking action potentials at ionotropic receptors, other compounds produce much slower alterations at metabotropic receptors (Panksepp, 1998). Synaptic transmission may also utilise secondary messengers for prolonged postsynaptic neuronal changes via GPCRs that can activate enzymatic activity or gene transcription (Guyton and Hall, 2006). By and large, as the production of neurotransmitters is energetically expensive, evolution has selected for organisms to recycle rather than waste such precious molecules. An imbalance in these evolved equilibria may cause neurological or psychiatric symptoms. For example, a disruption in the dopamine system results in Parkinson's disease. Dopamine–

glutamate dysfunction plays an important role in schizophrenia and bipolar affective disorder (Tomasetti et al., 2017). Serotonin seems to be involved in the pathophysiology of major depression and anxiety disorders (Jakobsen et al., 2017).

Neuropeptides are relatively simple protein molecules that can stimulate cells over larger distances, where they act as neurohormones. For example, enkephalins and endorphins act on the same receptors as morphine, thus attenuating pain perception. In vertebrates, the opioid receptor system emerged some 450 million years ago following genome duplications in the first jawed vertebrates (Dreborg et al., 2008). In addition to their roles in pain perception, enkephalins and endorphins are also involved in immune modulation (Wybran, 1985), control of pituitary hormone release and paracrine stimulation of cells in the pancreas and gonads (Petraglia et al., 1993). Thus, the opioid system is critical for pain perception, stress-coping responses, sexual behaviour and food intake. This explains why endorphin withdrawal may play a role in the pathophysiology of the premenstrual syndrome, postpartum depression (Halbreich and Endicott, 1981) and major depression.

Because chemical messengers are preserved between species and even between kingdoms (Roshchina, 2010), researchers can test drugs on multiple species before their introduction to humans. However, extrapolation of effects from other species is problematic, as some psychiatric conditions (e.g. schizophrenia) have no clear homologue in animals (Jones et al., 2011). Evolutionary perspectives on the universal roles of these systems should be indispensable for understanding psychopharmacology. Many psychoactive medications act on multiple neurotransmitters in many different organisms and systems, and almost none specifically act on humans or disease-specific neurons. This is because current psychiatric drugs are not truly disease specific, and in any case, psychiatric disorders generally involve multiple domains of aetiology, mechanism and dysfunction. For example, the multifaceted symptomatology of mania has not been reflected in any one of the large number of animal models, where locomotor activity remains the primary measure. In fact, this approach has resulted in numerous false positives for putative treatments (Young et al., 2011). Animal models for depression are also problematic (Belzung and Lemoine, 2011). Of the 18 potential models, it was concluded that only 6 have some potential predictive, face and construct validity. But despite best practice modelling, antidepressants have poor efficacy in many individuals (Kirsch, 2019). Furthermore, psychopharmacological treatments affect not only neurons but also somatic cells, as well as the gut microbiota, including commensals and pathogenic species (e.g. bacteria, viruses and fungi), which can have unintended consequences. Consequently, the prescription of psychopharmacological agents require complex cost–benefit calculations, as will be discussed later (Brüne, 2015).

An interesting evolutionary example illuminating the multiple and diverse functions of loosely related bio-mediators including neurotransmitters comes from demonstrating multiple drug effects as well as species cross-reactivity. In other words, we can examine the striking diversity of effects of closely related compounds. One example we use here is the multitude of actions and uses of psychotropic drugs and their activities against microorganisms (see Table 18.2).

We argue that a crossover of ideas from looking at other species and structure–function relationships is crucial for advancing psychopharmacology. Such an evolutionary perspective can expand the scope from looking only at the human mechanisms underlying attention, cognition and emotion to also looking at their phylogenetic origins and functional significance; in other words, it enables us to ask why such capacities exist in their current form.

It is important to note that genes, molecules, loci, emotions, attention and cognition interact in tangled causal pathways very different from those in any designed system. Understanding how molecules such as GABA or serotonin interact with multiple different receptors requires an integrative description of the mechanisms and their ontogeny, phylogeny and adaptive significance. Extreme complexity frustrates the understandable wish for simple models, but acknowledging this fact may suggest a route to new advances.

Evolutionary insights indicate that all organisms face broadly similar life challenges: to avoid predation and infection, to find food, to secure allies and status, to find mates, to reproduce and to care for offspring. The organism's fitness-enhancing efforts will produce various degrees of success or failure, and this explains why emotional states are positively or negatively valanced (Nesse and Ellsworth, 2009; Nesse and Stein, 2019) and why negatively valanced emotions (although aversive) can be adaptive and should only be diminished if it is safe to do so. Some studies have adapted methods for assessing emotions in humans and other animals to invertebrates, with intriguing results. Sea slugs, bees, crayfish, snails, crabs, flies and ants have all been shown to display various cognitive, behavioural and/or physiological phenomena that indicate internal states reminiscent of what we consider to be emotions. Given the limited neural architecture of many invertebrates and the powerful tools available within invertebrate research, these findings provide new opportunities for unveiling the neural mechanisms behind emotions and open new avenues towards the pharmacological manipulation of emotion and its genetic dissection, with advantages for disease research and therapeutic drug discovery (Perry and Baciadonna, 2017).

18.2.6 A Brief Evolutionary History of Psychopharmacology

Our evolutionary history of psychopharmacology starts with the ingestion of plants or specific plant parts, such as roots, buds, blossoms or fruits. Many plants evolved strategies to shield themselves against microorganisms by increasing the concentration of substances inhibiting bacterial, viral or fungal growth (Roshchina, 2010). Animals, particularly herbivores, evolved countermeasures against toxic plant products such as enzymatic degradation, and some ingestion of potentially toxic plant products may have helped keep the gut microbiota in healthy balance. Accordingly, 'pharmacophagy' became common among animals, including non-human primates (Fabrega, 1997; see also Chapter 12 of this volume). Palaeo-pharmacological studies demonstrate the use of medicinal plants in our evolutionary prehistory (Ellis, 2003). Medicinal plants were discovered in the Shanidar Cave, and remains of the areca nut were found in the Spirit Cave (Sneader, 2005). Geophagy (eating chemicals from the soil) was also part of the lives of our ancestors (Bender, 1965). There is in addition convincing evidence to suggest that Neanderthals possessed considerable knowledge about medicinal plants. One such individual found at the site of El Sidrón, now Spain, had apparently ingested

Table 18.2. Psychotropic diversity and antimicrobial reactivity (adapted from Kristiansen and Amaral, 1997; St John-Smith et al., 2013)

Drug name	Psychotropic group; function and some common clinical uses	Antimicrobial/anti-parasitic activity
Flurazepam	Benzodiazepine; anxiolytic, anticonvulsant, hypnotic, sedative and skeletal muscle-relaxant properties	Malaria *Toxoplasma gondii*
Diazepam	Benzodiazepine; anxiolytic, anticonvulsant, hypnotic, sedative and skeletal muscle-relaxant properties, used in anxiety and alcohol withdrawal	*Peptostreptococcus* spp.
Levomepromazine	Low-potency antipsychotic, strong analgesic, hypnotic and antiemetic properties	*Trypanosoma cruzi*
Amitriptyline	Antidepressant; pain syndromes, neuropathic pain, fibromyalgia, migraine, anxiolytic and anti-ulcer activity	*Bifidobacterium* spp. *Eubacterium* spp. *Proprionibacterium* spp. *Actinomyces* spp. *Peptococcus* spp.
Clonazepam	Benzodiazepine; seizures, panic disorder, akathisia	*Schistosoma mansoni*
Acetylcholinesterase inhibitors	Anti-dementia; myasthenia gravis, glaucoma, Alzheimer's disease, the Lewy body dementias and Parkinson's disease, cognitive impairments in patients with schizophrenia	Insecticides Nerve agents
Chlorpromazine	Antipsychotic; schizophrenia and bipolar disorder, severe behavioural problems, attention deficit hyperactivity disorder, nausea and vomiting, anxiety before surgery, hiccups	*Leishmania donovani, Candida albicans Staphylococcus aureus Enterococcus faecalis Escherichia coli Mycobacterium tuberculosis* Influenza virus Measles virus Herpes simplex virus
Phenothiazine	Antipsychotic; antihistamine	Insecticide Anti-helminthic *Bacteroides* spp. *Prevotella* spp. *Fusobacterium* spp.
Trifluoperazine	Antipsychotic; schizophrenia	*Shigella* spp. *Vibrio cholera Vibrio parahaemolyticus* Amoebiasis
Lithium	Mood stabiliser; schizoaffective disorder, bipolar disorder, resistant depression	Antiviral and antibacterial properties Herpes simplex virus
Isoniazid	MAOI/antidepressant	Mycobacterium
Linezolid	MAOI/antidepressant	Antibacterial *Staphylococcus aureus*
Levamisole	MAOI, stimulant; used to adulterate cocaine	Anti-helminthic
Bupranolol	Beta-adrenergic receptor antagonist	*Staphylococcus aureus Pseudomonas aeruginosa Bacillus subtilis Candida albicans*

Table 18.2. (cont.)

Drug name	Psychotropic group; function and some common clinical uses	Antimicrobial/anti-parasitic activity
Propranolol	Beta-adrenergic receptor antagonist; antihypertensive, antiarrhythmic, thyrotoxicosis, performance anxiety, essential tremors, migraine headaches	*Staphylococcus aureus* *Escherichia coli* *Pseudomonas aeruginosa*
Metronidazole	Disulfiram-like properties (N.B. disulfiram is active against *Staphylococcus aureus*)	Antibiotic
Diphenhydramine	Antihistamine; allergies, insomnia, tremor in parkinsonism, nausea	*Vibrio cholerae*
Haloperidol	Antipsychotic; schizophrenia, tics in Tourette's syndrome, mania in bipolar disorder, nausea and vomiting, delirium, agitation, acute psychosis, hallucinations in alcohol withdrawal	*Toxoplasma gondii* Rauscher murine leukaemia virus
Clomipramine	Antidepressant; obsessive-ompulsive disorder, panic disorder, major depressive disorder, chronic pain	*Leishmania donovani*
Imipramine	Antidepressant; Depression, anxiety, panic and bed-wetting.	Malaria
Valproic acid	Antiepileptic; epilepsy, bipolar disorder, migraine prevention	*Toxoplasma gondii* *Mycobacterium smegmatis* *Staphylococcus aureus*

MAOI = monoamine oxidase inhibitor.

plant material to treat a dental abscess (Hardy et al., 2012).

Alkaloids such as caffeine, nicotine and arecoline are anti-parasitic when orally ingested (St John-Smith et al., 2013; Sullivan and Hagen, 2002; see also Chapter 12 of this volume), but they also exert effects on the CNS, foremost the reward system (St John-Smith et al., 2013). Non-human animals and our hominin ancestors probably discovered how such substances can be used, their effects replicated and such plants recognised and used again to alter behaviour (e.g. induce trance-like states), as well as using them to enhance subjective well-being or help cope with hunger and famine (Huffman, 1997). We call this 'the dawn of psychopharmacology'. There are important cumulative cultural evolutionary processes involved in the transmission of knowledge regarding what effects various plants have (see Chapters 1 and 12). From the start of the Neolithic 12,000 years ago and with the proliferation of agriculture, new and greater quantities of psychoactive substances became available as by-products of farming. This process included the cultivation of plants containing opium and cannabis, as well as alcohol derived from the fermentation of cereals and fruits. From the beginning of history, societies began developing 'formularies' or lists of plants that were good for treating various physical and mental conditions, with Mesopotamia providing the earliest known record in around 2600 BCE (Sherratt, 1995).

Contemporary psychopharmacology begins with the deliberate production and use of drugs to treat psychological problems and psychiatric disorders. Barbiturates, although already synthesised in 1864, were first used medically in 1903 to anaesthetise dogs. Subsequently, barbiturates were used as hypnotics, sedatives, anticonvulsants and anaesthetics. They were used along with opiates for the management of acute behaviour. However, major issues with addiction, dependence and toxicity were recognised only by the 1940s (Galanter et al., 2014).

Amphetamine was first synthesised in Germany in 1887 (Edeleano, 1887) and was widely used as a stimulant by the German military until 1940, but its use was massively reduced after 1941 due to concerns over toxicity and abuse (Ulrich, 2005). The mid-twentieth century saw many medications for mental disorders synthesised or characterised (see Table 18.3).

Table 18.3. A brief chronology of 1950s' psychopharmacology (adapted from Owens, 1999)

1949: The anti-manic (and maintenance) effects of lithium salts identified

1950: Synthesis of chlorpromazine

1952: First systematic evaluation of Deniker chlorpromazine

1952: Mood-elevating effects of isoniazid identified

1954: Reserpine psychotropic effects identified

1954: Methylphenidate psychotropic effects identified

1955: Meprobamate psychotropic effects identified

1957: Introduction of monoamine oxidase inhibitors clinically

1957: First report of the antidepressant effect of imipramine

1957: Behavioural effects of 1,4-benzodiazepines identified

1958: Thioxanthenes introduced clinically

1958: Haloperidol introduced clinically

1959: Clozapine introduced clinically

1970s: Selective serotonin reuptake inhibitors introduced clinically

Chlorpromazine, a derivative from antihistamines, was synthesised in 1950 by Charpentier (López-Muñoz, 2005); lithium carbonate was used for mania in 1948 (Davies, 1999); and the antidepressants were developed in the 1950s. In 1952, iproniazid's antidepressant properties were discovered when researchers noted that the depressed patients given iproniazid experienced a relief of their depression (Ramachandraih, 2011). Imipramine, although synthesised in 1899, was only found to possess antidepressant effects in the mid-1950s. These latter two discoveries resulted in the establishment of monoaminergic drugs as antidepressants, ultimately resulting in the establishment of the monoamine theory of antidepressants (Healy, 1997).

The first benzodiazepine, chlordiazepoxide, was synthesised in 1955. The compound showed very strong sedative, hypnotic, anticonvulsant and muscle-relaxant effects. It was introduced clinically in 1960, and diazepam was introduced in 1963, which led to a decrease in the prescription of barbiturates (Shorter, 2005).

18.2.7 Cross-Reactivity

An illuminating consequence of evolutionary cross-reactivity due to evolutionarily conserved biological mechanisms and physiological systems can be demonstrated by the effects that human psychotropic agents can have on microorganisms (see Table 18.2; Kristiansen and Amaral, 1997; St John-Smith et al., 2013).

The remarkable similarity within the chemical basis of many psychotropic drugs has evolutionary roots in the closeness of structure and function of many natural bioactive chemicals including neurotransmitters and their receptors. Piperidine and its derivatives are an example of a class of related compounds that act on many seemingly biologically diverse systems. They are common building blocks in pharmaceuticals, and the piperidine structure is found in selective serotonin reuptake inhibitors (SSRIs), stimulants, nootropics, methylphenidate, ethylphenidate, selective oestrogen receptor modulators, vasodilators, minoxidil, antipsychotic medications, droperidol, haloperidol, risperidone, thioridazine opioids, dipipanone fentanyl and its analogues, loperamide, pethidine and cholinergic chemical weapons. Other derivatives have received attention due to their significant antimicrobial, antibacterial, antifungal, anti-HIV, anticancer, anti-tubercular, antitumor, antiinflammatory and other biological activities (Desai et al., 2016). Similarly, piperazine and its derivatives, initially marketed as antihelminthics, have a diverse range of applications (St John-Smith et al. 2013).

18.2.8 Controversy

Since the 1970s there have been voices of dissent who share concerns about psychiatric practice where and when it is heavily dependent upon formulaic diagnostic classification and the 'cookbook' use of psychopharmacology (Salzman, 2005). Expert guidelines remain an important contribution to evidence-based psychiatry. They are often used to teach the fundamentals of psychopharmacology. However, the guidelines are usually of limited applicability because of excessive reliance on Diagnostic and Statistical Manual of Mental Disorders (DSM) or International Classification of Diseases (ICD) diagnoses, especially for patients with atypical or comorbid disorders (McQueen and St John-Smith, 2009; Salzman, 2005).[2]

These concerns reflect the widespread heterogeneity and concerns around the construct validity of psychiatric diagnoses as well as scepticism about the effectiveness of antidepressants, mood stabilisers and antipsychotic agents (Moncrieff, 2008).

Notwithstanding these debates and arguments made by critics of psychopharmacological treatments, there is generally an acknowledgement of poor efficacy and slow progress, requiring the consideration of new approaches. We suggest that evolutionary psychiatry represents an additional basic science that poses new questions about why natural selection left us vulnerable to so many mental disorders (see Chapter 1) and brings new insights into how drugs work. Hence, the integration of psychopharmacology, neuropsychopharmacology, the neurosciences and evolutionary psychiatry is synergistic, going beyond the current pharmacological reductionism. An integrative evolutionary approach explains why agents that block useful aversive responses are usually safe and how to anticipate when they may cause harm. More generally, an evolutionary framework suggests novel practical strategies for finding and testing new drugs.

The optimal way to discover new treatments is to identify the cause(s) of any disorder. We suggest the use of Tinbergen's four questions (Tinbergen,

1963) to elucidate all such causes (see Chapter 1). Neurotransmitters, on which psychopharmaceuticals act, are clearly the basic mechanisms producing symptoms of psychiatric disorders, but they are not necessarily the primary cause of any disorder. Nevertheless, hopes of finding specific genetic or brain abnormalities have faded, even as a mountain of evidence demonstrates small average differences between people who do and do not have a mental disorder (Nesse and Stein, 2019). Attempts to map specific disorders to simplistic excesses or deficiencies of dopamine, serotonin and other neuroactive molecules have dissolved, despite ever-growing evidence for the relevance of these molecules in pathogenesis. The aspiration to characterise systems in reductionist terms is understandable, as is the wish that simple excesses or deficits of neurotransmitters could explain disorders. Evolutionary psychiatry proposes that the search for causes will progress more rapidly if it is recognised that organic complexity is different from complexity in designed systems. This perspective may also be particularly useful in psychopharmacological psychoeducation (Nesse and Stein, 2019; Stein, 1997, 2006).

One genetic avenue to pursue is to further the insight that psychiatric disorders and their related genes are the products of evolution and can be features that are maintained as by-products of selection. This can be further subdivided into those occurring (1) despite natural selection (e.g. mutation–selection balance and ancestral neutrality) and (2) because of natural selection (e.g. balancing selection, antagonistic pleiotropy, stabilising selection on continuous traits, alternating selection and functioning adaptations). These explanations are not mutually exclusive, and there may be multiple mechanisms maintaining some disorders in the population (Durisko et al., 2016). At another conceptual level, Gluckman et al. (2011) further categorises the possible evolutionary explanations and pathways that mediate the influence of evolutionary processes on disease vulnerability (see Box 1.1 in Chapter 1).

Appreciating this complexity is necessary, as traditional models of science that strive for single broadly applicable explanatory laws are ill suited to psychiatry and its treatments. Such models are based on the incorrect assumption that psychiatric illnesses can be understood from a single perspective at a single level of explanation. A more appropriate scientific model for psychiatry emphasises

---

[2] Guidelines are just that, not rules, nor complete statements of knowledge. They are dependent on choice and application of selection criteria and are subject to bias. They are based on a statistical abstraction of what happens in the 'population' with that diagnosis. They only apply to individuals in a probabilistic way – that is, insofar as one can extrapolate from the hypothetical statistical population to the concrete individual with their idiosyncrasies and individual histories. Individuals all differ from the population mean. Novice doctors base their prescribing decisions on guidelines, while senior doctors base their prescribing on a sophisticated holistic assessment of the individual patient that goes far beyond 'diagnosis'. Because of the impracticality of providing guidelines covering all of the important patient characteristics (independent variables), guidelines can only ever be highly generalised starting points. Expert doctors adapt guidelines to the individual patient in the consultation; this is a complex, partly automatic and unconscious activity that is developed through years of study, training and practice with unclear or complicated pictures.

the understanding of mechanisms, an approach that fits naturally with a multicausal (including evolutionary) framework and provides a realistic paradigm for scientific progress (Kendler, 2008). For instance, progress may accelerate when it is understood that aversive emotions are useful responses shaped by natural selection that are vulnerable to excess and dysregulation for several evolutionary reasons. Natural selection shapes mental mechanisms that maximise reproductive success, often at the expense of happiness or good health. The limits to what natural selection can do are substantial, with the inevitability of mutations, the frequent occurrence of genetic drift and the inability to start a design from scratch constraining optimality, as well as the risk of 'gene lag' and evolutionary mismatch in rapidly changing environments (Nesse, 2011).

18.2.9 Effects of Psychotropic Drugs Seen through the Lens of Evolution

Psychotropic drugs have desirable (therapeutic) and undesirable effects that need to be carefully monitored. The purpose of this section is to highlight some issues that often go under-recognised in clinical practice or are underestimated in their relevance.

As a general rule, no single drug exerts specific effects on neuronal signal transduction without impacting other somatic functions outside the CNS. This is so because the substances we conventionally call 'neurotransmitters' evolved hundreds of million years ago for very different biological functions – in fact, long before the first primitive nervous systems emerged. As the example of serotonin may illustrate, this substance is involved in the regulation of virtually all key body functions, including cell differentiation, defence, reproduction, locomotion, etc. It has been found in plants and unicellular animals, and it can be considered essential for maintaining homeostasis (see Table 18.1) (Azmitia, 2010). In higher animals, serotonin regulates food intake and digestion, sexual behaviour, aggression and explorative behaviour, in addition to the autonomic functions of the intestines, brain and sexual organs. Indeed, 95% of the body's serotonin is in the gut. With regards to the human brain, serotonin modulates the responses of neurons to other neurotransmitters rather than being excitatory itself, except in pyramidal

neurons in the cerebral cortex. Novel approaches such as receptor autoradiography have shown that the receptor densities of virtually all neurotransmitters, including the ones for acetylcholine, norepinephrine, dopamine, serotonin, glutamate and GABA, are heterogeneously distributed across the human neocortex and archicortex (Toga et al., 2006), such that different brain areas have distinct 'receptor fingerprints', with differences existing between primate species (Amunts and Zilles, 2015; Zilles, 2005). For example, there are at least 16 different types of serotonin receptors that evolved through a series of gene duplications. Their distribution across the human brain varies. The reuptake of serotonin from the synaptic cleft into the terminal axon is under the control of a serotonin transporter gene, which itself is controlled by a DNA promoter sequence that evolved in primates some 40 million years ago. Polymorphic variation of the promoter gene in humans has been associated with differences in personality traits such as anxiousness, impulsivity, hostility and proneness to depression.

Hence, in light of the manifold functions of serotonin in the body, it is unsurprising that enhancing serotonin transmission impacts multiple metabolic processes. Accordingly, SSRIs have many adverse effects on the intestines, the cardiovascular system and reproduction. While it is common knowledge that delayed ejaculation and reduction of sexual desire and arousal are side effects of SSRIs, it is less well known that SSRIs (as well as tricyclic antidepressants) can impair the motility, volume and morphology of sperm (Tignol et al., 2006), which may have profound interpersonal consequences. Taken together, not only does manipulating serotonin through drug treatment have profound effects on non-neuronal tissues across the whole body, there is also no evidence to suggest that the effects of SSRIs within the brain are specific to any one neuronal circuit. As serotonin is a precious molecule due to the sparse availability of its precursor tryptophan, the alteration of its availability in the synaptic cleft not only helps reduce depression and anxiety, it also changes regulation of body temperature, feeding, circadian rhythm, attention, memory formation and so forth. While it is clear that the treatment of severe depression and other psychiatric conditions with SSRIs can be beneficial, here we want to make the point that any decision about the prescription of these and other psychotropic medications deserves careful cost–benefit analysis. The same, we suggest, pertains to all other psychotropic drugs, though the reasons differ within each substance class.

18.3 Placebo Responses and Disorder Subgroups

Another major issue for psychopharmacology is the size of the so-called placebo responses in mood, anxiety and pain disorders. To overcome therapeutic signal to placebo noise issues, symptom profiles and genetic data have been used to identify subgroups of drug responders, but effect sizes tend to be small. An alternative approach is to create diagnostic subgroups based on the evolutionary situations and causal pathways that arouse low mood (e.g. Rantala et al., 2018). For example, depression arising from loss may be different from that arising from being trapped in a bad situation, and both are different from depression arising from a medication, infection or inflammation. Larger effect sizes might emerge if subgroups of patients are based on individual causal pathways and social contexts and if symptoms are analysed individually instead of as sum scores. Also, recognition of the function of emotions encourages measuring functional improvement as well as symptom relief.

Placebo effects do not represent random noise but may be considered as technical explanations of how healing and caring works (McQueen et al., 2013a, 2013b). The universality of placebo responses suggests a likely evolutionary basis to the underlying mechanisms. Placebo responses permit us to modify internal processes and behaviours. The stimuli for placebo responses are our perceptions of the internal and the external material and psychosocial environments. Adaptive advantages might result from the evolution of abilities to modify our internal environment in the light of positive evaluations of our external environments, social interactions and appraisals of the future. Nesse (2011) stresses that placebo responses primarily entail modification of the body's defences (e.g. pain, nausea, anxiety, depression, fever, itching, coughing, vomiting and diarrhoea) rather than altering disease processes. Hence, evolution has selected for mechanisms that defend against injury, infection or poisoning, and the regulation of these defences is influenced by appraisals of the environment.

From an evolutionary vantage point, it is striking to observe that 'placebo' healing rituals exist in virtually all known cultures, often tied to spiritual beliefs, and that healing rituals can indeed be helpful in coping with illness. Humans are particularly susceptible to 'medical information', which can be seen as either nocebo or placebo in relation to context. Indirectly, by positively influencing one's mood, the prospects of a cure may improve (Brüne, 2015).

From a psychological perspective, sickness behaviour emerges not only from biological dysfunction (disease), but also involves illness as a 'lived experience of distress' (Miller et al., 2009). The latter concerns an individual's attempt to integrate their subjective experience into something meaningful, which takes into account culture, social norms and values as well as personal preferences and attitudes. Reducing the aversive responses may be considered as an important component of placebo effects. In the study of therapeutic actions, we distinguish natural healing from technological and interpersonal healing, with placebo responses seeming mainly to be involved in the latter (see Box 18.1).

Box 18.1 Three types of healing (McQueen et al., 2013b)

Natural healing: The spontaneous responses of the body to disease or injury, such as fighting infection or tissue repair. This does not require awareness or even brain activity.

Technological healing: Any deliberate intervention that acts directly on the organism, such as pharmacology and surgery. Again, this does not require awareness or brain activity. The patient is essentially a passive recipient of the treatment.

Interpersonal healing: The art of medicine orientated towards the experience of illness and the relief of suffering. It includes providing meaning, reassurance, hope and support. It involves a relationship between the clinician and the patient that promotes healing, and it requires the participation – at some level, even if outside of conscious awareness – of the patient.

Much of the placebo effect can probably be traced back to attachment-related interpersonal factors that impact on the quality of therapeutic alliances. Psychoanalytic schools have recognised the relevance of these processes, termed 'containment', 'attunement' or 'holding' (McQueen and St John Smith, 2012; McQueen et al., 2013a). These considerations may explain why different psychotherapeutic interventions are practically indistinguishable with regards to efficacy, which is sometimes referred to as the 'equivalence paradox'. This suggests that placebo mechanisms play an important role in psychotherapeutic treatment. Thus, the quality of the patient–clinician relationship makes a significant contribution to the soothing of anxiety, which increases the success of healing and improves outcomes. These considerations suggest that it remains imperative in light of an increasingly technicalised medicine to safeguard medical care against anonymity, impersonality and unfriendliness (McQueen et al., 2013a).

18.4 Finding New Psychopharmacological Agents

Most early psychopharmacological compounds were discovered serendipitously, and even newer drugs were only discovered based on the short-term effects that the early drugs had on animal models. This process has become rather circular, and this explains why many early drugs were of the same chemical class or had similar actions for any disorder. This has been called 'pharmacological isomorphism' (Matthysse, 1986). Isomorphic models are useful for elucidating mechanisms of drug action, but they are not able to step outside of the existing class of therapeutic agents. Assessing potential new agents by their similarity to known effective molecules is a tried-and-tested method, but it rarely leads to fundamentally different drugs. Furthermore, many animal models for depression that have been used – such as the forced swim test, which is a major screening test for antidepressants (Petit-Demouliere et al., 2005) – are nowadays regarded as of dubious validity, although they are standard practice. An evolutionary perspective, however, can better inform the results of animal testing. For example, Nesse and Stein (2019) question the standard view that persistence in swimming is good. They note that when rats stop swimming, they don't drown; rather, they float with their noses just above the water. In the natural environment, this strategy is often superior to useless struggle, as demonstrated by increased rates of drowning in rats treated with antidepressants compared with those treated with placebo (Molendijk and de Kloet, 2015). Nesse and Stein (2019) suggest that such evolutionary insights can help improve animal studies. For example, studies that aim to identify new antidepressants may find it useful to focus on persistence time in pursuit of scarce foods or mates.

18.5 Evidence-Based Medicine and Good Practice Guidelines

Aside from a deeper understanding of where neurotransmitters come from (evolutionarily), how they were 'co-opted' for signal transduction among neurons and astroglia at the tripartite synapse and why their delicate balance in the CNS is vulnerable to dysfunction through accidental or deliberate ingestion of psychoactive substances, possible benefits of medication can be more properly understood by analysing why the symptoms of mental disorders exist in the first place (Brüne, 2015; Nesse and Stein, 2019). This rationale applies not only to psychiatry but also to medicine more generally. For instance, if the function of pain is to promote healing by disincentivising the use of an injured body part, pharmacological reduction of pain without dealing with the reasons it has occurred may be detrimental to an individual's long-term health.

By conceptualising sickness behaviours, pain mechanisms and mental disorders in relation to the problems that they evolved to solve, medical practitioners are in a better position to provide treatment options that are both more intelligent and more effective for ensuring a patient's long-term well-being (Rantala et al., 2018).

Of major concern to many clinicians is the risk of 'cookbook' prescribing according to a DSM or ICD diagnosis and an almost reflex use of guidelines for pharmacological treatment of symptoms no matter what the cause. Although we fully recognise the importance of evidence and evidence-based practice, we suggest that an evolutionary perspective can help diminish formulaic diagnosis and encourage greater appreciation of the complexity and multifaceted nature of mental disorder and the need to personalise interventions to suit individual patient needs. The central message of the evolutionary approach to affective disorders is that it is erroneous to equate distress with disorder, underlining the importance of understanding the individual's context when assessing the need for treatment (Abed and St John-Smith, 2021). Some evolutionists have expressed the concern that normal sadness is being medicalised and that antidepressants are being employed where they are neither useful nor effective (e.g. Horwitz and Wakefield, 2007). The grief response is an example of a distressing state involving low mood that is both universal and generally self-limiting. While it is agreed that grief is part of the human behavioural repertoire, there is no agreement as to whether or not it is an actual adaptation. Some have suggested that it is a by-product of the attachment system (Nesse and Ellsworth, 2009), while others have proposed that it is an adaptive and complex stress response shaped by selection that has a number of components, including: (1) an immune response, principally an energy-conserving state that is coordinated with enhanced immune activity; (2) a cognitive response, principally a reflective disposition characterised by more realistic situational appraisals, ultimately encouraging adaptive actions; and (3) a social response, minimally an appeal to halt aggression and, more broadly, an appeal for altruistic assistance (Huron, 2018).

The controversy as to whether antidepressants are helpful or harmful in dealing with bereavement was further ignited by the decision of the DSM-5 committee to remove the 'bereavement exclusion' present in DSM-IV, whereby depression was not diagnosed in the first two months after bereavement. The result is that under DSM-5 major depressive disorder can be diagnosed and treatment offered if the symptoms persist beyond two weeks (Kavan and Barone, 2014). The justification for the bereavement exclusion is that symptoms of grief and major depression can be indistinguishable and the risk of suicide is similarly elevated in both. However, these premises have been vigorously disputed, and a recent study specifically found no evidence of elevated suicide risk from the bereavement exclusion in DSM-IV (Wakefield and First, 2012; Wakefield and Schmitz, 2014).

Schiefenhövel (2000) has described how grief can be contained in ritual ceremonies, thereby providing social support for the grieving individual, which helps them recuperate from and integrate overwhelmingly strong emotions. Hence, evolutionists have suggested

that caution is warranted with regards to interfering with such behaviour regulation systems by means of pharmacological treatment alone (Brüne, 2015).

18.6 Conclusions

In conclusion, modern psychopharmacology originated from many serendipitous discoveries and has progressed only slowly even with better understanding of brain mechanisms. Hopes remain high that the neurosciences will identify specific biomarkers and specific causal abnormalities, but this now seems progressively unlikely as such discoveries have been slow in coming, and few advances have been translated from the laboratory to the clinic. However, this approach can usefully be supplemented by evolutionary theory. Evolutionary psychiatry perspectives not only bring together neurotransmitters and genes, but they also bring the environmental context into psychopharmacology research. This is new in the search for pharmacological agents. The evolutionary approach doesn't just fatalistically accept that psychiatric diagnosis and treatment are problematic; rather, it reconsiders how subcategories of disorders based on the functions of emotions and the life situations of patients may increase the researcher's ability to demonstrate efficacy. Evolutionary perspectives on psychopharmacology also suggest that many agents act by disrupting normal defensive systems and that the study of these systems in context may provide a new route to drug discovery. Conceptualising sickness behaviours, pain mechanisms and mental disorders in relation to the problems that they evolved to solve potentially encourages practitioners to provide treatment options that are both more enlightened and more effectively targeted, ensuring a patient's long-term well-being, though the patient's immediate best interests must always be regarded as paramount (Rantala et al., 2018). Evolutionary psychopharmacology is also concerned with the explanation of the side effects of psychoactive medication through the lens of evolutionary theory. This view is notably different from the common clinical perspective of side effects because it highlights the interference of drugs with evolutionarily relevant systems that may have negative consequences for the individual's ability to attain vital biosocial goals.

References

Abed, R. and St John-Smith, P. (2021). Evolutionary psychology and psychiatry. In: T. K. Shackleford (ed.), *The Sage Handbook of Evolutionary Psychology: Applications of Evolutionary Psychology*. London: Sage, pp. 24–50.

Allman, J. M. (1999). *Evolving Brains*. New York: Scientific American Library: distributed by W.H. Freeman and Co.

Amunts, K. and Zilles, K. (2015). Architectonic mapping of the human brain beyond Brodmann. *Neuron*, 88, 1086–1107.

Attwell, D. and Laughlin, S. B. (2001). An energy budget for signalling in the grey matter of the brain. *Journal of Cerebral Blood Flow & Metabolism*, 21, 1133–1145.

Azmitia, E. C. (2010). Evolution of serotonin: sunlight to suicide. In: C. P. Müller and B. L. Jacobs (eds.), *Handbook of the Behavioral Neurobiology of Serotonin*. London: Academic Press, Elsevier, pp. 3–22.

Belzung, C. and Lemoine, M. (2011). Criteria of validity for animal models of psychiatric disorders: focus on anxiety disorders and depression. *Biology of Mood & Anxiety Disorders*, 1, 1–14.

Bender, G. A. (1965). *Great Moments in Pharmacy*. Tucson: Arizona Medical Center Library.

Brüne, M. (2014). On aims and methods of psychiatry. A reminiscence of 50 years of Tinbergen's famous questions about the biology of behavior. *BMC Psychiatry*, 14, 364.

Brüne, M. (2015). *Textbook of Evolutionary Psychiatry and Psychosomatic Medicine: The Origins of Psychopathology*. Oxford: Oxford University Press.

Changeux, J.-P. (2005). Genes, brains, and culture: from monkey to human. In: S. Dehaene, J.-R. Duhamel, M. Hauser and G. Rizzolatti (eds.), *From Monkey Brain to Human Brain*. Cambridge, MA: MIT Press, pp. 73–94.

Chen, G. Q., Cui, C., Mayer, M. L. and Gouaux, E. (1999). Functional characterization of a potassium-selective prokaryotic glutamate receptor. *Nature*, 402, 817–821.

Davies, B. (1999). The first patient to receive lithium. *Australian & New Zealand Journal of Psychiatry*, 33, 366–368.

Desai, N. C., Makwana, A. H. and Senta, R. D. (2016). Synthesis, characterization and antimicrobial activity of some novel 4-(4-(arylamino) 6-(piperidin-1-yl)-1, 3, 5-triazine-2-ylamino)-N-(pyrimidin-2-yl) benzenesulfonamides. *Journal of Saudi Chemical Society*, 20, 686–694.

Dreborg, S., Sundström, G., Larsson, T. A. and Larhammar, D. (2008). Evolution of vertebrate opioid receptors. *Proceedings of the National Academy of Sciences of the United States of America*, 105, 15487–15492.

Durisko, Z., Mulsant, B. H., McKenzie, K. and Andrews, P. W. (2016). Using evolutionary theory to guide mental health research. *Canadian Journal of Psychiatry*, 61, 159–165.

Edeleano, L. (1887). Ueber einige Derivate der Phenylmethacrylsäure und der Phenylisobuttersäure. *Berichte der deutschen chemischen Gesellschaft*, 20, 616–622.

Edgar, N. and Sibille, E. (2012). A putative functional role for oligodendrocytes in mood regulation. *Translational Psychiatry*, 2, e109.

Ellis, L. (ed.) (2003). *Archaeological Method and Theory: An Encyclopaedia*. London: Routledge.

Emes, R. D. and Grant, S. G. N. (2012). Evolution of synapse complexity and diversity. *Annual Review of Neuroscience*, 35, 111–131.

Fabrega, H., Jr (1997). Earliest phases in the evolution of sickness and healing. *Medical Anthropology Quarterly*, 11, 26–55.

Faissner, A., Pyka, M., Geissler, M., Sobik, T., Frischknecht, R., Gundelfinger, E. D. and Seidenbecher, C. (2010). Contributions of astrocytes to synapse formation and maturation – potential functions of the perisynaptic extracellular matrix. *Brain Research Reviews*, 63, 26–38.

Fehm, H. L., Kern, W. and Peters, A. (2006). The selfish brain: competition for energy resources. *Progress in Brain Research*, 153, 129–140.

Fields, R. D., Araque, A., Johansen-Berg, H., Lim, S. S., Lynch, G., Nave, K. A., Nedergaard, M., Perez, R., Sejnowski, T. and Wake, H. (2014). Glial biology in learning and cognition. *Neuroscientist*, 20, 426–431.

Galanter, M., Kleber, H. D. and Brady, K. (eds.) (2014). *The American Psychiatric Publishing Textbook of Substance Abuse Treatment*. Washington, DC: American Psychiatric Publishing.

Gluckman, P. D., Low, F. M., Buklijas, T., Hanson, M. A. and Beedle, A. S. (2011). How evolutionary principles improve the understanding of human health and disease. *Evolutionary Applications*, 4, 249–263.

Guyton, A. C. and Hall, J. E. (2006). *Textbook of Medical Physiology*. Philadelphia, PA: Elsevier.

Halbreich, U. and Endicott, J. (1981). Possible involvement of endorphin withdrawal or imbalance in specific premenstrual syndromes and postpartum depression. *Medical Hypotheses*, 7, 1045–1058.

Hardy, K., Buckley, S., Collins, M. J., Estalrrich, A., Brothwell, D., Copeland, L., García-Tabernero, A., García-Vargas, S., De La Rasilla, M., Lalueza-Fox, C. and Huguet, R. (2012). Neanderthal medics? Evidence for food, cooking, and medicinal plants entrapped in dental calculus. *Naturwissenschaften*, 99, 617–626.

Haroon, E., Miller, A. H., and Sanacora, G. (2017). Inflammation, glutamate, and glia: a trio of trouble in mood disorders. *Neuropsychopharmacology*, 42, 193–215.

Healy, D. (1997). *The Antidepressant Era*. Cambridge, MA: Harvard University Press.

Herculano-Houzel, S., Avelino-de-Souza, K., Neves, K., Porfírio, J., Messeder, D., Mattos Feijó, L., Maldonado, J. and Manger, P. R. (2014). The elephant brain in numbers. *Frontiers in Neuroanatomy*, 8, 46.

Hofman, M. A. (2014). Evolution of the human brain: when bigger is better. *Frontiers in Neuroanatomy*, 8, 15.

Horwitz, A. V. and Wakefield, J. C. (2007). *The Loss of Sadness: How Psychiatry Transformed Normal Sadness into Depressive Disorder*. Oxford: Oxford University Press.

Huffman, M. A. (1997). Current evidence for self-medication in primates: a multidisciplinary perspective. *American Journal of Physical Anthropology*, 104, 171–200.

Huron, D. (2018). On the functions of sadness and grief. In: H. C. Lench (ed.), *The Functions of Emotions: When and Why Emotions Help Us*. Cham: Springer, pp. 59–92.

Jaiteh, M., Taly, A. and Hénin, J. (2016). Evolution of pentameric ligand-gated ion channels: Pro-loop receptors. *PLoS ONE*, 11, e0151934.

Jakobsen, J. C., Katakam, K. K., Schou, A., Hellmuth, S. G., Stallknecht, S. E., Leth-Møller, K., Iversen, M., Banke, M. B., Petersen, I. J., Klingenberg, S. L. and Krogh, J. (2017). Selective serotonin reuptake inhibitors versus placebo in patients with major depressive disorder. A systematic review with meta-analysis and trial sequential analysis. *BMC Psychiatry*, 17, 1–28.

Jerison, H. J. (1973). *Evolution of the Brain and Intelligence*. Cambridge, MA: Academic Press.

Jones, C. A., Watson, D. J. G. and Fone, K. C. F. (2011). Animal models of schizophrenia. *British Journal of Pharmacology*, 164, 1162–1194.

Kavan, M. G. and Borone, E. J. (2014). Grief and major depression – controversy over changes in DSM-5 diagnostic criteria. *American Family Physician*, 90, 693–694.

Kendler, K. S. (2008). Explanatory models for psychiatric illness. *American Journal of Psychiatry*, 165, 695–702.

Kirsch, I. (2019). Placebo effect in the treatment of depression and anxiety. *Frontiers in Psychiatry*, 10, 407.

Konstantinidis, K. T. and Tiedje, J. M. (2004). Trends between gene content and genome size in prokaryotic species with larger genomes. *Proceedings of National Academy of Sciences of the United States of America*, 101, 3160–3165.

Kristiansen, J. and Amaral, L. (1997). The potential management of resistant infections with non-antibiotics. *Journal of Antimicrobial Chemotherapy*, 40, 319–327.

Kudryavtsev, D., Shelukhina, I., Vulfius, C., Makarieva, T., Stonik, V., Zhmak, M., Ivanov, I., Kasheverov, I., Utkin, Y. and Tsetlin, V. (2015). Natural compounds interacting with nicotinic acetylcholine receptors: from low-molecular weight ones to peptides and proteins. *Toxins*, 7, 1683–1701.

Le Duc, D. and Schöneberg, T. (2019). Cellular signalling systems. In: M. Brüne and W. Schiefenhövel (eds.), *The Oxford Handbook of Evolutionary Medicine*. Oxford: Oxford University Press, pp. 45–76.

López-Muñoz, F., Alamo, C., Cuenca, E., Shen, W. W., Clervoy, P. and Rubio, G. (2005). History of the discovery and clinical introduction of chlorpromazine. *Annals of Clinical Psychiatry*, 17, 113–135.

Maeda, N. (2015). Proteoglycans and neuronal migration in the cerebral cortex during development and disease. *Frontiers in Neuroscience*, 9, 98.

Matthysse, S. (1986). Animal models in psychiatric research. *Progress in Brain Research*, 65, 259–270.

McQueen, D. and St John-Smith, P. (2008). What should clinicians do when faced with conflicting recommendations? *BMJ*, 337, a2530.

McQueen, D. and St John-Smith, P. (2012). Placebo effects: a new paradigm and relevance to psychiatry. *International Psychiatry*, 9, 1–3.

McQueen, D., Cohen, S., St John-Smith, P. and Rampes, H. (2013a). Rethinking placebo in psychiatry: how and why placebo effects occur. *Advances in Psychiatric Treatment*, 19, 171–180.

McQueen, D., Cohen, S., St John-Smith, P. and Rampes, H. (2013b). Rethinking placebo in psychiatry: the range of placebo effects. *Advances in Psychiatric Treatment*, 19, 162–170.

Miller, F. G., Colloca, L. and Kaptchuk, T. J. (2009). The placebo effect: illness and interpersonal healing. *Perspectives in Biology and Medicine*, 52, 518–539.

Molendijk, M. L. and de Kloet, E. R. (2015). Immobility in the forced swim test is adaptive and does not reflect depression. *Psychoneuroendocrinology*, 62, 389–391.

Moncrieff, J. (2008). The myth of the chemical cure. In: *The Myth of the Chemical Cure*. London:

Palgrave Macmillan, pp. 217–224.

Moroz, L. L. (2009). On the independent origins of complex brains and neurons. *Brain, Behavior and Evolution*, 74, 177–190.

Nedergaard, M., Ransom, B. and Goldman, S. A. (2003). New roles for astrocytes: redefining the functional architecture of the brain. *Trends in Neurosciences*, 26, 523–530.

Nesse, R. M. (2011). Why has natural selection left us so vulnerable to anxiety and mood disorders? *Canadian Journal of Psychiatry*, 56, 705–706.

Nesse, R. M. and Ellsworth, P. C. (2009). Evolution, emotions, and emotional disorders. *American Psychologist*, 64, 129.

Nesse, R. M. and Stein, D. J. (2019). How evolutionary psychiatry can advance psychopharmacology. *Dialogues in Clinical Neuroscience*, 21, 167.

Owens, D. C. (1999). *A Guide to the Extrapyramidal Side Effects of Antipsychotic Drugs*. Cambridge: Cambridge University Press.

Panksepp, J. (1998). *Affective Neuroscience: The Foundations of Human and Animal Emotions*. New York: Oxford University Press.

Perry, C. J. and Baciadonna, L. (2017). Studying emotion in invertebrates: what has been done, what can be measured and what they can provide. *Journal of Experimental Biology*, 220, 3856–3868.

Petit-Demouliere, B., Chenu, F. and Bourin, M. (2005). Forced swimming test in mice: a review of antidepressant activity. *Psychopharmacology*, 177, 245–255.

Petraglia, F., Comitini, G. and Genazzani, A. R. (1993). β-Endorphin in human reproduction. In: A. Herz (ed.), *Opioids II*. Berlin: Springer, pp. 763–780.

Ramachandraih, C. T., Subramanyam, N., Bar, K. J., Baker, G. and Yeragani, V. K. (2011). Antidepressants: from MAOIs to SSRIs and more. *Indian Journal of Psychiatry*, 53, 180.

Rantala, M. J., Luoto, S. and Krams, I. (2017). An evolutionary approach to clinical pharmacopsychology. *Psychotherapy and Psychosomatics*, 86, 370–371.

Rantala, M. J., Luoto, S., Krams, I. and Karlsson, H. (2018). Depression subtyping based on evolutionary psychiatry: proximate mechanisms and ultimate functions. *Brain, Behavior, and Immunity*, 69, 603–617.

Raven, P., Johnson, G., Mason, K., Losos, J. and Duncan, T. (2017). The nervous system. In: *Biology*. New York: McGrath-Hill Education.

Roshchina, V. V. (2010). Evolutionary considerations of neurotransmitters in microbial, plant, and animal cells. In: M. Lyte and P. E. Freestone (eds.), *Microbial Endocrinology*. Berlin: Springer, pp. 17–52.

Ryan, T. J. and Grant, S. G. (2009). The origin and evolution of synapses. *Nature Reviews Neuroscience*, 10, 701–712.

Salzman, C. (2005). The limited role of expert guidelines in teaching psychopharmacology. *Academic Psychiatry*, 29, 176–179.

Schiefenhövel, W. (2000). [Suffering without meaning? Illness, pain and death. Development of evolutionary medicine]. *Gesundheitswesen*, 62, S3–S8.

Sherratt, A. (1995). Alcohol and its alternatives: symbol and substance in pre-industrial cultures. In: J. Goodman (ed.), *Consuming Habits: Global and Historical Perspectives on How Cultures Define Drugs*. London: Routledge, pp. 11–45.

Shorter, E. (2005). *A Historical Dictionary of Psychiatry*. Oxford: Oxford University Press.

Sneader, W. (2005). *Drug Discovery: A History*. Hoboken, NJ: John Wiley & Sons.

Solms, M. (2021). *The Hidden Spring: A Journey to the Source of Consciousness*. London: Profile Books.

St John-Smith, P., McQueen, D., Edwards, L. and Schifano, F. (2013). Classical and novel psychoactive substances: rethinking drug misuse from an evolutionary psychiatric perspective. *Human Psychopharmacology: Clinical and Experimental*, 28, 394–401.

Stahl, S. M. (2000). *Essential Psychopharmacology. Neuroscientific Basis and Practical Application*. Cambridge: Cambridge University Press.

Stearns, S. C., Nesse, R. M., Govindaraju, D. R. and Ellison, P. T. (2010). Evolution in health and medicine Sackler colloquium: evolutionary perspectives on health and medicine. *Proceedings of the National Academy of Science of the United States of America*, 107, 1691–1695.

Steegborn, C. (2014). Structure, mechanism, and regulation of soluble adenylyl cyclases – similarities and differences to transmembrane adenylyl cyclases. *Biochimica et Biophysica Acta*, 1842, 2535–2547.

Stein, D. J. (2006). Evolutionary theory, psychiatry, and psychopharmacology. *Progress in Neuro-Psychopharmacology and Biological Psychiatry*, 30, 766–773.

Stein, D. J. and Bouwer, C. (1997). A neuro-evolutionary approach to the anxiety disorders. *Journal of Anxiety Disorders*, 11, 409–429.

Sullivan, R. J. and Hagen, E. H. (2002). Psychotropic substance-seeking: evolutionary pathology or adaptation? *Addiction*, 97, 389–400.

Tamames, J., Ouzounis, C., Sander, C. and Valencia, A. (1996). Genomes with distinct function composition. *FEBS Letters*, 389, 96–101.

Tasneem, A., Iyer, L. M., Jakobsson, E. and Aravind, L. (2005). Identification of the prokaryotic ligand-gated ion channels and their implications for the mechanisms and origins of animal Cys-loop ion channels. *Genome Biology*, 6, 1–12.

Tignol, J., Martin-Guehl, C., Aouizerate, B., Grabot, D. and Auriacombe, M. (2006). Social phobia and premature ejaculation: a case–control study. *Depression and Anxiety*, 23, 153–157.

Tinbergen, N. (1963). On aims and methods of ethology. *Zeitschrift für Tierpsychologie*, 20, 410–433.

Toga, A. W., Thompson, P. M., Mori, S., Amunts, K. and Zilles, K. (2006). Towards multimodal atlases of the human brain. *Nature Reviews Neuroscience*, 7, 952–966.

Tomasetti, C., Iasevoli, F., Buonaguro, E. F., De Berardis, D., Fornaro, M., Fiengo, A. L. C., Martinotti, G., Orsolini, L., Valchera, A., Di Giannantonio, M. and de Bartolomeis, A. (2017). Treating the synapse in major psychiatric disorders: the role of postsynaptic density network in dopamine-glutamate interplay and psychopharmacologic drugs molecular actions. *International Journal of Molecular Sciences*, 18, 135.

Ulrich, A. (2005). Hitler's drugged soldiers. *Der Spiegel*. Retrieved from www.spiegel.de/international/the-nazi-death-machine-hitler-s-drugged-soldiers-a-354606.html

Wakefield, J. and First, M. B. (2012). Validity of the bereavement exclusion to major depression: does the empirical evidence support the proposal to eliminate the exclusion in DSM-5? *World Psychiatry*, 11, 3–10.

Wakefield, J. C. and Schmitz, M. F. (2014). Uncomplicated depression, suicide attempt, and the DSM-5 bereavement exclusion debate: an empirical evaluation. *Research on Social Work Practice*, 24, 37–49.

Watson, C., Provis, J. and Herculano-Houzel, S. (2012). What determines motor neuron number? Slow scaling of facial motor neuron numbers with body mass in marsupials and primates. *The Anatomical Record: Advances in Integrative Anatomy and Evolutionary Biology*, 295, 1683–1691.

Wybran, J. (1985). Enkephalins and endorphins as modifiers of the immune system: present and future. *Federation Proceedings*, 44, 92–94.

Young, J. W., Henry, B. L. and Geyer, M. A. (2011). Predictive animal models of mania: hits, misses and future directions. *British Journal of Pharmacology*, 164, 1263–1284.

Zilles, K. (2005). Evolution of the human brain and comparative cyto- and receptor architecture. In: S. Dehaene, J.-R. Duhamel, M. Hauser and G. Rizzolatti (eds.), *From Monkey Brain to Human Brain*. Cambridge, MA: MIT Press, pp. 41–56.

What the Evolutionary and Cognitive Sciences Offer the Sciences of Crime and Justice

Brian B. Boutwell, Megan Suprenant and Todd K. Shackelford

Abstract

Science has become increasingly interdisciplinary, marked by the rapid expansion of social science fields melding with 'natural' sciences previously considered less relevant for the study of humans. Psychology in particular now depends heavily on insights from medicine, biology, sociology, genetics and cognitive science and has done so for years. By grounding itself in evolutionary theory, moreover, psychology has moved towards a more mature science of human mind and behaviour. The crime sciences – criminology and criminal justice – are poised to make similar progress. While already interdisciplinary fields, we make the case that the evolutionary and cognitive sciences can unify existing knowledge about crime and justice, can help to pose new and interesting questions to study and can push the fields forward in ways that will benefit not only the scientific world, but society in general as well.

Keywords

cognitive science, consilience, criminology, evolutionary psychology

Key Points

- The natural and social sciences have become tightly interlaced across the decades.
- Evolutionary theory has aided this process by serving as the shared foundation.
- In this context, the combination of the psychological and cognitive sciences has accelerated our understanding of the human brain and mind.
- The crime sciences have become similarly interdisciplinary; however, they have yet to take advantage of the insights offered by evolutionary theory and cognitive science.
- We propose a roadmap for consilience in the crime sciences moving forward.

Calls for consilience of knowledge, as described by Wilson (1999) decades ago, have at times evoked mercurial receptions across the social sciences, to put it mildly (Pinker, 2002). Still, the clarity of hindsight offers a more encouraging vista of how things have changed over time. Consider the field of psychology. By virtually any metric, this is an academic field in which consilience has flourished. Perhaps the largest 'social science' arena, various edges of psychology have become so tightly welded to medicine, genomics and neuroanatomy that bright boundaries are simply absent. Tracking all of the cross-pollination becomes tricky indeed. Various branches and sub-branches have natural affinities for each other, and they function to shed light on problems across fields that previously seemed intractable (Gazzaniga, 2009).

It seems fair to also say that the deeper animating force for this ongoing consilience, moreover, is evolutionary theory, a tool that gives psychological scientists the ability to best contextualise their results. It's hard to imagine how this could have worked differently, as Darwinian logic provides the foundation on which all knowledge about life on the planet can be grounded (Duntley and Shackelford, 2008a; Pinker, 2002). Returning to Wilson (1999) for a moment, his guiding assumption was that, like all animals, humans occupy a place in a branching tree of life. Darwin, of course, had beaten him to this conclusion over a century prior. Like every other species, our placement in life's branching tree was not immediately realised. Our existence is owed to a gradual and sometime glacial process of change, contributing to a slow physiological, cognitive and cultural departure from our primate kin.

Make no mistake, our evolutionary history sparked an ongoing cultural evolution as well. Our species has erected complex and complicated social milieus that shape and are shaped by us (Heinrich et al., 2008). It was only a matter of time before a field concerned almost exclusively with mental processes realised that to invoke the mental meant invoking the neurological. The neurological, in turn, demanded an understanding of the physiological, which compelled scholars to grasp on some level the evolutionary process that created it all. Consilience driven by evolutionary insights in any field interested in human beings, like it or not, is most likely a *fait accompli* (for a more in-depth discussion of this, see Pinker, 2002).

19.1 No Longer Islands unto Themselves

Though they, too, have been undergoing their own version of consilience, criminal justicians and criminologists remain comparatively more isolated in their work (Barnes et al., 2014; Duntley and Shackelford, 2008a, 2008b). The difference is simply one of degree. Insights from economics, sociology, social psychology and even behavioural and molecular genetics have made vital inroads into the criminological sciences proper (Barnes et al., 2014; Boutwell and Adams, 2020; Tanksley et al., 2020). This is a hallmark of scientific progress, and it simplifies our goal here. Instead of starting from scratch, what we're asserting is that just a bit more integration will knit together the knowledge flowing from all of the fields probing the worst behaviours of human beings. The logic of evolutionary psychology melded with the insights of cognitive science, we propose, constitutes the next logical and necessary step towards a mature science of crime.

19.2 Borrowing Some New Tools

Because we're not starting from scratch, there is no need to invent new tools or strategies, we can just borrow strategically from others. In fact, we can start with perhaps the most vital tool of evolutionary theorists. Reverse engineering something to divine its possible purpose, or lack thereof, is a broadly useful strategy in science (Pinker, 1997; Tooby and DeVore, 1987). Traits emerge and persist: (1) because they promoted fitness in our ancestors; (2) because they came along for the ride with other adaptive phenotypes; or (3) because of historical 'accidents' of a type more formally known as genetic drift (Buss, 2007; Pinker, 1997). Thinking about a phenotype and working backwards to understand its possible purpose in our past can yield invaluable insights (Duntley and Shackelford, 2008a).

Revisiting some prior work of Duntley and Shackelford (2008a, 2008b, among others) is helpful at this point, as it prompts us to ponder the fact that our ancestors faced a grab bag of recurrent problems. Many of these challenges had to do with dealing with other people. How does one navigate an encounter with a non-relative whose intentions cannot necessarily be readily discerned simply by looking at them (Buss, 2007)? What strategy is best for navigating a dispute over food or a possible mate? Simple physical force might suffice at times, but that strategy can fail stupendously when one encounters a larger, stronger individual. What constitutes 'fairness'? This is a deceptively complicated question, yet it was an unavoidable one if mixed groups of related and unrelated humans wanted to live together and cooperate with some degree of success.

The point, of course, is that human beings have had to solve the *cognitive* problems of 'each other' for a very long time, and natural selection has had the opportunity to design a mind with at least some capacity to meet this challenge (Pinker, 1997). This is precisely the reason why evolutionary psychologists have thought about human mental processes using a Darwinian lens for decades. And the relevance of this work for criminology and criminal justice should, at most, be only thinly veiled. Understanding why people take advantage of each other, sometimes violate social codes (laws), obey those codes, and ultimately understanding where those codes come from in the first place, all reside at the heart of the crime sciences (Black, 1976; Tyler, 1990). Moreover, it is worth mentioning again that the sheer number of scholars across fields taking advantage of evolutionary logic – including psychiatrists, cognitive scientists, anthropologists and even a small number of criminologists – testifies to its broad applicability (Kavish and Boutwell, 2018; Shackelford, 2020; Tielbeek et al., 2018).

The component parts of our anatomy offer immediate clues when we attempt to reverse engineer them to discern their purpose. Duntley and Shackelford (2008a, 2008b) mentioned a few of these, one of which included the obvious examples of the heart and lungs. On the one hand, the heart is an organ serving as a powerful pump used to circulate oxygenated blood throughout the body. On the other, the lungs represent a vital piece of hardware needed for extracting oxygen from the air and for releasing carbon dioxide from the body. Other examples could be listed *ad nauseam*. Far from a new point, it is nonetheless worth repeating here that the advantages of one design aspect over another need not be huge to be noticed by natural selection (Duntley and Shackelford, 2008a, 2008b; see also Falconer and MacKay, 1996). A trait offering the tiniest advantage, (or, more precisely, the genetic variants underlying that trait), can surge close to fixation in a population in only a few thousand generations (Duntley and Shackelford, 2008a, 2008b; Falconer and MacKay, 1996; Nilsson and Pelger, 1994).

Of course, we would be remiss not to mention some of the unfortunate design fallouts that arise from mindless, blind selection (Dawkins, 1996; Marcus, 2009). The passage of the male urethra directly through the prostate, protections from choking that were sacrificed for the production of speech and cell divisions that are essential but risk error and thus can yield cancer, are but a few of the starker examples (Dawkins, 1996; Marcus, 2009; Pinker, 1997). With the aid of a clever analogy, it has been convincingly argued that many of our 'design features' – including the design of human brains and minds – look a lot like a *kluge* – a clumsy, sometimes redundant, often inelegant solution to an engineering problem (Marcus, 2009).

Nonetheless, just as natural selection gradually sculpted physiological mechanisms with specific problem-solving functions, so too did it gradually sculpt the information-processing mechanisms that produce preferences, desires, emotions and attitudes (Pinker, 1997). Evolutionary processes, in other words, set in place a 'conspiracy' of

mental processes that work in the service of solving ancestrally recurrent problems (see Chapter 1). None of this should be controversial or even the least bit surprising. To endorse a Darwinian understanding of life necessitates that we endorse some version of what was just stated.

That said, the version of this logic that one accepts could manifest as a 'stronger' or 'weaker' variety. For instance, one might argue that the mind is full of specific modular adaptations, each designed to solve *specific* problems (Tooby and Cosmides, 1992). Alternatively, one may be more swayed by a version in which some number of more general modules exist that are capable of plying their problem-solving skills across various types of problems (concerning this debate, see Buss, 1991; Pinker, 1997). For our discussion here, where one lands on this spectrum is irrelevant. The point is that you cannot, on the one hand, ponder the evolution of physiological systems and, on the other hand, assert that the human brain was birthed fully formed, untouched by selective forces that have been – and are now – exerting influences on our species (Buss, 1991).

A key point already made by Duntley and Shackelford (2008a, 2008b) is quite relevant to this discussion, so we raise it at this point in our chapter. Humans, they remind us, do not have specialised physiological weaponry – something like long, pronounced fangs or sharp talons for when it's necessary to battle a rival. What we do have is a 'mind' produced by functioning in our brain. They argue – and we concur – that the mind houses information-processing adaptations. These 'modules' function to coordinate feelings, emotions and, ultimately, behaviours capable of solving the social interaction problems that humans have dealt with for so long.

So important is our use of cognitive toolkits to deal with each other that Tooby and DeVore (1987) went so far as to argue that our species occupies a 'cognitive niche' (see also Pinker, 2010). Any social interaction can run a spectrum ranging between easy cooperation to intense and possibly violent conflict. Strategies that coordinate cooperation whenever possible and avoid conflict were likely more beneficial than either trying to go it alone or attempting to kill every would-be rival that stumbled into your path (Trivers, 1971). Sometimes violence might be needed, of course (if one group is threatening another group, for instance), but in such cases coordination and cooperation are still essential if the hostile group is to be fended off by those under threat (Buss and Shackelford, 1997). What's essential to realise is that selective pressures were likely exerted around the need for strategies aimed at winning the near-constant competitions over scarce resources while also figuring out the motives and strategies of those you were in competition with (Buss and Shackelford, 1997; Duntley, 2005).

The contemplation about ancestral problems and their plausible solutions brings us to an intersection between topics that crime scientists care deeply about. To see what we mean, consider that when valuable resources are scarce injuring or incapacitating a rival makes sense in certain settings (Duntley and Shackelford, 2008a). The benefits of controlling contested resources, in such cases, can immediately plummet for the rival. If it becomes apparent that standing your ground will result in serious injury or death, discretion becomes the better part of valour. Put differently, when causing or giving a credible threat that you will cause pain or damage to a rival, their most prudent strategy becomes simply walking away (Duntley and Shackelford, 2008a, 2008b). The aggressive individual, in this instance, has won.

Circling this topic of credible threats a bit more, Pinker (2007) wryly noted that a mobster complimenting your store and then in the same breath noting that 'it'd be a shame if something happened to it' is not engaging in idle chit chat. The Mafioso has threatened something that you value. It's thinly veiled but also very credible, as you happen to know that this guy burnt down a neighbour's business not two weeks ago. So, unless you fork over some money (i.e. a valued resource), your store may burn down, maybe even with you in it! A collection of certain evolved adaptations, demented as they might seem in a modern world, can generate lifelong strategies for exploiting and abusing others. Indeed, some scholars have argued that these mental capacities represent the forerunners of the psychopathic tendencies disproportionately prevalent in some of the most chronic offenders in the population, hypotheses that warrant attention and empirical scrutiny (Lalumiere et al., 2001; Mealey, 1995; Pitchford, 2001).

What is hopefully becoming clear by now is that understanding the nature of recurrent conflicts in our evolutionary history can offer us useful insights into conflicts between people

today. These evolutionarily enduring conflicts and the adaptations produced by selection to navigate them afford the framework for an evolutionarily informed crime science. Stopping here, however, and not adding more meat to the bone of what we've described would be unsatisfying.

It is one thing (a useful thing) to describe a psychological architecture that contains tools for cooperation, exploitation, subversion and violence. Yet, to have a deeper understanding about these adaptations, evolutionary science requires the additional layer of cognitive science. To connect the dots necessitates that we more precisely describe terms like 'brain', 'module' and 'mind', something cognitive scientists have been thinking hard about for some time (Gazzaniga, 2005; Gazzaniga and Steven, 2005; Pinker, 2002).

It seems clear that natural selection shaped brains just as it did hearts and lungs, but the real reason why that's important is that it resulted in the mental modules that underpin the functioning of *minds* (Barkow et al., 1992; Pinker, 2007). When individuals contemplate an action, when we think about the pros and cons of doing something – say, stealing something or hurting someone – these are events in our minds. So far, we have not provided much discussion in the way of what minds do and how they operate when running the evolved cognitive software that we've been referring to as psychological adaptations. The next section fills some of this gap that we have created for the reader up until now.

19.3 Evolutionary Science Meets Cognitive Science

The best way to move the discussion forward here is by first moving back a little further in time. In the early days of evolutionary psychology, a frequent charge levelled at the field was one of unadulterated and unabashed 'reductionism' (Barkow et al., 1992; Pinker, 2002). Critics loudly and *correctly* noted that there is no specific brain region for 'mate selection' or 'rape' or any other specific behaviour (Duntley, 2005; Duntley and Shackelford, 2008a, 2008b; Pinker, 1997, 2002). Brains just aren't built like that. Conveniently, we are not aware of any well-informed evolutionary psychologists that argued for the existence of such mythical brain regions. Evolutionary psychologists have, in fact, argued *against* the likelihood of such specific brain regions for at least three decades (e.g. see Pinker, 1997; Symons, 1992; Tooby and Cosmides, 1992).

The interest of evolutionary psychologists was always largely been about *minds*, not necessarily brains. It has been long understood, at least in most quarters of science, that minds came from brains – that no 'ghosts' floated around in the skull (Pinker, 2002). But no serious scholar thought that brain scans or inspection at autopsy would reveal little neural enclaves where cooperation happened or where deception took place and nothing else. As it would happen, some key insights from cognitive science would provide clarity concerning the confluence of brains, minds, cognition and evolutionary purpose. Led primarily by Michael Gazzaniga along with others, the emergence of cognitive neuroscience – a field that also served to merge insights from neurology and neuroscience – would end up illuminating ideas from evolutionary psychology (Gazzaniga, 2008). In an interesting twist, work conducted under the auspices of cognitive neuroscience relied on key insights from within evolutionary psychology practically from the start. For crime scientists, the need to pay attention to this work stems from the simple fact that much of it deals directly with the topics of morality, justice and fairness, along with a cadre of topics encountered in the confines of traditional criminology and criminal justice research (Aharoni et al., 2008; Gazzaniga, 2008; Miller et al., 2010).

A thorough review is beyond our current scope, but such reviews have been published (see Aharoni et al., 2008; Goodenough and Tucker, 2010; Schacter and Loftus, 2013). What we can offer is a 'crash course' that, though incomplete, will reveal why the early revelations in the field are relevant for the science of crime and justice. In 1981, Roger Sperry was awarded[1] the Nobel Prize for his work with patients suffering from treatment-resistant epilepsy. The surgical intervention employed with these patients involved severing (fully or in part) the corpus callosum – a tract of fibres connecting the hemispheres of the brain (Bogen et al., 1965). In some but not all cases, the corpus callosum bisection also included

the patient's anterior commissure (Bogen et al., 1965; Gazzaniga, 1995). The intent of the procedure was to limit the ability of the seizures to spread across the hemispheres (Bogen et al., 1965; Gazzaniga, 1995).

The surgery was effective in that patients noticed no immediate ill effects and experienced marked reductions in seizures (Bogen et al., 1965; Gazzaniga and Sperry, 1967). To interact with a patient who had undergone either partial or complete commissurotomy would not immediately suggest evidence that they had undergone the procedure. General cognitive abilities were preserved, memory and recall abilities were left intact and personality traits were generally unaffected (Gazzaniga, 1995). The hidden effects of the surgery became apparent in the confines of specific lab tests, but once revealed, they were striking (Gazzaniga, 1995, 2005; Volz and Gazzaniga, 2017). It was known that visual information presented to the right visual field arrives in the left hemisphere for processing and visual information in the left visual field is dealt with by the right hemisphere (McGilchrist, 2010; for a more detailed depiction, see figure 2 in Volz and Gazzaniga, 2017).

Put a little differently, isolating visual information so that it is only processed by the right hemisphere, for example, leaves the left hemisphere functionally in the dark about what was seen and what is happening. Volz and Gazzaniga (2017) recount a particularly illustrative case of patient P. S. Patient P. S. was presented with a picture of a chicken claw but only to his left hemisphere. The patient's right hemisphere was shown a snowy image. P. S. was then asked to point to pictures related to what had been seen by either the left hemisphere (using the right hand) or the right hemisphere (using the left hand). The right hand pointed to a chicken and the left hand pointed to a shovel. When asked why he had chosen those pictures, P. S. informed the experimenter of his reasons, which must have felt completely logical. The claw belonged to a chicken, and shovels, P. S. asserted, are pretty necessary if you need to clean out the chicken shed (paraphrased from figure 4 in Volz and Gazzaniga, 2017).

This 'reason', as others have noted, was pure confabulation; it had to have been given that the speaking left hemisphere was not aware of why the left hand had pointed to the shovel

---

[1] David Hubel and Torston Wiesel shared in the Prize, honouring their work on the visual system.

(Gazzaniga, 1995). It had no idea what was shown to the right hemisphere (Volz and Gazzaniga, 2017). The left hemisphere *created* an explanation, albeit a plausible one, for what was going on (Gazzaniga, 1995). These early revelations would lead to a cascade of research across decades of time, work that would encompass topics ranging from causal inference to moral reasoning (Gazzaniga, 1995, 2005; Gazzaniga and Steven, 2005; Miller et al., 2010). Without cataloguing every study – there are too many to do so – a few broad points are relevant.

First, the brain has a type of 'modular' architecture, though not the variety that some of the critics of evolutionary psychology argued against (Clune et al., 2013; Gomez-Robles et al., 2014; Sporns and Betzel, 2016). Neuroanatomists provided what were at first rudimentary and then remarkably precise maps of various neural regions that contributed to a variety of different functions. The cerebellum, medulla, amygdala and neocortical layers, for example, processed information collaboratively in various instances when engaging in certain tasks (Gazzaniga, 1995). Still, modularity of brain structure was apparent (Gazzaniga, 1995). The ability to explore the functional roles of different regions was rapidly maturing during this time, further clarifying the overlap and distinctions between what different neurological regions did exactly (Gazzaniga, 2018). The amygdala does more than just one thing, as do the pons and prefrontal cortex. And while regions certainly work in a collaborative fashion, as we have noted, this need not always be the case (Gazzaniga, 2018). The cerebellum modulates motor movements but is largely and generally uninvolved with language processing, for instance (see Glickstein, 2007).

19.4 Modularity Redux

Years of rancorous palaver might have been avoided in psychology had two concepts not been conflated. Hopefully, dwelling on this a bit more will smooth the incorporation of evolutionary and cognitive insights into the crime sciences. Those oft-conflated concepts are (1) brain and (2) mind. As we have already pointed out in Section 19.2, evolutionary psychologists argued for the existence of *mental* modules, not modules of neurological tissue per se that have bright boundaries and serve a singular function. The 'mental'

qualifier here is crucial because it trains our focus on minds – what they do and what they are for (see Franklin, 1995). Minds are produced by brains, but to speak of minds is to speak of something distinct in key respects from brains (Franklin, 1995). Functioning in Broca's area coordinates aspects of language and speech. But speaking and reasoning with words are also mental processes that can create different mental states used to solve different types of challenges in real life (Gazzaniga, 1980, 2018).

Mental states do not correspond with fidelity to brain functioning in an isolated area (Gazzaniga, 2018; Sperry, 1976). In fact, even if one endorsed a view of the brain as an all-purpose 'module-less' organ (which is unsupported and outmoded), such an organ could still produce a modular mind. Mental states often inform the solving of real-world problems. The real-world challenge of courting a mate would involve different mental states from those needed when engaging in combat with a conspecific trying to kill you. So, even though neurological science has revealed the brain to have an architecture that is both 'layered' and 'modular' (paraphrasing Gazzaniga, 2018), had that not been the case modular minds could still abound.

When Gazzaniga and colleagues (for a review, see Volz and Gazzaniga, 2017) tested the split-brain patients, evidence of modularity was revealed yet again. Hemispheres were responsible for different tasks and possessed certain capabilities that appeared distinct unto them. To offer some general examples, the left hemisphere held the ability to speak and to perform certain types of causal inference analyses (Volz and Gazzaniga, 2017). The right hemisphere, among other things, seemed to handle tasks relevant to recognising human faces. Moreover, and especially relevant for our purposes here, it also seemed to be essential for engaging a 'module' used to probe the true intentions of other people – necessary information when doing the moral calculations that we humans use practically every day (Miller et al., 2010; Volz and Gazzaniga, 2017).

19.5 Creeping towards Cognitive Crime Sciences

As a thought experiment (loosely paraphrased from Miller et al., 2010), imagine observing a co-worker preparing coffee for a friend at work.

After adding what they honestly believed to be sugar, their friend dies because, as it would turn out, the sugar was in fact poison mistaken for sweetener. Now, imagine observing the same scenario but instead you know in this case that when the co-worker adds 'sugar' they genuinely believe it to be poison, even though it is in fact only sugar. The friend drinks the coffee and is fine. Who is the more loathsome, morally culpable person? When presented with a similar vignette, split-brain patients responded in an interesting manner. Miller et al. (2010: 2220) summarised their results thusly:

> The present study demonstrates that full and partial callosotomy patients fail to rely on agents' beliefs when judging the moral permissibility of those agents' actions. This finding confirms the hypotheses that specialized belief-ascription mechanisms are lateralized to the right hemisphere and that disconnection from those mechanisms affects normal moral judgments. Moreover, the neural mechanism by which interhemispheric communication occurs between key left and right hemisphere processes seems complex. Since the partial anterior callosotomy patients also showed the effect, it would appear the right TPJ [temporoparietal junction] calls upon right frontal processes before communicating information to the left speaking hemisphere.

Given the frequent social interaction of humans, the ability to 'read each other's minds' (known more formally as 'theory of mind'; see Miller et al., 2010; Premack and Woodruff, 1978) is essential. In other words, it's often quite useful and even necessary for us to be capable of inferring something about what a person was thinking when they violated a social norm. In modern contexts, did the person run over a child because they fell asleep at the wheel or because they were sending a text message? The result would be the same, but the mental state of the driver mitigates what we think about culpability. Pointing out the broader importance of understanding this process more fully, Aharoni et al. (2008: 148) observed that:

> Ultimately, a keen knowledge of why people break the law might gain leverage from understanding not how free agents make choices but how causal brains influence people to follow some rules and not others.

Such knowledge can lead us to a better understanding in general of how our minds – as well as conglomerate of minds, such as a jury – assess criminal culpability when we are asked to judge the moral responsibility of another's action.

As mentioned just above, these mind-reading skills – as clarified by the work with split-brain patients – seem to be a modular feature of the right hemisphere (Miller et al., 2010). When you disrupt the right hemisphere's ability to inform the left with this information, you disrupt the moral calculus that cues the typical assignment of culpability (Miller et al., 2010). Natural selection designed a brain capable of inferring intent in others (Baron-Cohen et al., 1985). These skills litter the arena of topics that crime scientists are interested in. They seem fundamental when pondering and describing how juries deliberate, how judges' reason and how law enforcement interacts with citizenry, along with a host of other research topics (Gazzaniga, 2008).

19.6 Where to Next?

Admittedly, readers may be dissatisfied at this point, as we are wrapping up our discussion having revealed no great insight into the causes of crime. This is just the reality of where things stand. We see all roads converging at the nexus of evolutionary and cognitive science and feel strongly that this will bolster an understanding of what is happening when individuals engage in fraudulent, aggressive and violent acts. Yet discussing the anticipated convergence of fields and the positive results that should follow represents the start of the pathway, but it doesn't get us to the end of it. There is much left to do.

Our arguments, we feel compelled to point out, do not minimise or obviate work already done by crime scientists. This work has revealed some well-replicated and robust results that will be vital moving forward. Consider one of the strongest correlates of crime: self-control (Pratt and Cullen, 2000; Vazsonyi et al., 2017). The ability to regulate impulses, behaviours and desires is a broadly important human trait, yet its precise cognitive nature is a topic in need of more work. Similarly, over five decades of research in behavioural genetics has unequivocally demonstrated that all quantitative traits are partly heritable, including antisocial, self-regulatory and aggressive behaviours (Barnes et al., 2014; Beaver et al., 2014; Polderman et al., 2015). The existence of trait heritability is no longer surprising, but neither is this particularly insightful at this point. If genetic variation indeed contributes to meaningful behavioural variation for criminogenic outcomes, it does so *indirectly* and by having at least some effects on neurological structure and functioning, which would then have some impact on cognitive processing and so on (Polderman et al., 2015). We have barely started exploring these causal pathways.

As work of this nature begins to proceed in earnest, though, likely to be most pressing for many in the public (and many criminal justice professionals) are the *perceived* implications it might have for choice and free will. In anticipation of this, the neuroscientist Sam Harris (2012: 1) observed:

> Without free will, sinners and criminals would be nothing more than poorly calibrated clockwork, and any conception of justice that emphasized punishing them (rather than deterring, rehabilitating, or merely constraining them) would appear utterly incongruous.

Concerns of this nature, it would seem, might be assuaged with some careful reasoning (see Dennett, 1984). For example, while certain causal processes can produce aggressive and violent behaviour, other causal processes can reduce or prevent the same behaviours (see Dennett, 1984; Harris, 2012; Volz and Gazzaniga, 2017).

To understand how and why this is the case, one need only consider that the broad goal of cognitive behaviour therapy, psychopharmacology or some combination of the two is to change cognition and behaviour in a causal fashion, but for the better (Harris, 2012). Talking about 'causation' does not mean abandoning ideas of responsibility or personal change (Dennett, 1984; Harris, 2012). An uninformed embrace of fatalistic determinism would dictate that trauma victims be abandoned to their post-traumatic stress disorder, a bizarre notion made more repugnant given the emergence of promising new therapies (Brown et al., 2022; Harris, 2012; Mitchell et al., 2021). In fact, we must retain meaningful ideas about causality – such as trauma *causing* a stress disorder – if we desire to embrace the idea of interventions *causing* positive change. Insights from evolutionary and cognitive science aid this process tremendously by assisting in the search for causal pathways and mechanisms (see also Duntley and Shackelford, 2008a). Far from a hindrance, these fields promise to be widely useful for building both a robust crime science and a more ethical and efficacious framework for aiding in the rehabilitation of those who have run afoul of societal mandates.

References

Aharoni, E., Funk, C., Sinnott-Armstrong, W. and Gazzaniga, M. (2008). Can neurological evidence help courts assess criminal responsibility? Lessons from law and neuroscience. *Annals of the New York Academy of Sciences*, 1124, 145–160.

Barkow, J. H., Cosmides, L. and Tooby, J. (eds.). (1992). *The Adapted Mind: Evolutionary Psychology and the Generation of Culture*. New York: Oxford University Press.

Barnes, J. C., Wright, J. P., Boutwell, B. B., Schwartz, J. A., Connolly, E. J., Nedelec, J. L. and Beaver, K. M. (2014). Demonstrating the validity of twin research in criminology. *Criminology*, 52, 588–626.

Baron-Cohen, S., Leslie, A. M. and Frith, U. (1985). Does the autistic child have a 'theory of mind'? *Cognition*, 21, 37–46.

Beaver, K. M., Barnes, J. C. and Boutwell, B. B. (eds.). (2014). *The Nurture versus Biosocial Debate in Criminology: On the Origins of Criminal Behavior and Criminality*. New York: SAGE Publications.

Black, D. (1976). *The Behavior of Law*. New York: Academic Press.

Bogen, J. E., Fisher, E. D. and Vogel, P. J. (1965). Cerebral commissurotomy: a second case report. *JAMA*, 194, 1328–1329.

Boutwell, B. B. and Adams, C. D. (2020). A research note on Mendelian randomization and causal inference in criminology: promises and considerations. *Journal of Experimental Criminology*, doi: 10.1007/s11292-020-09436-9.

Brown, R. L., Wood, A., Carter, J. D. and Kannis-Dymand, L. (2022). The metacognitive model of PTSD and metacognitive therapy for PTSD: a systematic review. *Clinical Psychology & Psychotherapy*, 29, 131–146.

Buss, D. M. (1991). Evolutionary personality psychology. *Annual Review of Psychology*, 42, 459–491.

Buss, D. M. (2007). *Evolutionary Psychology: The New Science of the Mind* (2nd ed.). New York: Allyn & Bacon.

Buss, D. M. and Shackelford, T. K. (1997). Human aggression in evolutionary psychological perspective. *Clinical Psychology Review*, 17, 605–619.

Clune, J., Mouret, J. B. and Lipson, H. (2013). The evolutionary origins of modularity. *Proceedings of the Royal Society of*

London. Series B: Biological Sciences, 280, 20122863.

Dawkins, R. (1996). *The Blind Watchmaker: Why the Evidence of Evolution Reveals a Universe without Design*. New York: W.W. Norton & Co.

Dennett, D. C. (1984). *Elbow Room: The Varieties of Free Will Worth Wanting*. Cambridge, MA: MIT Press.

DeVore, I. and Tooby, J. (1987). The reconstruction of hominid behavioral evolution through strategic modeling. In W. G. Kinzey (ed.), *The Evolution of Human Behavior: Primate Models*. Albany: State University of New York Press, pp. 183–237.

Duntley, J. D. (2005). Adaptations to dangers from other humans. In D. M. Buss (ed.), *The Handbook of Evolutionary Psychology*. New York: Wiley, pp. 224–249.

Duntley, J. D. and Shackelford, T. K. (2008a). Darwinian foundations of crime and law. *Aggression and Violent Behavior*, 13, 373–382.

Duntley, J. D. and Shackelford, T. K. (eds.). (2008b). *Evolutionary Forensic Psychology*. New York: Oxford University Press.

Falconer, D. S. and Mackay, T. F. C. (1996). *Introduction to Quantitative Genetics* (4th ed.). Harlow: Longmans Green.

Franklin, S. (1995). *Artificial Minds*. Cambridge, MA: MIT Press.

Gazzaniga, M. S. (1980). The role of language for conscious experience: observations from split-brain man. *Progress in Brain Research*, 54, 689–696).

Gazzaniga, M. S. (1995). Principles of human brain organization derived from split-brain studies. *Neuron*, 14, 217–228.

Gazzaniga, M. S. (2005). Forty-five years of split-brain research and still going strong. *Nature Reviews Neuroscience*, 6, 653–659.

Gazzaniga, M. S. (2008). The law and neuroscience. *Neuron*, 60, 412–415.

Gazzaniga, M. S. (2009). *The Cognitive Neurosciences*. Cambridge, MA: MIT Press.

Gazzaniga, M. S. (2018). *The Consciousness Instinct: Unraveling the Mystery of How the Brain Makes the Mind*. New York: Farrar, Straus and Giroux.

Gazzaniga, M. S. and Sperry, R. W. (1967). Language after section of the cerebral commissures. *Brain*, 90, 131–148.

Gazzaniga, M. S. and Steven, M. S. (2005). Neuroscience and the law. *Scientific American Mind*, 16, 42–49

Glickstein, M. (2007). What does the cerebellum really do? *Current Biology*, 17, R824–R827.

Gómez-Robles, A., Hopkins, W. D. and Sherwood, C. C. (2014). Modular structure facilitates mosaic evolution of the brain in chimpanzees and humans. *Nature Communications*, 5, 1–9.

Goodenough, O. R. and Tucker, M. (2010). Law and cognitive neuroscience. *Annual Review of Law and Social Science*, 6, 61–92.

Harris, S. (2012). *Free Will*. New York: Simon and Schuster.

Heinrich, J., Boyd, R. and Richardson, P. J. (2008). Five misunderstandings about cultural evolution. *Human Nature*, 19, 119–137.

Kavish, N. and Boutwell, B. (2018). The unified crime theory and the social correlates of crime and violence: problems and solutions. *Journal of Criminal Psychology*, 4, 287–301.

Lalumiere, M. L., Harris, G. T. and Rice, M. E. (2001). Psychopathy and developmental instability. *Evolution and Human Behavior*, 22, 75–92.

Marcus, G. (2009). *Kluge: The Haphazard Evolution of the Human Mind*. Boston, MA: Houghton Mifflin Harcourt.

McGilchrist, I. (2010). Reciprocal organization of the cerebral hemispheres. *Dialogues in Clinical Neuroscience*, 12, 503–515.

Mealey, L. (1995). The sociobiology of sociopathy: an integrated evolutionary model. *Behavioral & Brain Sciences*, 18, 523–599.

Miller, M. B., Sinnott-Armstrong, W., Young, L., King, D., Paggi, A., Fabri, M., Polonara, G. and Gazzaniga, M. S. (2010). Abnormal moral reasoning in complete and partial callosotomy patients. *Neuropsychologia*, 48, 2215–2220.

Mitchell, J. M., Bogenschutz, M., Lilienstein, A., Harrison, C., Kleiman, S., Parker-Guilbert, K., ... Doblin, R. (2021). MDMA-assisted therapy for severe PTSD: a randomized, double-blind, placebo-controlled phase 3 study. *Nature Medicine*, 27, 1025–1033.

Nilsson, D. E. and Pelger, S. (1994). A pessimistic estimate of the time required for an eye to evolve. *Proceedings of the Royal Society of London. Series B: Biological Sciences*, 256, 53–58.

Pinker, S. (1997). *How the Mind Works*. New York: W.W. Norton & Co.

Pinker, S. (2002). *The Blank Slate: The Modern Denial of Human Nature*. New York: Penguin.

Pinker, S. (2007). *The Stuff of Thought: Language as a Window into Human Nature*. New York: Penguin.

Pinker, S. (2010). The cognitive niche: coevolution of intelligence, sociality, and language. *Proceedings of the National Academy of Sciences of the United States of America*, 107, 8993–8999.

Pinker, S. (2011). *The Better Angels of Our Nature: Why Violence Has Declined*. New York: Viking Books.

Pitchford, I. (2001). The origins of violence: is psychopathy an adaptation? *Human Nature Review*, 1, 28–36.

Polderman, T. J., Benyamin, B., De Leeuw, C. A., Sullivan, P. F., Van Bochoven, A., Visscher, P. M. and Posthuma, D. (2015). Meta-analysis of the heritability of human traits based on fifty years of twin studies. *Nature Genetics*, 47, 702–709.

Pratt, T. C. and Cullen, F. T. (2000). The empirical status of Gottfredson and Hirschi's general theory of crime: a meta-analysis. *Criminology*, 38, 931–964.

Premack, D. and Woodruff, G. (1978). Does the chimpanzee have a theory of mind? *Behavioral and Brain Sciences*, 1, 515–526.

Schacter, D. L. and Loftus, E. F. (2013). Memory and law: what can cognitive neuroscience contribute? *Nature Neuroscience*, 16, 119–123.

Shackelford, T. K. (ed.). (2020). *The SAGE Handbook of Evolutionary Psychology* (vols 1–4). London: SAGE Publications.

Sperry, R. W. (1976). Mental phenomena as causal determinants in brain function. In G. G. Globus, G. Maxwell and I. Savodnik (eds.), *Consciousness and the Brain*. Boston, MA: Springer, pp. 163–177.

Sporns, O. and Betzel, R. F. (2016). Modular brain networks. *Annual Review of Psychology*, 67, 613–640.

Symons, D. (1992). On the use and misuse of Darwinism in the study of human behavior. In Barkow, J. H., Tooby, J. and Cosmides, L. (eds.), *The Adapted Mind: Evolutionary Psychology and the Generation of Culture*. New York: Oxford University Press, pp. 137–159.

Tanksley, P. T., Barnes, J. C., Boutwell, B. B., Arseneault, L., Caspi, A., Danese, A., Fisher, H. L. and Moffitt, T. E. (2020). Identifying psychological pathways to polyvictimization: evidence from a longitudinal cohort study of twins from the UK. *Journal of experimental criminology*, 16, 431–461.

Tielbeek, J. J., Barnes, J. C., Popma, A., Polderman, T. J., Lee, J. J., Perry, J. R., Posthuma, D. and Boutwell, B. B. (2018). Exploring the genetic correlations of antisocial behaviour and life history traits. *BJPsych Open*, 4, 467–470.

Tooby, J. and Cosmides, L. (1992). The psychological foundations of culture. In J. H. Barkow, L. Cosmides and J. Tooby (eds.), *The Adapted Mind: Evolutionary Psychology and the Generation of Culture*. New York: Oxford University Press, pp. 19–136.

Tooby, J. and DeVore, I. (1987). The reconstruction of hominid behavioral evolution through strategic modeling. In W. G. Kinzey (ed.), *The Evolution of Human Behavior*. Albany: State University of New York Press, pp. 183–238.

Trivers, R. L. (1971). The evolution of reciprocal altruism. *Quarterly Review of Biology*, 46, 35–57.

Tyler, T. R. (1990). *Why People Obey the Law*. New Haven, CT: Yale University Press.

Vazsonyi, A. T., Mikuška, J. and Kelley, E. L. (2017). It's time: a meta-analysis on the self-control–deviance link. *Journal of Criminal Justice*, 48, 48–63.

Volz, L. J. and Gazzaniga, M. S. (2017). Interaction in isolation: 50 years of insights from split-brain research. *Brain*, 140, 2051–2060.

Wilson, E. O. (1999). *Consilience: The Unity of Knowledge*. New York: Vintage.

Evolutionary Thinking and Clinical Care of Psychiatric Patients

Alfonso Troisi

Abstract

Psychiatric therapeutics is facing a major crisis that originates from its limited efficacy and dubious scientific credibility. Such a crisis requires a radical change in the paradigm that inspires psychiatric research and clinical practice. The new paradigm should integrate in a meaningful way all of the variables that mediate the aetiology and pathogenesis of psychiatric disorders: biological, psychological, developmental, behavioural and social. The essence of the evolutionary study of human psychology and behaviour is just such an integration. Therefore, evolutionary thinking has great potential to improve the clinical care of psychiatric patients. According to a modern view of medicine, the aims of therapy are not only to lessen symptoms and to reverse the pathogenic mechanisms, but also to restore the congruence between a patient's functional capacities and the conditions of the environment. Evolutionary thinking suggests replacing symptoms with functional capacities as the primary targets of psychiatric treatment. Most mental disorders are conditions of compromised functional capacities. Therapy should aim at improving patients' capacities necessary to enact behaviours associated with goal achievement. When treating patients, clinicians should distinguish between symptoms caused by dysfunctional mechanisms and symptoms that are adaptive reactions to environmental situations with negative cost–benefit outcomes.

Keywords

adaptive symptoms, biomedical model, brain–mind dichotomy, evolutionary psychiatry, functional capacities, placebo effect, psychiatric therapy, psychopharmacology, psychotherapy, symptomatic therapy

Key Points

- Therapy should primarily aim at improving the patient's functional capacities.
- Successful therapy restores the normal functioning of evolved behavioural systems.
- Symptoms can be caused by the direct action of aetiological agents (symptoms as defects) or reflect adaptive responses to environmental constraints (symptoms as defences). Targeting adaptive symptoms may lead to unwanted outcomes and harm patients.
- In patients with intact functional capacities, therapy should facilitate the development of revised models of the social environment and favour the implementation of behavioural strategies leading to goal achievement.

- In patients with suboptimal functional capacities, therapy should teach the use of alternative strategies. If this is impossible, patients should be advised to actively search for environments in which they are most likely to achieve high-priority goals.
- The acronym GOAL should inform the assessment of therapeutic outcomes: *give* less weight to symptoms, *observe* actual behaviour, *assess* functional capacities and *leave* your office (to observe patients' behaviour in their natural environment).

20.1 Introduction

Evolutionary psychiatry is a subfield of psychiatry and psychiatry is a subfield of medicine. The major goal of medicine is to prevent and cure human diseases. Devoid of therapy, medicine would become a different kind of science – a kind that the majority of patients and clinicians would consider as unsatisfactory or even useless. Medical knowledge needs to be related to therapy in one way or another. The relation can be distant as in the case of implementing successful preventative measures, relatively close as in the case of discovering modifiable pathophysiologic mechanisms or very close as in the case of treating patients with effective interventions. Yet, in any case, medical knowledge is expected to generate practical implications. Based on this premise, it is clear that the scientific status of evolutionary psychiatry is largely dependent on its capacity to take care of people with psychiatric disorders.

How is evolutionary psychiatry doing in the field of therapy? With few exceptions, the majority of psychiatrists believe that evolutionary psychiatry does not get on well in this field. Samuel Guze, one of the most influential educators and researchers in modern clinical psychiatry, wrote: 'Unless evolutionary explanations are tied directly to genetic and physiological knowledge of why some people get sick in certain ways while others do not, they are too vague and general to be *useful* in medicine' (1992: 92, emphasis added). Based on my personal experience, Guze's opinion reflects what most clinicians think. Some years ago, I was invited to give a lecture on evolutionary psychiatry at a major meeting of clinical psychiatrists. The audience was quite large and included clinicians who were engaged daily in diagnosing and treating patients with mental disorders. At the end of my talk, I submitted to the audience two questions and asked participants to reply through tele-voting. The first question was: does the evolutionary approach make an important theoretical contribution to clinical psychiatry? The great majority (87%) of the participants replied 'yes'. The second question was: is Darwinian psychiatry relevant for your clinical practice? Only 8% of the participants gave an affirmative response.

Interestingly, some of those who share a pessimistic view are psychiatrists with an evolutionary background. Reflecting on the fact that there are no evolutionary-based treatments for mental disorders, Randolph Nesse, one of the founders of evolutionary medicine, concluded that evolutionary biology's contribution to psychiatry is limited to offering a new conceptual framework for integrating findings from the many disciplines that study the human mind and behaviour (Nesse, 2005). The view of Jay Feierman, a former professor of clinical psychiatry at the University of New Mexico, is more drastic:

> I've been involved with this 'movement' of evolutionary psychiatry since its origins in the 1970s. It is very interesting but, unfortunately, just another version of rational therapeutics. There has not been a single evidence-based treatment that has come out of evolutionary psychiatry in the past 50 years. Most theories are not falsifiable. I don't see it much better than Freudian theory. I don't think Darwin himself would approve of the evolutionary psychiatry 'movement'. (Personal communication, 10 February 2021)

In this chapter, contrary to the belief of sceptics, I will try to convince the reader that evolutionary thinking has great potential to improve the clinical care of psychiatric patients. According to a modern view of medicine, the aims of therapy are not only to lessen symptoms and to reverse the pathogenic mechanisms, but also to restore the congruence between a patient's functional capacities and the conditions of the environment (Childs, 1999; Flaum, 2010; Klinkman, 2009). If therapy is conceived of in these terms, the therapeutic relevance of evolutionary psychiatry emerges clearly (Troisi, 2012). Evolutionary psychiatry can contribute more to the strategic aspects of therapy than to its tactical execution (i.e. the actual means used to achieve the therapeutic objectives).

This chapter is organised as follows: Section 20.2 consists of an evolutionary analysis of current psychiatric practice with a special focus on therapeutic goals. In this section, I will discuss how evolutionary thinking conceptualises successful therapeutic outcomes and to what extent the evolutionary view differs from clinicians' objectives and patients' expectations. The content of this section has practical implications because it suggests revising the priority of therapeutic goals and the methods for assessing therapeutic outcomes. Section 20.3 is more theoretical because it aims at understanding the origins of unsolved problems in psychiatric therapeutics through an evolutionary lens. I will discuss mind–body dualism and its implications for the choice between somatic and psychological therapies, the placebo effect, the harmful effects of some psychological interventions and the crisis of the biomedical model.

20.2 A Theory of Therapy

To decide whether evolutionary thinking can improve the clinical care of patients with mental disorders we should first define what are the goals of therapy. The question is deceptively simple. Saying that therapy aims at fighting disease and restoring health does not consider the complexity of psychiatric interventions and ignores the fact that patients' and clinicians' views can diverge.

20.2.1 What Patients Want

Experts in the treatment of depression have suggested that achieving remission should be viewed as the primary goal of therapy. Remission corresponds to complete or quasi-complete symptom resolution as measured by patients' scores on clinical rating scales (e.g. ≤ 7 on the Hamilton Depression Rating Scale). Yet patients seem to differ in their ranking of what is most important for cure in depression. In a study focusing on patients' perspectives, a brief questionnaire was distributed to 535 outpatients who were being treated for a major depressive episode (Zimmerman et al., 2006). They were asked to rate the importance of 16 statements in determining whether depression was in remission. The presence of positive mental health (optimism, vigour, self-confidence) got the highest ranking ahead of feeling like your usual self, return to your usual level of functioning, feeling in emotional control and participating in and enjoying relationships with family and friends. The alleviation of depressive symptoms was ranked only sixth.

According to patients' perspectives, normal functioning is an important criterion for defining remission in addition to positive affect. Zimmerman et al. (2012b) examined how many depressed patients in ongoing treatment who scored in the remission range on the 17-item Hamilton Depression Rating Scale did not consider themselves to be in remission from their depression. Approximately half of the patients scoring ≤ 7 on the rating scale did not consider themselves to be in remission. Compared to the self-described remitters, these disappointed patients reported significantly worse levels of functional impairment and coping ability. Conversely, some patients who do not meet symptom-based definitions of remission nonetheless consider themselves to be in remission if they regain satisfactory levels of functional capacity and coping ability (Zimmerman et al., 2012a).

These findings are very relevant to the discussion of how evolutionary thinking conceptualises the goals of psychiatric therapy. The discussion focuses on three interrelated features: the significance of subjective well-being, the risks of symptomatic therapy and the importance of functional capacities.

20.2.2 Don't Worry, Be Happy

The primacy given by depressed patients to positive affect is intuitive and in accord with common experience: we all want to be happy. However, it is also in accordance with the aims of positive psychology and psychiatry. The basic idea behind this new movement is that resolution of symptoms is not enough or, in the words of Martin Seligman, 'arriving at the good is a lot more than just eliminating the bad' (Seligman, 2019: 20). The hedonic view of well-being focuses on subjective happiness defined in terms of pleasure attainment and pain avoidance (Oades and Mossman, 2017). According to such a view, mental health professionals should work on building patients' well-being and not just on the traditional task of reducing their ill-being.

The new emphasis on well-being has prompted a wellspring of research into the neurobiological and psychosocial causes and consequences of positive emotions and affect (Alexander et al., 2021; Helliwell and Aknin, 2018). All of this research is about proximate mechanisms. It explicates the components and operation of the systems that modulate positive emotions from the level of molecular genetics and neurochemistry to the impacts of life events and personal relationships. What is omitted is an evolutionary explanation of positive emotions. Why does positive affect exist at all and what is its adaptive function? Reasoning about happiness (and related positive emotions) from an evolutionary perspective inevitably poses the same ultimate questions about depression (and related negative emotions). My friend and colleague Randolph Nesse has dedicated an entire book to answering those questions. His explanation is concise but exhaustive: '[E]motions are specialized states that adjust physiology, cognition, subjective experience, facial expressions, and behavior in ways that increase the ability to meet the adaptive challenges of situations that have recurred over the evolutionary history of a species' (Nesse, 2019: 54). From an evolutionary perspective, positive affect is not the goal. The goal is biological adaptation, and positive affect is just a rewarding signal elicited by (and designed for perpetuating) beneficial circumstances. By contrast, depression, like physical pain, is a warning signal elicited by (and designed for escaping) maladaptive circumstances.'

The therapeutic implications of the evolutionary view of emotions have been analysed by focusing mostly on the relief of mental pain (see Section 20.2.3). Much less has been said about positive affect. A major question concerns the possibility of decoupling mood change from the environmental circumstances that normally elicit emotions (see Chapter 12). If a therapeutic intervention makes a patient happy even if their life circumstances remain problematic, should we take such action? Drugs of abuse achieve this, but they are not considered therapeutic agents. To a lesser extent, antidepressant drugs can achieve this, as is suggested by studies of healthy volunteers and depressed patients. Single and repeated administrations of antidepressants across different pharmacological classes have been found to increase the relative recognition of positive over negative social cues in a facial expression recognition task in healthy people. Similarly, a single dose of a selective norepinephrine reuptake inhibitor facilitated the recognition of happy facial expressions and the recall of positive versus negative self-referent memories in patients with depression compared with the double-blind administration of placebo (Harmer et al., 2017). The discovery of new antidepressants (e.g. ketamine) is likely to further widen the gap between mood improvement and life changes: '[N]ovel rapid-onset drugs might be able to change or reduce memories of already encoded negative information, which would be predicted to have faster effects on mood because *there is less dependence on the environment*' (Harmer et al., 2017: 416, emphasis added).

In his book, Nesse (2019) has made it clear that the possible adaptive function of low mood does not mean that it should not be treated. Relieving pain – physical or mental – is a mandatory task for clinicians. However, in medicine, aetiological therapy (i.e. therapy aimed at removing the causes of the symptoms) is always preferable to symptomatic therapy (i.e. therapy aimed at relieving symptoms without impacting the pathogenic mechanisms). The argument can be extended to promoting positive affect. If we can make our patients happier by optimising their adaptive functioning, this is much better than giving them rose-tinted glasses. In this regard, the eudaimonic view of well-being (defined in terms of environmental mastery, self-realisation and optimal functioning; Oades and Mossman, 2017) is closer to evolutionary thinking than the hedonic view of well-being (defined in terms of pleasure attainment and pain avoidance), although there are important differences, as explained in Section 20.2.4.

20.2.3 Symptomatic Therapy: Don't Fire at the Wrong Target

Prevailing models of psychopathology consider psychiatric symptoms as products of one or more underlying dysfunctional processes (e.g. neurochemical imbalance, intrapsychic conflicts, learning distortions). The explaining metaphor is that of the body (brain) as a machine that the clinician is called upon to fix when it breaks. Within such a theoretical framework, the clinician's role is that of an engineer who uses technology (i.e. therapeutic tools) to reverse the pathways leading to machine malfunctioning (i.e. the pathogenic mechanisms of disease) or, if this is not possible, to alleviate the symptoms produced by the machine malfunctioning. Many psychiatric symptoms are best explained in this way (e.g. bizarre delusions, melancholic depression or agitated delirium). Yet not all symptoms are the same. Many manifestations of medical and psychiatric diseases are sophisticated adaptations, not just epiphenomena of a broken machine (Nesse, 2018). When classified from an evolutionary perspective, symptoms can be divided into two broad categories: symptoms as defects in the body's mechanisms and symptoms as useful defences. For example, seizures, jaundice, coma and paralysis have apparently no adaptive function and arise from defects in the organism. But many other manifestations of disease are defences. Vomiting eliminates toxins from the stomach. The low iron levels associated with chronic infection limit the growth of pathogens. Coughing clears foreign matter from the respiratory tract.

The distinction between defects and defences is of paramount importance for therapeutic decision-making. In Section 20.2.2, I raised the question of whether improving mood through symptomatic therapy is acting for the good of the patient. Although he titled his book *Good Reasons for Bad Feelings*, Nesse (2019) has maintained that the suppression of defensive symptoms is generally safe because the adaptive response is often excessive and/or useless under modern environmental conditions. Before arriving at such an optimistic conclusion we should prudently wait for the collection of more empirical data. I suspect that the scarcity of clinical evidence showing the risks of blocking adaptive symptoms depends largely on the selective blindness and under-reporting of contemporary psychiatric research. When research has focused on the suppression of adaptive symptoms, its findings have questioned the absolute safety of symptomatic therapy.

Post-traumatic stress disorder (PTSD) is a psychiatric disorder that may occur in people who have experienced or witnessed a traumatic event such as a natural disaster, a serious accident, a terrorist act, war/combat or rape or who have been threatened with death, sexual violence or serious injury. Since the distressing acute symptoms following traumatic experiences deserve effective and rapid alleviation, sedating and calming treatment in the post-stress acute phase is common. However, prospective studies have shown that there may be an increased incidence of PTSD in individuals treated with anxiolytics immediately after exposure to trauma (Guina et al., 2015). The deleterious effects of these acute-phase treatments are likely to be caused by their interference with the acute stress response, a set of physiological and psychological mechanisms that evolved to cope with traumatic events in the natural environment. The sedating and calming effects of benzodiazepines might interfere with fear extinction via reduced release of the stress hormones (i.e. glucocorticoids) that support extinction (Singewald et al., 2015). Matar et al. (2009) tested this hypothesis in a rodent model and found that a brief course with alprazolam (an anxiolytic drug) in the immediate aftermath of stress exposure is associated with less favourable responses to additional stress exposure later on. Drug treatment was associated with a significant attenuation of the corticosterone levels, suggesting a possible link between disruption of the initial hypothalamic–pituitary–adrenal axis (HPA) response and subsequent

unfavourable outcomes. The recent meta-analysis by Kothgassner et al. (2021) confirmed the efficacy of hydrocortisone in the prevention of PTSD in human subjects. The authors emphasised the utility of mimicking the adaptive reaction to acute stress: '[A]n appropriate release of glucocorticoids immediately after traumatic stress reboots the HPA axis and rapidly restores homeostasis' (p. 8).

The evidence against the use of benzodiazepines in the post-stress acute phase is unequivocal. By contrast, data on the possible adverse effects of antidepressant drugs are suggestive but not so clear in showing the risks of symptomatic therapy. Many studies reported unwanted interpersonal effects of antidepressant drugs (e.g. inhibition of natural sadness, caring less about self and others; Price et al., 2009; Read et al., 2014), often given verbatim: 'It makes me emotionally flat – for example, I had to stop taking them after a recent family bereavement to make sure I was able to cry at the funeral' (Read et al., 2017: 425). There is no doubt that antidepressant drugs can induce emotional indifference and apathy (Sansone and Sansone, 2010). Yet the open question is: can these psychoactive effects obscure a clear perception of environmental stressors and interfere with the implementation of life changes (Andrews et al., 2012)?

20.2.4 Focus on Functional Capacities

Sections 20.2.2 and 20.2.3 showed the limits of symptom-centred therapies. Evolutionary thinking suggests replacing symptoms with functional capacities as the primary targets of psychiatric treatment. Whatever else they are, most mental disorders are conditions of compromised functional capacities defined as those capacities necessary to achieve the short-term goals that, in the ancestral environment, correlated with enhanced genetic replication (Troisi, 2015). A non-exhaustive list of short-term goals include survival, self-protection, acquiring resources, making friends, developing social support networks, having high status, attracting a mate and establishing intimate relationships (McGuire and Troisi, 1998; Troisi, 2020b). Failure to achieve short-term goals elicits symptoms as adaptive reactions to maladaptive situations or situations with negative cost–benefit outcomes. Symptoms are expected to disappear if therapeutic intervention improves the patient's chances of achieving short-term biological goals and offsets negative cost–benefit outcomes.

The pathogenic model outlined in the previous paragraph requires some qualifications. First, not all psychiatric symptoms are adaptive reactions to maladaptive situations. Some symptoms are manifestations of pathophysiologic mechanisms (the metaphor of the 'broken machine'; see Section 20.2.3). Second, adverse environments can compromise the functionality of optimal capacities. This is the case where therapy should help the patient to identify the environmental and personal constraints that interfere with achieving short-term goals. This is also the case where symptom-centred treatment is strongly advised against. Third, the inability to achieve short-term goals is often due to suboptimal capacities and/or the incapacity to exit from adverse environments. These suboptimal traits are common features of a variety of psychiatric disorders (e.g. chronic depression, personality disorders, anxiety disorders, somatic symptom disorders) and usually originate from gene–environment interactions (Uher, 2014). Therapy should aim at improving the capacities necessary to enact behaviours associated with goal achievement. However, modifying suboptimal capacities is often extremely difficult. When patients are not able to develop and execute novel behavioural strategies in spite of therapeutic intervention, they should be advised to search actively for environments in which they are most likely to achieve priority goals (Troisi and McGuire, 2000).

The evolutionary model reverses the directionality of the causal relationship between symptoms and functional capacities postulated by prevailing models of psychopathology. Impaired functioning or disability is commonly viewed as a consequence of psychiatric symptoms (Üstün and Kennedy, 2009). This is certainly true in some psychiatric disorders (e.g. social withdrawal in psychotic patients with persecutory delusions). In other conditions, functional impairment comes first (e.g. depression and anger in patients with borderline personality disorder who fail in establishing rewarding intimate relationships). Symptoms follow functional impairment when they are evolved warning signals that biological goals have not been or are not being achieved.

The evolutionary model can explain some puzzling findings that have emerged from clinical studies of the relationship between symptoms and functional capacities. Using data from the Netherlands Study of Depression and Anxiety (NESDA), Saris et al. (2017) analysed social functioning in a large sample of patients with depressive and anxiety disorders. In addition to the expected finding that social functioning was compromised in all diagnostic subgroups, the authors found that functional impairment remained even after complete remission of symptoms. According to the authors, one possible explanation for this is that social disability precedes the onset of clinical symptoms and is minimally altered by therapy. In effect, they found that perceived social disability was the sole significant predictor of anxiety and/ or depressive disorders two years after the initial screening. The longitudinal correlation between symptoms and functional capacities is weak not only in anxiety and depressive disorders but also in bipolar disorder (e.g. Rosa et al., 2009) and schizophrenia (e.g. Ganev, 2000).

As already noted in Section 20.2.2, the eudaimonic view of well-being (Oades and Mossman, 2017) is closer to evolutionary thinking than the hedonic view of well-being because it emphasises the importance of functional capacities to achieve and maintain a stable condition of positive mood. However, the eudaimonic view overlaps with the evolutionary model of optimal functioning only to the degree that personal goals are framed within the natural hierarchy of biological goals. Obviously, cultural values and social learning interact with evolved inclinations in setting priorities among biological goals. Yet, there is a limit to individual and cultural relativism. Maladaptive changes in the hierarchy of life goals (e.g. dismissing self-protection) is one of the most reliable indicators of serious mental illness (Troisi, 2015).

20.2.5 Key Points

The key points of a theory of psychiatric therapy as conceptualised from an evolutionary perspective are summarised in the 'Key Points' section at the beginning of this chapter. An additional point that needs to be underscored is that, in medicine, therapy is closely linked to diagnosis. Changing the therapeutic approach requires a parallel change of the diagnostic approach. Elsewhere (Troisi, 2012), I have proposed the acronym GOAL to summarise which changes are necessary to conduct an evolutionary diagnostic evaluation of psychiatric disorders: *give* less weight to symptoms, *observe* actual behaviour, *assess* functional capacities and *leave* your office (to observe patients' behaviour in their natural environment). Accordingly, the evaluation of therapeutic effects should follow the same principles.

20.3 Controversies in Psychiatric Therapeutics

Psychiatric therapeutics presents several unsolved problems that impact the clinical care of patients in the 'real world' in spite of their apparently philosophical nature. Evolutionary thinking can contribute to the debate about these open questions by providing researchers and clinicians with a new theoretical perspective that is substantially different from the traditional view of mainstream psychiatry.

20.3.1 Brain and Mind

In clinical discourse, references to 'mind' and 'brain' have become a form of code for different ways to think about the aetiology of psychiatric disorders and their treatment. The aetiology and pathogenesis of 'biological' disorders would depend mainly on genetic predisposition and neural dysfunction, whereas environmental factors and interpersonal problems would be the main causal factors of 'psychological' disorders. Somatic therapies (e.g. pharmacotherapy) would be best indicated for biological disorders and psychotherapy would be the treatment of choice for psychological disorders (Lebowitz and Applebaum, 2019). As a practicing psychiatrist, I am often asked by my patients if their problem is physical or psychological: 'Is there a chemical imbalance in my brain?', 'Did I get the wrong genes from my parents?', 'Does it depend on the way my mother treated me when I was a child?', 'It's the effect of job frustration, isn't it?'. An all-encompassing answer ('all factors play a role in what is happening to you') is just a courteous trick to hide the fact that we do not know how biological, psychological and social factors should be combined to explain and treat mental disorders.

Despite countless attempts to promote an integrative model, the dualistic view continues to dominate psychiatric theory and practice (Miresco and Kirmayer, 2006). The biopsychosocial model introduced by George Engel more than 40 years ago (Engel, 1980; also see Chapter 2 of this volume)

has increasingly turned into an additive, eclectic framework that does not explain the conceptual relationship between its components (Henningsen, 2015). In psychiatry, as stated by Davies and Roache (2017: 3), 'the biopsychosocial paradigm is, in a sense, everywhere and yet nowhere'.

From an evolutionary perspective, the integration of biological, psychological and social factors is the inevitable consequence of interpreting all of these variables as proximate mechanisms that work and interact in the service of a common function. The unifying concept is that of a behavioural system. A behavioural system (e.g. the attachment system) can be defined as an integrated group of functionally related components consisting of specific psychological processes, physiological mechanisms, anatomical structures and genetic influences. To serve the adaptive function that increases (or increased in the past) the likelihood of survival and/or reproduction, a behavioural system needs: (1) a set of activating stimuli; (2) a set of behaviours that are enacted to attain the system's goal; (3) a specific set goal (i.e. a change in the person–environment relationship that terminates the system's activation); (4) genetic, anatomical and physiological substrates that allow it to function; and (5) cognitive and emotional processes that motivate and guide the system's activity. The fact that, in the course of evolution, all of these components were selected for serving a common adaptive function explains the conceptual relationship between them. No component has an intrinsic priority over the others and malfunctioning can originate anywhere in the system. When this happens, malfunctioning propagates to all of the components. From such a perspective, it does not make any sense to say that insecure attachment or excessive aggression (two major behavioural systems) is either a biological or a psychological condition. And, more generally, it does not make any sense to say that a psychiatric disorder is 'organic' or 'functional' (where 'functional' is used to indicate that there is no demonstrable somatic lesion).

Focusing on behavioural systems and functional capacities blurs the distinction between somatic and psychosocial therapies. All types of therapy are biological because, from an evolutionary perspective, biology is not only genes and neurological correlates but also evolved reactions to life stressors, adaptive symptoms and calibrated life history strategies (Troisi, 2019). Brain functioning is inseparably connected to a person's environment and life history. Viewing the brain as a social and historical organ designed to solve adaptive problems allows for the integration of biological, psychological and social mechanisms into a coherent framework (Fuchs, 2004).

The relative indications of pharmacotherapy and psychotherapy should not be based on the postulated aetiology (biological versus psychosocial) of the condition to be treated. Rather, the choice should be based on empirical data showing which type of intervention is more efficacious in causing a long-term improvement of functional capacities. Pharmacotherapy (and other somatic therapies) and psychotherapy (and other psychosocial interventions) are not simply equivalent forms of treatment that act on the same substrates through bottom-up or top-down mechanisms. Rather, they are likely to be specific ways of altering the proximate mechanisms that cause the dysfunctional operation of one or more behavioural systems. The therapeutic modification of proximate mechanisms (be they biological, psychological or social) is successful only to the extent that it causes a substantial increase in the patient's capacity to achieve adaptive goals. The superiority of psychotherapy over pharmacotherapy (or vice versa) is a false problem just like the question of whether the pathogenic mechanisms causing psychiatric disorders are biological or psychological. The real questions are: (1) to what extent do psychiatric therapies impact suboptimal capacities and functional impairment? And (2) what works for whom?

20.3.2 The Placebo Effect

The placebo effect has been defined as the beneficial effect that is attributable to the brain–mind response to the context in which a treatment is delivered rather than to the specific actions of the treatment itself. The placebo effect is mediated by multiple processes, including learning, expectations and social cognition, and it can influence various clinical and physiological outcomes related to health (Wager and Atlas, 2015).

The placebo response is an important and clinically relevant effect in psychiatry because it impacts the outcomes of both pharmacological and psychological therapies (Bracken et al., 2012). The placebo response in psychotropic drug trials has a relatively large effect size.

Approximately 30% of patients in antidepressant and antipsychotic trials respond to placebo treatment (Huneke et al., 2020). In psychotherapy, the 'equivalence paradox' (i.e. the observation that different specific techniques account for very little of the variance in outcome, far less than the non-specific effect of being in therapy) has been interpreted as indirect evidence that the placebo effect plays a major role in psychological therapies (Blease, 2018).

Awareness that the placebo effect is a powerful ingredient of successful therapy has stimulated a flurry of scientific interest in the proximate question of how it works. Yet, few studies have thought to ask the ultimate question of why it works. Why did natural selection favour the evolution of self-healing mechanisms that are closely linked to the context in which a treatment is delivered? More than 20 years ago, Michael McGuire and I advanced the hypothesis that regulation–dysregulation theory (RDT) could in part explain the placebo effect of psychological therapies (Troisi and McGuire, 2000). Our hypothesis was based on studies showing that specific types and frequencies of interpersonal relationships are essential for maintaining physiological regulation and contrasting pathogenic mechanisms. If a patient enters a therapeutic environment that is supportive, non-judgemental and minimally demanding, such an environment mimics the social milieu that, in the 'real world', correlates with a high probability of achieving biological goals. The therapeutic effects are physiological re-regulation and symptom reduction. Since the publication of our hypothesis, the database confirming the positive or negative impacts of social relationships on human health has grown at an impressive rate (Holt-Lunstad, 2018).

The RDT hypothesis of the placebo effect can be extended to any type of treatment where the doctor–patient relationship is key in activating beneficial placebo mechanisms. The well-established observation that specific features of the therapeutic relationship (e.g. empathy, collaboration and support) predict better outcomes can be explained by the evolution of healing behaviour. In a highly cooperative species like our own, natural selection favoured the evolution of behaviours aimed at helping group companions who were wounded or sick through two different mechanisms: kin selection and reciprocal altruism. For a long period of our evolutionary history, care of the sick followed the path of intimate and affectionate relationships; delegation to unfamiliar experts came much later. Today, our emotional brain takes over our rational mind and tends to view medical care as motivated by affection and compassion, although we are, in fact, interacting with a professional, not a relative or friend, whose main task is to solve our case by applying scientific knowledge. Being the recipient of care by others could activate physiological self-healing mechanisms through the modulation of a steering system that Humphrey and Skoyles (2012) have named the 'health governor'. They hypothesise that this system has evolved to perform a kind of economic analysis of what the costs and benefits of self-cure will be, taking account of how dangerous the situation seems to be right now and what can be expected to happen next. The health governor might detect that family and friends are present and forecast that tender loving care will be provided and so deploy costly healing resources.

The evolutionary interpretation of the placebo effect as a form of interpersonal healing (McQueen and St John-Smith, 2012) suggests that we need more investigations that aim to understand how psychiatrists should interact with patients to maximise the benefits of any intervention. Certainly training is important, but the person of the psychiatrist is inextricably intertwined with the outcome of therapy. For example, Norcross and Lambert (2018) reported on a large naturalistic study that estimated the outcomes attributable to 581 psychotherapists treating 6146 patients in a managed care setting. The finding was that about 5% of the outcome variation was due to therapist effects and 0% was due to specific treatment methods. In my book *The Painted Mind* (Troisi, 2017: 133), I addressed the issue of clinician's personality:

> ... education of future doctors should emphasize that scientific knowledge and the capacity to establish a good relationship with patients belong to the same conceptual domain, because the relationship is a powerful therapeutic (or anti-therapeutic) agent that can be analyzed from a scientific perspective. Such an ambitious educational program should not neglect personality traits of future physicians. Some medical students seem to have a natural talent for interacting with patients. Others shine when they treat clinical cases

as scientific puzzles. Current educational programs ignore these individual differences and thus fail to take advantage of human resources that could improve medical practice.

20.3.3 Harmful Psychotherapies

When discussing the risks of symptomatic therapy (see Section 20.2.2), I have mentioned the possible harmful effects of antidepressant drugs due to their potential interference with evolved mechanisms of adaptation. Whereas the harmful impacts of antidepressants (Andrews et al., 2012; Read et al., 2014) and other psychiatric drugs (Moncrieff et al., 2020) are still debated, the interference with evolved mechanisms of adaptation has been convincingly demonstrated for some types of psychological intervention.

Immediately after natural or human-made disasters, it is common to offer debriefing interventions to exposed people to protect them from developing PTSD. Debriefing is typically a single-session procedure that lasts three to four hours, although it is occasionally conducted across several sessions. It is usually performed in groups and administered within 24–72 hours of the traumatic event. Therapists strongly encourage group members to discuss and process their negative emotions, delineate the PTSD symptoms that group members are likely to experience and discourage members from discontinuing participation once the session has begun. Several studies have found that victims randomly assigned to debriefing report a higher prevalence of PTSD and overall anxiety symptoms in the months following the intervention compared to victims in an assessment-only control group (Locher et al., 2019). Lilienfeld (2007: 59) hypothesised that debriefing may cause long-term harmful effects 'perhaps by impeding natural recovery processes'. If such a hypothesis is correct, the iatrogenic effect of debriefing would be comparable with that exerted by benzodiazepine administration in the post-stress acute phase (see Section 20.2.2).

Harmful effects have also been reported for grief therapy with individuals who have suffered losses of loved ones and are experiencing normal bereavement reactions (Jordan and Neimeyer, 2003). The finding that these harmful effects are observed in individuals with 'normal' as opposed to 'traumatic' grief reactions suggests that the interference with evolved mechanisms of adaptation is the likely cause of unwanted therapeutic outcomes.

Both trauma debriefing and grief therapy force participants to focus on their negative emotions and painful memories. Such a therapeutic strategy may counteract adaptive psychological reactions consisting in temporarily taking one's attention away from traumatic experiences and in distorting reality through ego defence mechanisms (Nesse, 1990). We need to conduct further clinical research in order to decide whether the hypothesis based on the interference with evolved mechanisms of adaptation explains by itself the harmful effects of some psychological therapies. Yet, in general, we can confidently affirm that an accurate understanding of patients' natural needs and evolved reactions is essential for avoiding iatrogenic effects of psychiatric therapies.

20.3.4 The Crisis of the Biomedical Model

Recently, the former National Institute of Mental Health (NIMH) director Thomas Insel made a remarkable statement:

> I spent 13 years at NIMH really pushing on the neuroscience and genetics of mental disorders, and when I look back on that I realize that while I think I succeeded at getting lots of really cool papers published by cool scientists at fairly large costs – I think $20 billion – I don't think we moved the needle in reducing suicide, reducing hospitalizations, improving recovery for the tens of millions of people who have mental illness. (www.psychologytoday.com/us/blog/theory-knowledge/201705/twenty-billion-fails-move-the-needle-mental-illness)

Insel's strong stance reflects the growing awareness that the biomedical model has not made meaningful progress sufficient to affect the clinical care of psychiatric patients. As a result of this failure to deliver on its promises, biological psychiatry and its therapeutic arm, psychopharmacology, are increasingly being criticised.

The evolutionary perspective suggests some reflections on the limits of biomedical explanations of psychiatric disorders. First, it is wrong to equate the biology of psychiatric disorders with the biomedical model. Biology is not only genes, neurochemistry and neurophysiology but also psychological and behavioural mechanisms that have evolved to maximise adaptation. Second, in evolutionary biology, the environment is a crucial variable for explaining the functioning (or malfunctioning) of individual organisms. Such a postulate is in contrast with the 'bottom-up' approach of the biomedical model that can be summarised in this way: mental health problems arise from faulty brain mechanisms that occur within the individual and are not context-dependent. As a general rule of thumb, evolutionary thinking suggests just the opposite: most psychiatric conditions are context-dependent and environmental factors are decisive in triggering the onset of symptoms. Third, the evolutionary approach conceptualises psychiatric syndromes as composites of malfunctioning behavioural systems (e.g. attachment, aggression, social cognition, mating). Such a view contradicts the biomedical or drug-centred model that there is a specific link between a neurobiological alteration (e.g. serotonin deficit), a syndromal condition (e.g. depression) and the therapeutic action of certain drugs (e.g. selective serotonin reuptake inhibitors). In fact, convergent evidence shows that the drug-centred model is no longer tenable (Drukarch et al., 2020) and that this model is largely responsible for the crisis of psychopharmacology (Margraf and Schneider, 2016).

The drug-centred model relies on the assumption that homogeneous biological abnormalities (lesions) underlie specific clinical phenotypes (symptoms or syndromes) that can be identified through biomarkers and can become specific targets for pharmacological treatments. This model ignores the fact that the same biological abnormalities are seen in multiple disorders and that a single disorder is associated with multiple biological abnormalities. Evolutionary thinking suggests complementing (or replacing) the drug-centred model with a functional approach targeting evolved behavioural systems.

The Research Domain Criteria (RDoC) framework (Cuthbert, 2020) provides a useful starting point for this approach, whereby different psychobiological domains relevant to psychiatric disorders have been described within a framework that includes different levels of investigation ranging from genes to subjective experience. A point of convergence between the RDoC framework and evolutionary thinking is that psychiatric research and clinical practice should target transdiagnostic constructs, not symptoms or syndromes. However, there is a major point of divergence. The RDoC framework is organised around the concept of mechanism (i.e. 'proximate causation' in evolutionary terms). The basic idea is that both normal behaviour and mental disorders are mediated by brain circuits that can be studied using the tools of neuroscience and genomics. Its primary focus is on neural circuitry with levels of analysis moving in two directions: upward from physiological measures of the circuitry to clinically relevant behaviours and self-reports; and downward to the genetic and molecular/cellular processes that underlie the structure and function of the circuits.

The RDoC framework architects claim that the psychobiological domains have been chosen to reflect 'broad domains of function' (Insel et al., 2010: 749). This could suggest that the selection of the domains was based on an evolutionary analysis of human behaviour with a specific focus on evolved behavioural systems. In reality, the selection resulted from a consensus by a work group that determined that five major domains of functioning would serve as an organising system for subsuming various dimensions. Dimensions were included in the matrix if the work group members deemed that they met two stringent criteria: (1) there had to be evidence of a valid behavioural function; and (2) there had to be evidence for a neural circuit or system that plays a preponderant role in implementing the function (Cuthbert, 2020). I think that future revisions of the RDoC framework should include not only the findings of neuroscience but also evolutionary data on the functional organisation of human behaviour. Such a combination is likely to help identify new targets for psychiatric therapies and provide a better match between research findings and

clinical decision-making. With its limited focus on proximate causation as the only level of explanation for mental disorders, the RDoC project risks repeating the same errors of the biomedical model.

20.4 Conclusion

The view that evolutionary thinking is irrelevant for the clinical care of psychiatric patients is difficult to reconcile with two related facts. First, psychiatric therapeutics is facing a major crisis that originates from its limited efficacy and dubious scientific credibility. Such a crisis requires a radical change in the paradigm that inspires psychiatric research and clinical practice. The new paradigm should integrate in a meaningful way all of the variables that mediate the aetiology and pathogenesis of psychiatric disorders: biological, psychological, developmental, behavioural and social. The essence of the evolutionary study of human psychology and behaviour is just such an integration. Second, there is a long list of evolutionary phenomena that are ignored by contemporary psychiatry in spite of their importance for understanding the behaviour of people with or without psychiatric conditions. In this chapter, I have mentioned only a few of these phenomena. Here is a non-exhaustive list (also see Chapter 1) that I would suggest to treating psychiatrists for further study: adaptive symptoms, alternative strategies, behavioural systems, developmental plasticity, differential susceptibility, kin altruism, life history strategies, mating effort, mismatch hypothesis, non-verbal communication, parental effort, parental manipulation, reciprocal altruism, social attention-holding potential, social deception and vantage sensitivity (Troisi, 2020a).

References

Alexander, R., Aragón, O. R., Bookwala, J., Cherbuin, N., Gatt, J. M., Kahrilas, I. J., Kästner, N., Lawrence, A., Lowe, L., Morrison, R. G., Mueller, S. C., Nusslock, R., Papadelis, C., Polnaszek, K. L., Helene Richter, S., Silton, R. L. and Styliadis, C. (2021). The neuroscience of positive emotions and affect: implications for cultivating happiness and wellbeing. *Neurosci Biobehav Rev*, 121, 220–249.

Andrews, P. W,. Thomson, J. A., Jr, Amstadter, A. and Neale, M. C. (2012). *Primum non nocere*: an evolutionary analysis of whether antidepressants do more harm than good. *Front Psychol*, 3, 117.

Blease, C. R. (2018). Psychotherapy and placebos: manifesto for conceptual clarity. *Front Psychiatry*, 9, 379.

Bracken, P., Thomas, P., Timimi, S., Asen, E., Behr, G., Beuster, C., Bhunnoo, S., Browne, I., Chhina, N., Double, D., Downer, S., Evans, C., Fernando, S., Garland, M. R., Hopkins, W., Huws, R., Johnson, B., Martindale, B., Middleton, H., Moldavsky, D., Moncrieff, J., Mullins, S., Nelki, J., Pizzo, M., Rodger, J., Smyth, M., Summerfield, D., Wallace, J. and Yeomans, D. (2012). Psychiatry beyond the current paradigm. *Br J Psychiatry*, 201, 430–434.

Childs, B. (1999). *Genetic Medicine: A Logic of Disease*. Baltimore, MD: Johns Hopkins University Press.

Cuthbert, B. N. (2020). The role of RDoC in future classification of mental disorder. *Dialogues Clin Neurosci*, 22, 81–85.

Davies, W. and Roache, R. (2017). Reassessing biopsychosocial psychiatry. *Br J Psychiatry*, 210, 3–5.

Drukarch, B., Jacobs, G. E. and Wilhelmus, M. M. M. (2020). Solving the crisis in psychopharmacological research: cellular-membrane(s) pharmacology to the rescue? *Biomed Pharmacother*, 130, 110545.

Engel, G. L. (1980). The clinical application of the biopsychosocial model. *Am J Psychiatry*, 137, 535–544.

Flaum, M. (2010). Strategies to close the 'mortality gap'. *Am J Psychiatry*, 167, 120–121.

Fuchs, T. (2004). Neurobiology and psychotherapy: an emerging dialogue. *Curr Opin Psychiatry*, 17, 479–485.

Ganev, K. (2000). Long-term trends of symptoms and disability in schizophrenia and related disorders. *Soc Psychiatry Psychiatr Epidemiol*, 35, 389–395.

Guina, J., Rossetter, S. R., DeRhodes, B. J., Nahhas, R. W. and Welton, R. S. (2015). Benzodiazepines for PTSD: a systematic review and meta-analysis. *J Psychiatr Pract*, 21, 281–303.

Guze, S. B. (1992). *Why Psychiatry Is a Branch of Medicine*. Oxford: Oxford University Press.

Harmer, C. J., Duman, R. S. and Cowen, P. J. (2017). How do antidepressants work? New perspectives for refining future treatment approaches. *Lancet Psychiatry*, 4, 409–418.

Helliwell, J. F. and Aknin, L. B. (2018). Expanding the social science of happiness. *Nat Hum Behav*, 2, 248–252.

Henningsen, P. (2015). Still modern? Developing the biopsychosocial model for the 21st century. *J Psychosom Res*, 79, 362–363.

Holt-Lunstad, J. (2018). Why social relationships are important for physical health: a systems approach to understanding and modifying risk and protection. *Annu Rev Psychol*, 4, 437–458.

Humphrey, N. and Skoyles, J. (2012). The evolutionary psychology of healing: a human success story. *Curr Biol*, 22, R695–R698.

Huneke, N. T. M., van der Wee, N., Garner, M. and Baldwin, D. S. (2020). Why we need more research into the placebo response in psychiatry. *Psychol Med*, 50, 2317–2323.

Insel, T., Cuthbert, B., Garvey, M., Heinssen, R., Pine, D. S., Quinn, K., Sanislow, C. and Wang, P. (2010). Research Domain Criteria (RDoC): toward a new classification framework for research on mental disorders. *Am J Psychiatry*, 167, 748–751.

Jordan, J. R. and Neimeyer, R. A. (2003). Does grief counseling work? *Death Studies*, 27, 765–786.

Klinkman, M. S. (2009). Assessing functional outcomes in clinical practice. *Am J Manag Care*, 15, S335–S342.

Kothgassner, O. D., Pellegrini, M., Goreis, A., Giordano, V., Edobor, J., Fischer, S., Plener, P. L. and Huscsava, M. M. (2021). Hydrocortisone administration for reducing post-traumatic stress symptoms: a systematic review and meta-analysis. *Psychoneuroendocrinology*, 126, 105168.

Lebowitz, M. S. and Appelbaum, P. S. (2019). Biomedical explanations of psychopathology and their implications for attitudes and beliefs about mental disorders. *Annu Rev Clin Psychol*, 15, 555–577.

Lilienfeld, S. O. (2007). Psychological treatments that cause harm. *Perspect Psychol Sci*, 2, 53–70.

Locher, C., Koechlin, H., Gaab, J. and Gerger, H. (2019). The other side of the coin: nocebo effects and psychotherapy. *Front Psychiatry*, 10, 555.

Margraf, J. and Schneider, S. (2016). From neuroleptics to neuroscience and from Pavlov to psychotherapy: more than just the 'emperor's new treatments' for mental illnesses? *EMBO Mol Med*, 8, 1115–1117.

Matar, M. A., Zohar, J., Kaplan, Z. and Cohen, H. (2009). Alprazolam treatment immediately after stress exposure interferes with the normal HPA-stress response and increases vulnerability to subsequent stress in an animal model of PTSD. *Eur Neuropsychopharmacol*, 19, 283–295.

McGuire, M. T. and Troisi, A. (1998). *Darwinian Psychiatry*. Oxford: Oxford University Press.

McQueen, D. and St John-Smith, P. (2012). Placebo effects: a new paradigm and relevance to psychiatry. *Int Psychiatry*, 9, 1–3.

Miresco, M. J. and Kirmayer, L. J. (2006). The persistence of mind–brain dualism in psychiatric reasoning about clinical scenarios. *Am J Psychiatry*, 163, 913–918.

Moncrieff, J., Gupta, S. and Horowitz, M. A. (2020). Barriers to stopping neuroleptic (antipsychotic) treatment in people with schizophrenia, psychosis or bipolar disorder. *Ther Adv Psychopharmacol*, 10, 2045125320937910.

Nesse, R. M. (1990). The evolutionary functions of repression and the ego defenses. *J Am Acad Psychoanal*, 18, 260–285.

Nesse, R. M. (2005). Evolutionary psychology and mental health. In D. Buss (ed.), *Handbook of Evolutionary Psychology*. Hoboken, NJ: Wiley, pp. 903–927.

Nesse, R. M. (2018). The smoke detector principle: signal detection and optimal defense regulation. *Evol Med Public Health*, 2019, 1.

Nesse, R. M. (2019). *Good Reasons for Bad Feelings: Insights from the Frontiers of Evolutionary Psychiatry*. London: Penguin Random House.

Norcross, J. C. and Lambert, M. J. (2018). Psychotherapy relationships that work III. *Psychotherapy (Chic)*, 55, 303–315.

Oades, L. and Mossman, L. (2017). The science of wellbeing and positive psychology. In M. Slade, L. Oades and A. Jarden (eds.), *Wellbeing, Recovery and Mental Health*. Cambridge: Cambridge University Press, pp. 7–23.

Price, J., Cole, V. and Goodwin, G. M. (2009). Emotional side-effects of selective serotonin reuptake inhibitors: qualitative study. *Br J Psychiatry*, 195, 211–217.

Read, J., Cartwright, C. and Gibson, K. (2014). Adverse emotional and interpersonal effects reported by 1829 New Zealanders while taking antidepressants. *Psychiatry Res*, 216, 67–73.

Read, J., Gee, A., Diggle, J. and Butler, H. (2017). The interpersonal adverse effects reported by 1008 users of antidepressants; and the incremental impact of polypharmacy. *Psychiatry Res*, 256, 423–427.

Rosa, A. R., Reinares, M., Franco, C., Comes, M., Torrent, C., Sánchez-Moreno, J., Martínez-Arán, A., Salamero, M.,

Kapczinski, F. and Vieta, E. (2009). Clinical predictors of functional outcome of bipolar patients in remission. *Bipolar Disord*, 11, 401–409.

Sansone, R. A. and Sansone, L. A. (2010). SSRI-induced indifference. *Psychiatry (Edgmont)*, 7, 14–18.

Saris, I. M. J., Aghajani, M., van der Werff, S. J. A., van der Wee, N. J. A. and Penninx, B. W. J. H. (2017). Social functioning in patients with depressive and anxiety disorders. *Acta Psychiatr Scand*, 136, 352–361.

Seligman, M. E. P. (2019). Positive psychology: a personal history. *Annu Rev Clin Psychol*, 15, 1–23.

Singewald, N., Schmuckermair, C., Whittle, N., Holmes, A. and Ressler, K. J. (2015). Pharmacology of cognitive enhancers for exposure-based therapy of fear, anxiety and trauma-related disorders. *Pharmacol Ther*, 149, 150–190.

Troisi, A. (2012). Mental health and well-being: clinical applications of Darwinian psychiatry. In S. Roberts (ed.), *Applied Evolutionary Psychology*. New York: Oxford University Press, pp. 277–289.

Troisi, A. (2015). The evolutionary diagnosis of mental disorder. *Wiley Interdiscip Rev Cogn Sci*, 6, 323–331.

Troisi, A. (2017) *The Painted Mind: Behavioral Science Reflected in Great Paintings*. New York: Oxford University Press.

Troisi, A. (2019). The biology of mental disorders: what are we talking about? *Behav Brain Sci*, 42, e29.

Troisi, A. (2020a). Are we on the verge of Darwinian psychiatry? In L. Workman, W. Reader and J. Barkow (eds.), *The Cambridge Handbook of Evolutionary Perspectives on Human Behavior*. Cambridge: Cambridge University Press, pp. 409–418.

Troisi, A. (2020b). Social stress and psychiatric disorders: evolutionary reflections on debated questions. *Neurosci Biobehav Rev*, 116, 461–469.

Troisi, A. and McGuire, M. T. (2000). Psychotherapy in the context of Darwinian psychiatry. In P. Gilbert and K. G. Bailey (eds.), *Genes on the Couch: Explorations in Evolutionary Psychotherapy*. Philadelphia, PA: Taylor & Francis, pp. 28–41.

Uher, R. (2014). Gene–environment interactions in severe mental illness. *Front Psychiatry*, 5, 48.

Üstün, B. and Kennedy, C. (2009). What is 'functional impairment'? Disentangling disability from clinical significance. *World Psychiatry*, 8, 82–85.

Wager, T. D. and Atlas, L. Y. (2015). The neuroscience of placebo effects: connecting context, learning and health. *Nat Rev Neurosci*, 16, 403–418.

Zimmerman, M., Martinez, J., Attiullah, N., Friedman, M., Toba, C. and Boerescu, D. A. (2012a). Why do some depressed outpatients who are not in remission according to the Hamilton Depression Rating Scale nonetheless consider themselves to be in remission? *Depress Anxiety*, 29, 891–895.

Zimmerman, M., Martinez, J. A., Attiullah, N., Friedman, M., Toba, C., Boerescu, D. A. and Rahgeb, M. (2012b). Why do some depressed outpatients who are in remission according to the Hamilton Depression Rating Scale not consider themselves to be in remission? *J Clin Psychiatry*, 73, 790–795.

Zimmerman, M., McGlinchey, J. B., Posternak, M. A., Friedman, M., Attiullah, N. and Boerescu, D. (2006). How should remission from depression be defined? The depressed patient's perspective. *Am J Psychiatry*, 163, 148–150.

Index

Printed in the United States
by Baker & Taylor Publisher Services